EXCIMER LASERS IN OPHTHALMOLOGY
Principles and Practice

EXCIMER LASERS IN OPHTHALMOLOGY
Principles and Practice

Charles N J McGhee MB BSc(Hons) FRCS FRCOphth FRSA

Professor and Head
Department of Ophthalmology
University of Dundee
Scotland, UK

Hugh R Taylor MD FRACS FRACO FACS FAAO

Professor and Head
Department of Ophthalmology
University of Melbourne
Victoria, Australia

David S Gartry MD FRCS FRCOphth BSc(Hons) DO FCOptom

Consultant Ophthalmic Surgeon
Moorfields Eye Hospital
London, UK

Stephen L Trokel MD

Professor of Clinical Ophthalmology
Columbia-Presbyterian Medical Center
New York, NY, USA

Butterworth-Heinemann

Boston   Oxford   Johannesburg   Melbourne   New Delhi   Singapore

Cover pictures—acknowledgements:
Dr Paul van Saarloos and Mr Chris Barry, courtesy of the
Lions Eye Institute, Perth, Western Australia and Professor
Charles N J McGhee, University of Dundee, Scotland.

First published in the United Kingdom in 1997 by
Martin Dunitz Ltd
The Livery House
7–9 Pratt Street
London NW1 0AE

First published in the United States of America in
1997 by Butterworth-Heinemann

  A member of the Reed Elsevier group

Every effort has been made to ensure that the drug
dosage schedules within this text are accurate and
conform to standards accepted at the time of
publication. However, as treatment recommendations
vary in the light of continuing research and clinical
experience, the reader is advised to verify drug dosage
schedules herein with information found on product
information sheets. This is especially true in cases of
new or infrequently used drugs.

Library of Congress Cataloging-in-Publication Data
applied for

A CIP catalogue record for this book is available
from the British Library

ISBN 0-7506-9785-7

Composition by Scribe Design, Gillingham, Kent,
United Kingdom
Origination by Bright Arts, Hong Kong
Manufactured in Singapore by Imago

Contents

Contributors

Noel A Alpins MB BS DO(Melb) FRACO FRACS FRCOphth FACS
Medical Director of the Cheltenham Eye Centre, PO Box 7373, Melbourne 3004, Australia.

Con N Anastas MD
Corneal Research Fellow, Corneal Diseases and Excimer Laser Unit, Sunderland Eye Infirmary, Queen Alexandra Road, Sunderland SR2 9HP, UK.

David B Cano MD
Eye Physician and Surgeon, Intra Coastal Eye Assessment Clinic, 2601 North Flagler Drive, Suite 203, West Palm Beach, FL 33407, USA.

Deepak K Chitkara MB ChB DO FRCOphth
Consultant Ophthalmic Surgeon, Department of Ophthalmology, Aintree Hospitals Trust, Walton Hospital, Rice Lane, Liverpool L9 1AE, UK.

Geoffrey J Crawford MBBS FRACO FRACS
Consultant Ophthalmic Surgeon, Lions Eye Institute and Centre for Ophthalmology and Visual Science, University of Western Australia and Cornea Clinic, Royal Perth Hospital, Perth, Australia.

Jean-Pierre Danjoux MB BS FRCOphth
Senior Registrar, Sunderland Eye Infirmary, Queen Alexandra Road, Sunderland SR2 9HP, UK and Fellow in Corneal and Refractive Surgery at Sydney Refractive Surgery Centre.

Christine R Ellerton FRCOphth
Senior Registrar in Ophthalmology, Sunderland Eye Infirmary, Queen Alexandra Road, Sunderland SR2 9HP, UK.

Wallace S Foulds CBE MD ChM FRCS DO DSc FRACO FCMSA FRCOphth
Emeritus Professor of Ophthalmology at University of Glasgow and Consultant Ophthalmologist, Kinnoul Place, 68 Downside Road, Glasgow G12 9DL, Scotland, UK.

David S Gartry MD FRCS FRCOphth BSc(Hons) DO FCOptom
Consultant Ophthalmic Surgeon, Cornea Service, Moorfields Eye Hospital, London EC1V, UK.

Jose L Guell MD
Associate Professor of Ophthalmology, Institut de Microcirugia Ocular de Barcelona, Spain.

Jerry Jayamanne FRCOphth
Registrar in Ophthalmology, Sunderland Eye Infirmary, Queen Alexandra Road, Sunderland SR2 9HP, UK.

Lyn Jenkins MRCOphth
Ophthalmologist, Laser Vision Centre, Harley Street, London, UK.

Johannes Junger MSc
Director of Medical Application and Development, Chiron Technolas, Munich, Germany.

Brian A Kidd MB ChB MRCPsych
Consultant Psychiatrist, Mental Health Directorate, Central Scotland Health Care Trust, Scotland, UK.

Stephen D Klyce PhD
Professor of Ophthalmology and Anatomy, LSU School of Medicine and Adjunct Professor of Biomedical Engineering, Tulane University, New Orleans, LA 70112, USA.

Peter Koay FRCOphth
Consultant Ophthalmologist, Darlington Memorial Hospital, Darlington, UK.

Chris P Lohmann MD PhD
Consultant Ophthalmologist, University Eye Clinic, Regensberg, Germany.

Cathy A McCarty PhD MPH
Research Fellow, University of Melbourne Department of Ophthalmology and Head of Epidemiology, Research Unit, First Floor, 32 Gisbourne Street, East Melbourne 3002, Australia.

Marguerite B McDonald MD FACS
Director, Refractive Surgery Center of the South at EENT Hospital, New Orleans and Clinical Professor of Ophthalmology, Tulane University School of Medicine, New Orleans, LA 70115, USA.

Charles N J McGhee MB BSc(Hons) FRCS FRCOphth FRSA
Professor and Head of the Department of Ophthalmology, University of Dundee DD1 9SY, Scotland, UK. Formerly Consultant Ophthalmologist and Professor of Ocular Therapeutics, Corneal Diseases and Excimer Laser Unit, Sunderland Eye Infirmary, Sunderland, UK.

Paul G McMenamin BSc PhD MSc
Senior Lecturer, Department of Anatomy and Human Biology, Nedlands, Perth, Western Australia.

Christopher M Rogers MB BS FRACS FRACO
Director of the Sydney Refractive Surgery Centre and Chairman and Head of the Department of Ophthalmology, Royal North Shore Hospital, Pacific Highway, St Leonards, NSW 2065, Sydney, Australia.

Helmut Sachs MD
University Eye Clinic, Regensberg, Germany.

Michael K Smolek PhD
Research Associate in Ophthalmology, LSU Eye Center, Louisiana State University Medical Center School of Medicine, New Orleans, LA 70112, USA.

Grant R Snibson MBBS(Melb) DipRACOG FRACS FRACO FRCOphth
Senior Lecturer, Melbourne University School of Ophthalmology and Senior Ophthalmologist, Corneal Unit, Royal Victorian Eye and Ear Hospital, East Melbourne 3002, Australia.

Cameron Stark MB, ChB, MRCPsych, DPHM
Consultant Physician in Public Health, Department of Public Health, Ayrshire and Arran Health Board, Scotland, UK.

Ronald M Stasiuk MB BS FRACO FRACS
Clinical Associate, Melbourne University Department of Ophthalmology and The Royal Victorian Eye and Ear Hospital, 32 Gisborne Street, East Melbourne, Victoria 3002, Australia.

Christopher Steele BSc(Hons) MCOptom
Head of Optometry Services, Sunderland Eye Infirmary, Queen Alexandra Road, Sunderland SR2 9HP, UK.

Geoffrey C Tabin MA MD
Assistant Professor, University of Vermont Medical School and Director of Corneal and Refractive Surgery, Fletcher Allen Health Care, University of Vermont, Burlington, VT 05401, USA.

Hugh R Taylor MD FRACS FRACO FACS FAAO
Professor and Head, Department of Ophthalmology, University of Melbourne and Director of Eye Services and Head of Corneal Unit, Royal Victorian Eye and Ear Hospital, Victoria 3002, Australia.

Stephen L Trokel MD
Professor of Clinical Ophthalmology, Columbia-Presbyterian Medical Center, New York, NY 10032, USA.

Paul P van Saarloos BSc MSc PhD
Adjunct Senior Lecturer, The University of Western Australia and Director of Research - Lasers and Engineering, Lions Eye Institute of Western Australia, Perth 6009, Australia.

George O Waring III MD FACS FRCOphth
Professor, Department of Ophthalmology, Emory University School of Medicine, Atlanta, GA 30322, USA.

Suzanne K Webber FRCOphth
Registrar in Ophthalmology, Sunderland Eye Infirmary, Queen Alexandra Road, Sunderland SR2 9HP, UK.

Kathryn H Weed BSc(Hons) MSc MBCO
Senior Research Fellow, University of Dundee and Principal Optometrist, Ninewells Hospital and Medical School, Dundee DD1 9SY, Scotland, UK.

Preface

More than two thousand years ago the classical scientific writers such as MoTi, Euclid, and Claudius Ptolemy understood the reflection of light, and that light travelled in straight lines at such enormous speeds that, the very instant the eyes were opened, distant stars could clearly be seen. Aristotle also appreciated the association of large eyes and short-sight, and was first to use the term *myops*. However, refraction and the optical system of the eye took much longer to unravel. At the end of the first millennium the Arabian writer Al-Hazen transformed the science with *The Book of Optics*, considering reflection from plane, spherical, and parabolic mirrors in addition to studies of magnifying glasses. Nonetheless, it was not until the early seventeenth century that Kepler established the fundamental laws of the dioptrics of the eye, refraction by convex and concave lenses, and the optics of myopia. Finally, in 1704, Sir Isaac Newton consolidated the laws of optics, refraction, reflection and the dioptric system of the eye in his *Opticks*.

Although the inventor of spectacles to correct refractive error remains debatable, presbyopic spectacles certainly appeared in Venice around 1270 and myopic corrections were prescribed by Holerius about 1550. Whilst astigmatism was clinically described by Young in 1801 astigmatic spectacle lenses were not widely utilized until the latter part of the nineteenth century. The final piece of the refractive jigsaw, the clear distinction between hyperopia and presbyopia, was not fully elucidated until 1864 by Donders. Thus, although simple forms of spectacle correction have been with us for 700 years, the complete armamentarium of appropriate lenses has only been available in the last century.

Surgical attempts to alleviate myopia followed rapidly upon the widespread acceptance of spectacles, with Boerhaave suggesting clear lens extraction as early as 1708. The response to this suggestion is not recorded but generally the ophthalmic profession has been reserved in the acceptance of refractive surgery as a legitimate employment of surgical skills. Indeed, William Bates, perhaps best known for his seminal work on astigmatism (1894), was forced to leave the New York Post-Graduate Medical School because of his insistence that myopia could be corrected surgically. Over the subsequent forty years strategies to surgically correct myopia added little to the pioneering papers of Bates and Lans. In the late 1930s Sato developed a form of posterior radial keratotomy which he felt was 95% effective in the treatment of up to 5.00D of myopia without loss of visual acuity. Any scholar of refractive surgery will be well aware that his initial enthusiasm was misplaced, and subsequent follow-up studies demonstrated widespread corneal decompensation some 10–20 years later. The procedure was abandoned in 1960 and refractive surgery underwent a hiatus, punctuated only by the singular activities of Jose Barraquer, until Fyodorov and Durnev developed and popularized anterior radial keratotomy in the Soviet Union in the mid 1970s. This was the first refractive procedure to capture the attention of the general populous and is still widely referred to by the layman as the 'Russian operation.' However, PERK and other studies have highlighted the limitations and complications of RK in the attempted treatment of moderate to high myopia.

The advent of the Ruby laser in 1960 captured the imagination of the public and the precision and potential power of lasers has been a recurring theme in popular fiction from Ian Fleming to *Star Wars*. The reality has been no less exciting with lasers speeding information along optical cables, robotically etching metal with exquisite precision and being bounced from earth to moon, and back, to measure the distance to an accuracy within a few centimetres. At a more familiar level lasers now uncode music from CD-Roms and guide the ubiquitous laser printer. Within medicine lasers have enjoyed equally widespread acceptance in many branches of surgery; specifically, a few years after their invention lasers were adopted into ophthalmology to perform photocoagulation of the retina and are now common to most ophthalmic operating rooms and clinical settings.

In the light of the foregoing potted history of refractive surgery, and our familiarity with the relatively commonplace laser, the uninitiated might be forgiven for being surprised at the excitement generated by the arrival of excimer lasers in ophthalmology. However the advent of a laser which removes corneal tissue with submicron precision without appreciable thermal effect has ushered in a whole new era of interest in refractive surgery. From the early primate excimer laser studies in the mid eighties to FDA acceptance in 1995/1996, there has never been a refractive procedure which has been associated with such interest from public and practitioner alike. More than 500 000 individuals may have already been treated worldwide, although the facts are often difficult to sieve from the hype, and with only a year gone since FDA approval many overly enthusiastic practitioners are already heralding the demise of surface based excimer laser to be supplanted by LASIK.

However, analysis of refractive surgery involves a pedigree much longer than the last glossy review or most recent journal article. Our knowledge of the success or failure of any technique should build from established scientific principles, via practical and reproducible techniques, to an accumulation of incontrovertible clinical evidence upon which to base sound clinical policy. This book brings together 35 authors from diverse scientific and clinical backgrounds who pool extensive and unique experience in their respective fields to provide the latest information on the many forms of surface based and lamellar excimer laser procedures. This practical guide to excimer laser techniques is placed in perspective to alternative refractive procedures and in the context of the whole patient, not merely a refraction or unaided acuity. This text is extensively illustrated by clinical images of both normal and rare sequelae of excimer laser surgery, supported by critical review of published data, which should be useful to both the beginning and experienced excimer laser surgeon.

The development of refractive surgery has been a slow continuum over the last 300 years, but as we approach the second millennium the prospect of correcting most ametropias by excimer laser surgery, a prospect considered fanciful ten years ago and impossible 30 years ago, is indeed a genuine possibility.

Professor Charles NJ McGhee
Editor in Chief
March 1997

Dedication

This book is dedicated to all our families

Chapter 1 History of the excimer and other ophthalmic refractive lasers

Stephen L Trokel

INTRODUCTION

Ophthalmologists were already aware of keratomileusis and radial keratotomy (RK) when the Nd:YAG photodisruptor laser became widely available. The magic quality of the surgical action of the Nd:YAG photodisruptor laser and its ability to section strands and open capsules within the closed eye led to serious speculation that a laser system capable of performing refractive surgical procedures could be developed. The hope was that such a system would produce clinical results with greater accuracy and precision and fewer complications than was being achieved with conventional surgical technology, specifically RK and keratomileusis. Barraquer's creation of keratomileusis as a corneal refractive procedure was well known.[1] Less well known were his early experiments (Fig. 1.1) in which he attempted to alter the refractive power of the eye by

removing tissue directly from the corneal surface.[2] He abandoned this approach because, in his own words 'all the animal eyes developed severe scarring of their corneas'.[3] This corneal response led to development of a surgical procedure of removing tissue with a cryolathe from the undersurface of an excised corneal lamella. This experience of surface scarring and the improved results when tissue was removed from the undersurface of a stromal lamella led to the persistent view that the presence of Bowman's layer was, in some way, necessary to maintain corneal transparency. However, the cryolathe removed tissue with a lack of precision that produced a broad range of refractive change.

Efforts to alter the refractive power of the eye by direct removal of tissue from the corneal surface had preceded[4] Barraquer by many years and continued[5,6] after his development of keratomileusis. Neither Barraquer's nor any of the preceding or following efforts were sufficiently precise or accurate enough to create a smooth optically precise surface on the cornea. Furthermore, substantial corneal scarring similar to Barraquer's findings resulted from all these attempts at corneal reshaping.

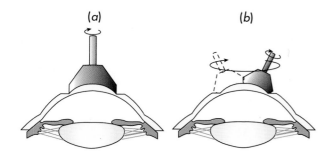

(a)　　　(b)

Figure 1.1 *Diagrammatic representation of surface grinding in an attempt to change the corneal optics. This was unsuccessful because all animals developed irregular astigmatism and corneal scarring.*

LASER TECHNOLOGY AND REFRACTIVE SURGERY

This was the background that led to efforts to develop laser technology that would be suitable for refractive surgery. In 1982 and 1983 a number of attempts were made to incise the cornea with photodisruption, first using existing neodymium: Yttrium Aluminium Garnet (Nd:YAG) lasers designed for anterior segment photodisruption, then with custom-designed photodisruptor laser systems. The initial interest was expressed in a commercial effort

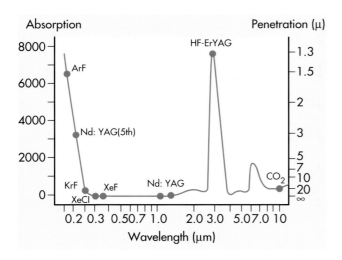

Figure 1.2 *Absorption of light by the cornea. Note that significant absorption occurs in the UV below 300 nm and above 2 μm in the IR.*

to develop a system that could incise the cornea either on the surface or within the stroma. A prototype was shown in 1985 at the American Academy of Ophthalmology, but was never successfully applied clinically. These efforts have continued and led to refractive laser systems based on photodisruption. The Intelligent Surgical Laser system has been used to remove tissue within the corneal stroma in limited human trials.[7]

A diagrammatic representation of corneal absorption of light is shown in Figure 1.2. The cornea is virtually transparent to light at wavelengths from 0.305 μm to 1.3 μm, a range that includes the visible and the near ultraviolet (UV) and infrared (IR) regions. Lasers emitting in the light IR B and C and the UV B and C regions that are absorbed by the cornea have been studied for their potential surgical applications. The first successful applications of lasers to alter the corneal curve used a thermal interaction based on the known absorption of CO_2 laser light by the cornea. Interest in thermokeratoplasty, first reported in the early- and mid-20th century,[8–10] has been cyclic with sporadic reports in the 1950s of heated corneal probes[11] used to flatten corneal cones. Various technologies have been used to heat the cornea in an effort to change its shape. This method relied initially on surface heating[12,13] with conduction of heat into the stroma, and reached its culmination with the development of microwave heating[14] and the insertion of an electrically heated wire deep within the cornea designed to heat the entire stromal thickness.[15]

Efforts were also made to use the continuous wave CO_2 laser as a source of heat for refractive corneal surgery[15] and the pulsed CO_2 laser to create incisions[16] as shown in Figure 1.3. Russian investigators[17] tried using the CO_2 laser instead of an electric wire to heat the cornea but quickly realized that the deposition of thermal energy was excessively superficial. In an attempt to create a better distribution of heat within the stroma, the investigators developed a prototype laser system that had deep penetration of the corneal

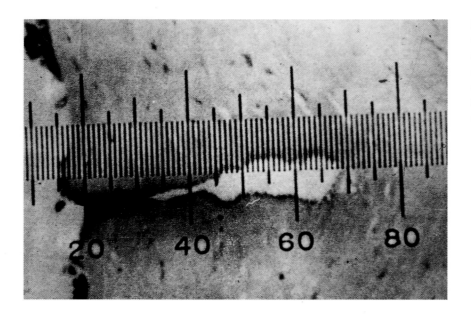

Figure 1.3 *Incision created with a CO_2 laser. Notice the irregularity of the incision and its edges. Thermal damage extends a considerable distance into the adjacent stromal tissues. (Reprinted with permission of R.J. Keates.)*

Table 1.1

Lasers used in refractive surgery

Laser type	Wavelength	Pulse width	Interaction	Depth
CO_2	10 μm	CW	Thermal	Superficial
CO_2	10 μm	0.05 sec	Thermal	Superficial, less thermal spread
Erbium	3 μm	200 μsec	Fast thermal	Superficial
Holmium	2.0 μm	200 μsec	Fast thermal	Deep
Thulium	1.9 μm	200 μsec	Fast thermal	Deep
Erbium:Glass	1.6 μm	200 μsec	Fast thermal	Deep
Solid state harmonic	213 nm	10 ns	Ablative photodecomposition	Very superficial
Argon–fluoride excimer	193 nm	10–15 ns	Ablative photodecomposition	Most superficial
Photodisruption	varied	femto- and picosecond pulses	Optical breakdown	Varies

stroma.[18] This laser, operating in the near IR region, was based on an Erbium Glass rod emitting laser light at 1.6 μm. The laser was delivered in single pulses, had a very slow repetition rate but was absorbed throughout the stromal thickness. The Russians applied single, double, or triple radial rows of laser applications to produce an increasing effect. The light energy was more deeply distributed in the cornea and investigators reported more favorable clinical results than when using the CO_2 laser. The current interest[19–21] in mid-IR lasers to treat hyperopia is a direct descendant of this clinical investigative work.

Table 1.1 summarizes the lasers that have been used extensively in an attempt to change the corneal refractive power. All attempts at refractive control using lasers to heat the cornea suffered from limited precision and accuracy, and inadequate long-term stability. Attempts to incise or excise tissue were accompanied by damage to adjacent tissues and a tissue removal process that was difficult to control. When excimer lasers became available and were applied to the corneal surface the effect that was observed was immediately perceived as unique and potentially revolutionary for corneal surgery of all kinds.

DEVELOPMENT OF THE EXCIMER LASER

The history of excimer lasers is quite short, with the possibility of UV laser action suggested in 1975 and commercial devices developed in 1981. Laser action was proposed in 1975 when it was calculated that xenon atoms would react with halogens to produce an unstable xenon halide compound that should emit a highly energetic UV photon as it decomposed.[22] A quote from the authors of this paper summarizes the origin of excimer laser systems: 'These bound-free emissions have considerable potential as ultraviolet laser systems for excitation of mixtures of xenon (or other rare gases) and halogen containing compounds.' Within a year of this publication, mixtures of xenon with fluorine, chlorine, bromine, and a mixture of krypton and fluorine, were shown to lase when excited in an electron beam,[23–25] and laser action at 193 nm from argon and fluorine was shown some months later.[26] The first demonstrations of lasing action used a Van der Graaf accelerator to excite the rare gas–halide combination and were of limited practical use for application experiments. By the end of 1976 laser action was shown to be possible[27] in a relatively compact device adapted from a CO_2 laser. This led to the development of commercial UV lasers in 1981, which were initially used to investigate potential hazards, followed by industrial and subsequently potential medical applications.

The term 'excimer' was based on a misconception of the physicists working with this new system who thought that the rare gas molecules in the lasers formed an 'excited dimer' when ionized. The word 'excimer', a contraction of 'excited dimer' was coined by physical chemists in 1960 to describe a short-lived energized molecule with two identical components.[28] This term has persisted to describe these lasers even

Table 1.2
Excimer lasers and their output.

Excimer laser type	Abbreviation	Wavelength	Photon energy
Fluorine	F_2	155 nm	7.90 eV
Argon fluoride	ArF	193 nm	6.42 eV
Krypton fluoride	KrF	222 nm	5.59 eV
Krypton chloride	KrCl	248 nm	4.99 eV
Xenon chloride	XeCl	308 nm	4.03 eV
Nitrogen	N_2	337 nm	3.68 eV
Xenon fluoride	XeF	351 nm	3.53 eV

though no excited dimer exists during the laser process. Alternative names in use include rare gas–halide lasers as a general descriptive term, and argon–fluoride laser to describe the specific system using argon and fluorine as the lasing medium. Pure nitrogen and fluorine will, when energized, form a true excited dimer and will emit UV light. Because of this, they are included in lists of excimer lasers although they are not rare gas–halide lasers. The output of the different excimer lasers is listed in Table 1.2.

Only those excimer lasers based on argon fluoride (ArF), krypton fluoride (KrF), xenon chloride (XeCl) and xenon fluoride (XeF) have substantial outputs of energy, and only ArF and XeCl have found medical applications. The 308 nm output of the XeCl laser can be transmitted through an optical fiber which has facilitated research into the potential for performing endarterectomy. The tissue interactions of the ArF laser have been actively studied and this is the most widely used excimer laser because of its unique application as a corneal surgical system. The UV output from these laser systems is in the form of an individual pulse of photons, which lasts about 10–50 nanoseconds, depending on the design of the cavity. Laser repetition rates to 100 Hz and energies to 1 J per pulse are typically available.

THE EXCIMER LASER AND THE EYE

In 1981, shortly after the commercial excimer lasers became available, publications in the health physics literature from the Laser Effects Branch of the Radiation Sciences Division at the United States Air Force School of Aerospace Medicine reported the first investigations of the interactions of these new lasers with the eye. The output of KrF and ArF excimer lasers were studied to analyze their effects on animal corneas and to determine damage thresholds. John Taboada reported the response of rabbit corneal epithelium to 248 nm radiation produced by the KrF laser.[29] This wavelength produced either an opacification or an area of the exposed cornea that would stain with fluorescein and which took the general shape of the laser beam distribution. In a later paper, Taboada reported the damage effects of 193 nm ArF on the cornea.[30] An ArF (193 nm) beam with an area of 0.1 cm^2 was used to search for damage similar to that found after exposure of the cornea to the KrF (248 nm) beam.

Taboada was an experienced investigator of ocular damage for the military and had investigated damage effects of mode-locked and Q-switched Nd:YAG laser pulses. At that time I was preparing a technical monograph[31] about high-powered pulsed Nd:YAG lasers and I invited Taboada to contribute a chapter describing damage effects of these lasers on ocular tissues. An unusual phrase that Taboada used to describe the effect observed after exposure of the cornea to more energetic ArF laser pulses caught my attention. While he described a range of damage effects, he noted that:[30] 'At the higher levels, exposures of 27.5 mJ/cm^2 or greater, an immediate indentation of the corneal surface appeared taking the shape of the beam. One hour later, the surface indentation would fill in.' Taboada postulated that the far-UV light was resonantly captured in random electromagnetic cavities formed by the microprojections of the anterior epithelial cell layer that may have caused a preferential temperature jump in this thin layer of tissue. However, his observation of an 'indentation' suggested to me that tissue was being removed and I sought access to an excimer laser to attempt to study this phenomenon.

The motivation was to bypass the technical limits of current corneal surgical technology by devising a laser technique that could create a perfectly predictable excision of tissue to achieve the long-sought goal of removing tissue from the corneal surface without inducing scarring or irregularities. It was clear to me that only experimentation could confirm the surgical potential of these laser systems. In early 1983 I was introduced to R. Srinivasan, a photochemist, who was working with the ArF excimer laser at the IBM TJ Watson Laboratories.

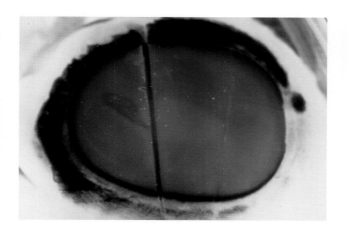

Figure 1.4 *Photograph of an eye after a 1 mm wide laser beam was exposed on the cornea. This groove was made deeper with increasing laser pulses and there was no visible deformation of adjacent corneal tissue.*

In June 1983, I reviewed Taboada's work with Srinivasan who showed me plastics that had been ablated using 193 nm laser light. With this example, the possibility of removing tissue from the corneal surface with optical precision to alter its refractive state seemed reasonable. In a preprint of a paper[32] describing the effect of 193 nm light on plastic Srinivasan had written, 'A threshold ... for ablative photodecomposition ... was measured at 10 mJ/cm². Thus, one pulse at 16 mJ/cm² gave an etch mark that was clearly visible in reflection, whereas 50 pulses at 4 mJ/cm² did not leave any etch mark ...' This explained the Taboada observation[39] of the corneal indentation and we planned experiments the following week.

Before these scheduled experiments, I travelled to California to perform test surgery on the new Nd:YAG laser system Munnerlyn was developing. I told him about the Taboada paper[30] and the Srinivasan work[32] with plastic, described the unusual nature of the excimer plastic interaction, and reviewed my planned experiments. Munnerlyn later told me that his interest in excimer lasers and his development of an excimer laser system began with this conversation. What I subsequently discovered[33] was that many unsuccessful efforts had been made using a variety of CO_2 lasers to remove tissue from the cornea.

On my return to New York, I obtained six bovine eyes and took them to Srinivasan's laboratory at IBM to study the interaction of the laser beam with corneal tissue. These eyes are ideal for this type of

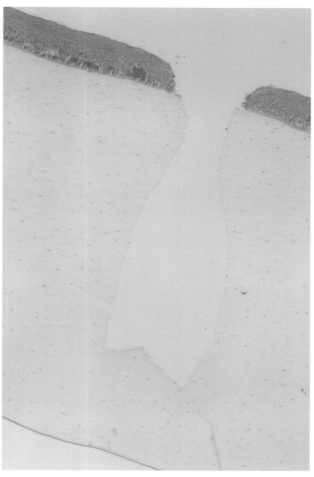

Figure 1.5 *Histologic analysis showed no damage to the stromal tissue adjacent to the area of excision. We calculated the depth per pulse and estimated it to be about 0.25 nm of corneal stroma per pulse. The lack of damage to the adjacent walls as well as the smooth and regular surface was impressive and unique in our experience in evaluating laser–cornea interactions.*

prototype investigation because of their large corneas. We shaped the beam for the first eye with a 1 mm wide slit and exposed the cornea to several different numbers of ablations. The ablations showed an unusual response as the exposed cornea seemed to melt away. The resulting crisply edged trench (Fig. 1.4), made deeper in successive ablations seemed to appear with no deformation in the adjacent corneal tissues. This was confirmed when histologic analysis showed no collateral damage (Fig. 1.5), and creation of a uniquely smooth surface with an optical shape

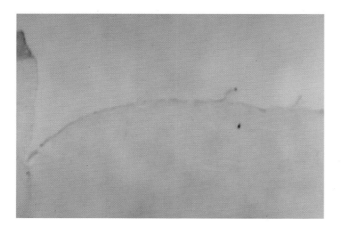

Figure 1.6 *The smoothness and optical contour of the ablated corneal surface encouraged further studies.*

(Fig. 1.6). It was these findings that immediately underpinned the potential for refractive surgical applications.

In 1983 the results of these early experiments were published[34] in a paper that contained the essentials of the far-UV light laser–cornea interaction. In this study, each pulse of laser light removed a fraction of a micron of corneal tissue, about 0.25 µm of tissue per pulse and the resulting surfaces were extremely smooth and uniform, with no collateral damage to adjacent unirradiated tissues. The experiments demonstrated that we could control the shape and pattern of tissue removal by adjusting the fluence and shape of the laser beam incident on the corneal surface. It was immediately apparent that the laser had possible surgical applications including the creation of incisions, and removal of large areas of tissue to form a controlled laser lamellar keratectomy. We stated, 'The laser can be used to reshape the corneal curvature in a manner similar to keratomileusis ... excising more tissue either centrally or peripherally. The net effect would be to flatten or steepen the cornea.'

Immediately after the initial experimental results in July 1983, the laser manufacturer, Lambda Physik in Germany explained to me the pattern of laser light emitted by the excimer laser and how it might be processed to achieve a large uniform circle. More importantly, they leased to me, for investigative purposes, an excimer laser for investigative use at the Columbia–Presbyterian Medical Center. I visited Reinhardt Thyzel, then the owner of Meditec Laser GmbH, and showed him the results of our experi-

ments and he believed that this laser interaction would be the technique for producing an improved radial keratotomy. Following this visit, he started development of a medical excimer system designed to cut slits into the cornea to improve the RK operation.

His enthusiastic initial reaction was typical as, after publication of first animal results, interest was centered around constructing a laser system to create improved radial keratotomy incisions. Many investigators enquired whether the depth of the incision could be better controlled using a laser, and if the finite width of excised tissue would have a greater central flattening effect than a simple diamond knife incision. Obviously, a great deal of investigative work was necessary to develop the knowledge that would guide clinical efforts. In planning experiments, it quickly became apparent that development of an effective delivery system would require industrial support and help. There were many questions about excimer laser functions and UV laser optics that required considerable technical assistance.

INVESTIGATIONS PRECEDING CLINICAL INVESTIGATIONS

The very first exposures of corneas to 193 nm laser light suggested that a direct laser keratomileusis could be performed by removing tissue from the anterior corneal surface to modify its curve, and hence control its optics. This was considered worthy of investigation in spite of the concerns about Bowman's layer, which had been considered sacrosanct because of the poor historical experience when direct surface corneal reshaping was attempted, and prior clinical experience with keratomileusis. We were encouraged in this because no previous surgical technology was able to provide accurate tissue removal to the standard of precision that would allow predictable optical properties. The corneal surgical potential of the ArF laser became increasingly apparent when we found that only 0.25 µm (less than half a wavelength of light) of tissue was removed with each pulse of laser light, and ultrastructural analysis showed no damage to adjacent unirradiated tissues.[35] For the first time, precision surgical technology that allowed optically precise 'machining' of tissue was available.

Attempts to alter the corneal refractive power by direct tissue removal from the corneal surface now seemed more feasible in spite of the failures of the past. When initially proposed, this was by no means a generally accepted hypothesis as there existed a strong presumption that Bowman's layer was essential for uniform corneal topography and transparency. Of all those whom I asked, only Dr. Herbert Kaufman questioned this conventional wisdom. When I queried him about preservation of optical function after smoothly removing Bowman's layer he replied that no one has ever been able to create a precise and smooth surface on a cornea. His advice was to 'try it!' When we subsequently showed that circular ablations of rabbit and monkey corneas healed with remarkable clarity, and smooth widely spaced mires, the way was open to investigation of clinical applications.[36]

EXPERIMENTS

One of the first (unreported) experiments we did was to remove a 9 × 9 mm square of corneal stroma from a rabbit cornea. We showed that the remnants retained a normal electrical potential across the remaining endothelial surface. This was heartening and we undertook a series of studies of narrow excisions and ablated 3 mm circular areas to study the ultrastructure of the ablation and healing of the cornea. Ronald Krueger, a young electrical engineer and at that time a medical student, helped study the physical nature of the laser–cornea interaction and

we determined thresholds, ablation rates, heating patterns, and ablation parameters for all available excimer wavelengths.[37,38] Further research quantitated the tissue removed[39] and described the histologic nature[40] of the laser interaction for each available excimer wavelength. Other investigators[41,42] confirmed that only the 193 nm wavelength produced the smooth even tissue removal that was so unusual in its appearance. Research in New York was carried out by Olivia Serdaravic,[43] Richard Darrell,[43] and Arthur Cotliar[44] who made important contributions in experimental applications of this new laser system. Particularly impressive were the results of studies in which we created[43] a fungal corneal ulcer (Fig. 1.7) and excised a 3 mm circular disc of tissue (Fig. 1.8) that healed the ulcer. This experiment, with its demonstration of clear healed corneas, did much to develop the concept that lamellar refractive surgery on the anterior surface would be possible.

Shortly after initial publication, Professor John Marshall, having read my initial paper, suggested we collaborate and study the ultrastructural properties of the ablated tissues. In the spring of 1984, I brought a number of specimens to the Institute of Ophthalmology in London for ultrastructural analysis. The animal corneas were exposed to the laser radiation in my laboratory at the Columbia–Presbyterian Medical Center. The specimens were prepared, placed in cacodylate solution and carried in insulated carriers packed with dry ice to London. The next morning was devoted to the excision of blocks and

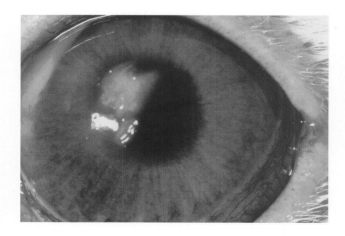

Figure 1.7 *A fungal corneal ulcer was induced in a rabbit cornea after corticosteroid pretreatment. (Courtesy of Olivia Serdaravic.)*

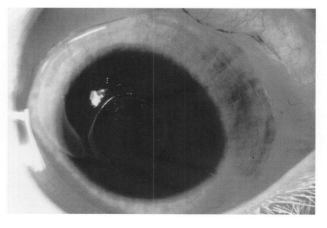

Figure 1.8 *View of the rabbit cornea after excision of the fungal ulcer. Notice the smooth surface of the 3 mm ablation and the transparency of the underlying tissue. (Courtesy of Olivia Serdaravic.)*

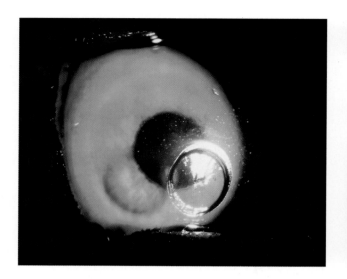

Figure 1.9 *A smooth optical surface was formed on a monkey cornea, which confirmed the potential for refractive surgical applications. We used a 3 mm circle on the end of a metal cone to define the beam adjacent to the animal cornea. This was held by a clamp, and positioned to select the most uniform part of the squared laser beam. The monkey was positioned with the cornea several millimeters from the aperture.*

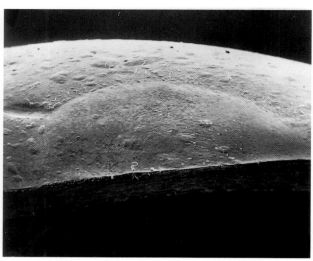

Figure 1.10 *SEM of healed corneal surface. The clarity of the healed cornea and the ultrastructural smoothness of the healed, epithelialized surface was strong evidence that we had removed tissue to standards of optical precision.*

viewing of the first scanning electron micrographs (SEMs). This work resulted in a series of publications over the next few years.[35–38] Using a crude delivery system we studied the texture of the ablated corneal surface (Fig. 1.9), the ultrastructural detail of each layer of the cornea, and the clinical and ultrastructural appearance of the healed cornea.

Marshall prepared scanning and transmission electronmicrographs of smoothly ablated surfaces prepared in our laboratory, first in rabbit, then monkey corneas, both acutely after exposure and after healing. Most impressive was the quality (Fig. 1.10) of the surface after ablation and the optical quality of the epithelialized healed surface. These specimens were presented at the Gordon Conference in July 1984, where the example of a healed corneal ulcer was less interesting to the audience than the transparent appearance of the healed cornea after ablation of a significant portion of its stroma. Charles Munnerlyn reviewed with me the quantitative relationships he had derived which calculated the amount of tissue that has to be removed to achieve a given optical result. I was impressed because his

calculation showed that for a 4 mm optical zone, only 5 µm of tissue had to be removed to flatten the cornea by 1D. Four millimeters seemed a reasonable diameter because RK surgeons had been using optical zones as small as 3 mm. Thus, the quantitative relationships between removal of central corneal tissue and the induced refractive change were derived as early as 1984[45] and prepared in a paper with illustrations of clear corneas after central ablation. In this paper, the term 'Photorefractive Keratectomy' (PRK) was coined and the relationship between tissue removal, optical zone size, and a given optical effect were detailed and diagrammed. However, it took four more years before it would be published[45] because it was deemed to be 'too speculative and of no practical value'.

To evaluate the corneal response to tissue removal, I ablated a series of progressively deeper 3.0 mm circles in rabbit corneas. Several weeks after the experiment, only the rabbit with the deepest ablation showed any haze. The others healed without discernible opacification when examined biomicroscopically. These experiments provided the impetus to proceed with the development of clinical excimer laser systems. During the early 1980s, my laboratory in New York continued to have the only excimer laser in the world dedicated exclusively to ophthalmic research. This situation changed rather abruptly in 1985 when interest in surgical applications of this technology exploded. New systems were in place at the Massachusetts Eye and Ear Infirmary in the laboratory of Steinert and Puliafito, a research prototype at the Free University in Berlin in Theo Seiler's laboratory, and a prototype system at the University of Connecticut organized by Francis L'Esperance, which developed into the Taunton system.

ArF, KrF, and XeCl lasers emit at wavelengths of 193 nm, 248 nm, and 308 nm, respectively, and all generate photons that are absorbed by and can ablate the cornea at sufficiently high irradiance. However, only the 193 nm photon was found to have the uniquely precise interaction and restricted damage zone that captured the imagination of ophthalmic surgeons. Every early investigator commented on this precision of tissue removal with limited damage in adjacent tissues seen after ablating with the ArF laser. One theory to explain this extreme localization suggests it occurs because the ablation arises from molecular bonds that are split by the pulse of the high-energy photons rather than by focal heating of a target volume of tissue. It is postulated that the molecular bond splitting is followed by a rapid, highly localized release of small molecular fragments without damage to remaining adjacent tissues.

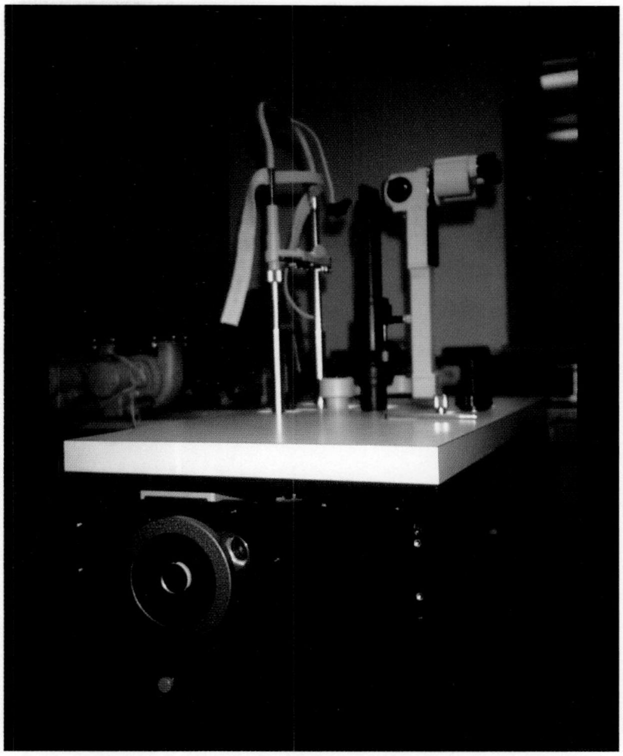

Figure 1.11 *First commercial prototype built by Meditec and shown at the American Academy of Ophthalmology meeting in the fall of 1985. This was designed to project a slit of excimer light on to the cornea of a seated patient using a slit lamp delivery system.*

EARLY EXCIMER LASER SYSTEMS FOR CORNEAL SURGERY

Meditec developed an instrument (Fig. 1.11), presented at the American Academy meeting in the fall of 1985, which was designed to project a slit-shaped excimer beam on to the cornea of a reclining patient using a slit lamp delivery system. This was soon converted to a microscopic delivery for a seated patient that became the archetype for the clinical Meditec systems. When it became apparent that large area ablation was having clinical success, Meditec converted their stationary projected slit into a slit that was rapidly scanned across the cornea. This was originally conceived as an expedient, but the clinical success of their early trials led to progressive refinement of the system.

Munnerlyn continued his system development at the Ophthalmic Laser branch of Cooper Vision and used development funds to build the clinical prototype pictured in Figure 1.12 that was designed to perform PRK with the beam shaping done by an expanding iris diaphragm. One of these prototypes was placed at Louisiana State University (LSU) with access to the primate colony of Tulane University. This prototype was shown at the American Academy meeting in 1986 as the first fully configured and operational excimer system for corneal refractive surgery.

Summit Technology had been developing an excimer system to perform angioplasty at 308 nm. When they became aware of the corneal surgical potential of this technology, they switched emphasis of their product development to a corneal surgical

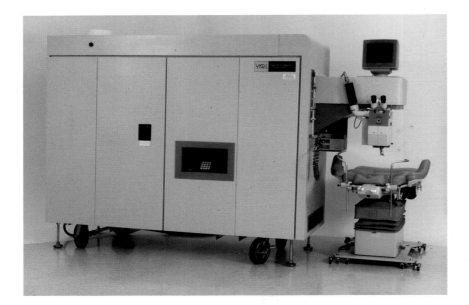

Figure 1.12 *First commercial prototype built by Cooper Vision lasers for large area ablation. This was tested by Marguerite McDonald in animals and blind eye studies. She performed the first successful PRK in a sighted myope in June 1988 using this equipment.*

system. The prototype system at the University of Connecticut became the Taunton system, with a commercial version available in 1987.

In the original generation of laser systems, the cavities used plastic insulators to support the electrodes and had fan bearings within the gas reservoir. The organic materials associated with these structures interacted with the UV photons and created contaminants that rapidly degraded the laser action. To counter this degradation and maintain satisfactory output, the gas mixture had to be either constantly cleansed with a cryogenic circulator or frequently replaced to maintain the extremely pure state of gas necessary for full laser output. Modern systems have improved laser cavity design with ceramic supports for their electrodes and magnetic coupling of circulating fans. These design features minimize the level of organic contaminants within the cavity and have created a substantially longer life for the laser gas. Adequate system performance can now be anticipated without the need for cryogenic purification or frequent gas refills during use. In addition to reducing cavity organic contamination, modern ophthalmic excimer laser systems are built to maintain their output by automatically adding gas or adjusting the laser discharge voltage whenever the laser output falls.

CLINICAL APPLICATIONS

The first[46] clinical work was done by Seiler using the Taunton system prototype when he excised superficial diseased corneal tissue in 1986 and created relaxing keratotomies in 1987 (Fig. 1.13).[47] The Meditec laser, designed to create linear keratotomies, was used in limited clinical trials in 1986 and 1987. The Munnerlyn commercial prototype was installed in LSU where the first human PRK studies were conducted in 1987 in blind eyes and in June 1988[48] in a sighted patient. Creating radial or transverse incisions to treat myopia or astigmatism has been shown to have no clinical advantages compared to using a diamond knife and this application is of historic interest only. Direct reshaping of the cornea remains the most important medical application of the excimer laser.

Tissue can be removed from large areas of the cornea in two ways and in two places. The location of the ablation can be the corneal surface or under a corneal flap, as described by Pallikaris.[49] The ablation pattern can be achieved with a number of large laser pulses, each of which has a varied energy distribution or shape, or the pattern can be formed by rapidly scanning a series of small laser pulses of uniform

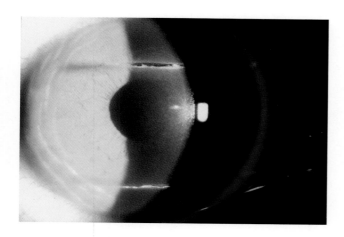

Figure 1.13 *Relaxing keratotomies for astigmatism. The first excimer application for refractive surgery created relaxing incisions to relieve astigmatism by flattening the steep meridian of the cornea. A contact lens was used to mask the beam, which allowed a narrow trench of tissue to be ablated from the stroma.*

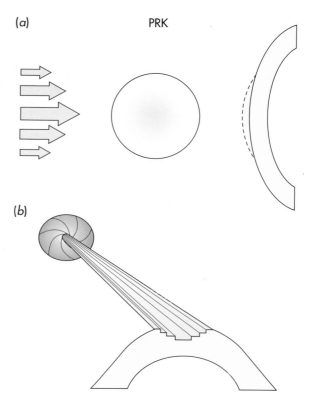

Figure 1.14 *(a) A diagram of a laser beam with more energy centrally than peripherally. This pattern is difficult to engineer and in practice is approximated by a series of circular pulses of increasing diameter (b) or a small scanning spot.*

energy over the surface. The possibility of prolonged exposures on a moving eye was an early concern and initial speculation was that exposure times would be minimized by simultaneous irradiation of a large area of the cornea. This reasoning supported the development of systems that quickly altered the cornea in the shortest time by using a beam with a large area as opposed to systems that scan a small beam over the corneal surface. Both systems have been developed and both produce results with no or minimal corneal haze. In Figure 1.14a, the center of the laser beam contains the highest concentration of energy, which decreases towards the beam periphery. This beam will remove more tissue centrally than peripherally with each pulse and produce a flattened, less strongly refracting cornea. Conversely, if the irradiance were made greater in the periphery, more tissue would be removed from the edges than the center, which would steepen the cornea. In principle, any contour can be transferred to the cornea by controlling the energy distribution within the beam incident upon the cornea. However, control of energy within the laser beam is technically difficult to achieve. It is far simpler to deliver more energy to the center by exposing the cornea to a series of circular beams (Fig. 1.14b) of increasing diameter. The center of the cornea receives more laser energy than the periphery, causing the cornea overall to become flatter. By controlling the

diameter and the size of the circular pulses, the amount of flattening and the resulting dioptric change can be controlled. Development of hyperopic algorithms generally has required introduction of scanning elements to create ablations that extend into the corneal periphery.

Scanning systems can be similarly configured to alter the corneal contour and were first developed by Meditec and Nidek, both of whom use a scanning beam in the shape of a slit. More recent developments using a small flying spot have been developed by LaserSight and Autonomous Technologies, using a scanning spot based on a small excimer laser, and by Novatec using a solid-state based system. The main advantage of a scanning system is that it requires a less powerful laser and each exposure has a minimal shock wave. Its disadvantage lies in the increased laser exposure time, with increased difficulties in stabilizing the alignment of the scanning beam during exposure and creating a smooth surface. The relative clinical efficacy and safety of these approaches has not yet been determined.

WHERE WE ARE

With the development of commercial interest in excimer laser systems for refractive surgery, attention and resources were diverted from the laboratory into development of apparatus suitable for clinical application. Even after the many hundreds of thousands of patients who have been operated upon by excimer technology, technical questions remain that have been incompletely answered and require more investigation. Among the most important of these is what is the optimal ablation pattern to recontour the optical surface of the cornea? What is the optimum fluence that should be used? Is the shape of the newly ablated corneal surface critical? How important is the tear film in healing? What about the blend or junction zone where the ablated and normal areas of the cornea meet? What are the limits of PRK and when should alternative technology be considered to correct refractive error?

As important as recognition of unanswered questions are the areas in which our clinical knowledge and testing of visual function is limited. The PRK procedure has galvanized the technique of videokeratography and moved a laboratory curiosity into the mainstream of ophthalmic practice. We have come up against the limits of measurement of refraction and visual function. We are concerned about possible degradation in night driving function yet we recognize that there is no simple test of visual function under these conditions. Clearly, a better understanding of the causes and natural history of refractive error is necessary if we are to understand the long-term stability of the patient who has undergone any refractive surgical procedure. The answers to most of these questions await the hand of time, clinical experience, and clinical investigation.

REFERENCES

1. Barraquer JI, Queratoplastia Refractiva, *Est e Inform Oftal* (1949) **2**:10: 15–64.
2. Barraquer JL, *Queratomileusis y Queratofaquia* (Bogota, Litografia Arco: Bogota, 1980) 88–123.
3. Barraquer JL, (Personal communication, 1994).
4. Weiner M, Meier's method of peeling of the cornea, *Ophthal Year Book* (1917):52.
5. Mueller OF, O'Neill P, Some Experiments on Corneal Grinding, *Exp Eye Res* (1967) **6**:42–47.
6. Olson RJ, Kaufman HE, Rheinstrom SD, Reshaping the cat corneal anterior surface using high speed diamond fraise, *Ophthalmic Surg* (1980) **11**:784–6.
7. Lasers systems marketed by Intelligent Surgical Lasers Inc., (San Diego, Ca) and Phoenix Lasers Inc., (San Francisco, Ca).
8. Wray (1914) cited by Tosti, E (see 10).
9. O'Conner R, Corneal cautery for high myopic astigmatism, *Am J Ophthal* (1933) **16**: 337–40.
10. Tosti E, Correxziones dell'astigmatismo corneale mediante diatermo coagulazione, Act Primus Latinus Congresses Ophthalmologiae (Arte della Stampa: Roma, 1953) 125–28.
11. Gasset AR, Shaw EL, Kaufman HE, Thermokeratoplasty, *Trans Am Acad Oph Otol* (1973) **77**:451–4.
12. Aquavella JA, Smith RS, Shaw EL, Alterations in corneal morphology following thermal keratoplasty, *Arch Ophth* (1976) **94**:2082–5.
13. Arentson JJ, Rodrigues MM, Laibson PR, Histopathologic changes after thermokeratoplasty for keratoconus, *Invest Ophthal Vis Sci* (1977) **16**:32–38.
14. Rowsey JJ, Electrosurgical keratoplasty: update and retraction, *Invest Ophthal Vis Sci* (1987) **28**:224.
15. Vasco Posada J, Queratocon; Electrocoagulacion circular de la corne para la adaptacion de lentes de contacto, *Arch Soc Amer Oftal Optom* (1981) **15**:159–64.
16. Keates RH, Pedrotti L, Weider H, Possel W, Carbon dioxide laser beam control for corneal surgery, *Ophthal Surg* (1981) **12**:117.
17. Fyodorov SN, Semyonov AD, Sorokin AS, et al, Laser correction of Hypermetropia and Hypermetropic Astigmatism. In: *Laser Methods of Treatment and Angiographic Investigations in Ophthalmology* (Moscow Scientific and Investigation Institute of Ocular Microsurgery: Moscow, 1984) 3–14.
18. Kanoda AN, Sorokin AS, Laser Correction of Hypermetropic Refraction. In Fyodorov SN, ed. *Microsurgery of the Eye: Main Aspects.* (Mir Publishers: Moscow, 1987) 147–154.
19. Horn G, Spears KG, Lopez Lopez O, et al, New refractive method for laser thermal keratoplasty with the $CO:MgF_2$ laser, *J Cat Refract Surg* (1990) **16**:611–16.
20. Seiler T, Matallana M, Bende T, Laser thermokeratoplasty by means of a pulsed holmium: YAG laser for hyperopic correction, *J Refract Corn Surg* (1990) **11**:325–9.
21. Moreira H, Campos M, Sawusch R, McDonnell JM, Sand B, McDonnell PJ, Holmium laser thermokeratoplasty, *Ophthalmology* (1993) **100**:752–61.
22. Velazco JE, Setser DW, Bound-free emission spectra of diatomic xenon halides, *J Chem Phys* (1975) **62**: 1990–1.

23. Searles SK, Hart GA, Bound free emission spectra of xenon halides, *Appl Phys Lett* (1975) **27**:243.

24. Ewing JJ, Brau CA, Untitled letter, *Appl Phys Lett* (1975) **27**:350.

25. Brau CA, Ewing JJ, Untitled letter, *Appl Phys Lett* (1975) **27**:435.

26. Hoffman JM, Hays AK, Tisone GC, High-power UV noble-gas-halide lasers, *Appl Phys Lett* (1976) **28**:538–9.

27. Burnham R, Djeu N, Ultraviolet-preionized discharge-pumped lasers in XeF, KrF, and ArF, *Appl Phys Lett* (1976) **29**:707–9.

28. Stevens B, Hutton E, Radiative lifetime of the pyrene dimer and the possible role of excited dimers in energy transfer processes, *Nature* (1960) **186**:1045–6.

29. Taboada J, Mikesell GW, Reed RD, Response of the corneal epithelium to KrF excimer laser pulses, *Health Phys* (1981) **40**:677–83.

30. Taboada J, Archibald CJ, An extreme sensitivity in the corneal epithelium to far UV ArF excimer laser pulses, Proceedings of the Scientific Program of the Aerospace Medical Association, San Antonio, Texas, 1981.

31. Trokel SL, *YAG Laser Ophthalmic Microsurgery.* (Appleton–Century Crofts: New York, 1983).

32. Srinivasan R, Kinetics of the ablative photodecomposition of organic polymers in the far ultraviolet (193 nm), *J Vac Sci Technol B1* (1983) **4**:923–6.

33. Munnerlyn CM (Personal communication, 1994)

34. Trokel SL, Srinivasan R, Braren B, Excimer Laser Surgery of the Cornea, *Am J Ophthalmol* (1983) **96**:710–15.

35. Marshall J, Trokel SL, Rothery S, Schubert H, An Ultrastructural Study of Corneal Incisions Induced by an Excimer Laser at 193 nm. *Ophthalmology* (1985) **92**:749–58.

36. Marshall J, Trokel S, Rothery S, Krueger R, Photoablative Reprofiling of the Cornea using an Excimer Laser, Photorefractive Keratectomy, *Lasers in Ophthal* (1986) **1**:21–48.

37. Marshall J, Trokel SL, Rothery S, Krueger R, A Comparative Study of Corneal Incisions Induced by Diamond and Steel Knives and Two Ultraviolet Radiations from an Excimer Laser, *Br J Ophthalmol* (1986) **70**:482–501.

38. Marshall J, Trokel SL, Rothery S, Krueger RR, Long term healing of the central cornea after photorefractive keratectomy using an excimer laser, *Ophthalmology* (1988) **95**:1411–21.

39. Krueger RR, Trokel SL, Quantification of Corneal Ablation by Ultraviolet Laser Light, *Arch Ophthalmol* (1985) **103**:1741–2.

40. Krueger RR, Trokel SL, Schubert HD, Interaction of Ultraviolet Laser Light with the Cornea, *Invest Ophthal Vis Sci* (1985) **26**:1455–64.

41. Puliafito CA, Steinert RF, Deutsch TF, Adler CM, Excimer laser ablation of the cornea and lens, *Ophthalmology* (1985) **92**:741–8.

42. Krauss JM, Puliafito CA, Steinert RF, Laser interactions with the cornea, *Surv Ophthal* (1986) **31**:37–53.

43. Serdarevic O, Darrell RW, Krueger RR, Trokel SL, Excimer Laser Therapy for Experimental Candida Keratitis, *Am J Ophthalmol* (1985) **99**:534–8.

44. Cotliar AM, Schubert HD, Mandell ER, Trokel SL, Excimer Laser Radial Keratotomy, *Ophthalmology* (1985) **92**:206–8..

45. Munnerlyn CR, Koons SJ, Marshall J, Photorefractive keratectomy: a technique for laser refractive surgery, *J Cat Refract Surg* (1988) **14**:46–52.

46. Berlin M, Bende T, Seiler T, Corneal resurfacing by excimer laser photoablation, ARVO abstracts, *Invest Ophthal Vis Sci* (1988) **29(Supp)**:310.

47. Seiler T, Bende T, Trokel S, Wollensak J, Excimer laser keratectomy for correction of astigmatism, *Am J Ophthalmol* (1988) **105**:117–24.

48. Mcdonald M, Kaufman HE, Frantz JM, Shofner S, Salmeron B, Klyce SD, Excimer Laser Ablation in a Human Eye, *Arch Ophthalmol* (1989) **107**:641–2.

49. Pallikaris IG, Papatzanaki ME, Stathi EZ, et al, Laser in situ keratomileusis, Lasers Surg Med (1990) **10**:463–8.

Chapter 2 Physical principles of excimer lasers

Paul P van Saarloos

BASIC LASER BACKGROUND

LIGHT AMPLIFICATION BY STIMULATED EMISSION OF RADIATION

What is light? Sometimes light behaves as if it is composed of waves and at other times as if it is composed of particles. For this reason, the nature of light is often a difficult concept to grasp. Light is a transverse electromagnetic wave; the energy 'waves' as it oscillates between an electric field and a magnetic field. (The collapsing electric field generates a magnetic field and vice versa.) For light to also have the properties of a particle, it is useful to consider these waves to come in packets of a limited size (photons).

When the electrons spinning around an atom are energized to a higher energy orbit and then decay back to a lower energy orbit, they can give off a photon of light. The wavelength of this light is inversely proportional to the energy lost by the electron, which in turn is dependent upon the type of atom. This process of light generation is called *spontaneous emission*, whereas *stimulated emission* occurs when this event is triggered by another photon that has an identical wavelength to that which the atom will produce. The *amplification process* is thus one photon triggering the release of two nearly identical photons. In a laser, each photon may then go on and trigger two more photons, and so on.

LASER PUMPS

Lasers need to consist of a 'pump' (a source of energy to energize the electrons), a 'medium' that contains the atoms that do the lasing, and a cavity consisting of mirrors to direct the light backwards and forwards through the energized media to allow the amplification process to grow to a useful level.

There are many different methods for pumping lasers, ranging from chemical reactions to electron beams. Probably two of the most common forms of pumping involve electrical discharge or current, and light energy produced by either flash lamps or another laser.

LASER MEDIA

The laser medium also comes in a large number of variations covering all the states of matter. Lasers with a gas medium include Co_2 lasers, excimer lasers and argon lasers; dye lasers have a liquid medium, while neodymium:YAG (Nd:YAG) and diode lasers are examples of solid medium lasers.

Ophthalmologists are usually familiar with the argon and Nd:YAG lasers. Argon lasers utilize a gas medium that is usually pumped by an electrical discharge through the gas, whereas Nd:YAG lasers are solid medium lasers that are usually pumped with flash lamps. In the latter, the medium is neodymium atoms. The YAG crystal holds the neodymium atoms in place and helps to transfer the flash lamp pump energy to the neodymium atoms.

It is vital that the pumped medium be in a state of *population inversion* for lasing to occur. Population inversion is when more than half of the atoms in the medium are energized to an excited state. An atom that is capable of being excited and then stimulated to emit a photon of light will also resonantly absorb a photon of the same wavelength when not excited. Hence, it is easy to perceive that unless there are more atoms in an excited state than in a non-excited state, then the absorption process will exceed the stimulated emission process and amplification will not occur.

COMMON PROPERTIES OF LASERS

If lasers are essentially just beams of light, why are they considered more useful than, for example, light from a torch? Light from a laser has a number of properties that make it different from other light sources. Firstly, the divergence of a laser beam is much, much lower than that of other light sources. This allows the laser beam to be confined to *very narrow beams* and to be focused to very small spot sizes. Secondly, laser light is usually *monochromatic*, that is, the light is of a single very pure colour (single wavelength). Thirdly, laser beam light is usually *coherent*, that is, all the waves of the photons are oscillating in phase with each other.

EXCIMER LASER HISTORY AND DEVELOPMENT

'Excimer' is a contraction of the term 'excited dimer'. Dimers are usually considered to be molecules made up of two identical atoms. However, the term 'excimer' has subsequently been extended to include other excited molecules (though usually diatomic). If two systems (atoms or molecules) do not form a strong chemical bond when they are in their ground states, but do form a strong chemical bond when one of them is in an excited state, then the bound excited state is called an excimer.

The fact that the excimer dissociates in the ground state has important consequences in a laser system, as this helps to maintain the population inversion necessary for lasing action. The lack of well-defined bonding electron energy levels in the ground state means that excimer lasers usually have a small tuning range (up to 1 nm). The early development and theory of excimer lasers has been reviewed by Rhodes,[1,2] Huestis,[3] and Hecht.[4]

Excimers and their continuous ultraviolet (UV) spectra have been studied since the 1930s. It was first proposed that excimers could be involved in laser action by Houtermans in 1960.[5] However, problems associated with the very high pump energies required meant that true stimulated emission was not observed until 1971. Basov et al[6] observed lasing action in condensed xenon (Xe), and a year later stimulated emission was observed from Xe in a gaseous state (a true excimer laser).[7] It was developments in the production of high-energy electron beams, to provide the pump energy, that facilitated the production of stimulated emission from excimer systems.

The first rare gas halide excimer laser was reported in 1975 by Searles and Hart.[8] This was closely

Table 2.1

Major wavelengths and pulse energies that can be generated by a Questek model 2820 excimer laser.

Gas	Wavelength (nm)	Pulse energy (mJ)
F_2	157	25
ArF	193	425
KrCl	222	200
KrF	248	750
XeCl	308	400
XeF	351	350

followed by a number of reports of other rare gas excimer lasers. Rare gas halide excimer lasers have since evolved into the most efficient and well-developed excimer lasers, and form the main work horses in many applications. The electron-beam sources used to pump these early excimer lasers were bulky and expensive, which limited their availability. Excimer lasers pumped by a transverse electric discharge were reported in 1976[9] and offered a solution to this problem. Commercial lasers based on this pumping scheme appeared on the market about a year later (see also Chapter 1).

EXCIMER LASER WAVELENGTHS

Excimer lasers are a rich source of new laser wavelengths. Table 2.1 shows the wavelengths that an early commercial excimer laser is capable of producing. These new laser transitions were considered to have many promising applications in photochemistry and isotope separation.[10,11] It was while the laser was being tested for applications in the microelectronics industry in 1982, that it was first reported as having been applied to organic polymers.[12,13] The very clean etching seen in these early polymer applications aroused interest in the excimer laser, that eventually led to testing this laser for cutting and 'sculpting' corneal tissue.

HOW EXCIMER LASERS WORK

Excimer lasers are relatively straightforward to construct. However, the technology to make these

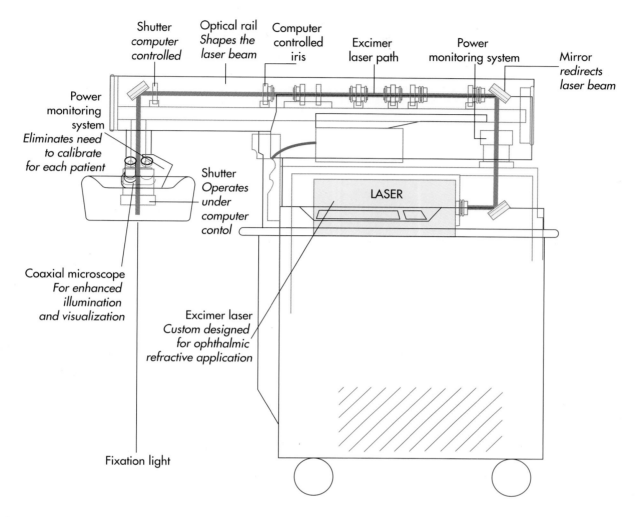

Figure 2.1 *Typical excimer laser beam path demonstrating the multiple optical components (Summit Omnimed laser). (Courtesy Summit Technology, Waltham, MA, USA.)*

lasers work efficiently and with reasonable component and gas lifetime is extremely complex.

Excimer lasers usually consist of a large, elongated aluminum box. This box is filled with the appropriate gas mixture. Running the full length of this box are two metal electrodes spaced about 2–3 cm apart. At one end of the box, aligned with the gap between the electrodes, a mirror is mounted and, at the other end, a window. The window is usually an uncoated optic. The small amount of reflection that normally occurs from each surface is enough to provide laser action.

Outside the box there is usually a large bank of capacitors, and these are charged using a high voltage power supply to several tens of kilovolts. A special switch (thyraton) is used to dump the energy stored in these capacitors across the electrodes inside the box. The electrical discharge through the gas between the electrodes ionizes the gas and allows the excimer molecules to form. Lasing action usually occurs within nanoseconds.

One of the first problems with making an excimer laser work is posed by the amount of energy involved and the rate with which it needs to be delivered across the electrodes. With voltages around 30 000 volts and currents of approximately 10 000 amps reached within 50 ns, the electrical characteristics are not unlike a bolt of lightning.

A thyraton is usually used as the switch to quickly initiate the discharge and carry the high currents. The thyraton is actually based on valve technology because contemporary solid state electronics do not cope well with the high current levels and very fast switching times (thyratons were developed initially to drive radar systems in airports). The 'valve'-like nature of the thyraton explains the 5–10 minute warm up required for the excimer lasers. Early excimer lasers often used thyratons at more than ten times their rated levels and used poorly designed discharge circuits that actively damaged the thyraton. Thyraton failures were common and, as these devices cost many thousands of dollars, excimer lasers gained a reputation of being expensive to maintain. However, modern excimer lasers, with improved discharge circuit designs and using techniques such as electrical pulse compression and insaturable inductors, have significantly reduced the load on those switches and thyraton failures are now relatively uncommon.

Another very important problem relates to maintaining the quality of the gas within the cavity. Excimer lasers are usually specified to run at purities of 99.99995% . The fluorine in the gas usually makes up only 0.1–0.2% of the gas volume. However, fluorine is an extremely reactive gas and can react with most materials that make up the components inside an excimer laser cavity and will also react with most impurities that have either entered with the gas or are out-gassed from the materials inside the laser cavity. These reactions not only use up some of the fluorine gas, so that the lasing action becomes very inefficient, but also create products that can absorb the laser radiation, interfere with the energy transfer process to the argon fluoride excimers and form deposits on the laser cavity optics. These processes can also significantly interfere with the lasing action. To make matters worse, the intense UV and hot plasma which is formed by the electrical discharge between the electrodes helps to initiate many of these reactions.

DELIVERY SYSTEMS FOR EXCIMER LASERS

Generally, delivery systems (Fig. 2.1) for excimer laser photorefractive keratectomy (PRK) systems can be divided into two groups: *scanning* and *large beam* (Figs 2.2a–c). Scanning systems have numerous advantages in that they are smaller and cheaper to purchase and are much simpler to design. However, there are a number of inherent problems with

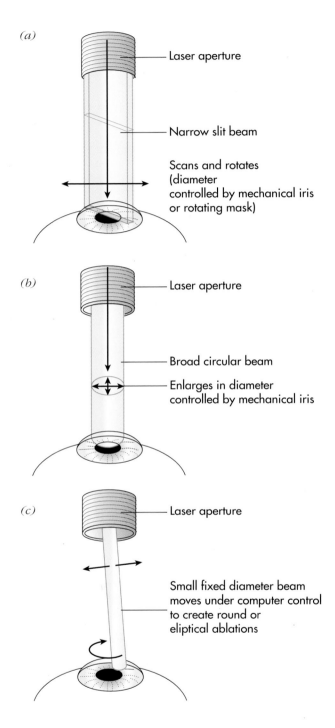

(a) — Laser aperture

— Narrow slit beam

Scans and rotates (diameter controlled by mechanical iris or rotating mask)

(b) — Laser aperture

— Broad circular beam

— Enlarges in diameter controlled by mechanical iris

(c) — Laser aperture

Small fixed diameter beam moves under computer control to create round or eliptical ablations

Figure 2.2 *Diagrams illustrating the three methods of excimer laser delivery to the corneal surface. (a) Slit scanning. (b) Large or broad beam. (c) Spot scanning.*

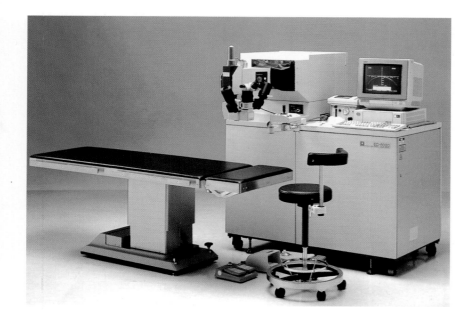

Figure 2.3 *The Nidek EC-5000 scanning excimer laser. (Courtesy Nidek.)*

scanning that suggest the optimum PRK laser system probably will not be a scanning system.

Scanning excimer lasers

One of the aspects that make scanning systems relatively simple to design is that the beam-shaping requirements are significantly lower. The beam need only be homogenous enough to ensure that the fluences at the corneal surface are outside the range that could damage the cornea, and that scanning the beam provides for a reasonably smooth ablated surface. In addition, because the beam does not need to be applied to the whole treatment area at once, the laser beam energy requirements for a scanning system are much less than a large beam system, hence much smaller and cheaper excimer laser units can be used. In theory, this should also relate to lower running costs (because of the smaller quantity of gas required). However, to date this has not been the case and, in any event, the cost of gas in running modern excimer lasers is fast becoming an insignificant proportion of the total running cost. Two laser systems in clinical use, the Nidek EC-5000 and Meditec lasers, utilize a scanning slit beam system (Figs 2.3, 2.4) and clinical results are discussed in Chapter 12.

Scanning systems are often stated to be 'gentler' to the cornea. This statement relates to the fact that a smaller beam generates a lower amplitude acoustic wave in the corneal tissue during ablation. Since the acoustic wave generated during normal large beam PRK procedures has not been shown to produce any damage to the corneal tissue, the 'gentleness' of an excimer laser ablation is probably irrelevant and may have no effect on the eye's healing response.

Although scanning provides a reasonably smooth ablated surface, it is not an optimally smoothed surface. Because of the alignment of the edges of the beam in a scanning system, a perfect scanning system will always produce a surface that is twice as rough as a perfect large beam system. In addition, if the beam being scanned is not smooth, then scanning can only go so far in producing a smooth surface, just as continuous rubbing (scanning) with a piece of coarse sandpaper will never produce a perfectly smooth result.

A major problem with scanning systems is that they are generally much slower in performing PRK procedures, which allows more time for eye movements and corneal hydration changes that could affect the clinical result. The treatment time for scanning systems using a small spot increases as the cube of the treatment zone diameter increases. If such a system worked with an adequate treatment time for

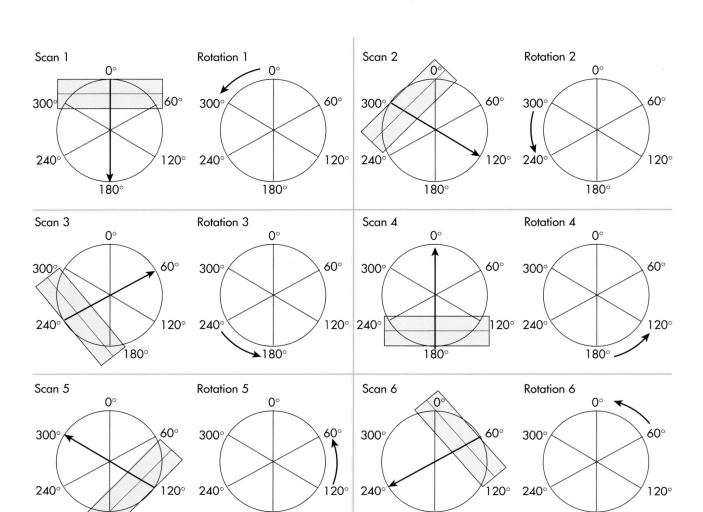

Figure 2.4 *Diagrammatic representation of pattern of scanning followed by the Nidek EC-5000 scanning excimer laser. The slit scans over the whole area back and forth once. During this scanning 10 laser pulses are delivered. After returning to the primary position the slit turns 60° to the left and makes a second scan back and forth. For the third scan, it turns a further 60° and so on, repeating six times on a full circle, i.e. 360°. (Courtesy Nidek.)*

a 5 mm ablation zone, it could become completely unusable for optical zones larger than 6 mm due to the extremely long treatment times. To overcome problems with fixation during lengthy spot scanning procedures, two systems are currently marketed with active eye tracking: the Autonomous Technologies T-PRK system, and the Chiron Technolas Keracor laser, which combines large beam and spot beam scanning (Figs 2.5, 2.6).

To partially compensate for the slow ablation rate, scanning systems are often run at very high pulse repetition rates. It has been shown that thermal damage to the remaining corneal tissue increases with increasing pulse repetition rate.[14] Because of the significant beam overlap and the need for a scanning system to dwell more in the centre of the cornea to remove more tissue from that area during myopic corrections, this effect is applicable to scanning laser systems. Although scanning laser systems are likely to induce more thermal damage to the corneal tissue, it is not known whether this has any effect on the clinical result.

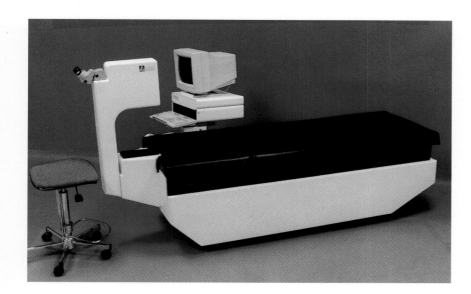

Figure 2.5 *The Autonomous Technologies T-PRK excimer laser system. In this spot scanning system, the excimer laser is integrated into the couch and an active tracking system follows the scanning spot beam, which takes nearly 20 s per diopter correction at a 6 mm ablation diameter. (Courtesy Autonomous Technologies.)*

Another problem with scanning systems relates to the difficulty in maintaining adequate and uniform corneal hydration. Since water evaporating through an ablated corneal surface can very quickly disrupt that surface, a scan pattern that leaves ablated tissue exposed to air for any length of time risks significantly damaging that tissue. The second point relating to corneal hydration is that the ablation rate of tissue is strongly related to its hydration level. The scan pattern that sweeps from left-to-right and then back from right-to-left will cut virgin tissue on the first path but on the reverse path will first cut tissue that is still dry from the recent ablation. At the other end of the right-to-left pass, the laser will be hitting tissue that has been left unexposed to the laser for a longer period; this tissue will be significantly more hydrated and will ablate at a much lower rate. This can lead to unpredictable keratectomy profiles, irregular astigmatism and/or corneal islands or central corneal depressions.

Large beam excimer laser systems

Large beam systems can be easily designed to maintain a uniform hydration over the whole treatment zone. A large beam treatment system can be simply built by placing a motorized iris in front of the output from an excimer laser. However, this type of

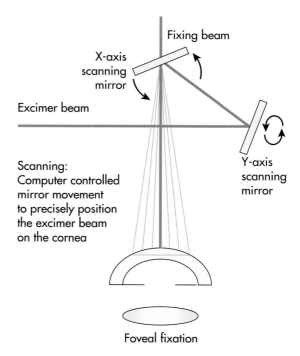

Figure 2.6 *The dual scanning mirror technique utilized in the Chiron Technolas excimer laser to move a small diameter beam precisely across the cornea. (Courtesy Chiron Technolas.)*

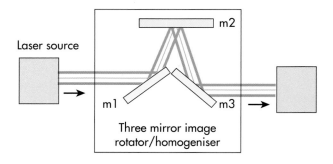

Figure 2.7 *Schematic of the delivery optics of an excimer laser utilizing a three-mirror system image rotator to smooth the beam, as used in the LE1200 system made by the Excimer Laser Company (TELCO).*

approach is not acceptable by today's requirements for small hyperopic shifts and low instances of corneal scarring. Producing a large beam system that is properly smoothed and homogenized is a more technically difficult problem than building a scanning laser system.

Smoothing large beams

Probably the two most common beam smoothing methods used in the excimer laser systems involve the use of *image rotators* or *optical integrators*. Image rotators come in two varieties, either 3 K mirror systems (Fig. 2.7) or dove prisms. These devices use three reflections to invert the beam. The axis by which the inversion takes place can be rotated by rotating the device and, hence, the image rotator effectively rotates the beam around its own central axis. This provides a beam smoothing mechanism similar to that provided by a scanning laser system, with the added advantage that the ablation becomes rotationally symmetrical, i.e. is astigmatically neutral.

Optical integrators work by using an optic that has multiple segments to divide the beam into many different beams (Figs 2.8, 2.9). Each of these beams is then made to overlap at the ablation site. Optical integrators have the advantage that they actually perform their beam smoothing on a single pulse, unlike scanning systems or image rotators that produce a smooth ablation by averaging the effect of many pulses. However, the use of optical integrators does not guarantee an homogenous beam, because the hot spots are merely moved around and are not

properly removed. In addition, after passing through an optical integrator, the laser beam loses much of its laser-like qualities, which places much higher constraints on the optical system that is placed after the optical integrator. For instance, one type of optical integrator may produce a spirograph-like flower pattern in the corneal surface when slightly defocused.

Another method of beam smoothing has been called the 'wobbling' mirror approach; this is, effectively, a mini scan of a large beam. Because the scan range is so small, the beam smoothing is probably not highly effective and provides no guarantee that an homogenous ablation will be performed.

A very common method of smoothing laser beams is *spatial filtering*. Although more difficult to apply to excimer lasers, this has been successfully done in at least one system (LE1200 system made by the Excimer Laser Company). This method has the advantage in that it smooths every pulse and is extremely effective in the high spatial frequency parts of the energy distribution (i.e. the worst hot spots). However, once again, this type of beam smoothing does not necessarily guarantee an homogenous beam.

Large homogenous beams have often been blamed for the formation of corneal islands. Although there are a number of possible reasons for the formation of corneal islands, some of these are related to the difficulty of producing a large homogenous beam. With a limited amount of laser energy available after smoothing, compromises sometimes need to be made to produce optical zones of at least 6.0 mm diameter.

One method is to deliberately misalign an image rotator so that it scans in a small circle (e.g. scanning a 5 mm beam in a 1 mm circle will cut a 6 mm zone). However, if the beam has a central hot spot (as is often the case) the resultant ablation will have a central island. Another likely cause of corneal islands is the central tissue being more hydrated than the peripheral tissue. Under these circumstances, the central tissue will ablate more slowly and a central island will form. This can also be caused by scraping the epithelium towards the centre of the cornea. Central islands may also be caused by fluid remaining on the corneal surface, or welling up from the ablated surface and being attracted to the centre of the ablation. This attraction process could, theoretically, be driven by the acoustic waves generated by the ablation process or by chemical changes on the ablated surface changing the surface tension of the fluid (see also Chapter 23).

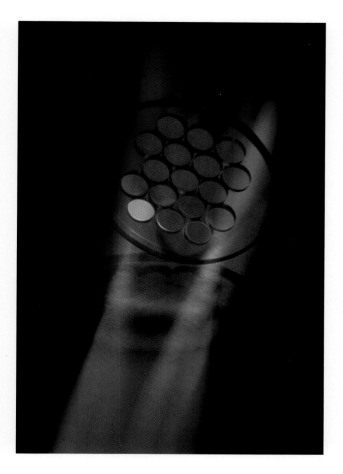

Figure 2.8 (*a*) *The optical integrator, which homogenizes the laser beam energy in the Coherent Schwind keratom, consists of an array of round prism palets made from synthetic quartz (Suprasil II) that is transparent for ultraviolet radiation. (Courtesy Coherent.)*

Figure 2.8 (*b*) *Schematic set-up of the laser beam delivery in the Coherent Schwind keratom. The original rectangular beam (8 × 24 mm) is expanded by a cylindrical lens system before being reflected by a mirror through 90° to pass through the optical integrator. The homogenized, expanded, but still rectangular beam then passes through a series of circular or oval beam stops on a steel band to create the intended dimensions of the laser beam. The beam passes to the cornea via a dicrotic beam splitter and a zoom lens system. (Courtesy Coherent.)*

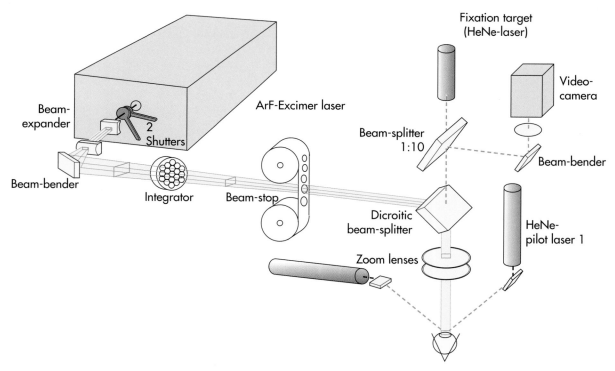

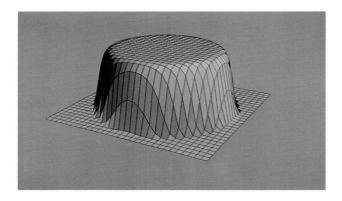

Figure 2.9 *After homogenization, hot or cold spots should have been removed and the normal Gaussian excimer beam profile should approach that of the perfect 'top hat' configuration illustrated. (Courtesy Coherent.)*

Large beam systems, in an effort to produce larger optical zones, often resort to using lower fluences. Low laser fluences do not cope well with either the differences in tissue hydration or fluid welling up from the ablated surface and, hence, are more likely to produce corneal islands in these situations.

SCANNING VERSUS LARGE BEAM

In conclusion, the fact that a laser is scanning or large beam does not indicate whether it is a good or bad laser. In the author's opinion, the ultimate excimer laser system would be a large beam system (with perhaps some scanning capabilities); however, scanning systems should be cheaper to purchase and even a poor-quality scanning system is likely to produce better results than the early unsmoothed large beam systems.

SOLID STATE OR GAS EXCIMER LASERS?

It is generally considered by most practitioners that the future belongs to solid state lasers. However, at this time, this statement is a long way from being fact. Ultraviolet solid state lasers usually start with a well-established and efficient solid state laser, for instance, the infrared Nd:YAG laser. The output from this laser

is passed through one or more non-linear crystals, which convert the infrared light into light of a shorter wavelength. A common non-linear technique is frequency doubling (second-harmonic generation).

In transparent crystals (that transmit the laser's wavelength) the electrons within the crystal are forced to move in phase with the light's electromagnetic wave. In non-linear crystals, the structure of the crystal does not allow the electron to move too far from its normal position without exerting additional forces on it. When the amplitude of the oscillating motion of the electron in the light's electromagnetic field gets too great, these additional forces cause the electron to oscillate at a different frequency from that of the light. One of the common ways that such electrons can obey the laws of physics is to oscillate at exactly twice the frequency they are being forced to oscillate at. These oscillating electrons therefore emit light at the frequency at which they subsequently oscillate, i.e. twice the frequency and half the wavelength of the input laser radiation.

There are a number of parameters that must be met before this frequency conversion will work efficiently. Firstly, the input laser radiation must be sufficiently intense to make the electrons oscillate at a high enough amplitude. This usually requires the input radiation to be focused to as narrow a beam as possible and sometimes pulsed with as short a pulse width as possible.

A second important parameter is called 'phase-matching'. With a large number of electrons oscillating at the new frequency, if the light produced by each of these electrons is not in phase, then the light produced by one electron could destructively interfere with the light produced by another. The net result would be practically no light at the new frequency.

In a perfect world, phase-matching would not be a problem because the input laser radiation would force the electrons to oscillate in phase with it, which would cause the frequency-doubled light also to be in phase. However, in the real world, light of different frequencies does not travel through crystals at the same speed and, hence, the frequency-doubled light will quickly become out of phase with the input light as the two beams travel through crystal. Phase-matching is then lost. The property of light of different frequencies travelling through crystals at different speeds is called *'dispersion'*. The solution to the problem of dispersion is usually related to another property of crystals called *'birefringence'*, when light of the same frequency, but of a different polarization, travels at different speeds through the crystal. Crystals that have a non-symmetrical atomic matrix are usually birefringent. The non-symmetrical atomic lattice structure may allow electrons to move more easily in one direction, e.g, up and down, than in another, e.g. side to side. Light with a vertical polarization would travel through the crystal at a faster speed than light with a horizontal polarization, and the crystal would be birefringent.

When the input laser beam is polarized, the second harmonic is generated in the polarization that is orthogonal to this input polarization. So, if a crystal can be found where the effect of birefringence on this frequency-doubled light exactly cancels the effect of dispersion, then the condition of phase-matching can be met and this frequency-doubled light will not cancel itself out over the length of the crystal.

Of course nature does not readily supply crystals with both the properties required for frequency conversion and for dispersion and birefringence to exactly cancel out. In practice, crystals with properties that are close to those required are fine-tuned to get their conditions exactly right. Sometimes birefringence or dispersion is temperature dependent, and the crystal can be fine-tuned by heating or cooling. Another technique to fine-tune a crystal is called 'angle tuning'. The amount of birefringence usually depends on the angle of propagation through the crystal, and so the crystal can be rotated with respect to the incoming laser beam until the birefringence exactly cancels the dispersion.

The requirements for both non-linear frequency conversion and phase-matching place stringent requirements on the quality of the crystals. Any defect in the crystal structure can cause the angle-tuning alignment to be imperfectly matched over the length of the crystal, and can cause local variations in the refractive index that cause the breakdown of the phase-matching condition. Small defects in the crystal may also absorb either of the laser wavelengths, which not only causes loss through the absorption process but also the local heating can cause the phase-matching condition to be lost.

Another non-linear process similar to frequency levelling is called optical mixing. Instead of applying one input laser wavelength to the crystal, two wavelengths can be applied. In this case, the electrons will be forced to oscillate under the influence of both the electromagnetic field frequencies. Again, when the amplitude of the electron oscillation reaches a level where the constraints of the crystal structure do not allow it to oscillate in phase with the input frequencies, the electron starts to oscillate at a higher frequency.

To match the laws of physics (e.g. conservation of energy), the wavelength of light generated by this higher frequency oscillation is given by the equation:

$$\lambda_3 = \frac{\lambda_1 \lambda_2}{\lambda_1 + \lambda_2}$$

Note that if: $\lambda_1 = \lambda_2$, then

$$\lambda_3 = \frac{\lambda_1}{2} \ ,$$

which is the frequency doubling situation.

Higher harmonics can also be generated in a similar fashion to frequency doubling or second-harmonic generation. However, it is generally very difficult to meet all the phase-matching requirements to generate these harmonics in a single crystal. Hence, it is usual for the higher harmonics to be generated in multiple steps.

For instance, to generate the third harmonic of a Nd:YAG laser, this could be initially frequency doubled in one crystal, which would generate 530 nm radiation that could then be mixed with the original 1066 nm radiation in a second crystal to generate the third harmonic at 353 nm. Although the crystals in both steps could be made of the same material, they would be set up differently to allow phase-matching for the appropriate stage.

To produce a wavelength close to the 193 nm from an excimer laser, a near infrared laser would need to be quintupled and a visible wavelength would need to be quadrupled. For instance, a Nd:YAG laser could be frequency doubled twice and then mixed with the original wavelength to produce the fifth harmonic at 213 nm.

Producing the fifth harmonic is a three-stage process. Although the first doubling stage can be more than 50% efficient, each of the final stages can be much less than 10% efficient. The high losses through this type of system mean that the Nd:YAG laser needs to be much more powerful and complex than the YAG lasers normally found in ophthalmology offices. To complicate matters, small temperature variations or very slight shifts in the alignment can cause large changes in efficiency.

One manufacturer has avoided using three steps by starting with a visible wavelength laser. However, this visible laser is very immature technology compared to that of Nd:YAG. Indeed, this laser is actually pumped by an argon ion gas laser, so the system is not genuinely a solid state system and will have all the problems associated with the old argon lasers used in ophthalmology (large amounts of water used for cooling, high maintenance, etc), as well as the problems associated with maintaining the frequency conversion crystals.

CONCLUSIONS – SOLID STATE EXCIMER LASERS

Solid state lasers have still not reached their theoretical low maintenance status. The crystals are exposed to extremely high laser radiation intensities that include UV wavelengths. This can damage and degrade the crystals over time, and they are expensive to replace. The alignment and temperature stability requirements are also very critical. In addition, solid state lasers are still not producing enough energy to compete with excimer lasers in scanning systems, let alone large beam systems.

Although solid state technology is improving at a very rapid pace, excimer laser technology is not standing still. There is at least one excimer laser system on the market (LE1200 system made by the Excimer Laser Company) that can be operated non-stop for more than 2 weeks on a single gas fill (without fluorine injection). This allows very low running costs and greatly simplifies use of the system. It will probably be many years before solid state lasers will be the optimum source of UV light around 200 nm for PRK procedures.

OTHER POTENTIAL REFRACTIVE LASERS

The excimer laser is not the only tool that can be used to reshape the anterior surface of the cornea to correct refractive errors. Both mechanical devices and other lasers have been tested. A review of other lasers that have been applied to the cornea was included in a report by Krauss et al.[15]

MECHANICAL DEVICES

The results of using a mechanical grinding tool to reshape the cornea were published in 1967 by Mueller and O'Neill.[16] A grinding cylinder, mounted in an engineer's drill, spun around two axes at speeds of up to 36 000 rpm. The central corneas of dogs were flattened with this device. It was reported that these corneas healed and remained transparent, and at 3 weeks were still clear. There was no sign of inflammatory response or vascularization. The only apparent problem with this technique is in accurately controlling the shape being cut.

In 1980, Olson et al reported using a diamond fraise, rotating at 30 000 rpm, to grind cat corneas.[17] The healing of these corneas was not as good as previously reported.[16] Significant scarring and vascularization were observed in some eyes. Keratometry revealed little change in the curvature of these corneas, and no change in the curvature of corneas that healed without scarring.

CO$_2$ LASERS IN REFRACTIVE SURGERY

The first laser with the ability to ablate the cornea was the CO$_2$ laser (10.6 μm wavelength). In 1967, Fine et al reported applying various powers of a 5 mm diameter CO$_2$ laser beam to the centre of rabbit corneas.[18] Healing was observed for 1 hour. An intense white opacity formed at the application site, with evidence of charring and inflammation. Higher intensities perforated the cornea. Campbell et al also observed very similar effects using CO$_2$ laser radiation.[19] Fine et al determined that the threshold for corneal damage was 0.15 W/cm^2 of continuous CO$_2$ laser exposure.[20] In this later experiment, rabbits with CO$_2$ laser burns were allowed to heal for up to 2 weeks. Clouding of the corneal stroma, well below the anterior surface, could be easily seen. Higher power levels (0.3 W/cm^2) produced deep corneal vascularization. Histopathology revealed considerable damage and repair activity in the superficial stromal layers and epithelial layer.

In 1969, Leibowitz and Peacock produced a more controlled corneal injury study, using 142 rabbits and varying both the laser power and the exposure time.[21] The healing was followed for a period of 2 months. Low radiation dosages caused damage within the epithelial layer only, which healed within a few days. Medium radiation dosages caused the epithelium and underlying stroma to have a grey, granular appearance. The epithelium took up to 10 days to return to a normal appearance, and the stromal haze cleared within 60 days. Dosages just below the level that ablated craters into the corneas caused endothelial changes and stromal haze that were still noticeable at 60 days. Most of the craters that were created by the CO$_2$ laser progressively increased in depth and spontaneously perforated 1 week later.

These early studies, applying continuous wave CO$_2$ laser radiation to the cornea, demonstrated that heat transfer during the exposure time produced significant damage to the eye. In 1971, Beckman et al reported testing a rapid firing (60–300 Hz) short-pulsed (1 μs) CO$_2$ laser on ocular tissues.[22] Arguing that the short pulse would not allow enough time for heat to be conducted to adjacent tissues, they used this laser to perform a number of ophthalmic procedures in rabbits. The pulsed CO_2 laser was used to perform limbectomies and circular keratectomies. The limbectomy procedures produced a 1 mm diameter drainage channel that was maintained as a filtering bleb in three of four treated rabbits for at least 1 month; an excellent result for rabbits. A circular keratectomy was performed that could penetrate the cornea and was potentially suitable for penetrating keratoplasty. It was noted that the edge of the cut was smooth and clean, although it was not straight. Non-penetrating keratectomies were allowed to heal. After 2 months these appeared as nebulous, circular scars. Histopathology showed charred damage zones, measuring 0.12 mm in width, at the edge of the cuts.

In 1981, Keates et al also tested a CO_2 laser for corneal surgery.[23] This laser could be Q-switched to produce pulses of only 500 ns in duration. It was reported that the Q-switched pulses produced cuts that appeared more uniform and less charred, than cuts made with longer pulse durations (> ms). It was suggested that this laser would make an ideal 'knife' for corneal procedures such as radial keratotomy, relaxing incisions and penetrating keratoplasty.

INFRARED LASERS

While the CO_2 laser does not appear to be suitable for large area keratectomies within the optical zone of the cornea, it does appear to have promise for making corneal incisions. The development of a number of other infrared lasers, closer to the absorption peaks of water, has shifted attention away from the CO_2 laser. Corneal tissue contains close to 80% water by weight, and water absorbs most of the infrared radiation directed at the cornea. Wavelengths around 3 μm are most strongly absorbed by water. High absorption is one of the most important parameters in reducing the damage zone around laser cut sites.

In 1986, Seiler et al reported testing the hydrogen fluoride (HF) laser (with multiple wavelengths from 2.6 to 3.0 μm) for corneal surgery.[24] Incisions were made in freshly enucleated rabbit eyes using 50 ns pulse durations. On gross examination, the incisions were bounded by a distinct white band. Histopathology showed damage zones, at the edges of the cuts, extending 5–20 μm into the stroma. This is similar to cuts made with the 248 nm excimer laser, but it is not as good as cuts made with the 193 nm wavelength.

Loertscher et al also observed similar results using an HF laser (200 ns pulse duration) to make incisions in human eye bank corneas.[25] A 10–15 μm coagulative damage zone was noticed at the incision sites. The superficial corneal tissue turned white when the laser was not well focused. It would seem that the large proportion of laser energy (about 40%) with wavelengths outside the main absorption peak of water, significantly increased the damage, compared to that expected to be caused by this laser.

In 1987, Peyman and Katoh published an investigation into the effects of a pulsed erbium:YAG, 2.94 μm wavelength laser, on various ocular tissues.[26] Freshly enucleated pig eyes were used, and it was reported that coagulative necrosis extended 10–15 μm around the incision sites in the cornea.

An extensive report by Stern et al, a year later, used laser wavelengths of 2.80–2.92 μm to make corneal incisions.[27] A Q-switched neodymium:YAG laser (normal wavelength 1.06 μm) with a pulse duration of 8 ns, was Raman shifted to 2.80 or 2.92 μm wavelengths. Incisions were made in the corneas of freshly enucleated bovine eyes or human eye bank eyes. The etch depth per pulse of the 2.8 μm radiation, plotted against fluence, resembled the same data for the 193 nm excimer laser in shape (sigmoidal), although the infrared wavelength was capable of removing much greater amounts of tissue per pulse. The corneal incisions appeared clean and smooth. Histopathology showed damage zones as small as 1.5 μm at low fluences, increasing to 10 μm at higher fluences. As the absorption at 2.9 μm is double that at 2.8 μm, it was expected that the 2.92 μm laser cuts would have a significantly smaller damage zone. However, the damage caused by each wavelength was very similar for the same fluence. The appearance of the damaged tissue was different to that seen at the edge of 193 nm laser incisions. Although the damage zone of these infrared laser incisions is at least five times greater than that of the 193 nm excimer laser, they may still heal with minimal scarring. Further healing studies are required to determine whether these infrared laser wavelengths will prove to be useful for refractive keratectomy procedures.

OTHER ULTRAVIOLET LASERS

Although infrared wavelengths do not appear to cut as cleanly as the UV wavelengths, it must be noted that the excimer laser is not the only laser capable of producing UV wavelengths. While the excimer laser remains bulky, difficult to use, and uses corrosive gases, there will be an active interest in other laser sources of ultraviolet radiation for corneal surgery. Berns and Gaster used the fourth harmonic (266 nm) of a Nd:YAG laser to produce clean cuts in a fresh human cadaver cornea.[28] The Nd:YAG laser output (normally 1.06 µm), was frequency doubled twice, to produce the 266 nm UV radiation. However, the frequency conversion process is not very efficient (less than 0.4%), hence the starting power must be very high.

An alternative method of using lasers to cut corneal tissue has also been investigated. When high-energy laser pulses of sufficiently short duration are focused to a point, optical breakdown occurs. When this is applied to the cornea, the tissue at the focus point is transformed into a plasma by the laser energy. The rapidly expanding plasma (explosion), also breaks up other tissue in the vicinity of the laser's focal point. This process is essentially non-thermal and does not depend on absorption of the laser radiation. While this technique should minimize thermal damage, shock wave damage will probably increase.

Recently Stern et al investigated this technique in enucleated bovine eyes.[29] Visible wavelengths (532 and 625 nm) with nanosecond, picosecond and femtosecond pulse widths were focused at the corneal surface. Shorter pulses require less energy to produce optical breakdown, and hence less tissue is disrupted per pulse and damage zones would be expected to be smaller. It was reported that incisions made with the 8 ns pulse duration had very ragged walls, with irregularities extending 10–30 µm into the stroma. However, on a submicron scale these walls appeared smooth. Picosecond (30 and 1 ps) and 100 fs pulse durations produced incisions with much smoother profiles. Denatured collagen was rarely seen more than 1 µm from the cut edges. The incision walls showed a strange mixture of denatured and disorganized collagen that probably reflects the extremely high pressures generated during plasma expansion. Reducing the pulse duration from 30 ps to 1 ps or 100 fs did not improve the cutting quality. In fact, these shorter pulses produced streaks of densely staining tissue radiating 20 µm away from the cut edges. This probably indicates increasing shockwave damage.

An interesting variation of this technique had been tried earlier. Troutman et al used 10 ps pulses of 595 nm from a dye laser to break up tissue within the stroma.[30] Because this wavelength is transmitted through the cornea, the laser could be focused into the stroma. Optical breakdown disrupted a small amount of tissue without damaging the epithelium, Bowman's membrane, or Descemet's membrane, or the endothelium. Precise control of the laser was used to create midstromal cuts in eye bank corneas, although it remains to be seen what range of refractive changes this intrastromal surgery can ultimately achieve.

REFERENCES

1. Rhodes CK, Review of ultraviolet laser physics, *IEEE J of Quantum Electronics* (1974) **10**(2), 153–74.
2. Rhodes CK, ed, *Excimer Lasers*, Topics in Applied Physics Volume 30, 2nd edn, (Springer Verlag: Berlin, 1984).
3. Huestis DL, The excimer age: Lasing with the new breed, *Optical Spectra* (1979) *June*: 51–55.
4. Hecht J, Excimer laser update, *Lasers and Applic* (1983) *Dec*: 43–49.
5. Houtermans FG, Uber maser-wirkung im optischen spektralgebiet und die moglichkeit absolut negativer absorption fur einege falle von molekulspektren (licht-lawine), *Helv Phys Acta* (1960) **33**: 933–40.
6. Basov Ngm Danilychev VA, Popov YM, Stimulated emission in the vacuum ultraviolet region, *Soviet J of Quantum Electronics* (1971) **1**(1): 18–22.
7. Koehler HA, Ferderber LJ, Redhead DL, Ebert PJ, Stimulated VUV emission in high-pressure xenon excited by high-current relativistic electron beams, *Appl Phys Lett* (1972) **21**(5): 198–200.
8. Searles SK, Hart GA, Stimulated emission at 281.8nm for XeBr, *Appl Phys Lett* (1975) **27**(4): 23–245.
9. Burnham R, Harris NW, Djeu N, Xenon fluoride laser excitation by transverse electric discharge, *Appl Phys Lett* (1976) **28**(2): 86–7.
10. Eden G, Burnham R, Champagne LF, Donohue T, Djeu N, Visible and UV lasers: Problems and promises, *IEEE Spectrum* (1979) *April*, 50–59.
11. Ruderman W, Excimer lasers in photochemistry. *Laser Focus* (1979) *May*, 68–69.
12. Kawamura Y, Toyoda K, Namba S, Effective deep ultraviolet photoetching of polymethyl methacrylate by an excimer laser *Appl Phys Lett* (1982) **40**(5), 374–75.
13. Srinivasan R, Mayne-Banton V, Self-developing photoetching of poly(ethylene terephthalate) films by far-ultraviolet excimer laser radiation, *Appl Phys Lett* (1982) **41**(6), 576–78.
14. Bende T, Seiler T, Wollensak J, Side effects in excimer corneal surgery: Corneal thermal gradients, *Graefe's Arch Clin Exp Ophth* (1988) **226**: 277–80.
15. Krauss JM, Puliafito CA, Steinert RF, Laser interactions with the cornea, *Surv Ophthalmol* (1986) **31**(1): 37–53.
16. Mueller FO, O'Neill P, Some experiments on corneal grinding, *Exp Eye Res* (1967) **6**:42–47.

17. Olson RJ, Kaufman HE, Rheinstrom SD, Reshaping the cat corneal anterior surface using a high-speed diamond fraise, *Ophthalmic Surg* (1980) **11**(11): 784–86.

18. Fine BS, Fine S, Peacock GR, Geeraets WJ, Klein E, Preliminary observations on ocular effects of high-power, continuous CO_2 laser irradiation, *Am J Ophthalmol* (1967) **64**(2): 209–22.

19. Campbell CJ, Rittler MC, Bredemeier H, Wallace RA, Ocular effects produced by experimental lasers. II Carbon dioxide laser, *Am J Ophthalmol* (1968) **66**(4): 604–14 .

20. Fine BS, Fine S, Friegen L, MacKeen D, Corneal injury threshold to carbon dioxide laser irradiation, *Am J Ophthalmol* (1968) **66**(1): 1–15.

21. Leibowitz HM, Peacock GR, Corneal injury produced by carbon dioxide laser radiation, *Arch Ophthalmol* (1969) **81** 713–21.

22. Beckman H, Rota A, Barraco R, Sugar HS, Gaynes E, Limbectomies, keratectomies and keratostomies performed with a rapid-pulsed carbon dioxide laser, *Am J Ophthalmol* (1971) **71**(6): 1277–83.

23. Keates RH, Pedrotti LS, Weichel H, Possel WH, Carbon dioxide laser beam control for corneal surgery, *Ophthalmic Surg* (1981) **12**(2): 117–22.

24. Seiler T, Marshall J, Rothery S, Wollensak J, The potential of an infrared hydrogen fluoride (HF) laser (3.0 µm) for corneal surgery, *Lasers in Ophthalmology* (1986) **1**(1): 49–60.

25. Loertscher H, Mandelbaum S, Parrish RK, Parel J, Preliminary report on corneal incisions created by a hydrogen fluoride laser, *Am J Ophthalmol* (1986) **102**(2): 217–21.

26. Peyman GA, Katoh N, Effects of an erbium:YAG laser on ocular structures, *International Ophthalmology* (1987) **10**: 245–52.

27. Stern D, Puliafito CA, Dobi ET, Reidy WT, Infrared laser surgery of the cornea. Studies with a Raman-shifted neodymium:YAG laser at 2.80 and 2.92 µm. *Ophthalmology* (1988) **95**(10): 1434–41.

28. Berns MW, Gaster RN, Corneal incisions produced with the fourth harmonic (26 nm) of the YAG laser, *Lasers Surg Med* (1985) **5**: 371–75 (1985).

29. Stern D, Schoenlein RW, Puliafito CA, Dobi ET, Birngruber R, Fukimoto JG, Corneal ablation by nanosecond, picosecond and femtosecond lasers at 532 and 625 nm, *Arch Ophthalmol* (1989) **107**: 587–92.

30. Troutman RC, Veronneau-Troutman S, Jakobiec FA, Krebs W, A new laser for collagen wounding in corneal and strabismus surgery: A preliminary report, *Trans Am Ophth Soc* (1986) **84**: 11–132.

Chapter 3 The development of excimer laser corneal surgery: beam tissue interactions

David S Gartry

ESSENTIAL PREREQUISITES OF CORNEAL SURGERY

From the description of the cornea's structure and function (Chapter 4) it is evident that a complex interplay of anatomical, biomechanical, and physiological factors exists to promote the strength, transparency, and refracting properties of the cornea. Any surgical intervention is likely to interfere with one or more of these factors leading to reduced function. Ten aims or prerequisites might characterize the ideal corneal surgical procedure (Table 3.1). and can be considered the, as yet elusive, 'Holy Grail' of corneal surgery.

Table 3.1

The essential requirements of corneal surgical procedures

1. No interference with corneal transparency by scarring or fibrosis
2. No endothelial damage in the short or long term
3. Maintenance of asphericity to minimize aberration
4. No induced corneal distortion leading to regular or irregular astigmatism
5. Maintenance of a perfectly smooth and stable epithelial surface
6. No reduction in corneal integrity and strength
7. The outcome of the procedure should be predictable
8. The outcome of the procedure should be stable
9. The procedure should have proven efficacy
10. The procedure must be safe with no risk of infection

REFRACTIVE CORNEAL SURGERY

INTRODUCTION

Since the cornea is the main refracting element of the optical system of the human eye, relatively small changes in its anterior curvature will produce relatively large changes in the patient's overall refraction. This principle has formed the basis for numerous surgical attempts to correct refractive error – most commonly myopia – but, as is the case with any condition for which a large number of alternative treatments exists, none of these techniques is problem-free. The underlying difficulty that pervades all forms of refractive corneal surgery is that of individual corneal/patient variation in response to the surgery. Where incisional keratotomy techniques are employed, such as radial keratotomy (RK) or astigmatic keratotomy (AK), a graded amount of corneal stroma is incised to a specified depth and the biomechanical properties of the cornea result in an altered (flatter) anterior corneal curvature. The wound healing that follows produces scars that are neither as strong nor as stable as the original stroma. Even if the incisions could be produced with an extremely high and repeatable precision, the complex changes that are likely to occur in the non-homogeneous corneal stroma, especially with regard to subsequent wound healing, could be expected to make the exact outcome impossible to predict.

In addition, it has been a traditional, and entirely reasonable, view that since a refractive error such as myopia is not a disease and the eye is in other respects entirely normal, refractive surgery of any type must be very safe. The 'Holy Grail' prerequisites are listed in Table 3.1 and, in summary, refractive surgery must be predictable, effective, and above all safe with a low or zero incidence of complications.

Those complications which might occur must be relatively minor when viewed in the context of what might be described as a 'cosmetic' procedure.

THE POTENTIAL OF LASERS IN CORNEAL SURGERY

Since one of the key elements contributing to the difficulty in predicting the outcome of refractive surgical procedures, such as incisional keratotomy, is the inevitable variation in surgical technique from surgeon to surgeon and from patient to patient, it was proposed that the use of lasers in refractive surgical procedures might eliminate these variables. It was also hoped that, by altering the corneal shape with laser radiation, greater control over the variability of the wound healing response might be possible. Finally, it was hypothesized that the successful use of laser energy to remove, for example, corneal tissue, could be a major step towards entirely automated or 'robotic' surgery that might find application in numerous clinical areas. Several lasers, selected on the basis of their beam–tissue interactions – principally their corneal absorption characteristics – have been investigated in relation to their 'corneal cutting potential' (Table 3.2).

INTERACTION OF LASER LIGHT WITH THE CORNEA

There are four ways in which laser light can interact with the cornea: transmission, scattering, reflection, and absorption. Which of these four predominates varies and depends upon the characteristics of the individual laser. Transmission of laser light through the normal human cornea occurs generally between 400 and 1400 nm. Laser light can also be scattered by the tissue, if a large area is exposed, with a concomitant reduction in efficiency as more energy is converted to heat. Reflection of the beam is insignificant and of no relevance in the context of surgical applications, while absorption lasers have been selected as potentially suitable for corneal surgery. The greater the absorption of laser radiation by tissue such as the cornea, the less the penetration into the tissue. Lasers ideally suited to corneal surgery are those in which absorption is high since, with limited penetration beyond the corneal surface, there is a large safety margin in relation to deeper ocular structures such as the corneal endothelium and crystalline lens. The greatest absorption in the cornea is by macromolecules in the far-UV portion of the electromagnetic spectrum (less than 300 nm) and by water in the middle (3000–6000 nm) and far (greater than 10 000 nm) IR regions (Figs 3.1, 3.2). Table 3.2

Table 3.2

Characteristics of some of the lasers potentially suited to corneal surgery. (Courtesy of Professor George Waring, MD.)

Laser type	Wavelength (nm)	Pulse duration (nsec)	Penetration depth (µm)
Excimer (ArF)	193	10–20	2–3
Excimer (KrF)	248	10–20	10
Excimer (XeCl)	308	10–20	300
Nd-YAG fifth harmonic	213	10	2
Holmium YAG	2060	20 000	330
HF	2870–2910	50	1.5
Erbium YAG	2940	20 000	0.75
Raman shifted YAG	2800	10	1.5
CO_2	10 600	–	–

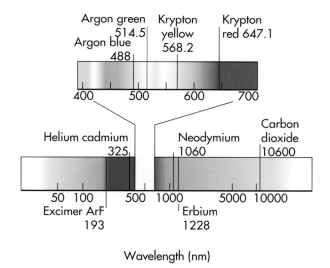

Wavelength (nm)

Figure 3.1 *The electromagnetic spectrum. The visible portion (approximately 400 nm to 700 nm) is 'exploded'. The argon fluoride excimer laser emits at 193 nm in the ultraviolet 'C' portion of the spectrum.*

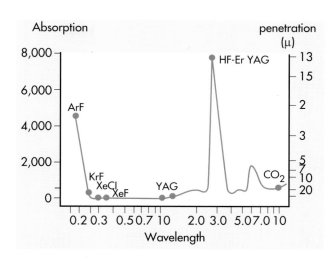

Figure 3.2 *Absorption versus wavelength (nm). Radiation from the argon fluoride excimer and Erbium-YAG lasers have high absorption within the corneal surface (therefore low penetration).*

defines lasers that have been used for superficial keratotomy in terms of the penetration depth of the emitted radiation and it can be seen that the argon fluoride (ArF) excimer (193 nm) laser and the fifth harmonic Nd-YAG laser have least penetration, or maximum absorption, and therefore would seem to be best suited, theoretically at least, to corneal surgery.

HISTORICAL OVERVIEW OF LASER CORNEAL SURGERY

The continuous wave (CW) carbon dioxide (CO_2) laser, which has an emission wavelength of 10 600 nm (10.6 µm), was the first laser to be investigated for its possible role in corneal surgery.[1] This followed from its original description in 1964 by Patel.[2] However, although it was shown to be capable of vaporizing corneal tissue, the amount of energy required to create incisions caused significant charring and burning of adjacent tissue. Pulsed exposures were then utilized to allow more dissipa-

tion of heat and hence less thermal damage[3] and the total energy exposure was then reduced further by Keates et al using Q-switching.[4] This restricted the unwanted charring at the incision site to a surrounding margin, which was only 25–30 µm in width. In spite of these improvements, however, the CO_2 laser was abandoned as a tool for corneal surgery and other lasers, such as the hydrogen fluoride (HF) laser and the Erbium-YAG laser, with higher absorption characteristics, less thermal damage and therefore greater accuracy, were evaluated.

The first application of the Erbium-YAG laser for corneal ablation was reported in 1986.[5] In the same year Loertscher and Seiler demonstrated that the pulsed HF laser (wavelength = 2.7–3.0 µm) could vaporize corneal tissue and produce well-defined incisions beyond which there was a zone of thermal damage only 1–15 µm wide.[6,7]

In the 1970s pulsed far-UV lasers (excimer lasers), capable of removal of material from an exposed surface with an unprecedented degree of accuracy, were developed for industrial use and, with their proposed clinical application in the mid-1980s, the role of lasers in corneal surgery entered a new era.

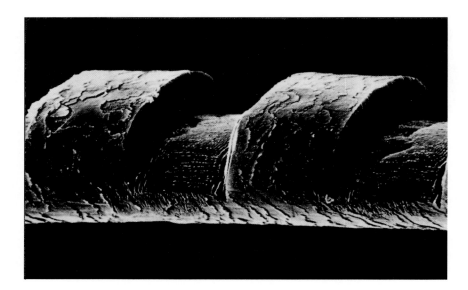

Figure 3.3 *The shaft of a human hair following repeated exposure to argon fluoride excimer laser radiation (rectangular beam profile). Blocks of keratin have been excised along the hair shaft with remarkable precision to leave smooth, perpendicular sides. The base of each cut segment has a similar contour to that of the surface of the hair. (Courtesy of Dr R Srinivasan.)*

THE DEVELOPMENT OF EXCIMER LASER CORNEAL SURGERY

BACKGROUND

Excimer lasers were first developed in the mid-1970s for use in the manufacture of printed circuitry and investigation into their potential use in ophthalmic surgery followed reports from scientists in both the health sciences and electronics fields.[8] It was noted that far-UV excimer laser radiation could be used to 'photo-etch' highly precise, well-defined, lines in plastic surfaces.[9–12] At lesser intensities, this excimer laser radiation could be used to produce surface markings in corneal epithelium[13] or even remove discrete blocks of tissue from, for example, the shaft of a human hair (see Fig. 3.3).[14,15] The first suggestion of their application in refractive surgery was made by Trokel, Srinivasan and Braren who argued that since excimer laser radiation could etch highly precise lines in plastics it might be possible to produce incisions in the cornea with an unprecedented accuracy.[16]

THE LASING MEDIUM AND BEAM–TISSUE INTERACTIONS

The nature of the emitted radiation at 193 nm provides the first of the two key elements of ArF

excimer laser radiation that make it eminently suitable for corneal surgery – the extremely high precision with which corneal tissue can be removed. The emission wavelength of 193 nm is in the UV C portion of the electromagnetic spectrum and at this wavelength the individual photons emitted have exceptionally high peak energy values – around 6.4 electron volts (eV). Since this value exceeds the binding voltages of carbon–carbon bonds, for example the bonds between biological molecules (which are of the order of 3 eV), on exposure to excimer laser radiation these molecular bonds in, for example, the corneal surface are broken and the resultant fragments are ejected away from the surface at speeds in excess of 2000 m/sec (Fig. 3.4).

Marshall and co-workers proposed that, since a single absorbed photon may lead to bond break-down, potentially the entire laser beam could be utilized in the 'tissue removal process' and the cornea might be reprofiled directly using *large area* photo-ablation rather than linear excisions.[17,18] In addition, UV radiation in this spectral domain does not propagate well in air and at any biological interface the high energy photons are virtually all absorbed within a few microns of the surface. Energy penetration into the tissues is, therefore, extremely limited to around only 3 μm, resulting in an extremely precise removal of tissue.[19,20] The average central corneal thickness is 520 μm by comparison. The process, which is one of photochemical or photoablative decomposition, has

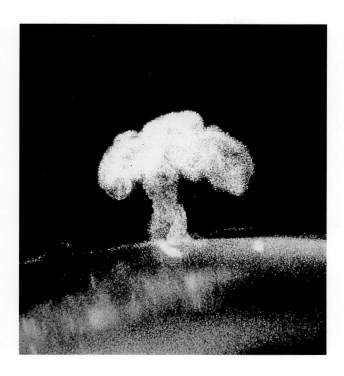

Figure 3.4 *The 'mushroom cloud' of ejected molecular fragments following photoablation of the surface of a cadaver cornea by a single pulse of excimer laser radiation. The fragments leave the surface at speeds in excess of 2000 m/s. (Courtesy of Dr Carmen Puliafito.)*

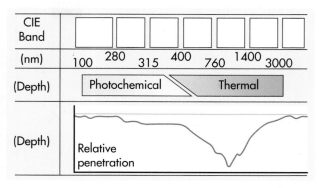

Figure 3.5 *Photochemical versus thermal tissue interactions defined by wavelengths. At shorter wavelengths beam–tissue interactions are characterized by photochemical processes (e.g. photochemical decomposition or* photoablation *in the case of the argon fluoride excimer laser at 193 nm. Penetration of energy into the tissue (depth) is severely limited at this end of the spectrum.*

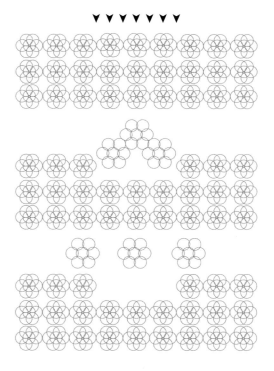

Figure 3.6 *Single photons of excimer laser radiation, represented here as solid arrows reach the surface of the target tissue. The high photon energy is absorbed and as bonds are broken the component molecular fragments expand apart. The resultant fragments can only move into free space and therefore leave the surface at high speeds (in excess of 2000 m/s). A surface layer of tissue is therefore removed with each pulse of radiation.*

been termed *photoablation* and the removal of tissue is restricted to an infinitesimally thin surface layer with each emitted pulse (Figs 3.5 and 3.6). Of equal importance is the fact that collateral damage to unexposed areas is strictly limited to a zone of thermal damage and condensate of only around 100–300 nm beyond the photoablated area.[20,21] Tissue removal from the corneal surface can be achieved therefore with an unprecedented precision.

The second key element of excimer laser radiation that makes it eminently suited to corneal surgery is its relatively wide beam, which can be configured in almost any cross-sectional shape, for example rectangular (Fig. 3.3) or circular (Fig. 3.7). Tissue removal induced by other clinical lasers is achieved by concentrating laser energy into a focused point. However, the excimer laser beam has a large cross-sectional area and since, as mentioned above, every

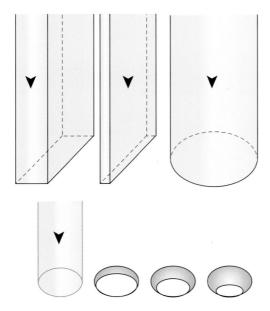

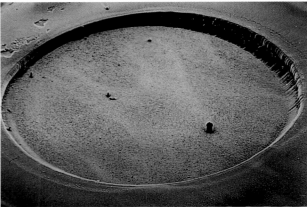

Figure 3.8 *This scanning electron micrograph shows a photoablated circular crater in a Petri dish. The smooth base of the crater is evident (with the exception of a few surface projections caused by debris in the path of the beam, which were more resistant to photoablation). (Courtesy of J Marshall, S Trokel, S Rothery and R Krueger.)*

Figure 3.7 *The excimer beam can be configured in any cross-sectional shape. Examples represented here diagrammatically are a rectangle, a slit, and a circle. With each successive pulse of, for example, a circular cross-section beam, a layer of surface molecules is removed. With repeated pulses over a period of time a circular 'crater' is produced.*

photon in the beam has the potential to produce tissue change the entire cross section of the beam can be utilized.[17,18] Thus, with each laser pulse, a layer of tissue only a few molecules thick will be photoablated from the surface. The initial 1×2 cm rectangular excimer laser beam profile is adjusted by cylindrical quartz lenses and the resultant square, or 'top hat' energy profile of the beam can be made circular by passing the emergent beam through an aperture.[17] This ability to photoablate large areas of cornea with great precision permits selective and graded removal of tissue to induce a refractive change. In practice, beam delivery is more easily configured to remove more tissue from the central cornea and progressively less towards the periphery, resulting in a flatter corneal surface profile. By reducing anterior corneal curvature, a treatment of myopia is possible. The reprofiling procedure has been termed photorefractive keratectomy (PRK).[18,22–25] Slit and rectangular

excisions can be achieved as well as the circular excisions presently used clinically for PRK. In addition, the term *excision* in relation to excimer laser photoablation is preferred since tissue is removed rather than pushed aside or 'incized', as would be the case if a diamond or steel scalpel blade was used.

HAZARDS OF EXCIMER LASER RADIATION

Above all, prior to the onset of clinical trials to evaluate excimer laser corneal surgery, it was essential for all possible problems relating to *safety* to be investigated fully. In assessing the safety of laser corneal surgery, the main concerns relate to the nature of and, in particular, the *penetration* of the wavelength under investigation. While it has been established that the principal beam–tissue interaction of excimer laser radiation at 193 nm is photoablative decomposition, or photoablation, of the corneal surface (see above), concern has been expressed in relation to *secondary fluorescence* since longer wavelengths would have increased penetration into the ocular tissues. Studies were undertaken, therefore, to assess the possible effect of excimer laser radiation on ocular structures deep to the corneal surface, such as the corneal endothelium and the lens. Damage to these structures would lead to *corneal decompensation* and *cataract formation*, respectively. In addition, potential problems in relation to the *acoustic shock waves* generated by the process of photoablation at each acoustic interface within the eye, the release of *toxic free-radicals* at the site of photoablation, and *mutagenesis* have been addressed.

PENETRATION OF EXCIMER LASER RADIATION AT 193 nm

It has been shown that the penetration depth of ArF excimer radiation with emission wavelength at 193 nm radiation is of the order of only 3–4 μm.[27] However, for excimer lasers emitting at 248 nm this value exceeds 25 μm[27] and at 308 nm it may be as high as 100 μm (Fig. 3.5).[28,29] These observations support previous studies using broad-band sources of radiation that showed that penetration depth increased with wavelengths between 100 nm and 400 nm.[30] This inverse relationship in the UV portion of the electromagnetic spectrum wavelength and absorption, and, in particular, the peak absorption at around 190 nm, would suggest that the argon fluoride excimer laser is ideally suited to corneal surgery.

MUTAGENESIS

During excimer laser corneal surgery, by definition, cell damage occurs as layers of surface molecules undergo photoablation and molecular fragments are ejected away from the anterior cornea at high speed. Where cell damage occurs it has been assumed that there must be the potential for damage to nuclear material with concomitant altered DNA or unscheduled, abnormal DNA synthesis. However, from several independent studies utilizing both unscheduled DNA synthesis (UDS) and tissue culture, along with enzyme poisoning techniques, it seems likely that there is little, if any, risk of mutagenesis at 193 nm.[31–38] This apparent lack of mutagenic response in cells deep to the ablation zone has been attributed to two aspects of the photoablation process. Firstly, that at the fluence used for clinical procedures the absorption of high energy photons results almost exclusively in corneal surface bond-breaking and virtually no photons penetrate beyond the zone of cells damaged by photoablation.[38] It has been estimated that the accumulated UV dose to the cornea and lens during PRK is less than that necessary to produce photokeratitis on exposure to an unguarded welding arc.[38] Secondly, the decreased cytotoxicity and mutagenicity of 193 nm radiation may be due to shielding of the nucleus by cytoplasmic and membrane components or to the formation of different DNA photoproducts.[32,33] It has been calculated, for example, that each micron of cytoplasm attenuates the incident radiation by around 99%.[36]

SECONDARY FLUORESCENCE AND CATARACTOGENESIS

Although complete absorption of 193 nm radiation occurs within only a few microns of the corneal surface, target fluorescence during photoablation generates longer wavelength photons, with deeper penetration characteristics. These photons are able, theoretically, to damage intraocular structures such as the crystalline lens. On inspecting the corneal surface during the procedure a faint 'bluish glow' is seen, which becomes much brighter when excess surface water undergoes photoablation. Since 193 nm radiation is in the 'C' portion of the UV part of the electromagnetic spectrum it would be completely invisible to an observer. The 'bluish glow' appearance must be due to secondary fluorescence or secondary radiation at around 450 nm. In addition, this glow potentially contains the more hazardous portions of the electromagnetic spectrum, between 250 and 350 nm, which are known to penetrate more readily into the eye, where they can generate phototoxic and cataractogenic effects.[39] A wavelength of around 320 nm seems to be the most cataractogenic.[39]

On biochemical analysis of the aqueous humour and lens of rabbits that had undergone PRK using a scanning laser delivery system (where several thousands of pulses are required) it was found that the concentrations of several markers for cataractogenesis were raised.[40] The energy thresholds for cataract formation at incident wavelengths of 300, 310, and 320 nm are 0.5, 1.5, and 15 mJ/cm², respectively.[39] In order to achieve optimal photoablation characteristics, ArF excimer laser systems are typically configured to deliver pulses to the corneal plane with energy densities of around 180 mJ/cm². It has been estimated that, maximally, only 10^{-5} of the incident energy will be transmitted into the eye as longer wavelengths generated by fluorescence or 'reradiation'.[41] Therefore, of a single excimer laser pulse only 0.0018 mJ/cm² is generated over a large range of the spectrum. Even if all of this reradiated energy was converted to wavelengths only approaching 320 nm, which is not the case, then the exposure levels are still far too low to cause a problem. The best available evidence therefore suggests that the fluorescence during a single PRK treatment, lasting on average 20 to 30 seconds, is associated with energy levels far below the threshold for UV damage to the lens. In addition, it is likely that this reradiated energy is insignificant when compared, for example, to a lifetime of exposure to the much higher levels, and broader spectrum, of radiation present in sunlight.

ACOUSTIC SHOCK WAVES

As emphasized above, UV radiation at 193 nm is absorbed within a few microns of the corneal surface; however, in addition to secondary phenomena such as fluorescence, the acoustic shock waves (generated at each acoustic interface) should be considered in relation to deeper ocular structures such as the corneal endothelium. It has been shown that linear laser excisions will cause endothelial damage when they are made to a depth of around 90% of the corneal thickness.[21,42] Wide area ablation, although only removing around 10% of the corneal thickness in order to achieve a refractive change, can also be followed by changes in the endothelium such as vacuolation, presumably induced by the acoustic shock waves, although these are short-lived and, at the present time, of doubtful clinical significance.[43]

THE GENERATION OF TOXIC FREE-RADICALS

Similarly, it has been demonstrated that potentially toxic free-radicals can be generated within bovine corneal stroma during excimer laser exposures, although these seem to be transient products, which have been demonstrated only in a cryogenic environment.[44] Although the clinical significance of these studies is yet to be elucidated, it has been hypothesized that these agents might have some effect on the wound-healing response following excimer laser PRK.

EARLY CLINICAL APPLICATIONS OF THE EXCIMER LASER

THE TREATMENT OF CORNEAL SCARS

Because of the potential of the excimer laser to remove thin layers of corneal tissue in a highly controlled manner, it was hoped that it might be used to treat selected corneal pathologies, thereby obviating the need for more complex and time-consuming traditional procedures. In 1984, Serdarevic and colleagues were the first to perform a series of successful excimer laser therapeutic lamellar keratectomies in rabbit models to treat experimental candida keratitis.[45] Their results confirmed that the technique of excimer laser phototherapeutic keratectomy (PTK) was not only feasible but could be used also to eradicate organisms from the cornea leaving the resultant smooth surface to re-epithelialize normally. The results of the first series of 25 sighted eye patients with superficial corneal pathology treated by excimer laser were reported by Gartry et al[46] and a description of the development of superficial keratectomy using the excimer laser (PTK) is given in Chapter 21.

EARLY 'INCISIONAL KERATOTOMY' WITH THE EXCIMER LASER

As noted above, one of the key advantages of ArF excimer laser radiation (193 nm) is the lack of significant damage beyond the exposed area. Ultrastructural examination of corneal excisions in animal models confirmed that these could be produced with a very high degree of accuracy and control. Damage to adjacent unexposed tissue was limited to a zone of only 100–300 nm beyond the boundary of the photoablated area.[20,21] In non-perforating excisions of varying depths, corneal endothelial damage was noted only when the base of the excision reached to within 40 μm of Descemet's membrane, which is similar to, but less extensive than, the effect on the endothelium of diamond knife incisions.[21,27,47,48] Furthermore, excimer laser excisions can be controlled precisely in terms of uniformity along the length of a single cut, reproducibility between cuts and in anticipated cut depth (accuracy ± 3%, diamond knife incisions ± 12%). The first clinical application was therefore the correction of astigmatism using T-cut excisions,[29,49–51] which have the same effect as paired arcuate keratotomies. In order to produce linear excisions with the laser it was necessary either to shield the cornea using a mask with slit apertures or limit the beam to a slit cross-section within the delivery system. The resultant 'excisions' were 'V-shaped' in profile rather than discrete linear cuts and were often filled with a 'plug' of corneal epithelial cells.[52] It was doubtful whether refractive changes arising from such wounds would be either predictable or stable and in any event masking proved too cumbersome to be practical. Moreover, it could be predicted that the use of excimer laser technology to perform what was essentially a radial keratotomy procedure would not obviate all of the problems of that particular technique. However, each photon within the relatively large cross-section of an excimer beam is capable of bond breakdown and the concept of refractive change by a computer-controlled, direct surface reprofiling, rather than by linear excisions, was put forward in 1986.[27] The descriptive term for this 'wide area ablation' – *photorefractive keratectomy* – was adopted at that time.[17]

AIMS IN THE EVALUATION OF EXCIMER CORNEAL SURGERY

As with any surgical procedure, for corneal surgery with the excimer laser to be accepted in clinical practice an understanding of the nature and quality of wound healing is essential. Complete epithelial wound healing is necessary to re-establish the outer osmotic barrier of the cornea and the optical brilliance of the refracting air/tear interface. Studies have been undertaken, therefore, to assess latency of wound healing, epithelial migration and adhesion properties, and the presence or absence of epithelial hyperplasia.[53,54] Stromal wound healing has been examined in relation to loss or disturbance of transparency, keratocyte infiltration, and scar formation.[18,23,53] The corneal endothelium has been assessed in relation to potential cell loss or long-term population changes.[42,53] Finally, as discussed above, the putative mutagenic effects of ultraviolet radiation on the cornea have been assessed.[31–38] None of these investigations highlighted areas of concern that would have precluded the commencement of clinical trials in patients.

REFERENCES

1. Fine BS, Fine S, Peacock GR, Geeraets WJ, Klein E, Preliminary observations on ocular effects of high power, continuous CO₂ laser irradiation, *Am J Ophthalmol* (1967) **64**:209–22.

2. Patel CKN, Interpretation of carbon dioxide optical laser experiments, *Phys Rev Lett* (1964) **12**:588.

3. Beckman H, Rota A, Barraco R, Limbectomies, keratectomies and keratotomies performed with a rapid pulsed carbon dioxide laser, *Am J Ophthalmol* (1971) **71**:1277–83.

4. Keates RH, Pedrotti L, Weichel H, Possel WH, Carbon dioxide laser beam control of corneal surgery, *Ophthalmic Surg* (1981) **12**:117–22.

5. Esterowitz et al, unpublished paper presented at the Conference on Lasers and Electro-Optics, San Francisco, 9–13 June, 1986.

6. Loertscher H, Mandelbaum S, Parrish RK, Parel JM, Preliminary report on corneal incisions created by a hydrogen fluoride laser, *Am J Ophthalmol* (1988) **102**:217–21.

7. Seiler T, Marshall J, Rothery S, Wollensak, The potential of an infrared hydrogen fluoride (HF) laser (3.0 microns) for corneal surgery, *Lasers Ophthalmol* (1986) **1**:49.

8. Searles SK, Hart GA, Stimulated emission at 281 nm XC, *Br Appl Phys Lett* (1975) **27**:243–5.

9. Srinivasan R, Mayne-Banton V, Self-developing photo-etching of polyethylene terephthalate films by far ultraviolet excimer laser radiation, *Appl Phys Lett* (1982) **41**:576–8.

10. Garrison BJ, Srinivasan R, Laser ablation of organic polymers: microscopic models for photochemical and thermal processes, *J Appl Phys* (1985) **57**:2909–14.

11. Rice S, Jain K, Direct high-resolution excimer laser photoetching, *Applied Physics A – Solids and Surfaces* (1984) **33**:195–8.

12. Deutsch TK, Geis MW, Self-developing UV photoresist using excimer laser exposure, *J Appl Phys* (1983) **54**:7201–4.

13. Taboada J, Mikesell GW, Reed RD, Response of the corneal epithelium to krypton fluoride excimer laser, *Heath Phys* (1981) **40**:677–83.

14. Dyer PE, Srinivasan R, Nanosecond photoacoustic studies on ultraviolet laser ablation of organic polymers, *Appl Phys Lett* (1986) **48**:445–7.

15. Sutcliffe E, Srinivasan R, Dynamics of the ultraviolet laser ablation of corneal tissue, *Am J Ophthalmol* (1987) **103**:470–1.

16. Trokel SL, Srinivasan R, Braren B, Excimer laser surgery of the cornea, *Am J Ophthalmol* (1983) **96**:710–15.

17. Marshall J, Trokel S, Rothery S, Krueger RR, Photoablative reprofiling of the cornea using an excimer laser: Photorefractive keratectomy, *Lasers in Ophthalmol* (1986) **1**:21–48.

18. Marshall J, Lasers in ophthalmology: The basic principles, *Eye* (1988) **2**:S98–S112.

19. Krueger RR, Trokel SL, Quantitation of corneal ablation by ultraviolet laser light, *Arch Ophthalmol* (1985) **103**:1741–2.

20. Puliafito CA, Steinert RF, Deutsch TF, Hillenkamp F, Dehm EJ, Adler CM, Excimer laser ablation of the cornea and lens. Experimental studies. *Ophthalmology* (1985) **92**: 741–8.

21. Marshall J, Trokel S, Rothery S, Schubert H, An ultrastructural study of corneal incisions by an excimer laser at 193 nm, *Ophthalmology* (1985) **92**:749–58.

22. Munnerlyn CR, Koons SJ, Marshall J, Photorefractive keratectomy: A technique for laser refractive surgery, *J Cataract Ref Surg* (1988) **14**:46–52.

23. Tuft SJ, Marshall J, Rothery S, Stromal remodelling following photorefractive keratectomy, *Lasers in Ophthalmol* (1987) **1**:177–85.

24. McDonald MB, Frantz JM, Klyce SD, et al, One year refractive results of central photorefractive keratectomy of myopia in the non-human primate cornea, *Arch Ophthalmol* (1990) **108**:40–7.

25. Gartry DS, Kerr Muir MG, Marshall J, Photorefractive keratectomy with an Argon Fluoride Excimer Laser: A clinical study, *Refract Corneal Surg* (1991) **7**:420–35.

26. Seiler T, Wollensak J, Myopic photorefractive keratectomy with the excimer laser. 1 year follow-up, *Ophthalmology* (1991) **98**:1156–63.

27. Marshall J, Trokel S, Rothery S, Krueger RR, A comparative study of corneal incisions induced by diamond and steel knives and two ultraviolet radiations from an excimer laser, *Br J Ophthalmol* (1986) **70**:482–501.

28. Berlin MS, Martinez M, Papaioannou T, Grundfest W, Goldenberg T, Laudenslager J, Goniophotoablation: Excimer laser glaucoma filtering surgery, *Lasers Light Ophthalmol* (1988) **2**:17–24.

29. Seiler T, Bende T, Wollensak J, Trokel SL, Excimer laser keratectomy for correction of astigmatism, *Am J Ophthalmol* (1988) **105**:117–24.

30. Seiler T, Bende T, Winckler K, Wollensak J, Side effects in excimer corneal surgery, *Graefe's Arch Clin Exp Ophthalmol* (1988) **226**:273–6.

31. Trentacoste J, Thompson K, Parrish RK, Hajek A, Berman MR, Ganjei P, Mutagenic potential of a 193 nm excimer laser on fibroblasts in tissue culture, *Ophthalmology* (1987) **94**:125–9.

32. Green H, Bold J, Parrish JA, Kochever IE, Oseroff AR, Cytotoxicity and mutagenicity of low intensity, 248 and 193 nm excimer laser radiation in the mammalian cell, *Cancer Research* (1987) **47**:410–3.

33. Green H, Margolis R, Boll J, Kochever IE, Parrish JA, Oseroff JR, Unscheduled DNA synthesis in the human skin after in vitro ultraviolet excimer laser ablation, *J Invest Dermatol* (1987) **89**:201–4.

34. Nuss RC, Puliafito CA, Dehm EJ, Unscheduled DNA synthesis following excimer laser ablation of the cornea in vivo, *Invest Ophthalmol Vis Sci* (1987) **28**:287–94.

35. Kochever IE, Cytotoxicity and mutagenicity of excimer laser radiation, *Lasers in Surg Medicine* (1989) **9**:440–4.

36. Kochever IE, Walsh AA, Green HA, Sherwood M, Shih MG, Sutherland BM, DNA damage induced by 193 nm radiation in mammalian cells, *Cancer Research* (1991) **51**:288–93.

37. Gebhardt BM, Salmeron B, McDonald MB, The effect of excimer laser energy on the growth potential of corneal keratocytes, *Cancer* (1990) **9**:205–10.

38. Sliney DH, Krueger RR, Trokel SL, Rappaport KD, Photokeratitis from 193 nm argon-fluoride laser radiation, *Photochemistry and Photobiology* (1991) **53**:739–44.

39. Pitts DG, Cullen AP, Hacker PD, Ocular effects of ultraviolet radiation from 295–365 nm, *Invest Ophthalmol Vis Sci* (1977) **16**:932–9.

40. Costagliola C, Balestrieri P, Fioretti F et al, ArF 193 nm excimer laser corneal surgery as a possible risk factor in cataractogenesis, *Exp Eye Res* (1994) **58**:453–7.

41. Muller-Stolzenburg NW, Muller GJ, Buchwald HJ et al, UV exposure of the lens during 193 nm excimer laser corneal surgery, *Arch Ophthalmol* (1990) **108**:915–6.

42. Dehm EJ, Puliafito CA, Adler CM, Steinert RF, Corneal endothelial injury in rabbits following excimer laser ablation at 193 nm and 248 nm, *Arch Ophthalmol* (1986) **104**:1364–8.

43. Zabel R, Tuft SJ, Marshall J, Excimer laser photorefractive keratectomy: endothelial morphology following area ablation of the cornea, *Invest Ophthalmol Vis Sci* (1988) **29**:390 (Abst).

44. Landry RJ, Pettit GH, Hahn DW, Ediger MN, Yang GC, Preliminary evidence of free radical formation during argon fluoride excimer laser irradiation of corneal tissue, *Lasers and Light in Ophthalmology* (1994) **6**:87–90.

45. Serdarevic O, Darrell RW, Krueger RR, Trokel SL, Excimer laser therapy for experimental Candida keratitis, *Am J Ophthalmol* (1985) **99**:534–8.

46. Gartry DS, Kerr Muir MG, Marshall J, Excimer laser treatment of corneal surface pathology: A laboratory and clinical study, *Br J Ophthalmol* (1991) **75**:258–69.

47. Yamaguchi T, Polacj FM, Kaufman ME, Endothelial damage after anterior radial keratotomy: An electron microscopic study of rabbit cornea, *Arch Ophthalmol* (1981) **99**:2151–8.

48. Bende T, Seiler T, Schilling A, Wollensak J, Reproduzierbarkeit von Exzisionstiefen bei der Laser-Hornhautchirurgie. In: Wollensak, J ed, *Laser in der Ophthalmologie* (ENKE Verlag: Stuttgart, 1988) 148–52.

49. Cotliar AM, Schubert HD, Mandel ER, Trokel SL, Excimer laser radial keratotomy, *Ophthalmology* (1985) **92**:206–8.

50. Aron-Rosa DS, Boerner CF, Bath et al, Corneal wound healing after laser keratotomy in a human eye, *Am J Ophthalmol* (1987) **103**:444–64.

51. Aron-Rose DS, Boulnoy JL, Carre F et al, Excimer laser surgery of the cornea: qualitative and quantitative aspects of photoablation according to the energy density, *J Cat Ref Surg* (1986) **12**:27–33.

52. Tenner A, Neuhann T, Schroder E et al, Excimer laser radial keratotomy in the living human eye: a preliminary report, *J Refract Surg* (1988) **4**:5–8.

53. Tuft SJ, Boulton ME, Marshall J, Assessment of corneal wound repair in vitro, *Curr Eye Res* (1989) **8**:713–9.

54. Tuft SJ, Zabel RW, Marshall J, Corneal repair following keratectomy: A comparison between conventional surgery and laser photoablation, *Invest Ophthalmol Vis Sci* (1989) **30**:1769–77.

Chapter 4 Cornea: anatomy, physiology and healing

Paul G McMenamin, Christopher Steele and Charles N J McGhee

DEVELOPMENT OF THE CORNEA

Around weeks six and seven of gestation, periocular mesenchyme, most likely derived from migrating mesencephalic neural crest, begins to condense around the optic cup (Fig. 4.1a).[1,2] The outer portion of this mesenchyme will form most of the fibrous coat of the eye, the sclera, and cornea. The inner portion, the inner vascular layer (uveocapillary lamina), will form the stroma of the uveal tract.

Following the formation of the lens the surface ectoderm seals over the lens pit.[3] This ectoderm forms the future corneal epithelium. At this stage (27 days) it is a stratified squamous epithelium 3–4 layers thick, the basal layer of which rests upon a thin basal lamina (Fig. 4.1b). Mesenchyme cells of neural crest origin pass over the optic cup margin and migrate centripetally in the space between the anterior surface of the lens and the surface ectoderm to form the presumptive corneal endothelium (around 33 days), which initially is composed of two layers. This is often described as the 'first wave' of mesenchyme, which contributes to the future cornea.[4]

Around day 49 a second 'wave' of mesenchyme commences migration from the optic cup margin and penetrates the space between the basal surfaces of the corneal epithelium and endothelium to form the corneal stroma (Fig. 4.1c).[1] By the eighth week the first evidence of loosely arranged collagen fibres can be detected amidst actively synthesizing fibroblasts, now known as keratoblasts. In subsequent weeks the endothelium is transformed into a simple cuboidal layer and ultimately a squamous layer resting upon a thick basal lamina – the precursor of Descemet's membrane (Fig. 4.1b). The intermediate layer of wing cells does not appear until the fourth or fifth month. By this time all the corneal layers are present with the exception of Bowman's layer, which becomes identifiable by 5 months as an acellular collagenous zone beneath the epithelium. The stromal collagen

bundles become organized into highly orientated lamellae with elongated flattened keratocytes interposed between the layers. This maturation process commences first in the posterior or deeper layers of the cornea and progresses anteriorly, thus the more anteriorly or superficially placed lamellae are those formed latest in embryonic/fetal life.[1,5,6]

Corneal thickness and diameter increase during development by both interstitial growth (thickening of lamellae) and appositional growth (addition of new lamellae). The glycosaminoglycan constituents alter during development from unsulphated forms to increasingly greater proportions of keratin sulphate after 6 months.[6] Corneal transparency is gradually attained prior to birth due to maturation of superficial lamellae and hydration activity of the endothelial cells, whose junctional complexes appear around month four. Innervation commences at 3 months and reaches the epithelium at 5 months' gestation.

In summary, the cornea is derived embryologically from both surface ectoderm and neural crest-derived mesenchyme. The former becomes the epithelium, while the latter gives rise to the deeper layers including Bowman's membrane, stroma, the endothelium and its thick basal lamina, Descemet's membrane.

GROSS AND SURGICAL ANATOMY

Whilst the transparency of the cornea is its most important property, the surface of the cornea (air–tissue interface) and associated tear film is responsible for most of the refractive power of the eye (approximately 44 D of 64 D total power).[7] Due to its highly exposed position, the cornea, like the sclera, must also present a tough non-compressible layer that can withstand considerable deformation and pressure and act as a physical barrier to trauma

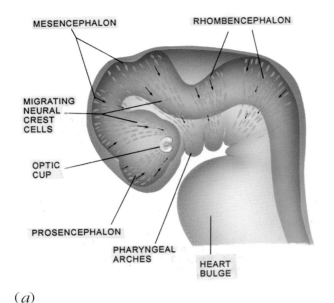

(a)

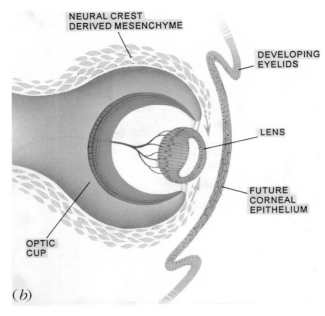

(b)

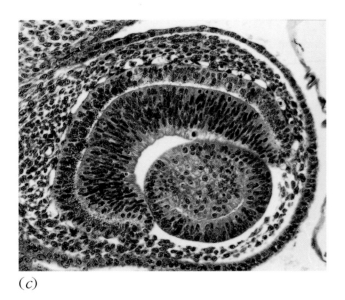

(c)

Figure 4.1 *(a) Diagram illustrating the manner in which mesencephalic and prosencephalic neural crest tissue migrates around the developing optic cup. (b) Diagram of the cornea showing the migration of the first 'wave' of neural crest-derived mesenchyme between the surface ectoderm and lens. This mesenchyme forms the corneal endothelium. (c) Black and white light micrograph showing the developing cornea after the second 'wave' of mesenchyme that has formed the primitive stroma. The cornea now has three basic layers.*

and infection. Most other tissues and cells in the body scatter and reflect light, thus rendering them opaque. Corneal transparency is due to a number of related factors: regularity and smoothness of the covering epithelium; its avascularity; and lastly the size and arrangement of the extracellular and cellular components in the stroma, which are dependent on the state of hydration, metabolism, and nutrition of the stromal elements.[6]

SHAPE

The cornea forms one-sixth of the circumference of the globe and has an average anterior surface radius of curvature of 7.8 mm, the remaining five-sixths of the circumference is formed by the sclera, which has a radius of 11.5 mm. The cornea meets the sclera at the limbus or corneoscleral junction. The cornea is smaller in vertical diameter (10.6 mm) than in

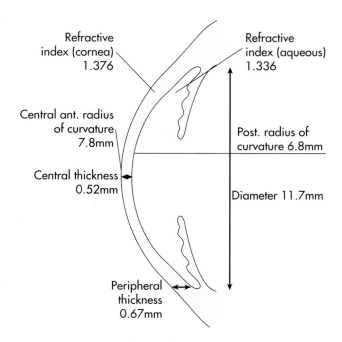

Figure 4.2 *Line diagram summarizing the major indices of the human cornea.*

horizontal diameter (11.7 mm); however, viewed from inside the eye the circumference is actually circular. The anterior corneal surface is aspheric with a central radius of 7.8 mm and a variably less steep peripheral corneal curvature; however, the posterior corneal surface is essentially spherical (Fig. 4.2). The cornea is thicker at the periphery (0.67 mm) than in the centre (0.52 mm).[8]

HISTOLOGICAL AND ULTRASTRUCTURAL ANATOMY OF THE CORNEA

The cornea is composed of five basic layers (Fig. 4.3a).

CORNEAL EPITHELIUM

The corneal epithelium is a stratified, squamous, non-keratinized epithelium that is 50–60 μm in thickness and consists of 5–6 layers of cells (Fig. 4.3b).

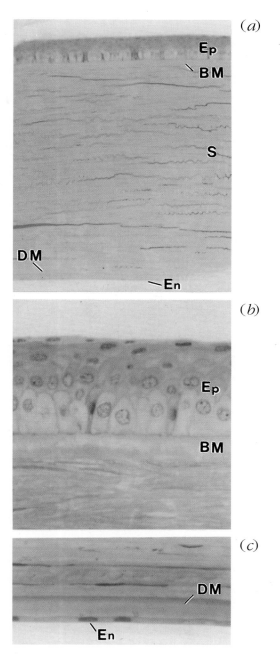

Figure 4.3 *(a) Low-power light micrograph of the normal human cornea demonstrating the five basic layers (1 μm thick section, toluidine blue, original magnification ×130). (b) High-power view of corneal epithelium and Bowman's layer (original magnification ×540). (c) High-power view of simple squamous corneal endothelium and Descemet's membrane. Note two distinct regions of Descemet's membrane visible even on light microscope sections (original magnification ×540). Ep, epithelium; BM, Bowman's layer or anterior limiting lamina; S, stroma or substantia propria; DM, Descemet's membrane; En, endothelium.*

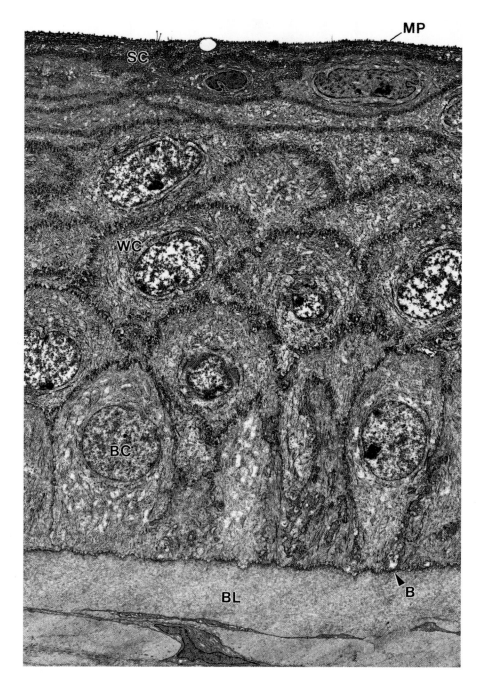

Figure 4.4 *Transmission electron micrograph of human corneal epithelium (original magnification ×3200). BL, Bowman's layer; B, basal lamina; BC, basal cell layer; WC, wing cell layer; SC, superficial cell layer; MP, microplicea. (Courtesy of D. Aitken.)*

Adjacent cells are held together by numerous junctions, including gap junctions (superficial cells), desmosomes (wing and adjacent basal cells), and to the underlying basal lamina by hemidesmosomes and anchoring filaments.[8] The superficial cells are flattened, nucleated and although morphologically they are classified as non-keratinized, they do in fact express a particular combination of paired 55/64 kDa keratins. The 55 kDa protein may have a role in inflammatory eye disease while the 64 kDa protein appears to be useful as a marker for differentiating cells of the central cornea from limbal stem cells. The anterior surface of the corneal epithelium is characterized by numerous microvilli and microplicae (ridges) whose glycocalyx coat interacts with, and helps stabilize, the precorneal tear film. Wing cells are irregular-shaped cells with oval nuclei that inter-digitate with superficial cells above, other wing cells, and with basal cells below (Fig. 4.4). The basal epithelial cells rest upon a thin, but prominent, basal lamina consisting of an apparently structureless lamina lucida (25 nm) and an electron-dense lamina densa (50 nm).[8]

Corneal epithelial cell adhesion is maintained by integrin receptors for basement membrane components such as fibronectin, laminin, and collagen. The basal epithelial–basement membrane interactions anchor the epithelium to Bowman's layer via a complex mesh of anchoring fibrils (type VII collagen) and anchoring plaques (type VI collagen) that inter-act with the lamina densa and the collagen fibrils of Bowman's layer in woven network.[6] The anchoring filaments may penetrate as far as 2 μm into Bowman's layer. In addition, transplasma membrane collagen type XVI supports firm adhesion in these basal cells. The basal lamina becomes multilaminar later in life.

The epithelium presents an effective barrier to fluid transport, which is achieved by extensive close contacts and junctional complexes between the basal cells, although true zonulae occludens type (tight) junctions have not been identified. Spot desmosomes are numerous and recent studies have revealed differences in the content of desmosomal proteins at this site: for instance, desmoglein and desmocollin are absent from basal limbal epithelial cells, which may have functional significance in relation to their role as putative stem cells. Corneal epithelial cells are strongly positive for VLA (Very Late Activating) integrins $-\alpha2$, $-\alpha3$, and less strongly for VLA$-\alpha4$, $-\alpha5$ and $-\alpha6$.[9] The ligands for the VLA integrins, which are part of the integrin superfamily, include leucocyte adhesion molecules, laminin (VLA$-\alpha3$ and $-\alpha6$), collagen (VLA$-\alpha2$ and $-\alpha3$) and fibronectin (VLA$-\alpha4$ and $-\alpha5$). Thus the expression by the epithelium of all the above integrins suggests they may be crucial to their adhesion to the underlying basal lamina and Bowman's layer.[9]

Corneal epithelium in the central two-thirds is effectively devoid of melanocytes and immune cells, including MHC class II-antigen bearing dendritic cells (Langerhans' cells). The absence of the latter cell type and the avascular nature of the cornea are of crucial functional significance in local immune responses and explain the less vigorous, or absent, host versus graft reaction following corneal transplantation, and minimal local inflammation following other forms of corneal surgery. The number of Langerhans' cells increases sharply near the limbus.[10]

The corneal epithelium presents the first refracting interface to transmitted light. Most of the light-absorbing properties of the cornea take place in this layer, mainly for short-wavelength light. However, the majority of the visible spectrum is transmitted through the epithelium.[7]

ANTERIOR LIMITING LAMINA: BOWMAN'S LAYER

Bowman's layer, contrary to popular opinion, is not a basement membrane but represents a modified acellular region of the collagenous stroma.[8] It is 8–12 μm thick and consists of fine, randomly arranged collagen fibrils of smaller diameter (20–30 nm diameter) than stromal collagen, and includes types I, V and VI with a high proportion of type III in a chondroitin/dermatan sulphate matrix. The anterior surface is well-delineated and separated from the epithelium by the epithelial basement membrane, whilst the posterior boundary is indistinct and merges with the stroma (Fig 4.4). Bowman's layer terminates abruptly at the limbus. It provides an important barrier to corneal invasion by tumours and pathogens. Bowman's layer is essentially restricted to the primate eye, although a thin layer has been described in the avian eye.[5]

SUBSTANTIA PROPRIA OR CORNEAL STROMA

The corneal stroma is a dense connective tissue of remarkable regularity. It comprises the vast majority of the corneal thickness and consists of 200–250 layers of flattened collagenous lamellae (2 μm thick) orientated parallel to the corneal surface and continuous with the less-regularly arranged collagenous lamellae of the sclera at the limbus.[8] The posterior lamellae are slightly thicker than the lamellae in the anterior one-third and have a more defined orientation parallel to the corneal surface. The collagenous lamellae form a highly organized orthogonal ply, adjacent lamellae being orientated slightly less than 90° to both anteriorly and posteriorly placed lamellae (Fig. 4.5a,b). In the anterior third of the cornea the lamellae display a more oblique orientation relative to one another in comparison to the posterior two-thirds, an orientation that becomes exaggerated in stromal oedema (Fig. 4.3a,c). Recent studies using X-ray diffraction techniques have shown that the parallel arrangement of the central corneal fibrils extends

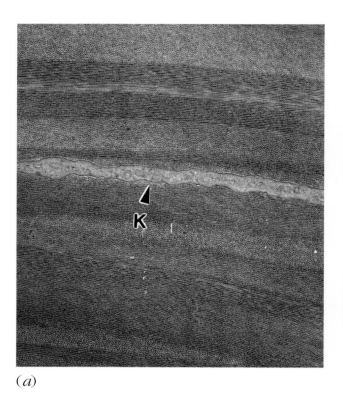

(a)

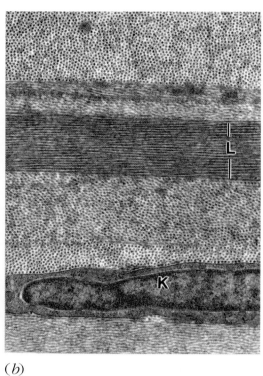

(b)

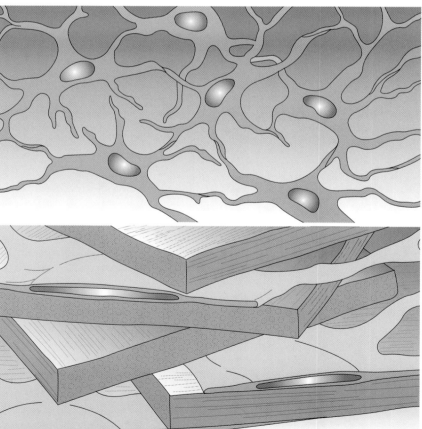

(c)

Figure 4.5 *Transmission electron micrograph of (a) corneal stromal lamellae (L) and keratocytes (K) at low magnification (original magnification ×8000) and (b) Higher magnification view of 3–4 adjacent stromal lamellae highlighting the regular spacing of collagen fibres (original magnification ×25 000). (c) Artist's impression of stromal lamellae alternating at less than 90°. Between the stromal lamellae lies a planar network of extremely flattened, stellate, modified fibroblasts known as keratocytes.*

to the periphery where the fibrils adopt a concentric configuration to form a 'weave' at the limbus. This imparts considerable strength to the peripheral cornea and permits it to maintain its curvature and thus its optical properties.

The collagen fibres are predominantly (50–55%) of type I (30 nm diameter, 64–70 nm banding) with some type III, V, and VI also present. Collagen type V (approximately 10%) and some type III (1–2%) collagen also exist in the corneal stroma while the remainder is made up of type VI collagen. Types I, III, and V collagen are fibrillar collagens, but type VI collagen has large non-helical, globular polypeptides at both the C– and N–termini of the helical protein backbone. It has been suggested that type V collagen is codistributed with type I and is implicated in regulating fibril formation and thus fibril thickness and interfibrillary distance. However, fibril thickness is also dependent on the nature of the stromal glycosaminoglycans (GAG) and proteoglycans.[11]

The corneal stroma is unusual in that it contains no hyaluronic acid (HA) except at the limbus where there is a gradual increase in HA concentration towards the sclera. The major corneal glycosaminoglycan is keratan sulphate. In the central cornea, non-sulphated chondroitin is also present while towards the periphery, chondroitin sulphate is the second major GAG. Chondroitin-4-sulphate and dermatan sulphate are chemically almost identical and many believe that the second major GAG may not be chrondroitin sulphate but dermatan sulphate.[11] Corneal GAG exists in the native state as proteoglycans, two forms of which are recognized: proteokeratan sulphate (PKS I and II) and proteodermatan sulphate (PDS I and II). Both corneal dermatan sulphate and keratan sulphate proteoglycan are considered to belong to the class of small, non-aggregating proteoglycans. Both dermatan sulphate proteoglycan-I and -II (DS-PG I and II) and keratan sulphate proteoglycan-I and -II (KS-PG I and II) bind to the collagen arrays at specific binding sites (one proteoglycan to one binding site) suggesting that these sites are essential to the spacing of the fibrils and to the width of the interfibrillar space.

Between the stromal lamellae lies a planar network of extremely flattened, modified fibroblasts known as keratocytes (Figs 4.5a,b,c).[8] These stellate-shaped cells, with thin-branched cytoplasmic extensions, contain conspicuously few distinctive organelles yet they are the source of stromal collagen and proteoglycans. They normally only express the common β1 chain of VLA integrins. Not much is known of collagen turnover in the adult cornea; however, it appears keratocytes are not highly metabolically active. They are more prominent in the posterior stroma. The corneal stroma normally contains no blood or lymphatic vessels but sensory nerve fibres course in the anterior layers 'en route' to the epithelium.

POSTERIOR LIMITING LAMINA: DESCEMET'S MEMBRANE

This is a thin, homogenous, discrete, periodic acid-Schiff (PAS) stain positive layer between the posterior stroma and the endothelium, from which it may become detached in pathological conditions. It is 8–12 μm in thickness and represents the modified basement membrane of the corneal endothelium (Fig. 4.3c). It consists of two parts: an anterior third which is banded and deposited in fetal life and consists of 30–40 compact lamellae in an hexagonal array; and a non-banded, homogenous posterior two-thirds that may contain occasional type I collagen fibres (Figs 4.6a,b). Disturbances in Descemet's membrane in gestation or in adult life often spare the anterior two-thirds. Descemet's membrane is rich in characteristic basement membrane glycoproteins, such as laminin, fibronectin and type IV collagen (mostly in the non-banded zone) and contains high levels of novel collagens, types V, VIII, IX, and XII in a lattice arrangement. This adds elasticity and deformability to the cornea while maintaining high levels of light transmission. Descemet's membrane also imparts strength and resilience to the corneal stroma, which aids the resistance to normal intraocular pressure. Collagen types V and VI may be involved in maintaining adherence at the interface of Descemet's membrane with the adjacent posterior lamellae of the stroma. Descemet's membrane can be traced peripherally and shares properties with the cortical zone of the trabeculae within the trabecular meshwork, including the tendency to thicken with advancing age. Microscopic wart-like protuberances (Hassall–Henle bodies or peripheral guttata) containing cell debris and 'long banded (100 nm)' deposits of an unknown nature (formerly thought to be collagen) appear in the periphery of Descemet's membrane with age. It is frequently thickened at its peripheral termination to form Schwalbe's line (or ring) at the anterior limit of the trabecular meshwork. If disrupted, Descemet's membrane tends to curl inwards towards the anterior chamber. It functions to provide mechanical support to the cornea and is more resistant than the stroma to destruction by trauma or inflammatory cells.

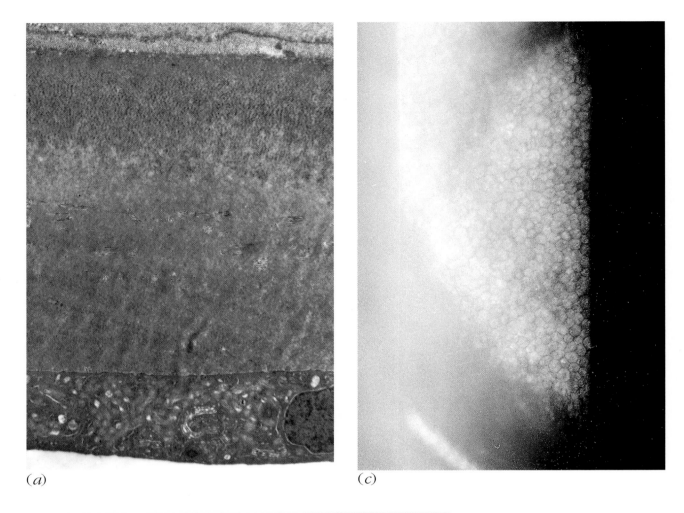

(a)

(c)

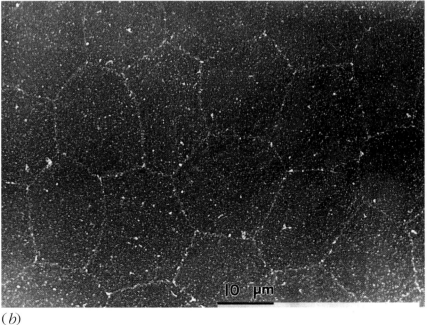

(b)

Figure 4.6 *(a) Low-power transmission electron micrograph of Descemet's membrane demonstrating anterior one-third banded and posterior two-thirds non-banded layers, with the adjacent cytoplasm and nucleus of an endothelial cell demonstrated inferiorly (original magnification ×7000). (b) Scanning electron micrograph of the inner corneal surface to reveal the regular hexagonal array of corneal endothelial cells (original magnification ×2700). (c) Specular micrograph of the endothelial mosaic.*

CORNEAL ENDOTHELIUM

Fluid is constantly being lost via evaporation at the ocular surface, a fact illustrated by increased corneal thickness after a night of lid closure or if an impermeable contact lens is placed over the epithelium. The corneal endothelium, a simple squamous epithelium or mesothelium, on the posterior surface of the cornea (Fig. 4.3c), performs the critical role of maintaining corneal hydration and thus transparency. Corneal endothelial cells rest upon Descemet's membrane and form a regular, uninterrupted polygonal or hexagonal mosaic that can be clearly seen in vivo with the aid of specular microscopy, which is also used to assess cell density, or ex vivo by scanning electron microscopy (Fig. 4.6b). The cells are 5–6 μm in height and 18–20 μm in diameter and have an average surface area of 250 μm². Their lateral surfaces are highly interdigitated and possess apical junctional complexes that together with the cytoplasmic organelles, such as abundant mitochondria, reflect their crucial role in active fluid transport. The corneal endothelium stains strongly for all VLA integrins.[9]

There are approximately 350 000 cells per cornea, approximately 3–4000 cells/mm² at birth, falling to 2500/mm² in mid-age and 2000/mm² in old age.[12] Consequently, with age the dense, regular, hexagonal arrangement of these cells, typical of young corneas, is replaced by fewer cells of more heterogeneous shapes and sizes. Damage to corneal endothelial cells and densities of below 800/mm² can rapidly lead to oedema and swelling of the stroma, with resultant loss of transparency, and a density of less than 1500/mm² generally renders a cornea unsuitable for transplantation. Occasional intracytoplasmic melanin granules in the endothelium indicate a weak phagocytic ability of these cells, a property more evident in trabecular meshwork cells to which they are closely related.

THE NERVE SUPPLY OF THE CORNEA

The cornea is richly supplied by sensory fibres derived from the ophthalmic division of the trigeminal nerve, mainly via the long ciliary nerves.[8] Branches radiate into the anterior corneal stroma from an annular plexus near the limbus, whereupon they lose their myelin sheaths and form a subepithelial plexus. From this latter plexus fine axons, devoid of Schwann cells, pierce Bowman's layer to form a terminal intraepithelial plexus (Fig. 4.7). There are apparently no specialized end-organs associated with these terminal axons, which are sensitive to pain and temperature. Larger

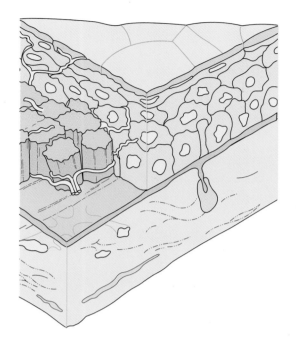

Figure 4.7 *Diagrammatic representation of the human corneal epithelial plexus. The unmyelinated axons lose their Schwann cell coverings as they enter the basal epithelium.*

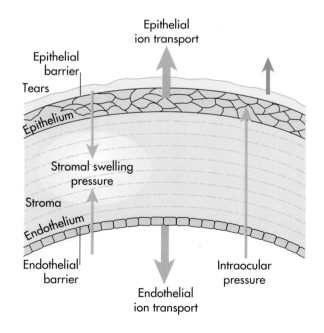

Figure 4.8 *Diagrammatic representation summarizing the mechanisms that maintain corneal hydration.*

myelinated nerve fibres can often be seen during slit-lamp examination as fine whitish fibres radiating into the cornea from the limbus. Damage to the corneal epithelium and intraepithelial nerve terminals causes a great deal of pain. Following deep excimer laser photoablation, although the epithelial plexus may fully regenerate within 3 months, the architecture of stromal nerves demonstrates abnormalities of morphology and function up to 12 months after treatment.[13] Reactivation of latent herpes simplex virus in the trigeminal ganglion may occur following damage to corneal nerve terminals, by e.g. cold, ultraviolet light exposure (including excimer laser), trauma, or corticosteroids, and activated virus is transmitted to the cornea leading to recurrent herpes simplex keratitis and superficial corneal ulceration.[14]

BASIC PHYSIOLOGY

The cornea is approximately 80% hydrated, which is higher than other tissues, including the sclera (70% hydrated). Despite this, the corneal stroma 'imbibes' water if it is placed in a solution of saline (this is well demonstrated by the injured, lacerated cornea, which swells and becomes opaque) and these water-attracting properties are due to its high content of GAGs. The cornea has been described as 'a slice of water stabilized in three dimensions by a meshwork of fibrils and soluble polymers'.[11] The cornea thus has a swelling pressure and a metabolic pump (the endothelium) designed to maintain it. The swelling pressure generates a level of interfibrillar tension and may be the biophysical mechanism whereby the fibrils are maintained in their normal arrangement.[6]

KERATOCYTES

Stromal keratocytes are important in maintaining transparency as they synthesize stromal collagens and proteoglycans. Although most of the changes that occur in the assembly of the matrix are post-translational, the enzymes that induce these changes are present in the keratocytes.

THE ENDOTHELIAL PUMP

Despite the higher than normal level of hydration of the corneal stroma, its water binding is unsaturated, a condition achieved by an endothelial pump that transports water out of the cornea towards the anterior chamber (Fig. 4.8). Na^+ and HCO_3^- are transported across the endothelium from the stroma to the aqueous, mediated by a Na^+/K^+-dependent ATPase and a HCO_3^--dependent ATPase, probably involving carbonic anhydrase. The Na^+/K^+-ATPase is located in the plasma membranes but the HCO_3^--dependent ATPase is present in the mitochondria, where its major role in ion transport may be to generate the ATP required for the Na^+/K^+-ATPase pump. Carbonic anhydrase may also be involved in the Na^+/H^+ antiport for maintaining intracellular pH. More recent evidence suggests that other mechanisms may be operative in the transport of fluid across the endothelium. These include a Na^+/H^+ exchanger protein that drives an electrogenic coupling between Na^+ and HCO_3^- ions. This 'antiport' is essential for the maintenance of the intracellular pH by exchanging Na^+ (in) with H^+ (out) in the cell.[6]

TWO-WAY TRANSPORT IN THE CORNEA

In addition to the transport of water from the stroma to the aqueous humour, there is a net flux of ions and water towards the epithelium and the tearfilm. Ion transport into the cornea, mediated by Na^+/K^+-ATPase and Ca^{2+}/Mg^{2+}-ATPase in the basolateral plasma membrane of the epithelium, is also operational in corneal ion shifts.[6] Na^+ movement from the tears into the epithelium is by passive diffusion down a concentration gradient, but from the epithelium into the stroma, active transport is required via the Na^+/K^+-ATPase to which Cl^- transport in the opposite direction is coupled.

OXYGEN HANDLING BY THE CORNEA

The epithelium obtains its oxygen from the preocular tear film at a rate of $3.5–4.0\,\mu l/cm^2/hr$. The endothelium, however, and the keratocytes in the deep stroma, receive their oxygen supply from the circulation via the aqueous humour. Corneal function and health is therefore dependent on local conditions at the surface of the eye and on systemic factors such as cardiopulmonary capacity.

CORNEAL TRANSPARENCY AND PHOTOREFRACTIVE KERATECTOMY

Two main theories compete to explain the unique transparency of the cornea and are essential to any discussion of post excimer laser haze. The first, by Maurice, suggests that the extremely uniform diameter (30–45 nm) of collagen fibrils and their exquisitely regular 'lattice' spacing within the corneal stroma, enables forward transmission of light with mutual destructive interference of any light scattered by adjacent individual fibres.[15,16] Indeed, the irregular distribution and size of collagen fibres (25–480 nm) in the opaque sclera stands in quite dramatic contradistinction to the regular lamellar arrangement of the cornea previously discussed. This theory concludes that as long as the distance between regularly arranged fibrils is less than one wavelength of light (400–700 nm) transparency is maintained, whereas, when this distance is greater, e.g. corneal oedema, mutual destructive interference no longer occurs due to light scattering, and transparency is lost.

However, the attraction of this lattice theory, in terms of geometric optics, as an explanation of corneal transparency is at variance with other (irregular) components of the same structure: Bowman's layer consists of small collagen fibres in an interwoven arrangement; and the layers of the corneal epithelium by definition are non-uniform.[17] Comparative anatomical studies have also shown that shark cornea, which maintains clarity at varying depths and salt concentrations, frequently contains areas of irregular collagen fibril arrangement.[18] Goldman and others have determined that refractive elements in tissues that are small (less than 200 nm) relative to the wavelength of light actually scatter considerably less light than might be predicted and corneal collagen fibrils are notably both small in diameter (30 nm) and closely spaced (approximately 55 nm). It is postulated that in structures with small refractile elements, as long as inhomogeneities in refractive index are separated by less than one-half wavelength of light (200–350 nm), light transmission is not affected.[19,20] The uniformity of corneal hydration (70–80%) and spatial separation of fibres is maintained to a large extent by the GAGs, which represent 4.5% of the dry weight of the cornea and have previously been outlined.[21,22] Interestingly, dermatan sulphate appears to be absent from the mature cornea in significant quantities but is present in the opaque sclera[23] and notably in mucopolysaccharide storage diseases (such as Hurler's and Scheie's syndromes) the abnormal accumulation of keratan and dermatan sulphate that occurs in the cornea in the first few years of life, is associated with loss of transparency and corneal 'cloudiness'.[24] Significantly, following full thickness or superficial

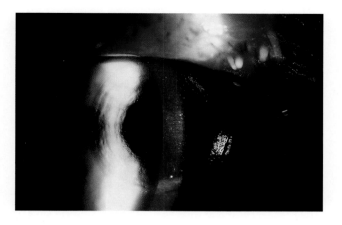

Figure 4.9 *Immediate post-operative slit lamp photograph of a 6 mm diameter, transepithelial PRK enhancement, demonstrating the circular 'steps' created in the corneal stroma by the excimer beam as the mechanical iris expands during treatment.*

corneal wounding, healing corneal scars contain abnormal GAGs and abnormally large proteoglycan filaments, with increased concentrations of dermatan sulphate, but as wounds mature and clear, keratan sulphate becomes the predominant GAG.[25–28]

Thus, the uniform small size of the refractive elements within the stroma and the close spacing of elements of differing refractive index, which is maintained in large part by the level of sulphation and relative proportions of GAGs, may be of greater importance in the maintenance of transparency in the normal cornea than the regularity of the lattice structure. Alteration of these complex relationships may be intrinsic to the development of haze and scarring in the post photorefractive keratectomy (PRK) cornea.[29,30]

CORNEAL WOUND HEALING AND PHOTOREFRACTIVE KERATECTOMY

In comparison to cutaneous wound healing, corneal wound healing is more complex, as a result of the greater differentiation and the strictly ordered organization of the corneal substructures. Much of our knowledge concerning corneal wound healing is derived from experimental work on animals such as rabbits and monkeys, although there have been

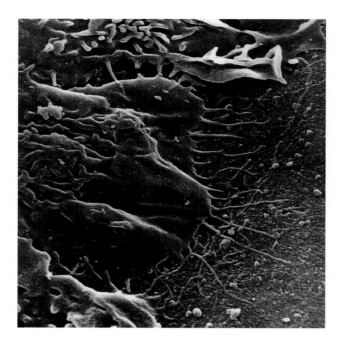

Figure 4.10 *Developing filopodia and lamellipodia during epithelial cell migration. (Reproduced with permission from* Acta Ophthalmologica.*)*

occasional studies reported involving human subjects. There are, however, certain anatomical differences between these species, in particular the absence of Bowman's layer in rabbits, and therefore caution should be exercised when extrapolating animal models to the human clinical situation.

Corneal wound healing, as in other parts of the body, is the end result of a sequence of events that is controlled by many factors. Wound healing at other sites culminates in scar formation and vascularization. One of the most crucial differences in corneal wound healing is how the healing processes aim to minimize these end results which would otherwise have serious visual consequences.

Photorefractive keratectomy uses the 193 nm excimer laser to photo-ablate Bowman's layer and anterior stromal tissue following mechanical removal of the epithelium, with negligible thermal effects to adjacent tissue.[31–34] Corneal wound healing following PRK can vary significantly with the smoothness of the ablation surface, which may in turn depend on the uniformity of the laser beam's spatial intensity profile and the number and size of corneal 'steps' (Fig. 4.9).

Following PRK, the ideal healing pattern would be: the epithelium perfectly adheres to the underlying stroma and retains its normal thickness. The subepithelial stroma shows no change from its normal architecture and shows no regeneration or scarring and the cornea retains its pretreatment mechanical stability without any deformation. There would also be no permanent changes to deeper lying stroma, and in particular, to the endothelium. In reality however, the healing phenomenon following PRK alters the biochemistry, morphological features and tissue functions of corneal tissue in a rather unpredictable fashion in some cases.

EPITHELIAL HEALING

The processes involved in the healing of corneal epithelial wounds can be described in three separate phases, which in reality are part of a continuous process. Animal studies (mainly rabbits and monkeys) have shown that these stages in epithelial healing can be described as the *latent phase, cell migration and adhesion*, and finally, *cell proliferation* (Table 4.1). There are many factors that will affect the healing process, including the size and depth of the wound and the causative agent. One very important factor is tear quality and integrity, as any tear deficiency may compromise the wound healing process.[35,36]

The latent phase

Following mechanical scraping the epithelium is normally healed within 3–4 days. Campos found that sharp instrument (surgical blade) de-epithelialization was more effective than that produced by blunt methods e.g. with a paton spatula.[37,38] Completeness of epithelial debridement may well influence the depth of ablation subsequently achieved. Immediately following PRK finely spaced concentric ablation 'steps' can be seen on the stromal surface.[31,39]

In the initial or latent phase, following corneal debridement in rabbits and monkeys, existing basal epithelial cells at the wound margin begin to slide and move within the 4–6 hours.[40] Throughout this phase polymorphonuclear leukocytes (PMNs), derived from tear fluid, are often seen at the wound margins removing necrotic cells and cell debris.[41–43] Due to this action these cells actually cause a microscopic enlargement of the epithelial defect; however,

Table 4.1
A summary of the major events in corneal epithelial wound healing.

Stage 1: The latent phase. Occurs within 4–6 hours	**Stage 2: Cell migration and adhesion. Lasts 24–36 hours**	**Stage 3: Cell proliferation. Lasts 36 hours to several months**
Epithelial debridement ↓ polymorphonuclear leukocyte invasion ↓ removal of necrotic cells/debris ↓ retraction/rounding of epithelial cells at wound edge ↓ reduction in hemidesmosome attachments 200 µm outward around wound margins ↓ commencement of lamellipodial and filopodial extensions	Intracellular formation of actin filaments (composed of fodrin, vinculin and ankyrin) ↓ formation of filopodial and lamellipodial extensions completed ↓ actin filaments accumulate at leading edges of lamellipodia and filopodia giving cytoskeletal support ↓ appearance of fibronectin usually within 1 hour ↓ temporary anchor formation cyclical process commences as cells start to advance ↓ centripetal migration of leading epithelial cells across stromal surface. Energy derived from glycogen metabolism ↓ formation of Y–X contact lines ↓ completion of epithelial monolayer covering wound area ↓ fibronectin disappears ↓ synthesis of new hemidesmosomes and other anchoring complexes ↓ appearance of type III collagen ↓ epithelial/stromal adhesion restored from 6 to 8 weeks although abnormalities can persist for up to 15 months	Activation of limbal stem cells ↓ stem cells produce transient amplifying cells (TACs) ↓ TACs give rise to postmitotic cells (PMCs) ↓ PMCs give rise to terminally differentiated cells (TDCs) ↓ further establishment of hemidesmosomes ↓ possible epithelial hyperplasia ↓ replacement of corneal nerve axon terminal endings ↓ hypersensitivity of corneal epithelial nerves for several months

PMN cells usually disappear once a monolayer of epithelial cells cover the wound area.[42] Rounding and retraction of epithelial cells at the wound edge, with loss of surface microvilli, can be observed before the basal cells start flattening and separating.[44,45] In rabbit studies it has been demonstrated that hemidesmosomal attachments between the basement membrane and the basal cells completely disappear to approximately 70 µm outward (i.e. towards the corneal periphery) from the epithelial defect margin, and are considerably reduced for a further 200 μm.[46,47] The final stage of the latent phase commences with the production of cellular processes on the basal edges of cells bordering the wound. These can be finger-like filopodia or wider shaped lamellipodia. Their appearance marks the beginning of the second phase of cell movement.[45,48,49]

Cell migration

The second phase involves the lateral migration of the epithelial cells across the wound area before mitosis commences, thus producing linear cell healing of the corneal wound. The movement of these cells is mediated by the intracellular formation and contraction of actin filaments[50] that are composed of proteins including fodrin, vinculin and ankyrin.[51-53] These actin filaments provide the cells with the cytoskeletal support required during this kinetic second phase (Fig. 4.11), and these are concentrated in the leading edges of the migrating cells, in particular lining the filopodia and lamellipodia.[50] The importance of actin filament synthesis to cell motion has been demonstrated by the negative effect of cytochalasin B, which inhibits actin filament formation.[54]

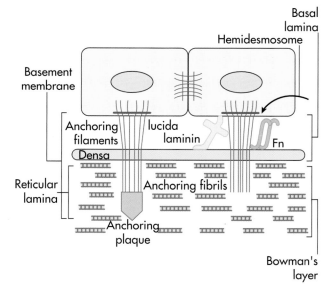

Figure 4.11 *Attachment of human corneal epithelium to stroma. (Adapted from Healing processes in the cornea,* Current Opinion in Ophthalmology.*)*

Soon after corneal wound healing, extracellular matrix proteins such as fibronectin, fibronectin/fibrin, laminin and tenascin appear on the wound surface.[55-62] There is evidence to suggest that the extracellular glycoprotein fibronectin plays an essential role, by providing a transient subepithelial matrix on to which the migrating epithelial cells can adhere during these frequent cyclical processes of cleaving and attaching of the migration. Fibronectin appears on the wound surface within 1 hour after injury[55] and demonstrates cell receptor sites in addition to binding sites for certain basement membrane components which include heparin sulphate and type IV collagen. Fibronectin stimulates epithelial cells to produce plasminogen activator which in turn converts plasminogen to plasmin which breaks down adhesions between cells and underlying subepithelial matrix.[53,64] In this way the filopodia and lamellipodial processes bind with and cleave from the underlying matrix during the cyclical process described above. Once corneal healing is complete fibronectin disappears.[55]

Only when migration of the epithelial monolayer is complete does it become more firmly anchored to the basement membrane and to Bowman's layer by newly synthesized hemidesmosomes and other anchoring filaments containing type VII collagen.[65] Prior to this stage adhesions are relatively weak allowing the new epithelium to be easily rubbed off. Although the precise process by which these anchoring complexes are formed is yet to be fully elucidated, various other protein molecules have also been identified in these anchoring complexes, including talin, fimbrin, integrins (i.e. heterodimeric transmembrane glycoproteins), laminin and kalinin.[60,66,67]

The regenerated epithelium re-establishes tight adhesion to the underlying stroma by completing the formation of hemidesmosomes, anchoring fibrils[68] and anchoring plaques (Fig. 4.11).[69-73] In monkey eye type III collagen, which is normally associated with scar tissue, has also been localized between 6 days and 18 months post PRK by immunofluorescence techniques.[69,70] In the rabbit model, it has been demonstrated that adhesion structures between corneal epithelium and stroma are fully restored approximately 6–8 weeks after injury (Fig. 4.12).[74-76] Although certain adhesion structures do regenerate, the overall architecture of the basement membrane is permanently altered in relation to the normal unoperated eye.[74]

Restoration of epithelial cell adhesion structures is a complex process which can proceed for many months following PRK. Abnormalities have been reported in the adhesion complexes of rabbits over 1

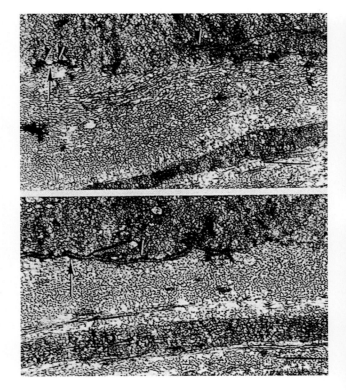

Figure 4.12 *Basement membrane zone of a 33-year-old patient after phototherapeutic keratectomy. Top: areas of absent and discontinuous basement membrane (arrow) are noted. Hemidesmosomes (arrowheads) are present in areas that correspond to basement membrane segments. Anchoring fibrils are absent. Bottom: Transmission electron micrograph of another treated region showing greater basement membrane (arrow) and hemidesmosome (arrowhead) reformation. Stromal keratocytes are noted in proximity to the epithelial basement membrane. (Reproduced with permission from Tamara R. et al, Reassembly of corneal epithelial adhesion structures after excimer laser keratectomy in humans, Arch Ophthalmol (1994)* **122***: 967–72.)*

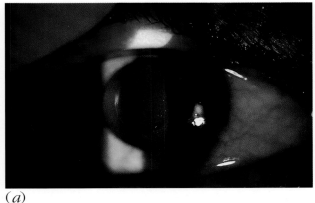

(a)

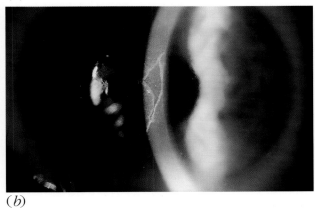

(b)

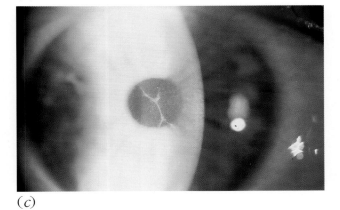

(c)

Figure 4.13 *Clinical photomicrographs of corneal epithelial healing following photorefractive keratectomy (PRK) using a 6 mm ablation zone and a 6.5 mm epithelial debridement zone. (a) 24 hours postoperatively centripetal movement of sheets of cells have already reduced the epithelial defect considerably. (b) Forty-eight hours post-PRK and the advancing epithelial edges have reduced the defect to less than 25%. (c) Seventy-two hours postoperatively. The epithelial defect has completely closed with the formation of an 'X' epithelial suture (confirming that the advancing epithelial sheets come from several regions of the epithelial wound edge).*

year after manual lamellar keratectomy.[75] In humans, adhesion complex abnormalities have been observed 6–15 months post PRK,[77] although in some other reports, it has been stated that adhesion complexes are complete 4 weeks after PRK.[78–80] The reappearance of anchoring fibrils and basal lamina has been shown to be directly proportional to wound healing duration, whereas hemidesmosome reformation occurs concurrently with basal lamina formation. Other factors that affect adhesion complex formation include the age, depth of keratectomy and the nature of any underlying condition.[77]

How quickly permanent hemidesmosomal attachments form is dependent on whether the basement membrane remained intact at the time of corneal wounding. Studies in monkey eyes, for example, have shown that despite their formation, fragmented regions of epithelial basement membrane can be devoid of type VII collagen anchoring fibrils even as long as 18 months after photorefractive keratectomy. This may help explain the symptoms of foreign body sensation, lacrimation or tenderness in some photorefractive keratectomy patients who suffer epithelial breakdown.[72]

Several studies have indicated that migration of cells occurs in a centripetal fashion from the limbus towards the centre of the cornea.[80,81] This occurs not only during normal epithelial regeneration but also in the wound healing process following PRK.[40] In the case of large central corneal abrasions, similar to those seen in PRK (Fig. 4.13), centripetal epithelial sheet movement occurs from more than one direction with the leading edges forming convex shapes. Eventually these various leading edges meet to close the wound forming Y- and X-shaped contact lines observable with the slit-lamp.[83] The rate of epithelial cell migration varies with species e.g. 17 μm/day in the mouse[81] and 64 μm in the rabbit.[44] Epithelial cells usually migrate *en masse* as a continuous sheet, with individual cells remaining in constant unchanging positions relative to each other.[46,82] Occasionally, small groups or columns of cells migrate independently giving rise to whorls of variable size, which can easily be observed with the use of fluorescein stain normally very close to the Y- and X-contact lines (Fig. 4.14).[84,85] This second, migratory and adhesive phase lasts for 24–36 hours.[40]

Epithelial cell proliferation

The final phase in the healing of an epithelial defect involves proliferation of the epithelial cells until normal epithelial thickness is resumed. The basal epithelial cells are the main participants in this proliferative process.[86] All self-regenerating tissues of the body have stem cells which are responsible for cell replacement and tissue regeneration. In the cornea these are located near the limbus, although not all the cells in this region are stem-cell types. Evidence to support this includes observations that large

corneal epithelial wounds near the limbus repair more quickly compared to smaller more central corneal defects.[87]

The two main categories of epithelial cell present in the cornea can be classified as the basal cells and the overlying suprabasal cells. Stem cells first produce rapidly dividing cells termed transient amplifying cells (TACs) which refer to corneal basal cells. These further divide into more differentiated cells termed postmitotic cells (PMCs). Similarly these cells produce the final fully differentiated corneal epithelial cells known as terminally differentiated cells (TDCs).[88] Both PMCs and TDCs have been described as the suprabasal cells of the corneal epithelium.[89]

Protuberances of underlying stroma are smoothed, producing a more regular corneal surface with proliferation of epithelial cells, and wound healing is completed with the formation of additional hemidesmosomes permanently anchoring the corneal epithelium to the underlying stroma. In extensive corneal wounds including the limbus and conjunctival epithelium, human studies have shown that conjunctival cells are capable of migrating centripetally into the cornea; however, these are poorly differentiated, irregular, and relatively thin.[83] In monkey studies, certain amounts of pigment have been observed in the central corneal region following PRK. This pigment could only have migrated from the relatively densely pigmented limbal conjunctiva.[90]

CORNEAL EPITHELIAL HEALING FOLLOWING EXCIMER LASER

Epithelial hyperplasia is seen histologically in monkey and human eyes in the early postoperative period after PRK, particularly non-tapered ablations.[91–93] Occasionally this persists and is related to regression of refraction.[39,90] Taylor reported transiently increased numbers of epithelial cells histopathologically by as much as 50% in a series of ablated human corneas,[39] although the actual number of epithelial cell layers was not specified. Indeed the actual number of cells is rarely given in any of the other studies but has been reported to increase up to 12 cells thick.[94] Epithelial hyperplasia has been shown to be thicker at the edge of an ablation than at the centre and may therefore alter the refractive effect of PRK.[95] Approximately 3–6 months post-PRK, normal epithelial maturation patterns can again be observed in humans.[72] Whilst the epithelium has a remarkable ability to heal without scarring in normal

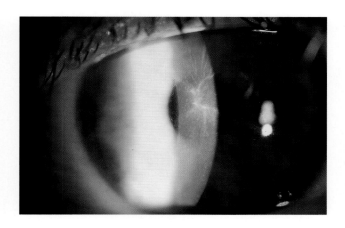

Figure 4.14 *Photomicrograph of the cornea of a 43-year-old female 72 hours after a −10.00 D PRK. Local proliferation of epithelium has produced a more vorticeal pattern of epithelial closure than the simple 'Y' or 'X' suture normally seen at 72 hours. Subsequent healing and refractive outcome was uneventful with a smooth epithelial surface and a maximum of grade 1 stromal haze.*

situations, significant structural alterations do occur once the PRK ablation area penetrates the basal cell membrane and basal lamina.

CORNEAL SENSITIVITY AND NERVE REGENERATION

Corneal nerve regeneration in rabbit eyes following PRK has been shown to be similar to that produced by other surgical procedures, except it is more intense after PRK.[96,97] Development of corneal hypersensitivity has been reported following excimer laser, although the reasons for this are not yet known. Compared with manual debridement, laser epithelial ablation results in an increase in networks of axons with terminal endings. Ishikawa[98] reported that laser ablated rabbit epithelia showed intraepithelial nerve increases of 45.8% at day 3, rapidly increasing to 116% at 1 month, and thereafter recovering to near normal levels by 7 months. This compared to a 39.2% increase at day 3, and thereafter gradually increasing to near normal levels at 7 months. These results have been used to support the current clinical practice of manual epithelial debridement prior to PRK.

STROMAL WOUND HEALING

Stromal regeneration depends upon a co-ordinated interaction between epithelial cells and keratocytes where polypeptide growth factors play an important role. Following stromal wounding, keratocytes undergo proliferation and migration stimulated by the release of certain cytokines (see Introduction to growth factors, below).[99,100]

Following epithelial debridement, stromal keratocytes die back in a 200 µm zone from the exposed wound surface. Subsequently, keratocytes migrate to the surface of the wound, which, in the absence of Bowman's layer,[101] normally consists of an irregular meshwork of filaments containing collagen types I, III, V and VI[102] and possibly IV.[103] This keratocyte activity does not occur until the corneal wound has been fully covered by new epithelium. Forty eight to seventy hours after injury the remaining keratocytes undergo fibroblastic transformation with resulting expansion of the fibroblast population by mitosis. This expansion and new production of connective tissue peaks between 3 and 6 days.[72,104] Keratocyte mitosis decreases with increasing keratocyte repopulation, created largely by mitotic division of cells peripheral to the epithelial defect rather than migration of keratocytes from the basal layers of the corneal stroma.[42,105,106] Interestingly, the initial keratocyte loss is also seen where the epithelial removal is performed by excimer laser, which mechanically is relatively atraumatic; thus keratocyte loss does not appear to be attributable to mechanical effects of epithelial debridement.[38,107] Furthermore, Campos showed that epithelial removal by excimer laser actually causes the greatest inflammatory response when compared to other mechanical methods.[38] The mechanism by which keratocytes initially disappear is not yet fully understood, although the fact that keratocytes disappear very quickly, with a lack of detritus, may indicate a mechanism of self-destruction rather than necrosis.[41]

Activated keratocytes (fibroblasts) produce collagens, glycoproteins, and proteoglycans, which form the new stromal extracellular matrix. In primate studies, the fibroblastic response was particularly intense at 3 months, with large numbers of activated keratocytes in the anterior 40–60 µm of the stroma. At 6–15 months the number of fibroblasts decreased as they developed into mature keratocytes.[78] The human corneal stroma contains collagen types I, III and V, all of which are now thought to copolymerize within the same fibrils throughout the stroma. Collagen type

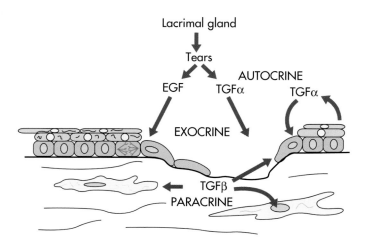

Figure 4.15 *Model of growth factor action in corneal wound healing.*

VI constitutes approximately 30% of the corneal stromal collagen content and is predominant in the connecting filaments interlinking stromal collagen fibrils.[108] This hybrid nature has led to the suggestion that fibril diameters in the cornea are controlled by the inclusion of one or more of these minor collagen types with type I collagen, which predominates in human corneal stroma.

In this early phase, the newly synthesized collagen fibrils are usually larger in diameter than normal, due to the higher concentration of chondroitin/dermatan sulphate which lasts for up to 3–4 months. This is in contrast to the normally low levels of dermatan sulphate in corneal stroma.[109,110] The resulting variation in collagen fibril diameter and interfibrillary distance may disrupt corneal transparency. Distortion of the regular lattice of the stromal architecture produces a vacuolated appearance, and this may produce subepithelial haze by scattering of incident light. In addition, newly formed collagen fibrils and extracellular matrix may well have differing refractive indices compared to the normal cornea where the refractive indices of these components are similar. In rabbits, abnormally large proteoglycans are present in newly deposited stromal matrix, and may persist for up to 45 weeks,[80] whereas Hanna reported that in monkeys, extracellular matrix disruption was greatest at 3 months, with marked vacuolation, but a more regular structure was observed by 6 months.[79] Normal ultrastructure was not seen in the epithelial

substroma for up to 15 months. With the passage of time, the composition of stroma gradually returns to more normal proteoglycan levels, similar to that found in undisturbed cornea,[109] although type III collagen levels remain elevated even at 18 months in monkeys.[79]

Stromal remodelling is thought to be controlled, in part at least, by various matrix metalloproteinases, e.g. collagenase, stromelysin, and gelatinase.[111] Removal of damaged collagen fibres is controlled by the activity of PMN cells and the proteolytic enzymes they contain.

A relationship between increasing depth of ablation and the level of subepithelial haze and fibrosis exists after excimer laser treatment (Chapter 23). This often persists for months or even years in deeper ablations. Goodman and co-workers noted that all corneas ablated to no more than 50 µm in depth were clear on clinical examination at 8 weeks.[112]

Durrie has suggested a clinical classification of corneal wounding following PRK that categorizes three groups.[113] Type I healing, the most common, is characterized by subepithelial haze and fibrosis that normally is maximal at between 2 and 6 months postoperatively and then dissipates, with the refraction tending to stabilize at about 6 months. Type II healing is characterized by minimal fibrosis and regression, resulting in permanent hypermetropic overcorrection. Type III healing produces marked fibrosis and significant regression of refraction to pretreatment levels.

ENDOTHELIAL WOUND HEALING

Damage to the corneal endothelium following various types of trauma has been well documented.[114] Endothelial cells in humans and primates have minimal or no capacity to replicate by mitosis and therefore endothelial wound repair is largely achieved by endothelial cells enlarging and sliding over the stromal/Descemet's surface, or more usually over a fibronectin submatrix. The endothelium is responsible for the deposition of a new Descemet's membrane throughout the wound area. Under certain circumstances a tissue layer forms posterior to the newly formed Descemet's membrane that also contains fibroblast-like cells, collagen fibrils, basement membrane proteins and junctional complexes. These have been termed retrocorneal fibrous membranes (RCFM).[71]

The reports specifically addressing corneal endothelial status following PRK have concluded that there are no short- to medium-term effects.[114–116] In addition to the effects of radiant exposure however, the endothelium may theoretically be damaged by shock waves produced by the impact of each laser pulse on the cornea.[91] The stromal matrix changes induced by PRK might also be associated with, as yet unrecognized, long-term metabolic sequelae,[117] which over the years might conceivably affect the endothelium resulting in cell loss and morphological alterations.

AN INTRODUCTION TO GROWTH FACTORS AND OCULAR WOUND HEALING

Growth factors are a heterogenous group of proteins capable of stimulating growth and multiplication of cells. There is mounting evidence that peptide growth factors have an important role by regulating many of the processes involved in normal corneal wound healing, including migration, mitosis, and differentiation of cells.

The eye is a target tissue for peptide growth factors from all of the major families of growth factors.[118–121] These include: epidermal growth factor (EGF);[122] fibroblast growth factor (FGF); platelet-derived growth factors (PDGF), insulin-like growth factors (IGF) and transforming growth factor beta (TGF β). Transforming growth factor beta is a potent inducer of lysyl oxidase mRNA levels of cultured scleral fibroblasts and these play a major role in the synthesis of corneal extracellular matrix components after injury.[120]

Epidermal growth factor is one of the most biologically potent growth factors and the best characterized, although its precise physiologic activity and clinical efficacy is yet to be fully elucidated.[119] Although EGFs stimulate wound healing, the efficacy is dependent on the nature of the wound sustained, e.g. as chemical, thermal or traumatic.[120] Epithelial wound healing rates in animal models have been reported to accelerate by as much as 25–45% in the presence of EGFs,[118,119,123–127] although the effect of EGFs in humans is less well documented.[128] EGFs are normally present in tear fluid whereas attempts to identify EGF in the anterior chamber have been relatively unsuccessful.[129]

Transforming growth factor alpha (TGFα) is also found in human tear fluid and also originates from the lacrimal gland.[131] This is another polypeptide hormone structurally very similar to EGF. These two main growth factors probably control spontaneous corneal wound healing by several pathways (Fig. 4.15) including an exocrine response produced by growth factors acting directly on epithelial cells; an autocrine pathway, where epithelial cells produce growth factors that act upon themselves, an example of a growth factor thought to act in this way is TGF; and a paracrine pathway that enables epithelial cells synthesizing growth factors to influence neighbouring cells (e.g. TGFα).[117]

Healing of stromal injuries is similar to epithelial injuries, with the major difference being the extensive production by stromal fibroblasts (activated keratocytes) of extracellular matrix components such as collagen.[120] Studies of dermal incision healing in skin have shown that TGF-β may be the factor most responsible for increased synthesis of collagen and therefore increased strength of stromal wounds.[132,133] Fibroblast growth factor and IGF are present, particularly in the stroma. Both FGF and EGF stimulate the proliferation of corneal epithelium, keratocytes and endothelium. As EGF is the more potent growth factor, however, it has superior properties in increasing tensile strength of corneal stromal wounds and even has a greater effect on endothelium than FGF. Insulin-like growth factor stimulates in particular the growth of keratocytes and enhances the effect of EGF on endothelial cells. Mesodermal growth factor (MGF) stimulates the proliferation of keratocytes and increases the healing rates of endothelial cells.[119,123]

Although growth factors are rapidly emerging as an exciting new generation of ophthalmic pharmaceuticals that will increasingly play a major role in wound healing management, none of these factors has presently gained an established role in clinical practice.

REFERENCES

1. Ozanics V, Jakobiec FA, Prenatal development of the eye and its adnexa. In: Jakobiec FA, ed, *Ocular Anatomy, Embryology and Teratology* (Harper and Row: Philadelphia, 1982) 97–119.

2. Noden D, Periocular mesenchyme: neural crest and mesoderm interactions. In: Jakobiec FA, ed, *Ocular Anatomy, Embryology and Teratology* (Harper and Row: Philadelphia, 1982) 97.

3. Mann I, The development of the human eye, 3rd edn. (Grune and Stratton: New York, 1964).

4. O'Rahilly R, The prenatal development of the human eye, *Exp Eye Res* (1966) **21**:93–112.

5. Hay ED, Development of the vertebrate cornea, *Int Rev Cyt* (1980) **63**:263–322.

6. Forrester JV, Dick AD, McMenamin PG, Lee WR, *The Eye: Basic Sciences in Practice*. (WB Saunders: London, 1996), 14–18, 101–2, 158–67.

7. Davson H, *Physiology of the Eye*, 5th edn (Pergamon Press: New York, 1990)

8. Rodrigues MM, Waring GO, Hackett J, Donohoo P, Cornea. In: Jakobiec FA, ed, *Ocular Anatomy, Embryology and Teratology* (Harper and Row: Philadelphia, 1982) 153–65.

9. Lauweryns B, van der Oord JJ, Valpes R, Foets B, Missoten L, Distribution of very late activation integrins in the human cornea, *Invest Ophthalmol Vis Sci* (1991) **32**:2079–85.

10. Van Buskirk EM, The Anatomy of the Limbus, *Eye* (1989) **3**:101–8.

11. Scott JE, Proteoglycan: collagen interaction and corneal ultrastructure, *Biochem Soc Trans* (1991) **19**:887–81.

12. Waring GO, Bourne WM, Edelhauser HF, et al, The corneal endothelium – normal and pathologic structure and function, *Ophthalmology* (1982) **89**:531–90.

13. Tervo K, Latval TM, Recovery of corneal innervation following photorefractive keratoablation, *Arch Ophthalmol* (1994) **112**(11):1466–70.

14. Vrabec MP, Anderson JA, Rock ME, et al, Electron microscopic findings in a cornea with recurrence of herpes simplex keratitis after excimer laser phototherapeutic keratectomy, *CLAO Journal* (1994) **20**(1):41–44.

15. Maurice DM, The structure and transparency of the cornea, *J Physiol* (1957) **136**:263–86.

16. Maurice DM, Physical properties of the cornea. In: Duke Elder S, eds, System of Ophthalmology, Vol IV. *The physiology of the eye and of vision* (Henry Kimpton: London, 1968) 343–7.

17. Klyce SD, Beuerman RW, Structure and Function of the Cornea. In: Kaufman HE, Barron BA, McDonald MB, Waltman SR, eds, *The cornea* (Churchill Livingstone: New York, 1988) 3–54.

18. Goldman JN, Benedek GB, The relationship between morphology and transparency in the non-swelling corneal stroma of the shark, *Invest Ophthalmol Vis Sci* (1967) **6**:574.

19. Goldman JN, Benedek GB, Dohlman CH, et al, Structural alteration affecting transparency in swollen human cornea, *Invest Ophthalmol Vis Sci* (1968) **7**:501.

20. Farrell RA, McCally RL, Tatham PER, Wavelength dependencies of light scattering in normal and cold swollen rabbit corneas and their structural implications, *J Physiol* (1973) **233**:589.

21. Borcherding MS, Blacik LJ, Sitting RA, et al, Proteoglycans and collagen fibre organization in human corneoscleral tissue, *Exp Eye Res* (1975) **21**:59.

22. Jain S, Azar DT, Extracellular matrix and growth factors in corneal wound healing, *Curr Opin Ophthalmol* (1994) **5**(IV):3–12.

23. Cornuet PK, Blochberger TC, Hassell JR, Molecular polymorphism of Lumican during corneal development, *Invest Ophthalmol Vis Sci* (1994) **35**:870–7.

24. Spencer WH, Cornea: Inherited Systemic metabolic diseases with corneal involvement. In: Spencer WH, ed, *Ophthalmic pathology, an atlas and textbook, 3rd edn* (WB Saunders: Philadelphia, 1985) 347–69.

25. Funderburgh JL, Chandler JW, Proteoglycan of rabbit corneas with non-perforating wounds, *Invest Ophthalmol Vis Sci* (1989) **30**:435–42.

26. Cintron, C, Covington HI, Kublin CL, Morphological analysis of proteoglycans in rabbit corneal scars, *Invest Ophthalmol Vis Sci* (1990) **31**:1789–98.

27. Cintron C, Gregory JD, Damle SP, Kublin CL, Biochemical analysis of proteoglycans in rabbit corneal scars, *Invest Ophthalmol Vis Sci* (1990) **31**:1975–81.

28. Rawe IM, Tuft SJ, Meek KM, Proteoglycan and collagen morphology in superficially scarred rabbit cornea, *Histochem J* (1992) **24**:311–8.

29. Rawe IM, Zabel RW, Tuft SJ, Chjen V, Meek KM, A morphological study of rabbit corneas after laser keratectomy, *Eye* (1992) **6**:637–42.

30. Rawe IM, Meek KM, Leonard DW, Takahashi T, Cintron C, Structure of corneal scar tissue: An X-ray diffraction study, *Biophysical J* (1994) **67**:1743–8.

31. Marshall J, Trokel S, Rothery S, Krueger RR, Photoablative reprofiling of the cornea using the excimer laser: photorefractive keratectomy, *Lasers Ophthalmol* (1986) **1**:21–48.

32. Seiler T, Kreigerowski M, Schnoy N, Bende T, Ablation rate of human corneal epithelium and Bowman's layer with the excimer laser (193), *Refract Corneal Surg* (1990) **6**(2):99–102.

33. Seiler T, Wollensak J, Myopic photorefractive keratectomy with the excimer laser: one year follow up, *Ophthalmology* (1991) **98**:1156–63.

34. Marshall J, Trokel S, Rothery S, et al, An ultrastructural study of corneal incisions induced by the excimer laser at 193 nm, *Ophthalmology* (1985) **92**:749–58.

35. Ohashi Y, Motokura K, Kinoshita Y, et al, Presence of epidermal growth factor in human tears, *Invest Ophthalmol Vis Sci* (1989) **30**:1879–82.

36. Pfister RR, Clinical measures to promote corneal epithelial healing, *Acta Ophthalmologica* (1992) **70**(suppl 202):73–83.

37. Campos M, Hertzog L, Wang XW, et al, Corneal surface de-epithelialization using a sharp and a dull instrument, *Ophthalmic Surg* (1992) **23**(9):618–21.

38. Campos M, Lee M, McDonald PJ, Keratocyte loss after different methods of de-epithelialisation, *Ophthalmology* (1994) **105**(5):890–94.

39. Taylor DM, L'Esperance FA, Del Pero RA, et al, Human excimer laser lamellar keratectomy. A clinical study, *Ophthalmology* (1989) **96**:654–65.

40. Dua HS, Gomes JAP, Singh A, Corneal epithelial wound healing: perspective. *Br J Ophthalmol* (1994) **78**:401–8.

41. Crosson CE, Cellular changes following epithelial abrasion. In: Beuerman RW et al, *Healing processes in the cornea*, (Gulf Publishing: London, 1989) 3–15.

42. Lee RE, Davison PF, Cintron C, The healing of non linear non perforating wounds in rabbit corneas of different ages, *Invest Ophthalmol Vis Sci* (1982) **23**:660–5.

43. Robb RM, Kuwabara T, Corneal wound healing. The movement of polymorphonuclear leukocytes into corneal wounds, *Arch Ophthalmol* (1962) **68**:636–42.

44. Crosson CE, Klyce SD, Beuerman RW, Epithelial wound closure in the rabbit cornea: a biphasic process, *Invest Ophthalmol Vis Sci* (1986) **27**:464–73.

45. Pfister RR, The healing of corneal epithelial abrasions in the rabbit: a scanning electron microscope study, *Invest Ophthalmol Vis Sci* (1975) **14**:648–61.

46. Buck RC, Cell migration and repair of corneal epithelium, *Invest Ophthalmol Vis Sci* (1979) **18**:767–84.

47. Kuwabara T, Perkins DS, Coggan DG, Sliding of the epithelium in experimental corneal wounds, *Invest Ophthalmol* (1976) **15**:4–14.

48. Brewitt H, Sliding of epithelium in experimental corneal wounds: a scanning electron microscope study, *Acta Ophthalmol* (1979) **57**:945–48.

49. Haik BC, Zimmy ML, Scanning electron microscopy of corneal wound healing in the rabbit, *Invest Ophthalmol Vis Sci* (1977) **16**:787–96.

50. Gipson IK, Anderson RR, Actin filaments in normal and migrating corneal epithelial cells, *Invest Ophthalmol Vis Sci* (1977) **16**:161–6.

51. Takahashi M, Toyoshi F, Honda Y, Ogawa K, Distributional change of fodrin in the wound healing process of corneal epithelium, *Invest Ophthalmol Vis Sci* (1992) **33**(2):280–85.

52. Soong HK, Vinculin in focal cell to substrate attachments of spreading corneal epithelial cells, *Arch Ophthalmol* (1987) **105**:1129–32.

53. Gipson IK, Kiorpes TC, Epithelial sheet movement: protein and glycogen synthesis, *Dev Cell Biol* (1982) **92**:259–62.

54. Soong HK, Cintron C, Disparate effects of calmodulin inhibitors on corneal epithelial migration in rabbit and rat, *Ophthalmic Res* (1985) **17**:27–33.

55. Gipson IK, Watanabe H, Zieske J, Corneal wound healing and fibronectin: review, *Int Ophthalmol Clin* (1993) **3**(4):149–63.

56. Nishida T, Nakagawa A, Fibronectin promotes epithelial migration of cultured rabbit cornea in situ, *J Cell Biol* (1983) **97**:1653–57.

57. Fujikawa LS, Foster CS, Harris TJ, et al, Fibronectin in healing rabbit wounds, *Lab Invest* (1981) **45**:120–29.

58. Suda T, Nishida T, Ohashi Y, et al, Fibronectin appears at the site of corneal stromal wounds in rabbits, *Curr Eye Res* (1981) **1**:553–56.

59. Murakami J, Nishida T, Otori T, Coordinated appearance of β_1 integrins and fibronectin during corneal wound healing, *J Lab Clin Med* (1992) **120**(1):86–93.

60. Paallysaho T, Williams DS, Epithelial cell substrate adhesion in the cornea. Localisation of actin, talin, integrin and fibronectin, *Exp Eye Res* (1991) **52**:261–67.

61. Fujikawa LS, Foster CS, Gipson IK, et al, Basement membrane components in healing rabbit epithelial wounds: Immunofluorescence and ultrastructural studies, *J Cell Biol* (1984) **98**:128–38.

62. Paallysaho T, Tervo T, Virtanen I, Tervo K, Integrins in normal and healing corneal epithelium, *Acta Ophthalmologica (suppl)* (1992) **202**:22–25.

63. Berman M, The pathogenesis of corneal epithelial defects. In: Beuerman RE, et al, *Healing processes in the cornea*, (Gulf publishing: London, 1989), 15–26.

64. Vaheri A, Bizik J, Salonen EM, et al, Regulation of the pericellular activation of plasminogen and its role in tissue-destructive process, *Acta Ophthalmologica* (1992) **70**:34–41.

65. Gipson IK, Spurr-Michaud SJ, Tisdale AS, Anchoring fibrils form a complex network in human and rabbit cornea, *Invest Ophthalmol Vis Sci* (1987) **28**:212–20.

66. Gipson IK, Spurr-Michaud SJ, Tisdale AS, et al, Hemidesmosomes and anchoring fibril collagen appear synchronously during development and wound healing, *Dev Biol* (1988) **126**:253–62.

67. Rouselle P, Lunstrum GP, Keene DR, et al, Kalinin: An epithelial-specific basement membrane adhesion molecule that is a component of anchoring filaments, *J Cell Biol* (1991) **114**(3):567–76.

68. Gipson IK, Adhesive mechanism of the corneal epithelium, *Acta Ophtlamologica* (1992) **70**:13–17.

69. Sunder Rai N, Geiss MJ, Fantes F, et al, Healing of excimer laser ablated monkey corneas: an immunohisto-chemical evaluation, *Arch Ophthalmol* (1990) **108**:1604–11.

70. Malley DS, Steinert RF, Carmen A, et al, Immunofluorescence study of corneal wound healing after excimer anterior keratectomy in the monkey eye. *Arch Ophthalmol* (1990) **108**:1316–22.

71. Assil KK, Quantock AJ, Wound healing in response to keratorefractive surgery, *Surv Ophthalmol* (1993) **38**(3):289–302.

72. Tuft SJ, Gartry DS, Rowe IM, Meek KM, Photorefractive keratectomy: implications of corneal wound healing, *Br J Ophthalmol* (1993) **77**:243–47.

73. Stock EL, Kurpakus MA, Sambol N, Jones JC, Adhesion complex formation after small keratectomy wounds in the cornea, *Invest Ophthalmol Vis Sci* (1992) **33**(2):304–13.

74. Khoudahoust AA, Silverstein AM, Kenyon KR, Dowling JE, Adhesion of regenerating corneal epithelium, *Am J Ophthalmol* (1968) **65**:339–48.

75. Gipson IK, Spurr-Michaud SJ, Tisdale AS, Hemidesmosomes and anchoring fibril collagen appear synchronously during development and wound healing, *Dev Biol* (1988) **126**:235–262.

76. Gipson IK, Spurr-Michaud SJ, Tisdale AS, Keough M, Reassembly of anchoring structures of the corneal epithelium during wound repair in the rabbit, *Invest Ophthalmol Vis Sci* (1989) **30**:425–34.

77. Fountain TR, de la Cruz Z, Green WR, et al, Reassembly of corneal epithelial adhesion structures after excimer laser keratectomy in humans, *Arch Ophthalmol* (1994) **112**(7):967–72.

78. Gipson IK, Spurr-Michaud S, Tisdale A, Reassembly of the anchoring structures of the corneal epithelium during wound repair in the rabbit, *Invest Ophthalmol Vis Sci* (1989) **30**:425–34.

79. Hanna KD, Pouliquen YM, Salvodelli M, Fantes F, et al, Corneal wound healing in monkeys 18 months after excimer laser photorefractive keratectomy, *Refract Corneal Surg* (1990) **6**:340–45.

80. Hanna KD, Pouliquen Y, Waring GO, et al, Corneal stromal wound healing in rabbits after 193 nm excimer laser surface ablation, *Arch Ophthalmol* (1989) **107**(6):895–01.

81. Buck RC, Cell migration in repair of mouse corneal epithelium, *Invest Ophthalmol Vis Sci* (1979) **18**:767–84.

82. Buck RC, Measurement of centripetal migration of normal corneal epithelial cells in the mouse, *Invest Ophthalmol Vis Sci* (1985) **26**:1296–99.

83. Dua HS, Forrester JV, Clinical patterns of corneal epithelial wound healing, *Am J Ophthalmol* (1987) **104**:481–89.

84. Lemp MA, Mathers WD, Corneal epithelial cell movement in humans, *Eye* (1989) **3**:438–45.

85. Dua HS, Watson NJ, Mather RM, Forrester JV, Corneal epithelial cell migration in humans: hurricane and blizzard keratopathy, *Eye* (1993) **7**:53–58.

86. Hanna C, O'Brien JE, Cell production and migration in the epithelial layer of the cornea, *Arch Ophthalmol* (1960) **64**:536–39.

87. Matsuda M, Ubels JL, Edelhauser HF, A larger corneal epithelial wound closes at a faster rate, *Invest Ophthalmol Vis Sci* (1985) **26**:897–00.

88. Tseng SCG, Concept and application of limbal stem cells, *Eye* (1989) **3**:141–47.

89. Schermer A, Galvin S, Sun TT, Differentiation-related expression of a major 64K corneal keratin in vivo and in culture suggests limbal location of corneal epithelial cells, *J Cell Biol* (1986) **103**:49–62.

90. Del Pero R, Gigstad JE, Roberts A, et al, A refractive and histopathologic study of excimer laser keratectomy in primates, *Am J Ophthalmol* (1990) **109**:419–29.

91. Marshall J, Trokel S, Rothery S, Krueger RR, Long term healing of the central cornea after photorefractive keratectomy using an excimer laser, *Ophthalmology* (1988) **95**:1411–16.

92. Fantes FE, Hanna KD, Waring GO, et al, Wound healing after excimer laser keratomileusis (photorefractive keratectomy) in monkeys, *Arch Ophthalmol* (1990) **108**:665–70.

93. Wu WC, Stark WJ, Green WR, Corneal wound healing after 193 nm excimer laser keratectomy, *Arch Ophthalmol* (1991) **109**(10):1426–32.

94. Hanna KD, Pouliquen YM, Waring GO, et al, Corneal wound healing in monkey eyes after repeated excimer laser photorefractive keratectomy, *Arch Ophthalmol* (1992) **110**(9):1286–91.

95. Sheih E, Moreira H, D'Arcy J, Clapham TM, McDonnell PJ, Quantitative analysis of wound healing after cylindrical and spherical excimer laser ablations, *Ophthalmology* (1992) **99**:1050–55.

96. Trabbuchi G, Brancato R, Verdi M, et al, Corneal nerve regeneration after excimer laser photorefractive keratectomy in rabbit eyes, *Invest Ophthalmol Vis Sci* (1994) **35**(1):229–35.

97. Terro E, Recovery of innervation and abnormal nerve structures, *Arch Ophthalmol* (1994) **112**:1466–69.

98. Ishikawa T, del Cerro M, Liang FQ, et al, Hypersensitivity following excimer laser ablation through the corneal epithelium, *Refract Corneal Surg* (1992) **8**(6):466–74.

99. Woost PG, Brightwell J, Eiferman RA, Schulz GS, Effect of growth factors with dexamethasone on healing of rabbit corneal stromal incisions, *Exp Eye Res* (1985) **40**:47–60.

100. Wilson SE, Lloyd SA, He YG, EFG, basic FGF and FGF beta 1 messenger RNA production by rabbit corneal epithelial cells, *Invest Ophthalmol Vis Sci* (1992) **33**:1987–95.

101. Matsuda H, Smelser GK, Electron microscopy of corneal wound healing, *Exp Eye Res* (1973) **16**:427–31.

102. Marshall GE, Kontas AG, Lee WR, Immunogold fine structural localisation of extracellular matrix components in ageing human cornea, Types I–IV collagen and laminin. *Graefes Arch Clin Exp Ophthalmol* (1991) **229**:157–63.

103. Benezra D, Foidart JM, Collagens and non-collagenous proteins in the human eye. Corneal stromal in vivo and keratocyte production in vitro. *Curr Eye Res* (1981) **1**:101–10.

104. Assil KK, Quantock AJ, Wound healing response to keratorefractive surgery, *Surv Ophthalmol* (1993) **38**(3):289–02.

105. Kratz-Owens KL, Hageman GS, Schanzlin DJ, An in vitro technique for monitoring keratocyte migration following lamellar keratoplasty, *Refract Corneal Surg* (1992) **8**:230–34.

106. Pedroza L, Beuerman RW, Klyce SD, Crosson CE, Keratocyte degradation following epithelial abrasion, *Invest Ophthalmol Vis Sci* (1986) **27**:31–6.

107. Nakayasu K, Stromal changes following removal of epithelium in rat cornea, *Jpn J Ophthalmol* (1988) **32**:383–07.

108. Marshall GE, Kontas AG, Lee WR, Immunogold fine structural localisation of extracellular matrix components in ageing human cornea. Collagen types V and VI, *Graefes Arch Clin Exp Ophthalmol* (1991) **229**:164–71.

109. Cintron C, Covington HI, Kublin CL, Morphologic analysis of proteoglycans in rabbit corneal scars, *Invest Ophthalmol Vis Sci* (1990) **31**:1791–98.

110. Hassell JR, Cintron C, Kublin C, Newsome DA, Proteoglycan changes during restoration of transparency in corneal scars, *Arch Biochem Phys* (1983) **222**:362–69.

111. Fini ME, Girad MT, Expression of collagenolytic/gelatinolytic metalloproteinases by normal cornea, *Invest Ophthalmol Vis Sci* (1990) **31**:1779–88.

112. Goodman GL, Trokel SL, Stark WJ, et al, Corneal healing following laser refractive keratectomy, *Arch Ophthalmol* (1989) **107**(12):1799–03.

113. Durrie DS, Cavanaugh TB, Vrabec M, Corneal topography with excimer laser photorefractive keratectomy. In: Sanders DR, Koch C, eds, *An atlas of corneal topography* (SLACK Inc; Thorofare NJ, 1993) 125–50.

114. Carones F, Brancato R, Venturi E, Morico A, The corneal endothelium after myopic laser photorefractive keratectomy, *Arch Ophthalmol* (1994) **112**(7):920–24.

115. Perez-Santoja JJ, Meza J, Moreno E, et al, Short term endothelium changes after photorefractive keratectomy, *J Refract Corneal Surg* (1994) **10**(2):194–98.

116. Amano S, Shimizu K, Corneal endothelial changes after excimer laser photorefractive keratectomy, *Am J Ophthalmol* (1993) **116**(6):692–94.

117. Scultz G, Chegini N, Grant M, et al, Effects of growth factors on corneal wound healing, *Acta Ophthalmologica* (1992) **70**:60–66.

118. Schultz G, Khaw PT, Oxford K, et al, Growth factors and ocular wounding, *Eye* (1994) **8**:184–187.

119. Tripathi BJ, Kwait PS, Tripathi RC, Corneal growth factors: a new generation of ophthalmic pharmaceuticals, *Cornea* (1990) **9**(1):2–9.

120. Bennet NT, Schultz GS, Growth factors and wound healing. I Biochemical properties of growth factors and their receptors, *Am J Surg* (1993) **165**:728–37.

121. Bennett NT, Schultz GS, Growth factors and wound healing. II Role in normal and chronic wound healing, *Am J Surg* (1993) **166**:74–81.

122. Cohen S, Isolation of a mouse submaxillary gland protein accelerating incisor eruption and eyelid opening in the new born animals, *J Biol Chem* (1962) **237**:1555–60.

123. Petroutsos G, Courty C, Guimares G, et al, Comparison of the effects of EGF, pFGF and EDGF on corneal epithelium wound healing, *Curr Eye Res* (1984) **3**:593–98.

124. Brightwell JR, Riddle SL, Eiferman RA, et al, Biosynthetic human EFG accelerates healing of neodecadraon-treated primate corneas, *Invest Ophthalmol Vis Sci* (1985) **26**:105–10.

125. Kitizawa T, Kinoshita S, Fujita K, et al, The mechanism of accelerated corneal epithelial healing by human epithelial growth factor, *Invest Ophthalmol Vis Sci* (1990) **31**:1773–78.

126. Pastor JC, Calonge M, Epidermal growth factor and corneal wound healing. A multicentre study, *Cornea* (1992) **11**(4):311–14.

127. Brazzell RK, Stern ME, Aquavella JV, Beuerman RW, et al, Human recombinant epidermal growth factor in experimental corneal wound healing, *Invest Ophthalmol Vis Sci* (1991) **32**(2):336–40.

128. Daniele S, Frati L, Fiore C, Santon G, The effect of the epidermal growth factor (EGF) on the corneal epithelium in humans, *Albrecht Von Graefes Arch Klin Exp Ophthalmol* (1979) **210**(3):159–65.

129. Rotatori DS, Kerr NC, Rapheal B, et al, Elevation of TGFα in aqueous humour of cats after endothelial injury, *Invest Ophthalmol Vis Sci* (1993) **35**:143–49.

130. Van Setten, Tervo T, Tervo K, Tarkkanen A, Epidermal growth factor (EGF) in ocular fluids: presence, origin and therapeutic considerations, *Acta Ophthalmologica* (1992) **70**:54–59.

131. Van Setten GB, Macauley S, Schultz GS, TGFα: presence in human tear fluid and in the lacrimal gland tissue, *Invest Ophthalmol Vis Sci* (1993) **34**:822–26.

132. Ishiwaka O, Yamakage A, LeRoy EC, Trojanowska M, Persistent effect of TGFβ1 on extracellular matrix gene expression in human dermal fibroblasts, *Biochem Biophys Res Commun* (1990) **169**:232–238.

133. Oxford KW, Balch KC, Schultz GS, et al, Effects of TGF-β on the re-epithelialisation and tensile strength of corneal wounds, *Invest Ophthalmol Vis Sci* (1993) **34**:1375–81.

Chapter 5 The natural history of myopia

Wallace S Foulds

INTRODUCTION

Myopia has been recognized since the time of the ancient Greeks, whose language gave rise to the term. Galen (quoted by Hirschberg[1]) defined myopia as a condition in which near objects are clearly defined but not distant ones. This definition, which takes no account of accommodation, is clearly inadequate and even today the definition of myopia remains somewhat controversial.[2] Usefully, myopia can be defined by its optical characteristics as a condition in which, with accommodation relaxed, the image of a distant object is focused in front of the retina (or more accurately the photoreceptor layer of the retina).

Myopia of even low degree has a significant deleterious effect on visual acuity and in the modern world, where many tasks are visually demanding, myopia can be economically disadvantageous. Additionally, a proportion of those with myopia, especially those with high myopia, suffer significant visual loss or even blindness from the degenerative changes that commonly accompany myopia. Thus, myopes are at risk of developing retinal detachment and may lose central vision from choroidoretinal atrophy. Myopes are prone to develop cataract and to suffer visual loss if the myopia is complicated by open-angle glaucoma.

The prevalence of myopia varies from one ethnic group to another and alters markedly throughout life. Thus, at birth there is a wide scatter of refractive errors from hypermetropia to myopia but during early childhood, as a result of the process of emmetropization, both hypermetropic and myopic errors reduce in severity and prevalence so that refractions tend to cluster around emmetropia. In late childhood, and especially around the time of puberty, an increasing minority of children becomes myopic but in most cases this myopia stabilizes by early adult life. Some young adults, however, develop myopia *de novo* in their early twenties and, in some, myopia continues to progress throughout adult life.

Historically there have been many theories to explain the causes of myopia and these have been in terms of either 'nature' or 'nurture'. In the 19th century it was commonly believed that myopia was the result of misuse of the eyes; accordingly it was thought myopia could be prevented or ameliorated by a suitable adjustment of the visual environment or the way in which the eyes were used.

In the early 20th century it became accepted that myopia was entirely the result of a genetic predisposition and largely brought about by a mismatch between the various optical components contributing to total refraction. Accordingly it was accepted that no therapeutic intervention would be of any benefit.

More recently, as a result of animal and human studies, it has become clear that modification of the visual environment in early life can have a significant effect on the process of emmetropization and in some circumstances lead to the development of ametropia, and myopia in particular. Visually induced changes in ocular refraction appear to reflect visually induced alterations in ocular biochemistry but whether these experimental models are of relevance to naturally occurring human myopia remains open to question. In the animal there appears to be a short critical neonatal period during which visual input can have a profound effect on ocular growth and refraction. In the human, plasticity of ocular growth may last longer than in some experimental animals and the quality of visual input in childhood may be of relevance to the normal growth of the eye and the achievement of emmetropia.

An interesting suggestion, for which there is some support, is that spectacle correction of myopia in early life might itself induce a worsening of the myopia that the spectacles were designed to correct.

In the belief that myopia might be the result of excessive accommodation during childhood, many attempts have been made to slow the rate of progression of myopia by the avoidance of near visual tasks, the use of bifocal glasses or the local administration of atropine in the eyes. The effects have been marginal, making a putative role for accommodation in the genesis of myopia somewhat doubtful. It does, however, appear that atropine and other muscarinic agents may have a direct effect on scleral growth. The potential efficacy of these agents in the control of myopia, and particularly the use of more specifically acting muscarinic antagonists with fewer side effects than atropine, is an area of interest that is currently being assessed in relation to the possible medical control of myopia.

Although the optics of the myopic eye can be made more emmetropic by the use of various surgical procedures, the natural history of the underlying myopia, especially in relation to accompanying degenerative changes in the choroid and retina, remains unaffected.

CLASSIFICATION OF MYOPIA

There are many classifications of myopia and their indiscriminate and often overlapping use has led to considerable confusion in the literature. Thus, myopia has been variously classified on the basis of its apparent underlying mechanism (axial, index, curvature, etc), by its severity (low, medium, high), by its associated clinical correlates (simple, degenerative, malignant), by its time of onset (congenital, juvenile, early adult, late adult, etc) or by terms that suggest a possible etiology (developmental, school myopia, etc).

A way out of the difficulty is to categorize the myopia purely in terms of the refractive error in diopters (D). When there is better understanding of the nature and etiology of myopia then will be the time to develop an appropriate classification.

Currently, there is some consensus that any myopia over 6 D should be regarded as high myopia.[1,3–5] The accuracy with which the refraction is determined, however, obviously depends on the sensitivity and specificity of the methodology used. In the case of emmetropia where theoretically there is no refractive error, an event that must be excessively rare, determination of refraction to an accuracy of ±0.5 D will give a very different prevalence to that obtained using a method with an error of ±1.0 D. In practical terms, emmetropia is often regarded as an error lying

within the range +1.0 D to −1.0 D and, in the adult population some 75% of subjects have refractions within this range.[6]

Most eyes demonstrate some degree of astigmatism and this complicates the statistical handling of refractive errors. In analysing prevalences or progression of myopia, devices such as the spherical equivalent, or the refraction in one chosen meridian have been used as a way out of the difficulty.

NATURE OF MYOPIA

The total refraction depends upon the individual contributions made by the various optical components of the eye in terms of their optical power and disposition (curvatures of corneal and lens surfaces, refractive indices of cornea, aqueous, lens and vitreous, axial length of the eye and, more particularly, the depth of the anterior chamber, the thickness of the lens and the length of the vitreous cavity).

The contributions of each component have been incorporated in various 'model' eyes, the most widely accepted being Gullstrand's 'exact' schematic eye[7] (Fig. 5.1). More recent modifications have sought to

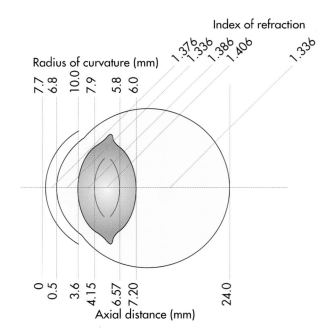

Figure 5.1 *Diagram to illustrate Gullstrand's exact schematic eye adapted from Gullstrand (1924).*[7]

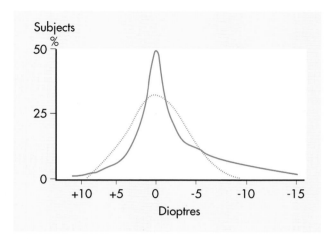
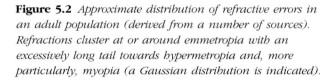

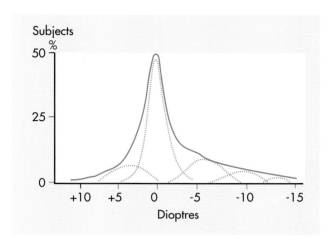

Figure 5.2 *Approximate distribution of refractive errors in an adult population (derived from a number of sources). Refractions cluster at or around emmetropia with an excessively long tail towards hypermetropia and, more particularly, myopia (a Gaussian distribution is indicated).*

Figure 5.3 *Possible explanation for the distribution of refractive errors in an adult population assuming that there is a series of overlapping ametropic populations.*

allow for optical aberrations[8] and changes brought about by accommodation.[9,10]

Refractive errors can be regarded as a chance mismatch among the many apparently independent variable components contributing to total refraction[11] but if refractive errors were entirely explicable on this basis one would expect them to have a normal Gaussian distribution. Among adults, however, the distribution of refractive errors is not Gaussian. There is an excess of refractions clustered at or around emmetropia so that the peak distribution is higher and narrower than in a normal distribution while, additionally, there is an excessively long tail towards hypermetropia and myopia, the distribution being significantly skewed towards myopia[12,13] (Fig. 5.2).

On the basis that there is a 'physiological' range of refractive errors around emmetropia, which is due to chance variation in the optical components contributing to total refraction and, additionally, a group of 'pathological' refractive errors representing high hypermetropia and, more particularly, high myopia, attempts have been made to uncover the basic physiological group by removing assumed pathological refractive errors from the distribution. Thus, removing refractive errors of over 6 D,[14] renders the remaining distribution more symmetrical, as does the elimination of myopes showing fundus abnormalities.[15,16] The remaining curve, however, still contains an

excess of emmetropes or near emmetropes and is still somewhat skewed towards myopia.

Attempts have also been made to explain the distribution of refractive errors by fitting a series of overlapping curves to the data,[17] based on the thought that there may be a large number of subgroups of myopia (and of hypermetropia) to explain the excessively long tails to the distribution curve (Fig. 5.3). The greater than expected number of refractions at or near emmetropia suggests that some control mechanism is acting to achieve emmetropization. Such a mechanism might operate by inducing a compensatory change in one or more components of refraction in response to the presence of an abnormality in another component and there is evidence that, far from being independent, the various optical compounds of the eye show a significant degree of interdependence.[16] Thus, changes in axial length of the eye tend to be compensated for by changes in corneal curvature and, to a lesser extent, by changes in lens power. Corneal power and lens power, however, appear to behave relatively independently. The effects of changes in the refractive indices of cornea or lens cortex appear to be much less than the calculated effects of such changes in the lens nucleus or the vitreous.[18]

The total refraction is, of course, greatly influenced by the anterior corneal curvature and the axial length of the eye or, more particularly, the axial length of the vitreous cavity.

The mechanisms underlying the process of emmetropization remain ill-understood but there is evidence that both environmental and genetic influences are important.

PREVALENCE OF MYOPIA

The calculated prevalence of myopia is obviously dependent on the definition of myopia adopted and is also influenced by the age composition and ethnicity of the sample investigated. Most studies have been restricted in terms of age group, source of subjects, and degree of myopia regarded as significant. As a result the true prevalence of myopia in various populations remains undetermined.

In Caucasians, a reasonable estimate for the prevalence of myopia of greater than 1 D, is 10–15% of the adult population[19] (8–14% with myopia of >1.00 D and 15–20% with myopia of >0.50 D). The prevalence among Chinese and Japanese appears greater,[20,21] and possibly as high as four times the rate in Caucasians.[22]

Apart from ethnicity, there is evidence that environmental factors may influence the prevalence of myopia. Thus, the prevalence of myopia among rural Chinese, is said to be similar to that in Caucasians, unlike that in urban Chinese of similar genetic origin, where the rate is much higher.[23]

In favor of an environmental influence is the accumulating evidence that the prevalence of myopia is increasing among populations where there has been a change in lifestyle, e.g., among the Inuit (Eskimo),[24–27] American Indians,[28,29] Kokar islanders in the Gulf of Finland,[30] and among Singaporean[31,32] and Taiwanese[33] school and university students. Apart from ethnicity and the possible influence of external environmental factors, the prevalence of myopia, and other refractive errors, alters significantly throughout life as the process of emmetropization gives way to maturation and, eventually, to age-related changes in refraction.

REFRACTION IN INFANCY AND CHILDHOOD

Early attempts to assess the refractive state of the newborn were rendered inaccurate from lack of cycloplegia and the use of the ophthalmoscope rather than the retinoscope as a measuring device. One early study[34] suggested that 78% of the newborn were myopic, a finding not supported by more recent studies using retinoscopy and cycloplegia.[35,36] It appears that at birth, refractions are distributed in a near normal fashion around a hypermetropic mean of some +2 D with a range of −6 D to +10 D. Some 20% of newborn infants are myopic.

Although the distribution of refractive errors among the newborn is symmetrical about the mean of +2 D, even at this early age the curve is more peaked around the mean than would be the case for a truly normal distribution,[19] suggesting that some control mechanism may already be operating at or before birth.

By the age of 6 years the scatter of refractions is greatly reduced by the virtual elimination of significant myopic errors and the higher degrees of hypermetropia so that the mean refraction is reduced from +2 D in the newborn to +1 D by the age of 6 years.[37] At this age the distribution is markedly peaked and the range of refractive errors runs from −1 D to +4 D, the distribution being somewhat skewed towards hypermetropia. Some 90% of refractions lie within 1 D of the mean, indicating that a significant degree of emmetropization has taken place during the first years of life. (Fig. 5.4).

Longitudinal studies[38,39] have confirmed that the dispersion of refractive errors is greatest shortly after birth and least at the age of 6 years. The spherical equivalent at 1 year appears to be a good predictor

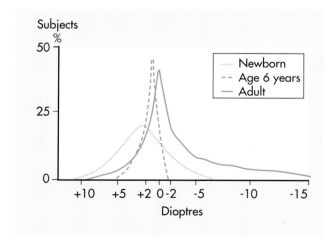

Figure 5.4 *The distribution of refractive errors at various ages (from various sources).*

of the refraction at a later age. Additionally, in the first 2 years of life there is a high prevalence of against-the-rule astigmatism, which declines and becomes with-the-rule by the age of 4 years.

For the majority of children, refraction remains stable from the age of 6 years onwards but an increasing proportion of children become myopic, particularly around puberty, so that the distribution of refractive errors, which was slightly skewed towards hypermetropia at the age of 6 becomes symmetrical by the age of 9 or 10 years and thereafter increasingly skewed towards myopia.[40] After puberty the adult pattern, with a marked skew towards myopia, is established.[16,19,41] There is some evidence for the existence of a very small group of children who have a high degree of myopia at birth but within this group there appears to be a very variable pattern in terms of severity and rate of progression.[42,43]

Apart from age differences in the prevalence of myopia there appear also to be sex differences. Many studies have confirmed that among schoolchildren myopia is significantly commoner among girls than boys.[44–46] It appears, however, that up to the age of 7 years and after the age of 15 years, there is little difference between the sexes with regard to the prevalence of myopia.[19] For both boys and girls a small proportion demonstrate a significant incidence or a worsening of myopia around the time of puberty and, as this occurs some 3 years earlier in girls than boys, it explains to a large extent the higher prevalence of myopia among schoolgirls as compared with schoolboys.

ADULT MYOPIA

For the majority of myopic adults the age range from 25 to 55 years is one of stability as regards the severity and prevalence of myopia. Most of those who are myopic in adult life develop their myopia during childhood, especially around the age of puberty, and the earlier in childhood the myopia appears the more severe is the refractive error in adult life.[47]

Childhood myopia tends to stabilize in the late teens and approximately a year earlier in girls than boys. Thus, myopia progression, which averages 0.5 D per year during childhood ceases in the majority by the age of 18 years in boys (mean 16.66 years ± 2.10), and 17 years in girls (mean 15.21 years ±1.74).[48] Cessation of myopia progression correlates well with cessation of bodily growth.[49]

There is, however, considerable variation in the behavior of myopic errors in early adult life. In the majority (87% of women and 68% of men) myopia stabilizes in early adult life.[50] In 25% of males and 13% of females, myopia continues to progress during adult years but at a slower rate than in childhood, while in a small number of males (6%) progression of myopia accelerates in early adult life.

Additionally, a small but significant number of emmetropic 17–18-year-olds develop myopia, usually of low degree, by the age of 22 or 23 years. Statistics supporting these data have usually been derived from studies of university students, military cadets, and so on[51] and an etiological role for intensive close work has been postulated.

In a meta-analysis of some 500 papers[52] it was concluded that some 20% of non-myopes entering an academic environment in the late teens developed significant myopia during the subsequent 4 years. In a study of airline pilots,[53] 24% became myopic after the age of 21 years and a similar finding was reported in a study of naval officers.[54]

The stability or otherwise of the refractive error in early adult life is of obvious concern to those undertaking refractive surgery and the mechanisms underlying young adult myopia are also important in this regard, but the data are conflicting. Thus, some studies[55,56] have suggested that young adult myopia is associated with a significant steepening of corneal curvature, while others[57,58] have concluded that this form of myopia is entirely explicable by increasing axial length of the eye.

Whatever the explanation, from the point of view of the refractive surgeon, the fact that some myopes continue to progress after the age of 21 years makes it important to identify in which subjects this is likely to occur. Currently, however, there appears to be no identifying feature that will predict which young adult myopes will progress other than serial measurements of refraction to try to establish when stability has been achieved.

One other aspect of adult myopia is of interest. High myopia of over 6 D is commoner among women than men, while for lower degrees of myopia men slightly outnumber women.[19]

REFRACTION AND AGEING

After the age of 60 years the distribution of refractive errors again changes, with a gradual decrease in the number of emmetropes and an increased prevalence of both hypermetropia and myopia,[59] the change being even more marked after the age of 70 years.[60] Most of the altered refraction is lenticular in origin, associated with an increased thickness, a lack of plasticity and an increase in refractive index of the lens. Thus, at birth, there is a wide spread of refractive errors from hypermetropia to myopia. By the age of 6 years the distribution of refractions is peaked around low hypermetropia with a slight skew towards hypermetropia. By the age of 9 years the distribution is symmetrical around near emmetropia but from this age until adulthood the distribution contains an increasing number of myopes so that the distribution is significantly skewed towards myopia.

During adult life, refractions mostly remain stable although progressive myopia does affect a small proportion. In old age, as with the newborn, the scatter of refractions again becomes wide and the number of emmetropes declines.

In childhood and young adulthood, myopia is mainly due to axial elongation of the globe but, while there may be some compensatory flattening of the corneal curvature in childhood, in adult-onset myopia steepening of the corneal curvature may be a significant contributor to the refractive error, which remains, however, mainly the result of axial elongation of the globe.

ETIOLOGY OF MYOPIA

From birth to adult age it has been remarked[61] that although the eye enlarges three-fold its components are so finely regulated that the image of a distant object continues to be in focus on the retina. Myopia can be considered as a failure of this regulatory process and genetic, humoral and environmental factors have been variously implicated in its pathogenesis.

In Victorian times it was taken for granted that myopia resulted from abuse of the eyes and, in particular, excessive close work in poor illumination. This view was based on extensive studies of refractive errors in schoolchildren in the mid-19th century[62,63] in which a correlation between the prevalence and severity of myopia and close work was first identified. As a result the Victorians set up 'sight-saving schools' in the hope of preventing or ameliorating myopia. These schools minimized close work and maximized illumination but eventually they were abandoned as ineffective. In the early 20th century an alternative theory was propounded, namely that refractive errors were primarily the result of a statistical mismatch in the optical components contributing to total refraction.[64]

Thus was set the main etiological arguments for the causation of myopia, i.e., that it was the result of adverse environmental factors or, alternatively, an in-built and presumably genetically determined mismatch in ocular optical components. The environmental theory allowed the possibility of therapeutic intervention, while the genetic theory maintained that refraction was, as it were, preordained and not amenable to intervention.

There is no doubt, that there is a strong association between myopia and formal education. Thus, 30% of Danish male conscripts educated to university entrance level showed myopia in excess of 1.5 D,[65] whereas only 3% of unskilled workers did so. Similar findings have been reported from the USA.[66] Moreover there is an association between near work and myopia.[67,68]

A major problem with the environmental theory is that most studies have interpreted correlations between myopia and environmental factors, such as close work, as indicative of causation, a well-recognized statistical fallacy. An equally plausible explanation of the correlation is that myopes find close work easier than do hypermetropes, so that the former tend to spend more time on reading and similar activities, while the latter might favor more outdoor activities.

As has already been indicated, however, there is persuasive evidence that the prevalence of myopia has increased significantly among populations where there has been a change from a rural to an urban lifestyle. A recent study[69] compared the severity of myopia in Jewish boys receiving a 'religious' education, involving up to 16 hours per day of demanding close work, with the prevalence and severity of myopia affecting boys (and girls) of similar genetic background undergoing a less rigorous form of education involving 4 hours of close work per day. Myopia was significantly more common and of greater severity in the boys undergoing 'religious' education, suggesting that prolonged close work was an etiological factor in their myopia.

As has already been noted, at birth the almost normal distribution of refractive errors around a low hypermetropic mean suggests that there is an in-built mechanism tending to match optical components and produce near emmetropia. The subsequent disappearance of all myopic errors and of most of the hypermetropic errors by the age of 6 years and the marked peaking of refractions in the neighborhood of emmetropia, indicate that refraction is not merely a chance distribution of optical components around emmetropia for, if that were the case, the distribution of refractive errors would remain Gaussian. The great excess of emmetropes from the age of 6 years onwards, and the compensatory changes that occur in some optical components in response to deviations in others, indicate an underlying control mechanism acting to achieve emmetropization. Whether myopia can be considered as a defect in this postulated control mechanism remains conjectural.

GENETIC INFLUENCES

If the process of emmetropization and the final refractive state were genetically determined one might expect a clear-cut pattern of inheritance but such a pattern is not readily discernible.

In terms of the optics of the eye, very small deviations from the mean can have significant effects on refraction, a 1 mm change in axial length, for example, inducing an error of 3 D.[70] The genetic contribution to such small differences is difficult to study.[71] Myopic parents have an increased chance of having myopic offspring. Thus, in one study 10–11% of children were myopic when neither parent was myopic, the incidence rising to 16–25% when one parent was myopic, and to 33–46% when both parents were myopic.[72]

These values, however, do not support a single gene inheritance although such a mode of inheritance may underlie a proportion of high ametropic errors.[73]

Offspring–parent and sibling–sibling (sib–sib) resemblances in refractive error favor a polygenic mode of inheritance but a meta-analysis of published data[73] suggests that such a mode of inheritance, coupled with random variations in environment, would only account for half the observed ametropia. Sib–sib resemblances in refraction tend to be stronger than offspring–parent resemblances and this might be due either to siblings sharing a similar environment or, possibly, some genetic alleles influencing refraction being recessive while others are dominant.

Monozygous twins are more likely to have similar refractions than dizygous twins.[74–76] Twins, however, are exposed to similar environmental influences and monozygous twins, for example, may have more similar reading habits than dizygous twins.[73]

Offspring–parent resemblances in ocular axial length have been studied[77] and found to be marked where parents had axial lengths in the emmetropic range but not where one or other parent had an increased axial length. This suggests that genetic control of emmetropization is tight but that ametropia associated with increased ocular axial length may be the result of other than genetic factors.

Thus, a few types of high myopia and myopia associated with systemic abnormalities may be inherited as a single gene trait. Low degrees of ametropia due to variation in the optical components underlying refraction may be inherited as polygenic traits, while for higher degrees of ametropia a combined effect of polygenic inheritance and environmental influences appears best to fit the available data.

ANIMAL STUDIES

Modification of the visual input in early life can have a profound effect on ocular growth and refraction. Although there appear to be in-built, and presumably genetically driven, mechanisms that guide the developing eye towards approximate emmetropia, animal studies (and clinical observation) suggest that regulation of ocular growth during childhood is a visually dependent phenomenon.

The observation that young primates[78] or cats[79] reared in conditions only allowing near vision, tend to become myopic, is an experimental demonstration that the quality of visual input in early life is an important factor in determining the refraction of the eye during postnatal development.

As already indicated refraction tends to remain fairly constant during ocular growth, the natural increase in ocular axial length being compensated for by a relative flattening of the cornea and by compensatory changes in other optical components of the eye.

Where a refractive error develops, it correlates well with the axial length of the eye,[80] suggesting that refractive errors result from a failure of ocular growth regulation. In animals of many species, deprivation of form vision in early life causes axial elongation of the eye and consequent myopia which can be extreme.[81–83] Human infants are also responsive to visual deprivation in early life. Lid hemangiomas,[84] ptosis[85] and opacities in the ocular media,[86] can all cause myopia.

Experimentally, lid suture in early post-natal life results in axial myopia in monkeys,[87–90] tree shrews,[91,92] cats,[93,94] rabbits and chickens.[95,96] There are interspecies differences in susceptibility and in the rate at which abnormal ocular growth occurs. Chickens and tree shrews, which mature quickly, are particularly prone to the rapid development of axial myopia in response to visual deprivation.

The ocular elongation associated with lid suture does not occur if the animal is reared in the dark,[97,98] indicating that the physical effects of lid suture, such as mechanical deformation of the eye or temperature elevation,[99] are not responsible for the altered ocular growth pattern and, additionally, that light is required to induce the increased axial length.

When animals are reared in total darkness, refractions tend to remain widely scattered around a mean that lies significantly to the hypermetropic side of emmetropia.[97,100,101] The pattern to some extent resembles that seen in newborn humans who might reasonably be considered to have been dark reared prior to birth.

The relatively random pattern of refractive errors with a peak at low hypermetropia that is seen in dark-reared animals suggests that, on their own, genetic influences guide eye growth towards near emmetropia in a rather inaccurate fashion. Accumulating evidence suggests that an appropriate visual input in early life is necessary to fine tune ocular growth to achieve emmetropia and that myopia and other refractive errors may well be due to a failure of this growth regulation, possibly as a result of an inappropriate visual environment in early life acting on a genetically predisposed visual system.

Anything that degrades the visual image in early life can lead to myopia. Thus, the wearing of translucent goggles[102] or the intrastromal injection of latex into the cornea,[103] which allow light transmission but not form vision, are effective ways of producing myopia in experimental animals.

The earlier the visual deprivation is induced and the longer it is maintained the greater the effect on ocular growth and refraction.[104] Visual deprivation, however, has to be near continuous to affect ocular growth in this way for as little as 20 minutes per day of form vision, even under anesthesia, is sufficient to allow normal ocular growth and emmetropization.[105]

In most animals, restoration of form vision after a period of visual deprivation is followed by a rapid normalization of ocular growth.[106] The ocular axial length, which grows at a greater than normal rate in the visually deprived eye, slows its growth rate when normal vision is restored and compensatory changes also occur in the corneal curvature, and possibly other optical components, to achieve emmetropization. The ametropia developed during visual deprivation occurs more slowly than the normalization after form vision has been restored. A possible explanation is that visual deprivation induces ametropia by acting against genetic factors trying to achieve emmetropia, whereas after restoration of normal vision the genetic factors and the now appropriate visual input act together in the direction of emmetropization.

Initially, it was believed that form-deprivation myopia was likely to be mediated through central connections with the brain and possibly involve accommodation. It has been found, however, that in many animals (e.g. rhesus monkey, chicken) form-deprivation myopia still occurs when the optic nerve has been sectioned[107] and retinal ganglion cells allowed to degenerate.[108] There are species differences in the response to visual deprivation and in the stump-tailed macaque monkey, for example, an intact optic nerve appears to be a prerequisite for the development of form-deprivation myopia.[108] Form-deprivation myopia can also develop in animals where accommodation has been abolished by destruction of the Edinger-Westphal nucleus or removal of the ciliary ganglion.[108,109]

In most species, atropinization has little effect on the development of form-deprivation myopia but visual-deprivation myopia does not occur in the atropinized stump-tailed macaque monkey whereas it does occur in other species of monkey.[108] This, however, is not really evidence that accommodation is contributing to the development of form-deprivation myopia in this species, for atropine has widespread effects in the eye apart from its obvious mydriatic and cycloplegic effects. An additional difficulty in ascribing a role to accommodation in the genesis of form-deprivation myopia is that in monocular form-deprivation myopia, accommodation would have to be abnormal in one eye and not in the other.

If form-deprivation myopia needs neither central connections nor accommodation in its pathogenesis it would appear that it is a purely ocular phenomenon, suggesting that the eye itself can recognize an appropriate or inappropriate visual image and alter its growth pattern accordingly. The evidence is that the retina itself is able to generate signals that affect the growth of the eye locally in response to the visual input in early life.

Somewhat surprisingly, it is not necessarily the whole retina and the whole eye that need be involved. If animals are reared so that only part of the retina is deprived of form vision while the rest retains a normal visual input, only that part of the eye related to the visually deprived portion of the retina grows abnormally so that the eye develops an increased dimension in one direction while retaining a normal growth pattern in other areas.[110,111] This visually induced local deformation of growth is particularly well seen in birds (chickens, pigeons) in which the cone density in the extrafoveal retina is high. The phenomenon may be a correlate of the normally occurring situation in ground-living birds like the pigeon, the eyes of which grow asymmetrically so that they are myopic in the lower field and emmetropic horizontally and above. This ensures that the ground and potential food is kept in clear focus, as is distance vision above the horizontal from where predators are likely to appear.[112] Attempts have been made to determine which retinal elements are important in growth regulation of the eye. Destruction of photoreceptors by specifically acting neurotoxins[113] not unexpectedly prevents the development of form-deprivation myopia and, as already noted, the condition can occur in the absence of viable ganglion cells. It appears likely that one class of amacrine cell is the source of cell signalling affecting ocular growth in early life, while the growth pattern can be significantly altered by neurotoxins with specific actions on particular classes of amacrine cell.[114] Form-deprivation myopia is associated with a decrease in retinal dopamine levels and an increase in vasoactive intestinal peptide levels.[115,116] Interestingly, lid-suture myopia can be prevented by the local application of the dopamine agonist, apomorphine.[117] It would seem that dopamine/melatonin concentrations in the retina can be affected by alterations in visual input and in some way, not at present understood, this can have an effect on the growth pattern of the immediately subjacent sclera.

To have an effect on scleral growth, signals from the retina would have to traverse the retinal pigment epithelium (RPE) and the choroid. It is known that there is a molecular movement from the intraocular compartment to the choroid and sclera, either via the anterior chamber and the uveo-scleral outflow pathway,[118] or across the posterior blood–ocular barrier.[119,120]

Apart from acting directly on the sclera, retinal signals might initiate a molecular cascade inducing the RPE or choroid to release growth factors, which might in turn affect scleral growth.[121]

There has long been an argument as to whether the increased ocular dimensions in myopia are the result of stretch or active growth. In favor of the former is the fact that the myopic sclera is thinner than normal and that myopes tend to have slightly higher, albeit normal, intraocular pressures than do non-myopes.[122] Attempts to influence the development or progression of myopia by reducing the intraocular pressure pharmacologically have, however, been ineffective.[123]

In support of active scleral growth is the fact that the myopic sclera is of increased volume and weight,[124] albeit thinner than normal sclera, and that, additionally, there is evidence of increased cellular proliferation in the myopic sclera[125] and an increased synthesis of protein and other extracellular constituents of the sclera as compared to the normal eye.[124]

Apart from the effects of form deprivation it has been found that if animal eyes are rendered ametropic during infancy by the use of plus or minus spectacles or contact lenses they grow to compensate for the ametropia[126] even in the absence of accommodation. Thus, plus lenses, which induce a myopic error, cause the eye to limit its axial growth so that after the spectacle lens has been removed the eye is significantly hypermetropic. Minus lenses, on the other hand, induce myopia. Whether this is of relevance to refraction in human children is an interesting speculation. It has been suggested that children habituated to prolonged detailed close work may 'emmetropize' to reading distance, i.e. become myopic.[127] It has also been suggested that correcting myopia in early life with minus lenses may in itself induce a worsening of the myopia and set up a vicious circle of progressive deterioration in the refractive error.[128]

Again, there appear to be species differences in 'compensatory' ametropia. In the marmoset, for example,[129] minus lenses of any strength induce myopia but, whereas plus lenses up to 6 D induce hypermetropia, the use of lenses in excess of 6 D results in myopia. It is possible that higher strengths of lens irrespective of sign induce form deprivation while lower strengths induce compensatory hypermetropia or myopia according to the sign of the lens. 'Compensatory' myopia in response to induced ametropia in animals appears to require central connections and its underlying mechanisms may be different to those resulting in form-deprivation myopia. An unanswered problem is how the visual system is able to detect whether an induced ametropic blur is hypermetropic or myopic. Suggested mechanisms have included chromaticity clues and temporal aspects of ametropia.[130] Currently, however, there is no generally accepted responsible mechanism.

A difficulty in extrapolating from animal work to myopia in humans, apart from the obvious species difference, is the rather short critical period during which myopia can be induced in young experimental animals. Thus, in monkeys, lid-suture myopia can be induced up to the age of 2 years or so,[110] while in chickens and tree shrews the critical period is much shorter.

Although in most species restoration of normal visual input results in a regression of induced myopia, in some monkeys myopia continues after visual deprivation is discontinued[131] and, indeed, may worsen. Such animals eventually may develop the degenerative fundus abnormalities that characterize high myopia in humans.[132] In experiments in which monkeys watched television for a year, only subsequently did myopia develop.[133]

Although it has commonly been believed that visual deprivation in human infants only leads to myopia if the deprivation is acting during the first 3 years of life, there is some evidence that the critical period during which the human visual system may remain responsive to visual input may be quite long, perhaps up to the age of 9 years.[134]

THERAPEUTIC INTERVENTIONS IN MYOPIA

Various surgical procedures have been developed to modify the effects of myopia but consideration of surgical manoevers designed to reduce the refracting power of the eye or to reinforce an abnormally thin posterior sclera are not the remit of this chapter, nor is the reduction in the myopic error that can be achieved temporarily by the wearing of contact lenses which, especially if fitted flatter than the corneal curvature, can reduce corneal refracting power without having any lasting effect on the natural history of the underlying myopia.[135]

Attempts have, however, been made to modify the natural history of myopia by interventions designed to reduce the putative abnormal accommodative effort thought to be of etiological importance in the genesis of myopia.

The main approaches have been to paralyze accommodation by the use of atropine locally in the eye or to relieve the accommodative system of its load by the use of optical aids such as bifocal glasses.

As far as atropinization is concerned, there is evidence that atropine applied locally in the eyes can reduce the rate at which myopia progresses.[136] The effect is not great, however, typically treated eyes being about 1 D less myopic than untreated eyes after some years of treatment.[137] In a study of myopic anisometropia[138] the application of atropine to the more myopic eye for 1–2 years allowed equalization of the refraction in the two eyes.

Atropine is a muscarinic antagonist and it is noteworthy that muscarinic receptors are widespread in the eye, being present in the retina, iris, ciliary body and in scleral cells. M1 muscarinic agonists promote growth of scleral fibrocytes in culture while M2 agonists inhibit growth of these cells.[139] Atropine is a non-specific muscarinic antagonist and can prevent the development of form-deprivation myopia in some species.[110,140,141] Atropine is only one representative of a class of muscarinic agonists and antagonists, some of which have actions restricted to specific subtypes of muscarinic receptor.

A number of observations suggest that any effect that atropine may have on the progress of myopia may be mediated by mechanisms other than accommodation. Thus, although form-deprivation myopia in the chick can be prevented by the intravitreal injection of atropine,[142] the chick ciliary muscle is striated, has nicotinic receptors and is unresponsive to atropinization. M1 muscarinic antagonists can prevent form-deprivation myopia in some mammals while M2 and M3 antagonists fail to do so.[141] Mammalian ciliary muscle receptors, however, are said not to be of the M1 subtype.[143] Additionally, parasympathetic stimulation of accommodation does not facilitate the development of lid-suture myopia.[144]

There is, thus, a growing body of evidence that atropine and more specific M1 receptor antagonists, such as pirenzepine, may affect ocular axial enlargement in both experimental and naturally occurring myopia, by acting either directly on the cells in the sclera or by blocking muscarinic receptors in the retina, and so inhibiting the retina-generated inappropriate signals for eye growth, which appear to underlie the development of myopia.

If excess accommodation were a significant factor in the genesis of myopia, one would anticipate that abolishing the need for excess accommodation by optical means would have a significant effect on the rate at which myopia progresses. Neither undercorrection of myopia, however, nor the use of bifocal glasses designed to relieve accommodative effort have been shown to be of any significant value when tested in randomized controlled trials in which subjects were matched for age and severity of refractive error.[135] As with the experimental work on the effects of muscarinic antagonists on myopia, clinical studies involving a reduction in accommodative effort suggest that accommodation has little, if any, role in the genesis of myopia.

CONCLUSION

It appears that both genetic factors and visual experience in early life determine the final refraction of the eye. Visual input appears to influence the axial length of the eye in various ways, depending upon whether light deprivation, form deprivation or induced ametropia is the active stimulus. Changes in axial length, in turn, may induce compensatory alterations in corneal curvature and other optical components of the eye, but these changes may be insufficient to nullify the refractive effect of changes in axial length.

Animal work has illustrated graphically how visual input can affect ocular growth and maturation and suggests that human myopia may have a similar multifactorial pathogenesis with genetic predisposition and visual experience in the formative years equally responsible for the ametropia.

Fortunately for the refractive surgeon, refraction in the majority of young adult myopes, remains stable. Unexpected progression, which does occur in a small proportion of cases, indicates the need to establish the stability of refraction before embarking on measures designed permanently to alter the refracting power of the eye. The significant changes that affect refraction in later life in many patients must also be considered when refractive surgery is being contemplated.

REFERENCES

1. Hirschberg J, *The Treatment of Short Sight* (G Lindsay Johnson Trans), (Rebman Co: New York, 1912).
2. Weymouth FW, Hirsch MJ, Theories, Definitions and Classifications of Refractive Errors. In: Grosvenor T & Flom MC, eds, *Refractive Anomalies: Research & Clinical Applications* (Butterworth-Heinemann: Boston, 1990), 6–12.
3. Jackson E, *Manual of the Diagnosis & Treatment of the Diseases of the Eyes* (Saunders: Philadelphia, 1900).
4. Duke-Elder WS, *The Practice of Refraction* (Brackiston Co: Philadephia, 1943).
5. May CH, *Diseases of the Eye, 17th Edition* (Williams & Wilkins: Baltimore, 1949).
6. Hirsch MJ, Changes in Refractive State after the Age of 45, *Amer J Optom, Arch Amer Acad Optom* (1958). **35**:564–73.
7. Gullstrand A, Appendices to Part I. In: Southall JPC, ed. *Helmholtz's Treatise on Physiological Optics, Vol 1*, (Optical Society of America: New York: 1924), 261–482.
8. Lotmar W, Theoretical Eye Model with Aspherics, *J Opt Soc Amer*, (1971), **61**:1522–29.
9. Erickson P, Mathematical Model for Predicting Dioptric Effect of Optical Parameter Changes in the Eye, *Amer J Optom Physiol Opt*, (1977) **54**:226–33.
10. Blaker JW, Towards an Adaptive Model of the Human Eye, *J Opt Soc Amer*, (1980) **70**:220–3.
11. Straub M, Uber die Aetiologie der Brechungsanomalien des Auges und den Ursprung der Emmetropie, *Graefes Arch*, (1909), **70**:130–99.
12. Sorsby A, Sheridan M & Leary GA, Vision, visual acuity and ocular refraction of young men. Findings in a sample of 1,033 subjects, *Brit Med J*, (1960), **1**:1394–8.
13. Sorsby A, Biology of the eye as an optical system. In: Duane T, ed, *Clinical Ophthalmology*, (Harper & Row: Hagarstown, 1980).
14. Tron EJ, Th Optical Elements of the Refractive Power of the Eye. In: Ridley F, Sorsby A, eds, *Modern Trends in Ophthalmology*, (Paul B Hoeber: New York, 1940).
15. Betsch A, Uber die mensliche refractionskurve, *Klin Mbl f Augenheilk, (1929)* 365–79.
16. Strenstrom S, Investigation of the Variation and the Co-Variation of the Optical Elements of Human Eyes (Trans D Woolf), *Amer J Opt & Arch Amer Acad Optom*, (1948) **25**:218–504.
17. Hirsch MJ, An Analysis of Inhomogeneity of Myopia in Adults, *Amer J Opt Arch Amer Acad Optom*, (1950) **27**:562–71.
18. Erikson P, Optical Components Contributing to Refractive Anomalies. In: Grosvenor T, Flom M, eds, *Refractive Anomalies, Research & Clinical Applications*. (Butterworth-Heinemann: Boston, 1990), 199–217.
19. Hirsch MJ, Weymouth FW, Prevalence of refractive anomalies. In: Grosvenor T, Flom M, eds, *Refractive Anomalies Research & Clinical Applications*, (Butterworth-Heinemann: Boston, 1990), 15–37.
20. Sato T, *The Cause and Prevention of School Myopia*. (Excerpta Medica, Amsterdam, 1993): pp 7–11.
21. Majima A, Nakajima A, Ichikawa H, *et al*, Prevalence of Ocular Anomalies among Schoolchildren, *Amer J Ophthalmol*, (1960) **50**:139–46.
22. Trevor-Roper T, *The Eye and its Disorders*. (Blackwell: Oxford, 1974).
23. Lam CSY, Goh SH, Millodot M, (1995). Prevalence of Refractive Errors among Young Adults of Southern China. In: Chew SJ, Weintraub J, eds, *Proceedings Vth International Conference on Myopia*, (Myopia International Research Foundation Inc: New York-Singapore), 93 (abst).

24. Young FA, Leary GA, Aldwin WR, *et al*, The Transmission of Refractive Errors within Eskimo Families, *Amer J Optom Arch Amer Acad Optom*, (1969) **46**:676–85.

25. Morgan RW, Speakman JS, Grunshaw SE, Inuit Myopia: An Environmentally Induced 'Epidemic'?, *Canad Med Assoc J*, (1975) **112**:575–77.

26. Johnson GJ, Matthews A, Perkins ES, Survey of Ophthalmic Conditions in a Labrador Community: I. Refractive Errors, *Brit J Ophthalmol, (1979)* **63**:440–8.

27. Alward WM, Bender TR, Demske JA, *et al*, High Prevalence of Myopia among Young Adult Yupik Eskimos, *Canad J Ophthalmol* (1985) **20**:241–5.

28. Boniuk V, (1973). Refractive Problems in Native Peoples (the Sioux Lookout Project), *Canad J Ophthalmol*, (1973) **8**:229–33.

29. Woodruff ME, Samek MJ, A Study of the Prevalence of Spherical Equivalent Refractive States and Anisometropia in Amerind Populations in Ontario, *Canad J Public Health*, (1977) **68**:414–24.

30. Forsius H, Erickson AW, Fellman J, Change of Refraction in the Same Population and in the Same Subjects Studied 1960–62 and 1991–92. In: Chew SJ, Weintraub J, eds, *Proceedings Vth International Conference on Myopia*. (Myopia International Research Foundation Inc: New York-Singapore, 1995), 98–104.

31. Rajan V, Foh TT, Chan TK, *et al*, Changing Prevalence of Myopia in Singapore Schoolchildren. In: Chew SJ, Weintraub J, eds, *Proceedings Vth International Conference on Myopia*. (Myopia International Research Foundation Inc (New York-Singapore, 1995), 41–8.

32. Chew SJ, Chia SC, Lee LKH, The Pattern of Myopia in Young Singaporean Men, *Singapore Med J*, (1989) **29**:201–11.

34. Lin LLK, Tsai CB, Shi HY, *et al*, Myopia in Students of National Taiwan University. In: Chew SJ, Weintraub J, eds, *Proceedings Vth International Conference on Myopia*, (Myopia International Research Foundation Inc: New York-Singapore, 1995), 40 (abst).

35. Jaeger E, *Uber die Einstellung des Dioptrischen Apparates im Menschlicten Augen*, (LW Seidel, UV Sohn Wasson: Wien, 1861).

35. Cook RC, Glascock RE, Refractive and Ocular Findings in the Newborn, *Amer J Ophthalmol*, (1951) **34**:1407–13.

36. Goldschmidt E, Refraction in the Newborn, *Acta Ophthalmol*, (1969) **47**:570–8.

37. Kempf GA, Collins SD, Jarman EL, Refractive Errors in the Eyes of Children as Determined by Retinoscopic Examination with Cycloplegic, *Public Health Bulletin No 182* (Government Printing Office: Washington DC, 1928).

38. Gwiazda J, Thorn F, Bauer F, *et al*, Emmetropization and the Progression of Manifest Refraction in Children followed from Infancy to Puberty, *Clin Vision Sci*, (1993) **8**:337–44.

39. Gwiazda J, Scheiman M, Mohinder I, *et al*, Astigmatism in Children—Changes in Axis and Amount from Birth to Six Years, *Invest Ophthal Vis Sci*, (1948) **25**:88–91.

40. Hirsch MJ, The Changes in Refraction between Ages 5 and 14. Theoretical and Practical Consideration, *Amer J Optom Arch Amer Acad Optom*, (1952) **29**:445–52.

41. Kronfeld PD, Devney C, Ein Beitrag zur Kenntnis der Refractions Kurve. *Graefes Arch Ophthalmol*, (1952) **126**:487–96.

42. Bartels M, Hohe Myopie in den ersten Lebensjahren, *Klin Mbl Augenbeilk*, (1931) **86**:536.

43. Bruckner A, FRanceschetti A, Myopie in Kindersalter, *Arch Augenheilk*, (1931) **105**:141.

44. Boselli A, *La Ametropie Nelle Scuole Elementori di Bolona*, (Regia Tipografia: Bologna, 1900) 27–38.

45. Nicholls JVV, A Survey of the Ophthalmic Conditions among Rural Schoolchildren, *Canad Med J*, (1940) **42**:553–6.

46. Wilson JA, Emmetropia and Sex. *Brit J Ophthalmol* (1935) **19**:613–4.

47. Goss DA, Cox VD, Trends in the change of clinical refractive error in childhood, *J Amer Optom Assoc*, (1985) **56**:608–13.

48. Goss DA, Winkler RL, Progression of myopia in youth: age of cessation, *Amer J Optom Physiol Opt*, (1983) **60**:651–8.

49. Goss DA, Erickson P, Herrin-Lawson GA, *et al*, Refractive error, axial length and height as a function of age in young myopes, *Optom Vis Sci*, (1996) **67**:332–8.

50. Goss DA, Childhood myopia. In: Grosvenor T, Flom MC, eds, *Refractive Anomalies: Research & Clinical Applications*, (Butterworth-Heinemann: Boston, 1990), 94.

51. Baldwin WR, Adams AJ, Flatteau P, Young adult myopia. In: Grosvenor T, Flom MC, eds, *Refractive Anomalies: Research & Clinical Applications*, (Butterworth-Heinemann: Boston, 1990), 104–20.

52. National Research Council Committee on Vision *Myopia Prevalence and Progression*. (National Academy Press: Washington DC, 1988).

53. Diamond KS, Acquired myopia in airline pilots, *J Aviation Med*, (1957) **28**:559–68.

54. Kent PR, Acquired myopia of maturity, *Amer J Optom Arch Amer Optom*, (1963) **40**:247–56.

55. Baldwin WR, Some relatonships between ocular, anthropometric and refractive variables in myopia. PhD thesis, (1964), Indiana University, Bloomington.

56. Goss DA, Erickson P, Meridional corneal components of myopia progression in young adults and children, *Amer J Optom Physiol Opt*, (1987) **64**:475–81.

57. Adams AJ, Axial elongation not corneal curvature as a basis of adult onset myopia, *Amer J Optom Physiol Opt*, (1987) **64**:150–2.

58. McBrien NA, Millodot M, A biometric investigation of late onset myopic eyes. *Acta Ophthalmol*, (1987) **65**:518–23.

59. Jackson E, Norms of refraction, *JAMA* (1932) **98**:132–40.

60. Tassman IS, Frequency of various kinds of refractive errors, *Amer Ophthalmol*, (1932) **15**:1044–53.

61. Raviola E, Wiesel TN, Neural control of eye growth and experimental myopia in primates. In: Bok GR, Widdows K, eds, *Myopia & the Control of Eye Growth*, (J Wiley & Sons: Chichester, 1990), 22–38.

62. Cohn H, (1866). Unter der augen von 10,060 schulkindern nebst vorsehlungen zur verbesesserung der augen nachteiligen schuleinrichtungen. *Ein Aetiologische Studie*, (Leipzig, 1866).

63. Donders FC, (1864). *On the anomalies of accommodation and refraction of the Eye*. Trans: Moore WD, (New Sydenham Society **22**:London, 1864).

64. Steiger A, *Die enstehung der spharischen refractionen des menslichen auges*. (Berlin, S Karger: Berlin, 1913).

65. Goldschmidt E, On the etiology of myopia, *Acta Ophthalmol (1968)* **46**(Suppl 98): 1–172.

66. Sperduto RD, Siegel D, Roberts J, *et al*, Prevalence of myopia in the United States. *Arch Ophthalmol*, (1983) **101**:405–7.

67. Angle J, Wissman DA, Age, reading and myopia, *Amer J Optom Physiol Opt*, (1978) **55**: 302–8.

68. Richler A, Bear JC, Refraction, near work and education. A population study in Newfoundland, *Acta Ophthalmol*, (1980) **58**:468–78.

69. Zylberman R, Landau D, Berson D, The influence of study habits on myopia in Jewish teenagers, *J Pediatr Ophthalmol Strabismus*, (1993) **30**:319–22.

70. Duke Elder WS, Abrams D, *System of Ophthalmology, Vol V, Ophthalmic Optics and Refraction*. (CV Mosby Co: St Louis, 1970).

71. Vogel F, Motulsky AG, *Human genetics: problems and approaches*. (Springer Verlag: New York, 1979).

72. Ashton GC, Segregation analysis of ocular refraction and myopia, *Hum Hered*, (1985) **35**:232–9.

73. Bear JC, Epidemiology & genetics of refractive anomalies. In: Grosvenor T, Flom MC, eds, *Refractive Anomalies: Research & Clinical Applications*. (Butterworth-Heinemann: Boston, 1990), 57–80.

74. Sorsby A, Sheridan M, Leary GA, Refraction and its components in twins, *Medical Research Council Special Reports*, Series No. 303, (HMSO: London, 1962).

75. Sorsby A, Fraser GR, Statistical note on the components of ocular refraction in twins, *J Med Genet*, (1964) **1**:47–9.

76. Chen CJ, Cohen BH, Diamond EL, Genetic and environment effects on the development of myopia in Chinese twin children, *Ophthal Pediat Genet*, (1985) **6**:113–9.

77. Sorsby A, Benjamin B, Mode of inheritance of errors of refraction, *J Med Genet*, (1973) **10**:161–4.

78. Young FA, The effect of restricted visual space on the primate eye, *Amer J Ophthalmol*, (1961) **52**:779–806.

79. Belkin M, Yinon U, Rose I, *et al*, Effect of visual environmental on refractive error of cats, *Doc Ophthalmol*, *(1971)* **42**:433–7.

80. van Alphen GWHM, On emmetropia and ametropia, *Ophalmologia* (1961) **142**(Suppl): 1–92.

81. Goss DA, Criswell MH, Myopia development in experimental animals—a literature review, *Amer J Optom Physiol Opt*, (1981) **58**:859–69.

82. Criswell MH, Goss GA, Myopia development in non-human primates—a literature review, *Amer J Optom Physiol Opt*, (1983) **60**:250–68.

83. Yinon U, Myopia induction in animals following alteration of the visual input during development: a review, *Curr Eye Res*, (1984) **3**:677–90.

84. Robb RM, Refractive errors associated with haemangiomas of the eyelids and orbit in infancy, *Amer J Ophthalmol*, (1977) **83**:52–8.

85. O'Leary DJ, Millodot M, (1979). Eyelid closure causes myopia in humans, *Experientia*, (1979) **35**:1478–9.

86. Curtin BJ, *The Myopias: Basic Science and Clinical Management*, (Harper & Row: Philadelphia, 1985).

87. Wiesel TN, Raviola E, Myopia and eye enlargement after neonatal lid fusion in monkeys, *Nature (Lond)*, (1977) **266**:66–8.

88. von Noorden GK, Crawford MLJ, Lid closure and refractive error in macaque monkeys, *Nature (Lond)*, (1978) **272**:53–4.

89. Thorn F, Doty RW, Gramiak R, Effect of eyelid suture on development of ocular dimensions in macaques, *Curr Eye Res*, (1982) **1**:727–33.

90. Troila D, Judge SJ, Ridley R, *et al*, (1990). Myopia induced by brief visual deprivation in a new world primate—the common marmoset (Cullithrix jacchus), *Invest Ophthal Vis Sci* (1990) **31**(ARVO Suppl): 1246 (abst).

91. Sherman SM, Norton TT, Casagrande IA, Myopia in the lid sutured tree shrew (Tupaia glis), *Brain Res*, (1977) **124**:154–7.

92. Marsh WL, Norton TT, (1983). Measures of refractive state, ocular length and axial curve in experimentally myopic tree shrews, *Invest Ophthal Vis Sci* (1983) **24**,(ARVO Suppl): 226 (abst).

93. Kirby DW, Sutton L, Elongation of cat eyes following neonatal lid suture, *Invest Ophthal Vis Sci*, (1982) **22**:274–7.

94. Nathan J, Crewther SG, Crewther DP, *et al*, (1984). Effects of retinal image degradation on ocular growth in cats, *Invest Ophthal Vis Sci*, (1984) **25**:1300–6.

95. Wallman J, Turkel J, Trachtman J, Extreme myopia produced by modest changes in early visual experience, *Science*, (1978) **201**:1249–51.

96. Yinon V, Koslove KC, Lobel D, *et al*, Lid suture myopia in developing chicks. Optical and structural considerations, *Curr Eye Res*, (1978) **2**:871–82.

97. Raviola E, Wiesel TN, Effect of dark rearing on experimental myopia in monkeys, *Invest Ophthal Vis Sci*, (1978) **17**:485–8.

98. Gottlieb MD, Wallman J, Retinal activity modulates eye growth: evidence for recovery in stroboscopic illumination, *Soc Neurosci Abstr*, (1987) **13**:1297.

99. Hodos W, Rezvin AM, Kuenzal WJ, Thermal gradients in the chick eye: a contributory factor in experimental myopia, *Invest Ophthal Vis Sci*, (1987) **28**:1859–66.

100. Regal DM, Boothe R, Tellor DY, *et al*, Visual acuity and visual responsiveness in dark reared monkeys (Macaca nemestrina), *Vis Res*, (1976) **16**:523–30.

101. Yinon V, Koslove EC, Rassin MI, The optical effects of eyelid closure on the eyes of kittens reared in light and dark, *Curr Eye Res*, (1984) **3**:677–90.

102. Hodos W, Kuenzal WJ, Retinal image degradation produces ocular enlargement in chicks, *Invest Ophthal Vis Sci*, (1984) **25**:652–9.

103. Wiesel TN, Raviola E, Increase in axial length of the macaque monkey eye after corneal opacification, *Invest Ophthal Vis Sci*, (1979) **18**:1232–6.

104. Smith EL, (1990). Experimentally induced refractive anomalies in mammals. In: Grosvenor T, Flom MC, eds, *Refractive Anomalies: Research & Clinical Applications*, (Butterworth-Heinemann: Boston, 1990), 248–9.

105. Wilbert AI, Wallman J, Brief daily visual experience even under anaesthesia can alter refractive error of chicks. In: Chew SJ, Weintraub J, eds, *Proceedings Vth International Conference on Myopia*, (Myopia International Research Foundation Inc: New York-Singapore, 1995) 130(abst).

106. Wallman J, Adams JI, Developmental aspects of experimental myopia in chicks: susceptibility, recovery and relation to emmetropia, *Vis Res*, (1987) **27**:1139–63.

107. Troilo D, Gottlieb MD, Wallman J, Visual deprivation causes myopia in chicks with optic nerve section, *Curr Eye Res*, (1987) **6**:993–9.

108. Raviola E, Wiesel TN, Neural control of eye growth and experimental myopia in primates. In: Bock GR, Widdows K, eds, *Myopia & the Control of Eye Growth*, (J Wiley & Sons: Chichester, 1990), 22–38.

109. Troilo D, Experimental studies of emmetropia in the chick. In: Bock GR, Widdows K, eds, *Myopia & the Control of Eye Growth*. (J Wiley & Sons: Chichester, 1990), 89–102.

110. Gottlieb MD, Fugate-Wentzek LA, Wallman J, Different visual deprivations produce different ametropias and different eye shapes, *Invest Ophthal Vis Sci*, (1987) **2**:1225–35.

111. Wallman J, Gottlieb MD, Rajavan V, *et al*, Local retinal regions control local eye growth and myopia, *Science*, (1987) **237**:73–7.

112. Fitzke FW, Hayes BP, Hodos W, *et al*, (1985). Refractive sectors in the visual field of the pigeon eye, *J Physiol*, (1985) **369**:33–4.

113. Oishi T, Lauber JK, Chicks blinded with formoguanamine do not develop lid suture myopia, *Curr Eye Res*, (1988) **7**:69–73.

114. Ehrlich D, Sattayasai J, Zappia J, *et al*, Effects of selective neurotoxins on eye growth in the young chick. In: Bok GR & Widdows, eds, *Myopia & the Control of Eye Growth* (J Wiley & Sons: Chichester, 1990), 63–84.

115. Stone RA, Lin T, Laties AM, *et al*, Retinal dopamine and form deprivation myopia, *Proc Nat Acad Sci USA*, (1989) **86**:704–6.

116. Stone RA, Laties AM, Raviola E, *et al*, Increase in retinal vasoactive intestinal polypeptide after eyelid fusion in primates, *Proc Nat Acad Sci USA*, (1988) **85**:257–60.

117. Stone RA, Lin T, Laties AM, *et al*, Apomorphine blocks axial elongation of the visually deprived chick eye, *Invest Ophthal Vis Sci* (1989) **30**(ARVO Suppl): 31 (abst).

118. Bill A, Conventional and uveo-scleral clearance of aqueous humour in the Cynomologous monkey, Macaca Irus, at normal and high Intraocular pressures, *Exp Eye Res*, (1966) **5**:45–54.

119. Foulds WS, Mosley H, Eadie A, *et al*, Vitreal, retinal and pigment epithelial contributions to the posterior blood ocular barrier, *Trans Ophthal Soc UK*, (1980) **100**:341–2.

120. Moseley H, Johnson NF and Foulds WS, Vitreo scleral fluid transfer in the rabbit. *Acta Ophthalmol*, (1979) **56**:769–76.

121. Wallman J, Retinal influences on sclera underlie visual deprivation myopia. In: Bock GR, Widdows K, eds, *Myopia and the Control of Eye Growth*, (J Wiley & Son: Chichester, 1990), 126–41.

122. Tomlinson A, Phillips CI, Applanation tension and axial length of the eyeball. *Brit J Ophthalmol* (1970) **54** :548–53.

123. Goldschmidt E, Myopia in humans: can progresson be arrested? In: Bok GR, Widdows K, eds, *Myopia & the Control of Eye Growth*. (J Wiley & Son: Chichester, 1990), 222–34.

124. Christenson AM, Wallman J, (1989). Increased DNA and protein synthesis in scleras of eyes with visual-deprivation myopia, *Invest Ophthal Vis Sci* (1989): **30**(ARVO Suppl): 402 (abst).

125. Gottlieb MD, Joshi HB, Wallman J, Local changes in the sclera of chick eyes made myopic by form deprivation, *Invest Ophthal Vis Sci* (1988), **28**(ARVO Suppl): 32 (abst).

126. Schaeffel F, Troilo D, Wallman J, *et al*, Developing eyes lacking accommodation grow to compensate for induced defocus, *Vis Neuro Sci*, (1990) **4**:177–83.

127. Wallman J, Nature and nurture of myopia, *Nature (Lond)*, (1994) **371**:202.

128. Duke-Elder S, Abrams D, Pathological refractive errors. In: Duke-Elder S, ed. *System of Ophthalmology (Volume 5)* (Henry Kimpton, London, 1970) 334–62.

129. Troilo D, Primate models of refractive development. In: Chew SJ, Weintraub J, eds, *Proceedings VTH International Conference on Myopia*. (Myopia International Research Foundation Inc: New York-Singapore, 1995), 133 (abst).

130. General Discussion II, What are the signals for defocus? In: Bok GR, Widdows K, eds, *Myopia & the Control of Eye Growth*, (J Wiley & Son: Chichester, 1990), 201–5.

131. Troilo D, Judge SJ, Ocular development and visual deprivation myopia in the common marmoset (Callithrix Jacchus) *Vis Res*, (1993) **33**:1311–24.

132. Tokoro T, Funata M, Akazawa Y, *et al*, A clinico-pathological study of experimentally myopic monkeys with a long-term follow-up. In: Chew SK, Weintraub J, eds, *Proceedings Vth International Conference on Myopia*. (Myopia International Research Foundation Inc: New York-Singapore, 1995), 134 (abst).

133. Shih F cited by Wallman J, Nature and nurture of myopia, *Nature (Lond)*, (1994) **371**:202.

134. Renda I, Metge P, Maurin JM, Unilateral high myopia and deprivation. In: Chew SJ, Weintraub J, eds, *Proceedings Vth International Conference on Myopia*. (Myopia International Research Foundation Inc: New York-Singapore, 1995), 82 (abst).

135. Grosvenor T, Management of myopia: functional methods. In: Grosvenor T & Flom MC, eds, *Refractive Anomalies: Research and Clinical Applications*, (Butterworth-Heinemann: Boston, 1990), 345–69.

136. Goldschmidt E, Management of myopia: pharmaceutical agents. In: Grosvenor T & Flom MC, eds, *Refractive Anomalies: Research and Clincal Applications* (Butterworth-Heinemann: Boston, 1990), 371–83.

137. Kennedy RH, Dyer J, Kennedy MA, *et al*, Atropine treatment for myopia. In: Chew SJ, Weintraub J, eds, *Proceedings Vth International Conference on Myopia*. (Myopia International Research Foundation Inc: New York-Singapore, 1995), 230 (abst).

138. Chew SJ, Wong PK, Atropine in the treatment of myopic anisometropia in children. In: Chew SJ, Weintraub J, eds, *Proceedings Vth International Conference on Myopia*. (Myopia International Research Foundation Inc: New York-Singapore, 1995), 247(1)–247(16).

139. Chu E, Chew SJ, Thompson RB, *et al*, Muscarinic antagonists inhibit normal and epidermal growth factor induced cell proliferation, *Invest Ophthal Vis Sci* (1992) **33**(ARVO Suppl), 820 (abst).

140. McKanna JA, Casagrande VA, Chronic cycloplegia prevents lid suture myopia in tree shrews. *Invest Ophthal Vis Sci* (1985) **26**(ARVO Suppl): 331 (abst).

141. Stone RA, Lin T, Laties AM, Muscarinic antagonist effects on experimental chick myopia. *Exp Eye Res*, (1991) **52**:755–8.

142. McBrien NA, Moghaddam HO, Reeder AP, Atropine reduces experimental myopia and eye enlargement by a non-accommodative mechanism, *Invest Ophthal Vis Sci*, (1993) **34**:205–15.

143. Honkanen RE, Howard EF, Abdel-Latif AA, M3 muscarinic receptor subtype predominates in the bovine iris sphincter smooth muscle and ciliary processes, *Invest Ophthal Vis Sci*, (1990) **31**:590–3.

144. Raviola E, Wiesel TN, An animal model of myopia *N Engl J Med*, (1985) **312**:1609–15.

Chapter 6 The principles of computerized videokeratoscopy

Michael K Smolek and Stephen D Klyce

INTRODUCTION

Modern corneal topographic analysis is said to be one of the most important diagnostic advances in ophthalmology in recent times; it has played a seminal role in the evaluation and development of modern refractive surgical procedures. Over the last decade there have been numerous advances, and today there are a growing number of videokeratoscope designs available to clinicians. While numerous instruments are based on well-established principles, and their measurements have been experimentally verified by independent laboratories, for others, there remain unanswered questions. This chapter will briefly review the development of modern videokeratoscopy – its basic principles, terminology, limitations, and potential in precisely measuring the complex shape of the normal, pathological, and surgically modified human cornea.

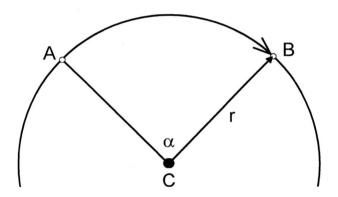

Figure 6.1 *Curvature of a surface is defined as the angle, α, in radians divided by the arc length of the distance AB, where C is the center of curvature of the surface. The angle α is equal to the arc length AB divided by the radius r. Therefore, the curvature is equal to the reciprocal of r.*

CORNEAL OPTICS AND SHAPE

CURVATURE

The cornea is the most effective focal component of the eye, providing nearly three-quarters of its total dioptric power. Because of this, even small changes in its curvature have pronounced effects on the eye's refractive state, making the corneal surface a potentially good site for surgical vision correction. The power of an optical surface is determined by its relative curvature and by the difference in the refractive index of the media separated by the surface. Curvature, R, of a spherical surface is defined as the angle, α, in radians that encompasses a corresponding unit of surface arc length in meters (Fig. 6.1):[1]

$$R = \alpha \; / \; arc \; AB \qquad \text{(Equation 1)}$$

Angle alpha is defined as:

$$\alpha = arc \; AB \; / \; r \qquad \text{(Equation 2)}$$

where r is the radius of curvature of the surface. Therefore curvature is the reciprocal of the radius of curvature of the surface:

$$R = 1/r \qquad \text{(Equation 3)}$$

In optical calculations, r is always expressed in meters. However, for descriptive applications, the radius of curvature of the cornea is normally expressed in millimeters.

POWER

The optical or focal power, F, of a simple, spherical surface is the product of the change in index of refraction at the surface (refractivity) and its curvature as shown by the equation:

$$F = (n' - n) * R \qquad \text{(Equation 4)}$$

where n' is the index of refraction of the material within the surface and n is the index of refraction of the surrounding medium.[1–4] This equation has been referred to by numerous terms including dioptric power, surface power, and optical power, as well as focal power, by some of the predominant texts in the field of visual optics. Generally, all of these terms are synonymous, and are descriptive of the application in which the basic formula is applied. However, as we shall see in this chapter, power can be calculated by other formulae, which may provide better estimates of the optical function of the cornea.

The power unit in visual optics is defined by the diopter, D. It is both a measure of the total magnitude of convergence or divergence of light per unit distance of one meter relative to the medium in which the light travels, and a measure of the inherent ability of an optical surface to alter the vergence of light.[1] The total dioptric power of the human eye is approximately +60 D, with the anterior surface of the cornea alone accounting for about 48 D.

Calculating the power of a surface using Equation 1 is valid only for the central paraxial rays where the sagittal depth is approximately proportional to the curvature.[1] For rays parallel to the axis but increasingly distant from the paraxial region (i.e. non-paraxial rays), power is increasingly underestimated.[5–8] It is difficult to establish guidelines by which one can decide at what optical diameter the formula produces unacceptable error for non-paraxial rays, because the amount of error varies with the shape of the surface. In the living eye, the contribution of the peripheral cornea is modulated by the entrance pupil diameter and attenuation by the Stiles–Crawford effect.[9] Roberts calculated this error using model corneas,[8] and for a typical cornea with an eccentricity of 0.5 and an axial power of 45 D, the calculated power would decrease by approximately 3 D at 3.25 mm from the axis.

SPECIFIC CALCULATIONS OF POWER

There has been debate concerning the method by which corneal power should be calculated. At least four methods have been presented in the literature, and these have been previously reviewed by Mandell,[5] Klein,[6,7] and Roberts.[8]

The first form of power calculation uses a non-fixed center of curvature determined by the local radius of curvature as described by Klyce.[10] This is the Instantaneous Power:

$$F_{inst} = (n' - 1) / r_{inst} \qquad \text{(Equation 5)}$$

where $n' = 1.3375$ and r_{inst} is the radius of curvature for any given point on the cornea. The instantaneous power is also referred to as sagittal power and is Roberts' paraxial power approximation #2.[8]

The index of refraction currently used in corneal topography analysis is an approximate value for the entire optically reduced cornea, and not that of the actual corneal stroma which is approximately 1.376. Historically, an index of refraction of 1.3375 was chosen to produce a calibration power of 45 D with a 7.5 mm radius of curvature, because keratometers (ophthalmometers) of the late 1800s required conversion tables to determine power from the radius of curvature. The instantaneous radius, r_{inst}, is typically determined from curvature analysis of videokeratoscope mire ring images adjacent to and including the ring in question.

The second of the four methods uses a fixed center of curvature on the videokeratoscopic axis for calculating the power at all points on the corneal surface. Thus, the radius of curvature varies with the surface position. This is called the Axial Power Method:

$$F_{axial} = (n' - 1) / r_{axial} \qquad \text{(Equation 6)}$$

where $n' = 1.3375$ and r_{axial} is the distance from the corneal surface to a point of intersection on the videokeratoscopic axis. The radius, r_{axial}, can be calculated from the height, y, of the corneal surface point of analysis from the videokeratoscopic axis (as determined from the mire image) and the sine of the angle theta (θ), which is the angle subtended between the surface intercept at height y and the videokeratoscopic axis relative to the center of curvature:

$$r_{axial} = y / \sin \theta \qquad \text{(Equation 7)}$$

Calculating corneal power using the mire image typically is done in an iterative fashion starting from the center of the cornea where errors tend to be small, and progressing toward the more peripheral regions. Thus, as each mire ring image is encountered, the power at that location is determined based on knowledge about the previous ring's position and power calculation. In order to initiate the iterative process of analyzing the mire images, the average radius of the innermost ring image can be used to determine radius at the vertex normal. This fixes the distance from the surface to the origin (i.e. center of curvature) from which angle θ is measured for more peripheral points.

The surface slope is the tangent of the angle θ. Therefore, this method also has been called slope-based power or tangential power, and is Roberts' paraxial power approximation #1.[8] Note that the first two equations both utilize variations of the generic optical power formula, Equation 4.

It has been pointed out that to better account for spherical aberration and analysis with non-paraxial rays, calculations based on focal lengths are more appropriate.[5–8] Thus, the third formula for power is based on the Second Principal Focal Point:

$$F = n' / f' \qquad \text{(Equation 8)}$$

where n' is 1.3375 and f' is the distance from the vertex normal to the secondary focal point located in image space approximately at or near the retina. Similarly, the fourth power formula is based on the First Principal Focal Point:

$$F = n / f \qquad \text{(Equation 9)}$$

where n is 1.00 for air and f is the distance to the primary focal point of the cornea located in object space. The formula for the Second Principal Focal Point is preferred because it corresponds to distant, parallel light entering the cornea and focusing on the retina.

Unlike the formulae based on the optical power method of Equation 4, the calculation of power using focal lengths is based directly on the principle of Snell's law of refraction for any given ray striking the corneal surface:

$$\sin(\theta_i) / n_{air} = \sin(\theta_r) / n_{cornea} \qquad \text{(Equation 10)}$$

where (θ_i) is the angle of incidence, (θ_r) is the angle of refraction, n_{air} has a value of 1.0 and n_{cornea} is assumed to be 1.3375. For aspherical surfaces, but disregarding skew rays that are not parallel to the axis, the focal point will be constrained to vary along the videokeratoscopic axis for rays striking different locations on the surface. The value of f' for increasingly peripheral rays can be determined from the equation:

$$f' = z + y \cot (\theta_i - \theta_r) \qquad \text{(Equation 8)}$$

where y is the height of the corneal location from the videokeratoscopic axis, z is the dimension along the videokeratoscopic axis with the origin at the vertex normal of the cornea, and θ_i and θ_r are the angles of incidence and refraction respectively. It should be noted that in order to successfully calculate corneal power using the focal length method, the local shape or slope of the cornea must be known a priori in order to calculate the angles of incidence and refraction.

Another power calculation that can be made on the cornea is that of circumferential power. In the preceding discussion, corneal curvature was always measured along meridians. The reason for doing this is simple convenience. Power has also been calculated circumferentially on the cornea across meridians. Doing so does not offer any particular advantage over meridional power calculations. In fact, when considering a small patch of corneal surface as part of an ellipsoid, there is no reason why either of the principal axes of the patch would orthogonally align with a meridional axis. Furthermore, from a practical standpoint, sampling Placido disk mire ring positions along a meridional axis may be more accurate than attempting to sample discrete points distributed circumferentially along a given ring when using a videokeratoscope.

Which of the methods is best for calculating the corneal power? The Instantaneous or Sagittal Power formula (Equation 5) produces inaccurate power values for peripheral portions of the cornea; however, the method does have the advantage of being very simple and direct. The Axial or Tangential Power formula (Equation 6) attempts to offer a more realistic representation of the peripheral corneal topography by determining corneal power from the local slope. This method produces significantly better estimates of the peripheral corneal power than Equation 5. Secondary focal length power analysis (Equation 8) is both theoretically valid and provides realistic values for corneal power in the periphery.

Perhaps the best representation of corneal power might come from averaging powers obtained from multiple meridians centered on each small patch of cornea under analysis (Craig Rousch, personal communication). Doing so would provide a composite power map closely approximating the local spherical equivalent power.

POWER VERSUS CURVATURE

Modern optics textbooks and historical treatises show that curvature and power are regarded as two separate entities of a single optical surface. Refracting surfaces such as the cornea have both a physical shape and an optical nature; however, the term 'diopter' should be used to describe only the cornea's refractive ability, and not its curvature. Historically,

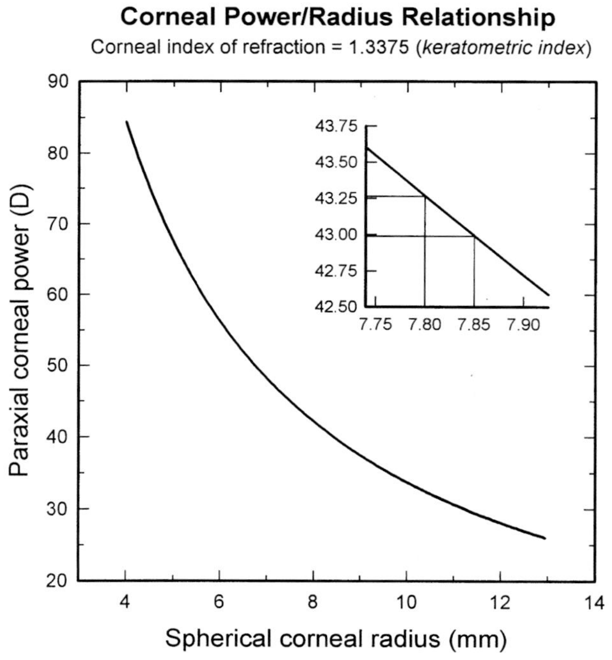

Corneal Power/Radius Relationship

Corneal index of refraction = 1.3375 (*keratometric index*)

Figure 6.2 *Paraxial corneal power as a function of corneal radius using the Instantaneous Power formula (Equation 5). Note the non-linear relationship that must be taken into account when computing large changes in corneal power, such as with some keratorefractive surgical procedures. The smaller inset graph is an expanded scale of a portion of the main graph. Note that even a 50 micron change in radius of curvature can elicit a clinically significant power change of one-quarter diopter.*

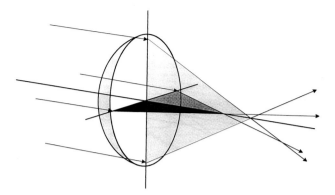

Figure 6.3 *Example of astigmatic error. When parallel rays of light interact with a toric lens surface, the resulting vergence will differ with the meridian angle. A meridian with a radius of curvature that is relatively short (horizontal meridian in example) will come to a focus in front of a meridian with a longer radius of curvature (vertical meridian). The caustic surfaces near the region of best focus may be rather complex forms, particularly when considering light rays that enter the eye at oblique angles.*

the term 'dioptric curvature' has been reserved for defining the optical vergence of a light wavefront independent from an optical element, or applied to describing the vergence change produced by curved mirrors.[1] Placido disk videokeratoscopes do use the mirror properties of the cornea to acquire data, but their algorithms are designed to measure refractive power of the total cornea and not surface reflective power. Therefore, videokeratoscope corneal power displays are scaled in diopters, although the results may be displayed in terms of the radius of curvature in millimeters by removing the refractivity component $(n'-1)$, from the equation used to calculate power. Recently the term 'dioptric curvature' has been used to describe videokeratoscope power maps;[11,12] however, this use of the term appears to be incorrect by current and historical definitions.

Measurement of curvature requires a high degree of accuracy. As shown in Figure 6.2, a 50 micron change in radius of curvature for a spherical surface from 7.8 mm to 7.85 mm will induce more than a one-quarter diopter shift in power (43.27 to 42.99 D). Because the functional relationship between power and radius of curvature is non-linear, care must be taken when estimating the power shift for a change in corneal radius, such as with certain keratorefractive procedures. The powers present on a pathological or surgically altered cornea may have a range of 30 D or more, and can vary appreciably across even relatively small distances on the cornea, e.g. near wound margins.

BASIC SHAPE OF THE CORNEA

Historically, corneas have been referred to with spherical, ellipsoidal, parabolic, and hyperbolic profiles, although in reality, these surfaces can only approximate the complex shape of an actual cornea. Nevertheless, surfaces modeled with these conic sections are quite useful for designing and testing corneal topography algorithms.[13]

Since the late 1800s, normal corneas have been said to have a spherical 'apical cap' (also referred to

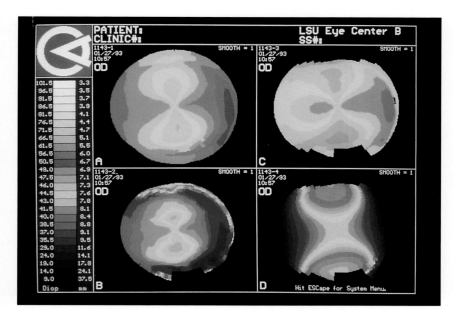

Figure 6.4 *Videokeratograph of with-the-rule astigmatism. Custom display with absolute color scale derived from the Computed Anatomy TMS-1 instrument. Upper left map: normal TMS-1 dioptric power display; lower left map: instantaneous radius of curvature algorithm; upper right: refractive power algorithm; lower right: elevation algorithm.*

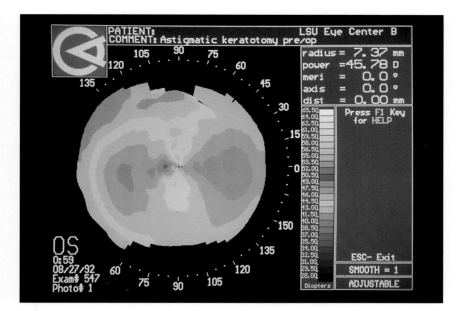

Figure 6.5 *Videokeratograph of against-the-rule astigmatism. Computed Anatomy TMS-1 display in the absolute scale showing a typical case of astigmatism with cylinder power oriented along the horizontal axis.*

as the corneal cap or apical zone) approximately 4 mm in diameter,[14–16] which roughly corresponds to what we refer to as the optical zone of the cornea under normal lighting conditions. The term optical zone has not been consistently applied, but historically it is the corneal region encompassing the cone of rays passing from the point of fixation and through the entrance pupil.[2,17–20] In recent years, the term optical zone also has been used to define the clear zone in radial keratotomy procedures, and the region demarcated by the treated ablation zone in photorefractive keratectomy procedures.[21–23]

MERIDIONAL SHAPE

Corneal toricity is the primary source of ocular astigmatism (Fig. 6.3).[1–4] Astigmatism tends to become an important refractive problem when the cylinder component has a magnitude of 1.5 D or greater. The

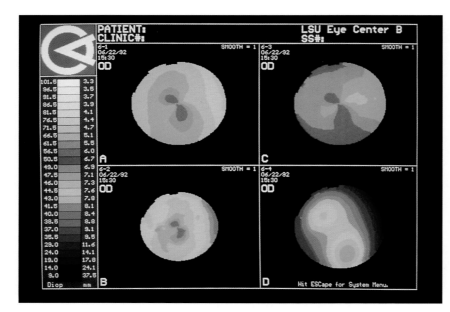

Figure 6.6 *Videokeratograph of irregular astigmatism in a mild keratoconus case. Note the evidence of cylinder power; however, the form has a lazy-8 appearance in the contour map, rather than a true orthogonal orientation of the axes. (Custom display with absolute color scale derived from the Computed Anatomy TMS-1 instrument). Upper left map: normal TMS-1 dioptric power display; lower left map: instantaneous radius of curvature algorithm; upper right: refractive power algorithm; lower right: elevation algorithm.*

most common form of corneal astigmatism is the regular form,[3] with the high- and low-powered principal axes orthogonally arranged, and with either the steep axis within ±15 degrees of the vertical axis (with-the-rule), or within ±15 degrees of the horizontal axis (against-the-rule) (Figs 6.4 and 6.5). Oblique astigmatism occurs with an orthogonal arrangement of the axes and meridional orientations approaching ±45 degrees.

Meridional astigmatic change from with-the-rule to against-the-rule appears to be age dependent, with the newborn exhibiting a large range of astigmatic errors that settle into with-the-rule astigmatism lasting into the fourth decade of life.[24–26] Older adults beyond the age of 50 tend to exhibit increasing amounts of against-the-rule astigmatism.[24–26] The mechanism for this change remains unknown; however, external forces such as eyelid pressure, have been shown to affect corneal toricity.[27–29] For these reasons, manipulating the eyelids during videokeratoscopy should be avoided.

While regular corneal astigmatism can be corrected by cylindrical optics, irregular astigmatism with non-orthogonally arranged axes cannot. Also, some forms of irregular astigmatism exhibit refractive variation along any given meridian, as well as a loss of axial symmetry. Irregular astigmatism is often a consequence of corneal disease, ocular trauma, penetrating keratoplasty, refractive surgical procedures, or corneal warpage from an improperly fitted contact lens (Fig. 6.6).

CONSEQUENCES OF AN OFF-AXIS VISUAL SYSTEM

Corneal topography analysis has been complicated by the aspherical/asymmetrical shape of the eye in which the nasal hemisphere is smaller than the temporal half.[30] This alone may impart the need for a flatter nasal corneal periphery often seen in videokeratographs (Fig. 6.7). In the typical human eye, the fovea is offset approximately 1 mm temporally relative to the posterior pole and 1.8 mm inferiorly to compensate for the nasally oriented insertion of the optic nerve (Fig. 6.8).[30]

Consequently, the major axis of symmetry of the normal cornea's anatomical or optical profile is not coincident with any axis of sight which can be defined to pass from the fixation point to the fovea. This also raises the question concerning the frame of reference by which corneal topography should be defined: centered with respect to a foveal vision-related axis, or centered with respect to an anatomical or optical axis of symmetry. Psychophysical studies have shown that because of the Stiles–Crawford effect of retinal photoreceptor orientation, visual performance is optimized for rays traveling near the center of the pupil.[9,31,32] Therefore, surgical procedures should be centered with respect to the line of sight which passes through the center of the entrance pupil as defined in the following section.[17] Logically, it follows that corneal topographic analysis that involves an evaluation of

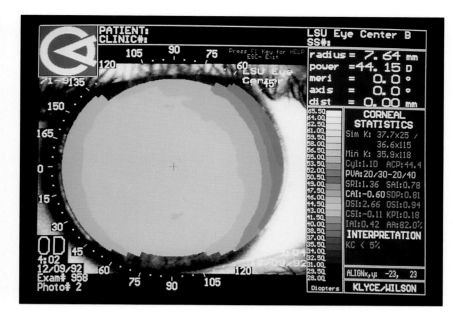

Figure 6.7 *Videokeratograph of a typical normal cornea. Computed Anatomy TMS-1 display in the absolute scale. Note the tendency for cooler contour colors at the extreme nasal edge of the map.*

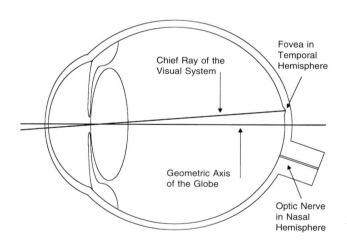

Figure 6.8 *Highly schematic cross-sectional view of the right eye (as seen superiorly). The lateral offset of the fovea relative to the geometric axis of the globe and the optic axis of the eye (schematically identical to the geometric axis) causes the chief ray or line of sight of the visual system to lie along a different axis and intersect the cornea at a slightly nasal position.*

visual potential should similarly be analyzed at or near the line of sight. In order to understand this issue more fully, a brief review of the cardinal points and axes of the eye, and their relationship to videokeratoscopy, is presented in the following section.

AXES OF THE EYE AND VIDEOKERATOSCOPY

The *optic axis* of the eye is defined as the best-fitting, theoretical line coincident with the centers of curvature of the anterior and posterior surfaces of the cornea and crystalline lens (Fig. 6.9).[33] In the theoretical schematic eye, this is an easily definable line, but in reality, the optic axis cannot be readily determined.

The optic axis of the eye may be estimated by the optic axis of the anterior corneal surface alone. However, the optic axis of a single spherical surface is undefined unless the center of the system's aperture is also specified.[4] Thus, in the case of the cornea, the optic axis can be defined by the line from the center of curvature of the surface and the center of the entrance pupil. The entrance pupil is the virtual image of the real pupil when viewed by refraction through the cornea and, consequently, it appears larger and closer to the cornea than the real pupil.

This definition of the optic axis of the anterior corneal surface is identical to that used for the pupillary axis (Fig. 6.10).[19,33] In fact, the *pupillary axis* is often used to estimate the optic axis of the eye; however, one should be cautious about applying this definition with decentered pupils. Normally, the orientation of the pupillary axis does vary slightly with dilation of the pupil,[34,35] and perhaps with the accommodative state of the eye due to unequal

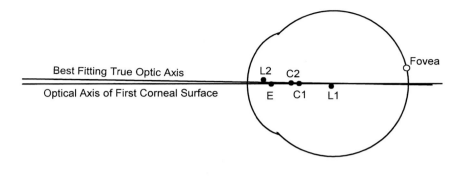

Figure 6.9 *Schematic illustration of the true optic axis of the eye which is a best-fitting line passing through the centers of curvature of the anterior and posterior corneal surfaces (C1, C2, respectively) and the anterior and posterior crystalline lens surfaces (L1 and L2, respectively). The optic axis of the eye can be estimated by the line passing through the center of the entrance pupil, E, and C1, which would make the axis perpendicular to the anterior corneal surface.*

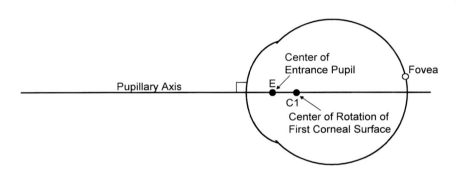

Figure 6.10 *Schematic illustration of the pupillary axis. The definition of the pupillary axis is the same as the estimated optic axis using the center of the entrance pupil, E, and the center of curvature of the anterior corneal surface, C1. Note that it does not pass through the fovea at the retina.*

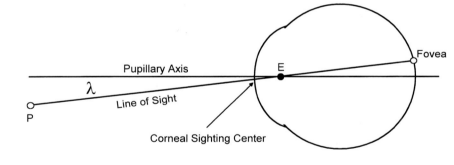

Figure 6.11 *Schematic diagram of the line of sight and its relationship to the pupillary axis. The line of sight is the line passing from the fixation point (P) to the center of the entrance pupil (E). It is assumed that if the subject is normally fixating, the line extends to the fovea. The intersection with the anterior corneal surface is the corneal sighting center. The angle between the pupillary axis and the line of sight is angle lambda (λ).*

torsional forces placed on the iris through the actions of the ciliary muscle.

The *line of sight* joins the center of the entrance pupil with the point of fixation, and therefore is the chief ray formed when a patient aligns a fixation point image onto the fovea (Fig. 6.11).[33] Consequently, a blur circle image formed at the fovea will have the line of sight passing through its center. The intersection of the line of sight with the anterior corneal surface has been called the *corneal sighting*

center.[5] The angle formed between the line of sight and the pupillary axis is angle lambda (λ).

The eye's *geometric axis* is defined as the line passing through the anterior and posterior poles of the eye (Fig. 6.12).[33] As the posterior pole is inaccessible in vivo, the axis can be defined as the line passing through the anterior pole and perpendicular to the best-fitting episcleral plane; however, this is more akin to a definition for the geometric axis of the cornea alone. Normally, the anterior pole is deter-

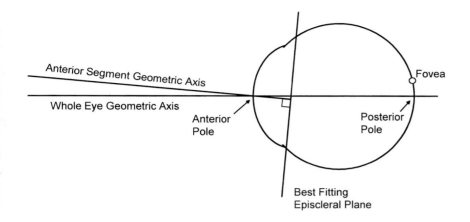

Figure 6.12 *Determining a geometric axis for the eye. Some corneal survey instruments may be aligned with an axis other than the line of sight. The geometric axis of the eye is defined as the line passing through the anterior and posterior poles of the eye. As the posterior pole is inaccessible in the living eye, the axis may be estimated by the line perpendicular to the best-fitting episcleral plane (here greatly exaggerated as being tilted), and passing though the anterior pole. The geometric axis does not align with the fovea.*

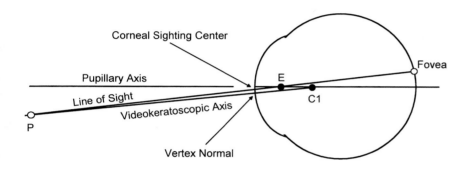

Figure 6.13 *Alignment of the videokeratoscope to the cornea. The videokeratoscopic axis is the optical axis of the video system and central point of the mire pattern for Placido-disk targets. When the patient fixates on point P in the videokeratoscope, the line of sight tends to be slightly lateral to the videokeratoscopic axis. This is because for even illumination of the mire image, the videokeratoscopic axis must pass through the center of curvature of the anterior corneal surface (C1) and not the center of the entrance pupil (E). The intersection of the videokeratoscopic axis with the cornea is the vertex normal.*

mined by the corneal apex which has been variously defined as the point of maximum corneal curvature,[36] the anterior-most point of the cornea when the eye is in the primary anatomic position,[30] and the geometric center of the apical cap.[37]

Whichever definition is chosen for the apex, if it is decentered toward a peripheral location as in cases of advanced keratoconus, defining the geometric axis becomes problematic. This may be significant in future videokeratoscope algorithms that attempt to use a frame of reference situated about the geometric axis or a similar axisymmetric point of the cornea, rather than a sight-based axis.

The geometric center of the cornea has been defined as the point where the longest horizontal and vertical surface arc lengths intersect;[37,38] however, this point does not necessarily correspond to the geometric center of the apical cap, to the corneal apex, or to the intersection of the geometric axis with the cornea. It is obvious that due to the multitude of definitions and the confusion of terms, one must be explicit when communicating new analytical methods in videokeratoscopy.

The *videokeratoscopic axis* is defined by the optical axis of the videokeratoscope camera when it is aligned normal to the cornea (Fig. 6.13).[5] Typically this is done in conjunction with the subjective align-

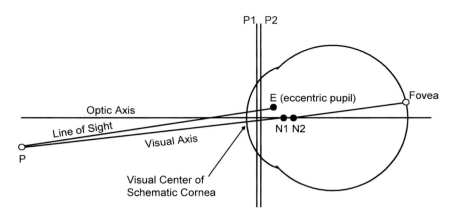

Figure 6.14 *Schematic illustration of the visual axis used exclusively for ray tracing. The visual axis is defined as the line connecting the fixation point (P) to the fovea, and passing through the nodal points (N1, N2) of the entire reduced optical system of the eye. The line may be segmented if N1 and N2 are not coaligned, which depends on the parameters chosen for the optical elements of the eye. The nodal point positions are determined by the location of the principal planes for light entering or leaving the eye (P1, P2), and the unskewed line passing from the fixation point to the fovea (the line may be broken at the nodal points, but the segments are parallel in space to one another). The intersection with the schematic anterior corneal position is called the visual center. The visual axis is not co-linear with the line of sight.*

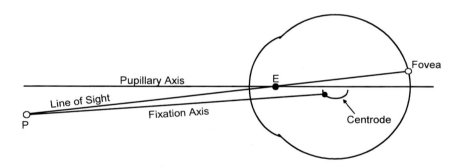

Figure 6.15 *Schematic diagram of the fixation axis. The fixation axis is defined by the fixation point (P) and the instantaneous center of rotation of the globe. As the eye traverses different visual directions in space through the actions of the extraocular muscles, the globe translates slightly in space. If a corneal measurement is fixed relative to space but the eye is free to translate, locations on the corneal surface could be erroneously calculated. This effect is not significant with videokeratoscopes, but historically, topogometers and similar devices analyzed corneal topography using eye rotations.*

ment of the patient's line of sight with the instrument fixation point. Note that the center of curvature of the cornea does not ordinarily coincide with the center of the entrance pupil. Therefore, the line of sight will tend to be slightly displaced temporally from the videokeratoscopic axis.[5] The significance of this in clinical use is probably minor[39] and may be within the range of acceptability of clinical accuracy. The point at which the videokeratoscopic axis intersects the cornea has been called the *vertex normal*.[40]

The *visual axis* is a theoretical line derived for ray tracing with schematic eye models having Gaussian (spherical) optics. It is defined as a line connecting the fixation point with the first nodal point of the eye's reduced visual system, and continuing from the second nodal point to the center of the fovea (Fig. 6.14).[4] Correct application of the visual axis depends on whether rays are being traced into or out of the schematic eye. The two nodal points may or may not be coincident, depending on the dimensions of the ocular parameters chosen in the model. The point at which the visual axis intersects the schematic cornea has been called the *visual center*.[4] Angle kappa (κ) designates the angle formed between the visual axis and the pupillary axis.

Use of the visual axis is generally irrelevant for issues dealing with videokeratoscopy or refractive procedures in real eyes, with the exception of ray tracing based on corneal topography data. Unfortunately, the term visual axis has, in recent years, taken on a generic meaning, and has been used in reference to any number of axes associated with the eye, including the optic, pupillary, geometric, and videokeratoscopic axes, as well as the line of sight. Often, this incorrect usage leads to erroneous conclusions.

The *fixation axis* joins the point of fixation and the center of rotation of the globe (Fig. 6.15).[41] The center of rotation is defined by a centroid or locus of points referred to historically as a centrode, which is determined by the transverse slippage of the globe in the orbit during rotational eye movements. This slippage may induce analytical errors when off-axis keratoscopy or topogometry is used (i.e. patient fixation of peripherally displaced targets), unless some trigonometric compensation is applied to the shifting center of rotation.

VIDEOKERATOSCOPE ALIGNMENT

Some users of videokeratoscopes, particularly those with instruments based on elevation measurement, have suggested that topographic analysis be displayed or acquired relative to the geometric or optic axis of the eye, or the corneal apex. While the corneal sighting center of the line of sight is closely estimated by the location of the vertex normal of the videokeratoscopic axis, transposing the topographic map from the vertex normal to the corneal apex or any other location needs careful verification of the accuracy of this extrapolation. Furthermore, besides the difficulty of determining the true location of the

apex, the issue of the best definition of the apex remains unresolved. Whichever definition is used, analysis of grossly asymmetrical corneas, as in advanced non-central keratoconus or with postoperative keratoplasty must be dealt with in a consistent and thoroughly reliable manner.

Furthermore, whichever method is adopted for topographical analysis, the corneal surgical procedures require proper centration of the clear optical zone with respect to the center of the entrance pupil. This centration is best achieved using the definition of the line of sight, which can be objectively determined in a clinical situation. The visual axis cannot be objectively determined, as it is a theoretical axis that can only be estimated with difficulty for a living eye. Uozato and Guyton have clearly and carefully reviewed the methods by which centration can be determined in a surgical setting, and have provided useful recommendations.[19]

MEASUREMENT TECHNIQUES

DEFINITIONS

All measurements can be defined by their resolution, accuracy, precision, and in some instances, repeatability or reproducibility. *Resolution* is the ability to discern the relative location of two discrete data points. In the case of videokeratoscopy, this typically entails spatially resolving the location of mire image points along ring edges or centers. The success of this operation depends in large measure on the quality of the video camera optics and the pixel density of the charge-coupled device (CCD) camera. Image processing techniques also can be applied to improve the detectability of mire reflections, and it is generally necessary to interpolate mire image point co-ordinates with subpixel resolution.

Videokeratoscopic resolution also refers to the scaled, transduced measure of the cornea expressed in diopters of power, millimeters of radius of curvature, or micrometers of surface elevation. These values may reflect contamination by mathematically amplified processing errors. Thus, a system touted as having high-resolution video sampling is not a guarantee that the system also has an accurate display.

Accuracy is the correspondence of the measured result to physical reality. Determining the accuracy of a system requires validating the obtained value against an independent standard, preferably by a different measurement principle. For example, interferometry-based systems may be useful in establishing the surface profiles of calibration targets with high precision.

Verifying the accuracy of videokeratoscopes requires aspherical calibration targets with curvatures spanning a range of corneal powers and eccentricities, and made to precise standards in testing.[42–45] In some cases, algorithms are tested using computer-generated files that represent mathematical models of corneal surfaces.

Precision is the exactness of a dimensional measure. The more significant digits we can confidently associate with a measure, the higher the precision. Care must be exercised to avoid overestimating precision by mathematical manipulation of the data. The level of precision that can be expressed is limited in large part by the resolution of the measurement standard. Whether or not high precision can be achieved depends on many factors including the focal length of the videokeratoscope optical system, the dimensions of the mire image, and the resolving power of the camera, as well as a number of other factors.

Although the ability to measure precision is limited by the resolution of the system, precision theoretically can be improved by statistical means using multiple measures of the same surface to account for measurement noise.[43–46] However, there are no commercially available instruments that use *repeatability* of videokeratoscopic measures as a means to improve precision and accuracy in a clinical setting.

NOISE

Measurement noise can come from a number of sources in videokeratoscopy, but generally these are of minor importance provided care is exercised in acquiring the image. A high ambient light level in the examination room can lower image contrast of the mire pattern and thus its detectability. This may be particularly true for some non-Placido videokeratoscopes that directly image diffuse reflections from the corneal surface, and for patients with lightly pigmented irides. Measurement noise also can be introduced by patient eye movements or by the operator's incorrect focusing and alignment technique. Operators should visually verify the quality of the analysis to screen out potential noise problems. Poorly engineered or maintained instruments may be more prone to wear of their mechanical parts, and thus more difficult to align and focus

over time. Interferometric systems such as holographic-based instruments tend to be particularly suspectable to motion due to the high degree of precision needed in the wavefront transduction process.[47–48]

Instruments also can lose calibration, or perhaps were never correctly calibrated by the manufacturer or operator prior to being put into service. Unfortunately, due to the numerous variations in videokeratoscope design and because many aspects of the algorithm designs are proprietary, an in-depth discussion of errors in transduction from the captured video image into corneal curvature or power is not possible here.

DIRECT MEASUREMENT OF THE CORNEA

A healthy cornea is a tissue that is highly transparent to wavelengths between 400 and 700 nm. As the cornea is normally a specular surface with little diffuse scattering of incident light, the surface is difficult to view directly. The term *specular* refers to the tendency of reflected light rays to be directed away from the surface normal at an angle equal in magnitude and opposite in direction to that traveled by the incident ray. Therefore, very precise orientations of an external light source (or mire) and the viewer's eye (or camera) must be arranged in accordance with the principle of optical reflection in order to visualize the virtual image of the surface. This method is the principle behind the Placido disk technology that projects a known mire pattern onto the corneal surface and analyzes the reflected image for distortions that can be attributed to surface shape.

Due to the clarity of the corneal tissue, some non-Placido disk methods that use direct measurement of surface position are difficult to apply. For example, holography may require a long-duration exposure due to the inefficiency of the recording medium.[47–48] This is in contrast to the transparency of the cornea and the need for short exposure times due to the motion sensitivity of a wavefront interference technique. One argument used in favor of holography and other direct surface imaging techniques has been that direct imaging of the corneal surface can be used even with diffusely reflecting corneas or corneas lacking an intact epithelium.[47–53] Because of the weak diffuse reflectance of the corneal surface, many direct imaging techniques also require the addition of a diffusing agent to the tear film, such as topical fluorescein.[49–53] It has been assumed that fluorescein instilled in the tear film layer has the same

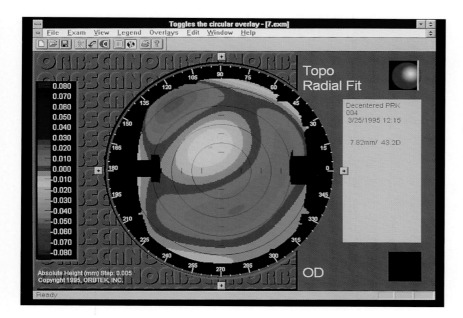

Figure 6.16 *ORBSCAN analysis of a postoperative photorefractive keratectomy cornea. The display shows absolute height in 0.005 mm color scale steps, relative to a base sphere with a 7.82 mm radius of curvature. Depressions are indicated by warm colors. (Courtesy Orbtek Inc.)*

surface cohesion and produces the same topography characteristics as the normal tear film layer; however, a study using artificial tears before videokeratoscopy has shown statistically significant changes in surface regularity in both normal and postoperative keratoplasty corneas.[54]

ELEVATION MEASUREMENT

An emerging area of topography analysis has been the use of surface elevation maps, which have been said to be a true representation of corneal topography as opposed to a derivative form (Fig. 6.16).[55] However, pure elevation cannot be used to display most clinically significant information, because elevation is relatively insensitive to optically significant surface features. Consequently, all systems that use elevation actually must display a map of the *relative change in elevation* by subtracting a spherical component from the data. There are currently no standards by which one selects a best-fit sphere component; presumably it might be based on the mean power over some predetermined surface area, such as the area encompassed by the optical zone, or based on the entire analyzed area.

Important issues about standardizing the color-coded scale of elevation maps remain subject to debate and change. If color is standardized to eleva-

tion relative to a mean sphere, and the scale is normalized to the residual range, then the scale will not be consistent from map to map. This is similar to the comparison difficulties that occur with user-adjustable or self-adapting normalized scales with dioptric maps, as opposed to a fixed scale. Thus, it may be necessary to standardize multiple absolute elevation scales if we wish to compare maps: one that is color-coded to specific elevation change independent of the mean elevation, and one that tracks change, but is also color-coded to the mean elevation.

Another potential problem is standardizing the elevation maps to be somewhat more consistent with expectations derived from the color spectrum displayed on dioptric maps. At least one current elevation display shows depressed areas with hot colors and elevated regions with cool colors.[55] This may be confusing when comparing the display to a dioptric power map in which hot colors refer to steep areas and cool colors to relatively flat areas. Although slope is not the same as elevation, it can seem odd to users of slope-based videokeratoscopes that a keratoconus cone may appear blue in an elevation map rather than red.

One interesting characteristic of the elevation map is that it appears to be very useful for acquiring surface-shape-related indices, although whether there will be any significant advantage over the current

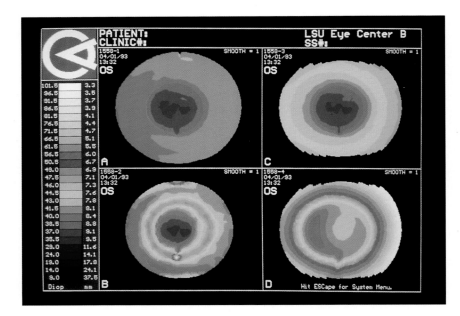

Figure 6.17 *Postoperative photorefractive keratectomy cornea on a custom display with absolute color scale derived from the Computed Anatomy TMS-1 instrument. Upper left map: normal TMS-1 dioptric power display; lower left map: instantaneous radius of curvature algorithm; upper right: refractive power algorithm; lower right: elevation algorithm.*

Placido disk-based indices remains to be determined. Furthermore, if the elevation map is transposed away from the corneal sighting center to the corneal apex or some other axis reflecting corneal symmetry, there may actually be some decrement in the performance of the vision-related indices that have proven useful for clinical applications. However, again this is speculative and remains subject to experimental verification.

Despite the obvious utility of elevation maps in some important applications, such as contact lens fitting and keratoconus shape analysis, general clinical use demands that dioptric power map displays remain available. Dioptric power maps provide an excellent means of assessing potential visual performance, particularly when the map is centered at or near the line of sight.

MODERN VIDEOKERATOSCOPE TECHNOLOGY

Radial keratotomy was the primary driving force in the early development and production of videokeratoscopy. In 1988, the first true videokeratoscope, the

Computed Anatomy Corneal Modeling System (CMS) was made commercially available[56–57] using the color-coded map display developed at LSU Eye Center.[58] This implementation revolutionized the entire field of corneal topography analysis. The Computed Anatomy CMS was the predecessor of the more powerful TMS-1 videokeratoscope (Tomey Technology, Cambridge, Massachusetts) introduced in 1990. The Computed Anatomy videokeratoscope was soon followed by the EyeSys (EyeSys Technologies, Houston, Texas)[43] and Visioptic (now the EH-290 Eyemap, Alcon Labs, Fort Worth, Texas)[59] systems in 1989. A rasterstereographer made its debut as a research instrument in 1988,[53] but this technique, which uses direct imaging and triangulation of grid patterns projected onto the cornea, has never enjoyed the popularity of the Placido disk systems. A commercial unit is available as the PAR Corneal Topography System from PAR Vision Systems Corporation, New Hartford, New York. Similarly, holography based topography systems have not proven as popular as the Placido disk instruments, possibly due to the way topography is displayed as a wavefront error, which differs considerably from the displays of most commercial instruments. A commercial holographic system, the KM-CLAS-1000, is available from Kera-Metrics Inc, Solana Beach,

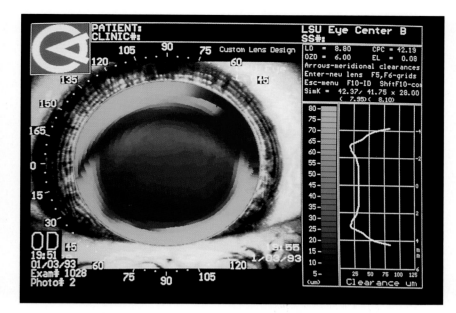

Figure 6.18 *Fluorescein staining modeled on the Computed Anatomy TMS-1 videokeratoscope. The clearance map is on the left of the figure with the staining hue scale adjacent to the main map. Note the significant amount of prior contact lens-induced warpage on this cornea, with a significant edge effect from the 9 o'clock to 3 o'clock positions.*

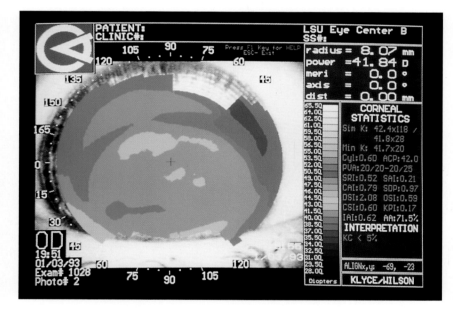

Figure 6.19 *Contact lens-induced corneal warpage. This Computed Anatomy TMS-1 videokeratoscope map was produced from the cornea shown in Figure 6.18. Note that the prior wear of a low-riding contact lens produced a flattening effect from the 9 o'clock to 3 o'clock positions. The irregular astigmatism index (IAI) has a high value of 0.75.*

California. The ORBSCAN is a relatively new instrument available from Orbtek, Inc., Salt Lake City, Utah. The ORBSCAN uses a scanning slit technology coupled to eye tracking to derive surface elevation and pachymetry. This methodology appears promising, particularly if more analytical features are incorporated into the device, such as precise tracking of the entrance pupil margin location.

Videokeratoscopes have undergone considerable refinement since their introduction, with greatly improved speed, algorithms, and user add-on utilities of clinical and surgical interest now available. The expansion of keratorefractive procedures into laser-based methodologies, such as photorefractive keratectomy (Fig. 6.17), has further expanded the marketplace. Whereas contact lens fitting made do

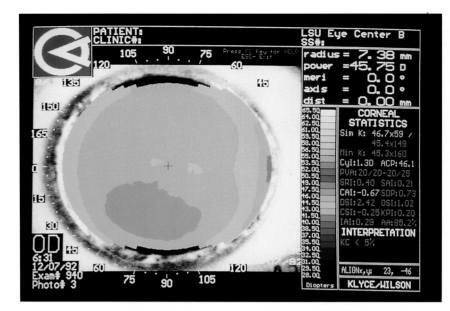

Figure 6.20 *Contact lens-induced corneal warpage. This Computed Anatomy TMS-1 videokeratoscope map shows a different form of lens-induced warpage with a localized high-powered region situated inferiorly. Note that only the center-surround index (CSI) is slightly non-normal with a cautionary yellow indicator.*

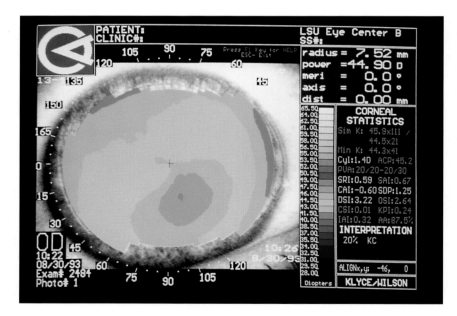

Figure 6.21 *Mild keratoconus. Compare this map to the one shown in Figure 6.20. Note the localized region of high corneal power situated inferiorly. Unlike the contact lens-induced corneal warpage case, this map shows a number of cautionary and abnormal corneal statistics. The keratoconus interpretation package of the TMS-1 videokeratoscope indicates a 20% likelihood of similarity to a typical case of keratoconus.*

with the simple keratometer in the past, some videokeratoscopes now provide simulation of fluorescein patterns for contact lens fitting (Fig. 6.18).[60] The videokeratoscope has also been found to be an excellent means of determining whether contact lens-induced corneal warpage exists, and observing its regression with the cessation of lens wear (Fig. 6.19).[61,62] Some forms of lens warpage resemble early keratoconus, and serial videokeratoscopy helps to make the distinction between keratoconus suspects and corneal warpage (Figs 6.20, 6.21).[62–64] Videokeratoscopy now makes extensive use of map-derived numerical indices to interpret a variety of corneal conditions for a higher success rate in clinical and surgical management.[65–67]

CONCLUSIONS

Videokeratoscopy is a continuously evolving technology which has yet to achieve its final form. Important issues remain unresolved in the minds of many users, and whether the non-Placido image instruments will achieve the same popularity as the Placido image instruments may be determined over the next several years. Controversies concerning the preferred method of analysis and display may never be resolved, and it appears likely that multiple analytical techniques and displays will be incorporated into these instruments.

Future uses of videokeratoscopy may include improved methods for contact lens fitting, expert systems for surface pattern interpretation, and real-time instruments that allow topographic analysis during surgical procedures. Research into topographic change over time in diseased, contact lens warped, and surgically altered corneas may provide new insight into surface anomalies. In 1995, Smolek introduced time-lapse videokeratoscopy to generate animations of the changing shape of the cornea based on historically acquired data.[68] This technology showed, for example, the stability of the cone apex position in keratoconus progression, and the instability of the ablation zone shape in postoperative photorefractive keratectomy corneas, even years after the procedure. It is clear that the science and technology of videokeratoscopy is still on the move and open to fresh ideas, and will involve ever-expanding roles and enhanced technology for many years to come.

REFERENCES

1. Fincham WHA, Freeman MH, Curvature: refraction at a curved surface, In: Fincham WHA, Freeman MH, eds, *Optics*, 9th edn (Butterworths: London, 1980) 61–83.
2. Gullstrand A, Optical imagery, In: Southall JPC, ed, *Helmholtz's Treatise on Physiological Optics*. Vol. I , Appendix I, (Dover Publications: New York, 1962) 261–300.
3. Michaels DD, Geometric Optics, In: *Visual Optics and Refraction, A Clinical Approach*, (CV Mosby: St. Louis, 1985) 25–55.
4. Bennett AG, Francis, Optical systems in general, In: Davson H, ed, The Eye, Vol 4, *Visual Optics and the Optical Space Sense*, (Academic Press: New York, 1962) 57–74.
5. Mandell RB, The enigma of the corneal contour, *CLAO J* (1992) **18**:267–73.
6. Klein SA, A corneal topography algorithm that produces continuous curvature, *Optom Vis Sci* (1992) **69**:829–34.
7. Klein SA, Mandell RB, Shape and refractive powers in corneal topography, *Invest Ophthalmol Vis Sci* (1995) **36**:2096–109.
8. Roberts C, The accuracy of 'power' maps to display curvature data in corneal topography systems, *Invest Ophthalmol Vis Sci* (1994) **35**:3525-32.
9. Stiles WS, Crawford BH, The luminous efficiency of rays entering the eye pupil at different points, *Proc R Soc Lond (Biol)* (1933) **112**:428–50.
10. Klyce SD, Computer-assisted corneal topography: high resolution graphical presentation and analysis of keratoscopy, *Invest Ophthalmol Vis Sci* (1984) **25**:1426–35.
11. Salmon TO, Horner DG, Comparison of surface elevation, dioptric curvature and refractive power maps of an elliptical cornea, *Invest Ophthalmol Vis Sci* (1995) *Suppl* **36**:s1032.
12. Chan WK, Carones F, Maloney RK, Corneal topographic maps: A comparison of axial curvature with true instantaneous curvature, *Invest Ophthalmol Vis Sci Suppl* (1995) **36**:s1032.
13. Roberts C, Cui D, Comparison of axial and instantaneous curvature topographic reconstructions on surfaces with complicated curvature profiles, *Invest Ophthalmol Vis Sci Suppl* (1995) **36**:s379.
14. Soper JW, Sampson WG, Girard LJ, Corneal topography, keratometry, and contact lenses, *Arch Ophthalmol* (1962) **67**:753–60.
15. Mandell RB, St Helen R, Stability of the corneal contour, *Am J Optom* (1969) **45**:797–806.
16. Clark BA, Mean topography of normal corneas, *Aust J Optom* (1974) **57**:65–9.
17. Waring GO, Making sense of keratospeak II: Proposed conventional terminology for corneal topography, *Refract Corneal Surg* (1989) **5**:362–7.
18. Duke-Elder S, Abrams D, The dioptric imagery of the eye, In: Duke-Elder S, ed, *System of Ophthalmology, Vol V, Ophthalmic Optics and Refraction*, (Henry Kimpton: London 1970) 93–152.
19. Uozato H, Guyton DL, Centering corneal surgical procedures, *Am J Ophthalmol* (1987) **103**:264–75.
20. Roberts CW, Koester CJ, Optical zone diameters for photorefractive corneal surgery, *Invest Ophthalmol Vis Sci* (1993) **34**:2275–81.
21. Cavanaugh TB, Durrie DS, Riedel SM, et al, Topographical analysis of the centration of excimer laser photorefractive keratectomy, *J Cataract Refract Surg* (1993) **19**:136–43.
22. Cavanaugh TB, Durrie DS, Riedel SM, et al, Centration of excimer laser photorefractive keratectomy relative to the pupil, *J Cataract Refract Surg* (1993) **19**:144–8.
23. Klyce SD, Smolek MK, Corneal topography of excimer laser photorefractive keratectomy, *J Cataract Refract Surg* (1993) **19**:122–30.
24. Vihlen FS, Wilson G, The relation between eyelid tension, corneal toricity, and age, *Invest Ophthalmol Vis Sci* (1983) **24**:1367–73.
25. Hayashi K, Matsumoto M, Fujino S, Hayashi F, Changes in corneal astigmatism with aging, *Nippon Ganka Gakkai: Zasshi* (1993) **97**:1193–96.
26. Kame RC, Jue TS, Shigekuni DM, A longitudinal study of

corneal astigmatism changes in Asian eyes, *J Am Optom Assoc* (1993) **64**:215–19.

27. Nisted M, Hofstetter HW, Effect of chalazion on astigmatism, *Am J Optom Physiol Opt* (1974) **51**:579–82.

28. Mandell RB, Bilateral monocular diplopia following near work, *Am J Optom Physiol Opt* (1966) **43**:500–4.

29. Knoll HA, Bilateral monocular diplopia after near work, *Am J Optom Physiol Opt* (1974) **52**:139–40.

30. Hogan MJ, Alvarado JA, Weddell JE, Eyeball, In: Hogan MJ, Alvarado JA, Weddell JE, eds, *Histology of the Human Eye*, (WB Saunders: Philadelphia, 1971) 45–54.

31. Van Loo JA, Enoch JM, The scotopic Stiles–Crawford effect, *Vision Res* (1975) **15**:1005–9.

32. Enoch JM, Laties AM, An analysis of retinal receptor orientation II. Prediction for psychophysical tests, *Invest Ophthalmol* (1971) **10**:959–70.

33. Cline D, Hofstetter HW, Griffin JR, *Dictionary of Visual Science*, 3rd edn, (Chilton Book Company: Radnor, 1980).

34. Fay AM, Trokel SL, Myers JA, Pupil diameter and the principal ray, *J Cataract Refract Surg* (1992) **18**:348–51.

35. Walsh G, The effect of mydriasis on the pupillary centration of the human eye, *Ophthal Physiol Opt* (1988) **8**:178–82.

36. Mandell RB, Corneal topography, In: Mandell RB ed, *Contact Lens Practice: Basic and Advanced*, (Charles C. Thomas: Springfield, 1965) 35–51.

37. Girard LJ, Nomenclature of corneal contact lenses, In: Girard LJ, Soper JW, Sampson WG, eds, *Corneal Contact Lenses* 2nd edn, (CV Mosby: St. Louis, 1970) 1–11.

38. Rowsey JJ, Corneal topography, In: Dabezies OH, ed, *Contact lenses — The CLAO Guide to Basic Science and Clinical Practice*, (Grune and Stratton: Orlando, 1984) 4.1–4.8.

39. Mandell RB, Klein CS, Chiang LY, Alignment effects in videokeratography, *Invest Ophthalmol Vis Sci Suppl* (1995) **36**:S379.

40. Maloney RK, Corneal topography and optical zone location in photorefractive keratectomy, *Refract Corneal Surg* (1990) **6**:363–71.

41. Alpern M, Specification of the direction of regard, In: Davson H, ed, *The Eye. Vol. 3, Muscular Mechanisms*, (Academic Press, New York, 1969) 5–12.

42. Hannush SB, Crawford SL, Waring GO III, et al, Accuracy and precision of keratometry, photokeratoscopy, and corneal modeling on calibrated steel balls, *Arch Ophthalmol* (1989) **107**:1235–39.

43. Koch DD, Foulks GN, Moran T, Wakil J, The corneal EyeSys system: accuracy, analysis and reproducibility of first generation prototype, *Refract Corneal Surg* (1989) **107**:1235–9.

44. Koch DD, Wakil JS, Samuelson SW, Haft EA, Comparison of the accuracy and reproducibility of the keratometer and the EyeSys Corneal Analysis System Model 1, *J Cataract Refract Surg* (1992) **18**:342–7.

45. Wilson SE, Verity SM, Conger DL, Accuracy and Precision of the Corneal Analysis System, and the Topographic Modeling System, *Cornea* (1992) **11**:28–35.

46. Hannush SB, Crawford SL, Waring GO III, et al, Reproducibilty of normal corneal power measurements with a keratometer, photokeratoscope, and video imaging system, *Arch Ophthalmol* (1990) **108**:539–44.

47. Baker PC, Holographic contour analysis of the cornea, In

Masters BR, ed, *Noninvasive Diagnostic Techniques in Ophthalmology* (Springer–Verlag: New York 1990) 82–98.

48. Friedlander MH, Mulet M, Buzard K, et al, Holographic interferometry of the corneal surface, *SPIE 1991; Ophthalmic Technologies* (1991) **1432**:62–9.

49. Berlin MW, Cambier JL, Nabors JR, PAR Corneal Topography System, In: Gills JP, Sanders DR, Thornton SP et al, *Corneal Topography The State of the Art*, (Slack: Thorofare, 1995) 105–22.

50. Berlin MW, Litoff D, Strods SJ, et al, The PAR Technology Corneal Topography System, *Refract Corneal Surg* (1992) **8**:88–96.

51. Arffa RC, Warnicki JW, Rehkopf PG, Corneal topography using rasterstereography, *Refract Corneal Surg* (1989) **5**:414–7.

52. Belin MW, Intraoperative raster photogrammetry — the PAR Corneal Topography System, *J Cataract Refract Surg Suppl* (1993) **19**:188–92.

53. Warnicki JW, Rehkopf PG, Curtin SA, et al, Corneal topography using computer analyzed rasterstereographic images, *Appl Opt* (1988) **27**:1135–40.

54. Pavlopoulos GP, Horn J, Feldman SJ, The effect of artificial tears on computer-assisted corneal topography in normal eyes and after penetrating keratoplasty, *Am J Ophthalmol* (1995) **119**:712–22.

55. Snook RK, Pachymetry and true topography using the ORBSCAN system, In: Gills JP, Sanders DR, Thornton SP et al, *Corneal Topography The State of the Art*, (Slack: Thorofare, 1995) 89–103.

56. Gersten M, Mammone RJ, Zelvin J, Illuminated ring projection device, *United States Patent 4772115* Sept 20, 1988.

57. Gormley DJ, Gersten M, Koplin RS, Lubkin V, Corneal modeling, *Cornea* (1988) **7**:30–5.

58. Maguire LJ, Singer DE, Klyce SD, Graphic presentation of computer-analyzed keratoscope photographs, *Arch Ophthalmol* (1987) **105**:223–30.

59. El Hage SG, A computerized corneal topographer for use in refractive surgery, *Refract Corneal Surg* (1989) **5**:418–24.

60. Klyce SD, Estinopal HA, Gersten M, Gormley DJ, Moore JW, Fluorescein exam simulation for contact lens fitting, *Invest Ophthalmol Vis Sci Suppl* (1992) **33**:697.

61. Wilson SE, Lin DTC, Klyce SD, Reidy JJ, Insler MS, Topographic changes in contact lens-induced corneal warpage, *Ophthalmology* (1990) **97**:734–44.

62. Smolek MK, Klyce SD, Maeda N, Keratoconus and contact lens-induced corneal warpage analysis using the keratomorphic diagram, *Invest Ophthalmol Vis Sci* (1994) **35**:4192–204.

63. Wilson SE, Lin DTC, Klyce SD, Corneal topography of keratoconus, *Cornea* (1991) **10**:2–8.

64. Maguire LJ, Bourne WM, Corneal topography of early keratoconus, *Am J Ophthalmol* (1989) **108**:107–112.

65. Dingeldein SA, Klyce SD, Wilson SE, Quantitative descriptors of corneal shape derived from computer-assisted analysis of photokeratographs, *Refract Corneal Surg* (1989) **5**:372–8.

66. Wilson SE, Klyce SD, Quantitative descriptors of corneal topography, *Arch Ophthalmol* (1991) **109**:349–53.

67. Wilson SE, Klyce SD, Screening for corneal topographic abnormalities before refractive surgery, *Ophthalmology* (1993) **101**:147–52.

68. Smolek MK, Klyce SD, Maeda N, Time-lapse videokeratography using computer morphing, *Invest Ophthalmol Vis Sci Suppl* (1995) **36**:s380.

Chapter 7 Computerized videokeratography in clinical practice

Charles N J McGhee and Kathryn H Weed

INTRODUCTION

The clinical practice of ophthalmology continues to evolve rapidly as yesterday's new treatments and investigational techniques quickly become today's best practice. This is particularly so in the field of refractive surgery and recent advances in refractive and cataract surgery have necessitated more detailed analysis of corneal contour and power. Although keratoscopes have been available in some form for more than 150 years, and 'grabbing' and storage of resulting images by photographic means was first established 100 years ago, it has been the development of the personal computer and the reawakened interest of the ophthalmic community in refractive surgery that has fuelled the rapid developments in computerized videokeratography (CVK) over the last decade. In the era of photorefractive keratectomy (PRK), photoastigmatic keratectomy (PARK), laser in situ keratomileusis (LASIK) and incisional refractive surgery, a CVK system is an essential tool for the ophthalmologist undertaking refractive surgery.

THE DEVELOPMENT OF KERATOSCOPY

The word topography – from the Greek 'topos' meaning place and 'graphien' meaning to write – can be defined as the science of describing or representing the features of a particular place in detail. The history of measurement of corneal shape and refractive power is a fascinating tale, evolving into a coherent analysis that over the last four centuries has involved some of the greatest minds in physics, mathematics and ophthalmology.[1-4] Kepler produced the first accurate scientific treatise on the refraction of the cornea and the dioptric system of the eye in 1611. The contemporary Jesuit scientist, Christopher Scheiner (1619), who had previously confirmed the focusing role of the crystalline lens by experiment, was the first to attempt measurement of the anterior corneal curvature. He sat subjects in front of a window with crossbars and by holding up a series of graduated marbles (convex mirrors) of varying radii he determined which produced an image size identical to the reflected image of the cornea under examination. In 1704, Sir Isaac Newton consolidated the knowledge of optics with a series of experiments covering reflection, refraction, the formation of images and the dioptric system of the eye.

The catoptric images of a candle flame formed by the cornea and crystalline lens were first accurately described by Purkinje (1823) and subsequently redescribed by Sanson (1838), and thus are commonly described as Purkinje–Sanson images. The anterior corneal surface creates the first of these images, which is an erect, bright and slightly diminished virtual image lying approximately 3–4 mm behind the anterior corneal surface. The principle of keratometry (von Helmholtz, 1856) makes use of this first Purkinje–Sanson image, with the cornea acting as a convex mirror, such that the size of a reflected image varies with the radius of curvature; thus, if the image of a luminous object of known size, at a known distance from the cornea, is accurately measured, the radius of curvature of the cornea can be calculated. The ophthalmometer (keratometer) of Helmholtz was subsequently modified by Javal and Schiotz (1881) into an instrument essentially indistinguishable from the keratometer used today. Unfortunately, as instruments to describe the corneal curvature, keratometers have several limitations, including the presumption that the cornea is spherical or spherocylindrical (the cornea is actually a toroidal asphere), astigmatism is presumed to be orthogonal, and only the central 3–4 mm of the cornea is measured, whilst it has been established for some time that the peripheral cornea is flatter than the central cornea (Helmholtz, 1856). Keratoscopy may have originated with the original observations of Brewster (1827) who noted the variations in, and distortion of, the candle-flame image created by the cornea. Ferdinand Cuignet coined the term 'keratoscopy' in descriptions during the 1820s of a basic keratoscopy technique, complicated by difficulties in alignment of light, target, patient and observer, and compounded by the limitation of viewing the image at a one-to-one ratio. Viewing the cornea from the side, Henry Goode (1847) utilized a luminous square to derive qualitative information about corneal curvature; however, it was the major improvement of this technique by the Portuguese oculist Antonio Placido (1880) that brought keratoscopy into more popular usage. Placido's keratoscopic disc of alternating black and white circles, with a central perforation to observe the reflex, remains in essence the basic component of photokeratoscopy and CVK. However, due to the purely qualitative nature of keratoscopy, despite Placido's major advance, it did not gain wide popularity.

Gullstrand (1896) introduced the concept of 'image capture' by applying photographic techniques to keratoscopy. Apparently following advice from Javal, Gullstrand developed a measuring microscope which, although very laborious and labour intensive, allowed translation of these qualitative 'keratographs' into measurements of radii of curvature.

MODERN PHOTOKERATOSCOPY AND COMPUTERIZED VIDEOKERATOGRAPHY

Although several attempts have been made at quantifying keratoscopic data in the 20th century, until the last 10 years most equipment has remained essentially qualitative. Instruments such as the Nidek photokeratoscope have been used with some success in assessment of corneal disease processes[5] and the management of postkeratoplasty astigmatism but have seldom left the rarefied environment of the specialist referral centre (Figs 7.1, 7.2). Two important advances, the digital video camera and the advent of relatively inexpensive personal computer technology, allowing rapid measurement and analy-

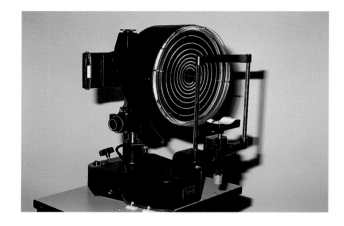

Figure 7.1 *A Nidek photokeratoscope demonstrating eight illuminated rings in a Placido arrangement.*

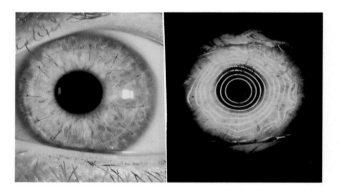

Figure 7.2 *An eye demonstrating a recent penetrating keratoplasty (left) and a photokeratoscopic image of the same eye (right) obtained with the Nidek photokeratoscope shown in Fig. 7.1. Selective suture removal has already been performed to reduce astigmatism; however, the very regular, round mires of the keratoscopic image fail to highlight residual astigmatism of +2.50 D at 95°.*

sis with increasing accuracy, have led to the rapid technical advances in keratoscopy during the past decade. Computers are now able to digitize a Placido image and apply complex mathematics (algorithms) to calculate curvature, and hence power, by utilizing a conversion factor (Standard Keratometric Index or SKI). This is the essence of the modern day CVK[6] system.

Whilst based upon the long-known principles of Placido imaging, CVK applies contemporary technol-

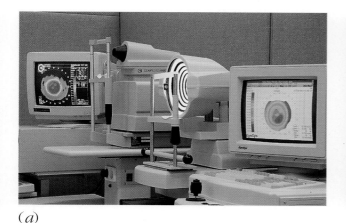

(a)

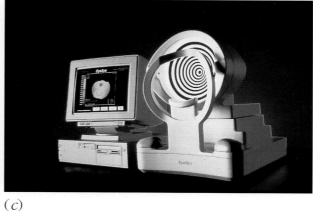

(c)

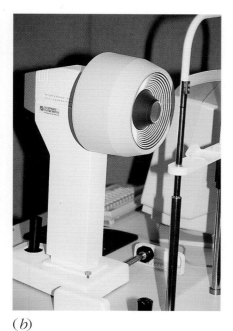

(b)

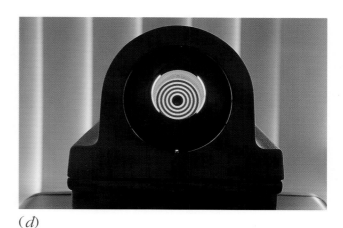

(d)

Figure 7.3 (a) Visual displays and Placido sources of the Computed Anatomy (Tomey) TMS-1 (rear) and Eyesys Technologies (foreground) CVK units. (b) Placido source of the Mastervue dual camera CVK system. (c) Placido source of the new Eyesys 2000 CVK system. (Courtesy of Eyesys Technologies.) (d) Close-up view of the small cone Placido source of the Computed Anatomy (Tomey) TMS-1 CVK system.

ogy[7,8] to enable a previously unparalleled interpretation of corneal topography (Fig. 7.3a). An illuminated Placido-type target source is projected onto the cornea (Figs 7.3b–d), following which the resultant virtual image formed by the cornea is displayed by a video camera with alignment and fine focusing determined by the observer. Single frames are captured by a video 'frame grabber' and subsequent digitization and analysis by proprietary computer software can

achieve accuracy and reproducibility in the range of ±0.20 D.

A multitude of commercial systems are now available, all sharing common basic principles, but varying substantially in the size, construction and coverage provided by the Placido source and the method of presenting the analyzed images. The accuracy[6] of any particular instrument is determined by the resolution achieved at each stage between the

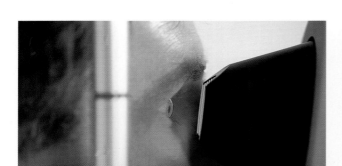

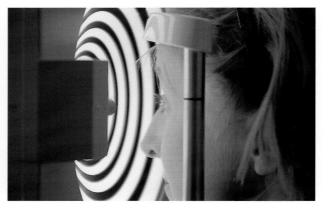

Figure 7.4 *The close working distance of the Computed Anatomy (Tomey) TMS-1 system theoretically prevents shadow from the nose and brow from compromising the peripheral corneal imaging.*

Figure 7.5 *Many CVK systems, such as the Eyesys Technologies units, utilize a working distance from the corneal vertex of approximately 90 mm that should, theoretically, minimize the effect of focusing errors.*

Table 7.1

Comparative data for four popular CVK systems

Company	Eyesys Technologies	Tomey Technology	Humphrey Instruments	Alcon Surgical
CVK system	System 2000	TMS-2	Mastervue	Eyemap
Modelling type	Placido	Placido cone	Placido	Placido
Number of rings	18	28 or 34	20	23
Data points per ring	360	256	180	360
Data points per exam	6480	8704	8000	8280
Corneal coverage (min–max diameter)	0.5–10.0 mm	0.38–11.0 mm	0.3–10.3 mm	0.46–10.0 mm
Average working distance	90 mm	40 mm	105 mm	117 mm
Average image processing time	5 sec	10 sec	5 sec	10 sec
Calibration (clinic/factory)	both	clinic	clinic	both
Operating system	Windows	DOS/Windows	Windows	DOS/Windows
Image storage format	BMP or others	PCX	BMP & others	BMP

generation of the mire pattern and the presentation of the data, with a general sensitivity of about 0.20–0.25 D or better within the central 70% of the surface area.[6,9,10] The average working distance of the instruments varies from 25 mm to 117 mm, being approximately 40 mm for the Tomey TMS 1 system (Fig. 7.4) and 90 mm for the Eyesys Technology system (Fig. 7.5), the two CVK systems in greatest widespread use. The hardware of most systems incorporates sophisticated fixation and focusing devices and, by the use of 15–38 illuminated Placido-type mires, enables coverage of almost the entire cornea, ranging from as little as 0.3 mm centrally to 11 mm diameter peripherally (Table 7.1). The great advantage of CVK systems over earlier methods of analyzing corneal power is the ability to measure the major part of the central cornea in detail and present the mathematical data in easily assimilated and interpreted display formats.

CVK DISPLAY FORMATS

PRESENTING THE POWER MAP

Corneal topographic data can be expressed in a number of ways, including a keratoscopic image (Fig. 7.6), a numerical chart (Fig. 7.7), a colour-coded contour map (Figs 7.8a,b) or a three-dimensional wire map. In 'absolute' scale colour maps identical colours represent the same corneal power in all corneal maps created with that scale. Such scales vary in their incremental value from 0.5 D to 1.5 D increments. Regardless of the incremental value, the greatest asset of such standardized scales is the facility to easily compare maps of an individual cornea chronologically, or even from different subjects, with the benefit of identical colours representing the same corneal power within each map.

In 'normalized' maps a standard set of colours, usually warm colours such as reds and oranges to represent greater dioptric power, and cool colours such as blues and greens to represent lesser dioptric power, are employed in every map. Since the range of colours is limited, in corneas with a larger range of power the steps or divisions represented by each colour will be greater, e.g. 0.8 D, than in corneas with a smaller range of power, in which case each colour will represent a smaller increment, e.g. 0.4 D. Therefore, in normalized maps, although the use of colours often maximizes the visual impact of the map and may provide greater apparent detail (if the incremental steps are small), chronological maps are less easily compared since the same colour in each map does not necessarily represent the same power, and dissimilar ranges and incremental steps may have been employed. Thus, if normalized colour-coded maps are used the clinician has constantly to consult the reference scale on each map.

Of course, the benefits of a fixed colour-to-power scale and incremental steps of the clinician's chosen magnitude can be combined in most topography systems by creating a personal, default, *adjusted* dioptric scale (Figs 7.8c–e).

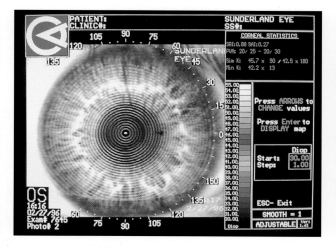

Figure 7.6 *A computerized videokeratographic image demonstrating coverage from central to peripheral cornea by Placido mires. However, in this unprocessed form the CVK image provides very limited information and allows minimal visual analysis.*

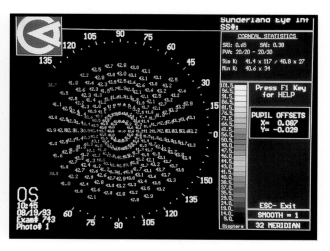

Figure 7.7 *The grabbed video image of a Placido display, as shown in Fig. 7.6, can be analyzed and converted to numerical values rather than the traditional colour maps. This information can be rather unwieldy and difficult to interpret quickly in a busy clinical setting.*

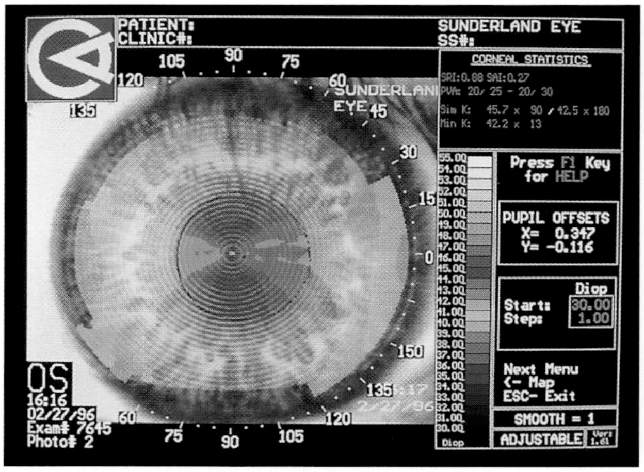

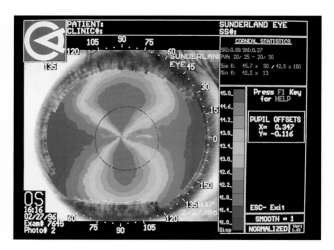

Figure 7.8a *Processing of the image displayed in Fig. 7.6 allows conversion to an overlayed transparent colour or power map. These are maps of corneal power rather than corneal shape and the incremental power of each step is highlighted by the vertical colour scale to the right of the corneal image. (Scale: 30.00–55.00 D using 1.00 D incremental steps.)*

Figure 7.8b *By utilizing a normalized or automatically adjusted scale most CVK systems will select incremental dioptric steps, such that areas of greatest corneal power are highlighted by warm colours, for example reds and oranges, and areas of least power are delineated by cool colours, such as greens and blues. This figure demonstrates the same cornea shown in Figs 7.6 and 7.8a; however, unlike Fig. 7.8a, the range of the dioptric scale is much smaller, being 41.00 D–45.00 D, with correspondingly smaller incremental steps of 0.40 D rather than 1.00 D. Using a solid colour option removes unnecessary background detail from the map.*

SUBTRACTION OR DIFFERENCE MAPS

These can be invaluable to the keratorefractive practitioner. Most contemporary CVK systems will allow comparison of topographic maps of the same eye, such that chronological changes can be identified. This information can be important in terms of assessing:

*   resolution of corneal warpage
*   comparing preoperative and postoperative topography
*   following myopic regression
*   establishing ablation zone centration[11] and
*   differentiating between focal undertreatment, focal regression and decentration.

SURFACE ELEVATION OR TANGENTIAL MAPS

All corneal topography presentations previously described have been maps of corneal power, rather than true corneal shape. Although dioptric power and shape are intimately related, it would be erroneous to infer accurate corneal shape in the peripheral cornea from a power map.[12] Peripheral asphericity of the cornea can be mathematically calculated from computerized corneal topography, but this peripheral corneal flattening does not appear to have a significant impact on the prediction of corneal refractive procedures such as radial keratotomy.[13]

Although, conceptually, the facility to report true corneal shape is attractive, the practical usefulness of maps of true shape to ophthalmologists, who generally work in dioptres, is limited (see Chapter 6). However, some of the currently available corneal topography systems are beginning to offer this facility by providing a two- or three-camera system, with one camera behind the Placido source and one or two cameras temporal (tangential) to the cornea, which allows accurate identification of the corneal profile (Figs 7.9–7.11). The addition of a temporal image grabbing facility provides several advantages: the corneal apex can be accurately aligned in three

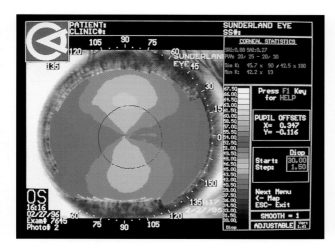

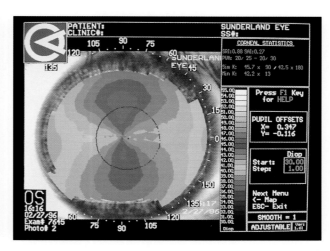

Figure 7.8c *The developers of CVK systems have advocated a variety of default scales with fixed incremental steps from 0.50 D to 1.50 D, utilizing fixed colours to represent the same power range in all maps produced using such absolute scales, with upper and lower limits sufficient to encompass extremes of corneal power. This image illustrates the same cornea shown in Figs 7.8a,b and 7.9. These images highlight the way in which different dioptric scales can greatly influence the appearance of a topographic map. (Scale: 30.00–67.50 D using 1.50 D incremental steps.)*

Figure 7.8d *This image illustrates the same cornea shown in Figs 7.6, 7.8 and 7.9a, using the author's preferred personalized default scale for keratorefractive surgery, with a range of 30.00–55.00 D using 1.00 D incremental steps. This has the advantage of a fixed colour to power relationship in the assessment of chronological changes in a cornea, whilst using sufficiently small steps to highlight significant refractive changes on a single dioptric scale.*

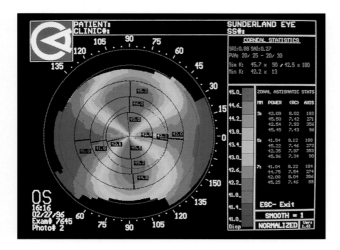

Figure 7.8e *The topographic image can be used to highlight astigmatic data. In this image a default normalized scale is utilized with the background video image omitted. In addition to the corneal statistics, which are routinely provided in the top right corner (SRI, SAI, PVA, Sim K and Min K), this map also illustrates zonal astigmatic data on the topographic map and in three columns to the right of the dioptric scale. (Scale: 41.00–45.00 D using 0.40 D incremental steps.)*

dimensions, a true vertical profile of the entire cornea can be deduced, accurate sagittal height measurements can be made and accuracy and reproducibility improved to <±0.1 D. Theoretically, unlike a topographic power map, an elevation map provides a true representation of the aspheric shape and peripheral flattening of the normal cornea; however, it must be remembered that these corneal shape

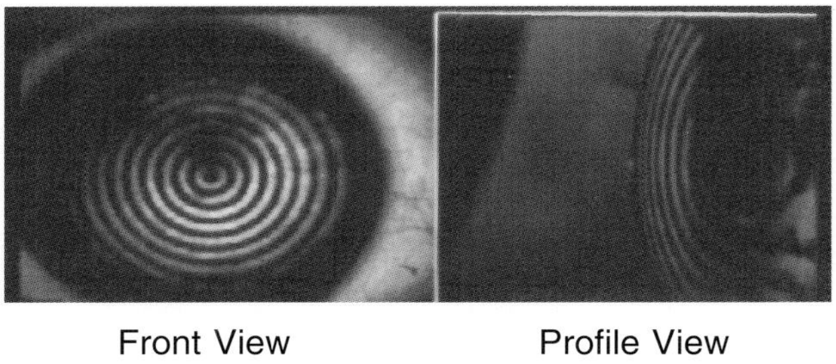

Figure 7.9 *A profile view of the cornea obtained by the temporal camera in the Eyesys 2000 CVK system. A red square on the computer screen highlights the corneal apex ensuring accurate focusing and a true sagittal height measurement from apex to limbus. (Courtesy Eyesys Technologies.)*

Front View   Profile View

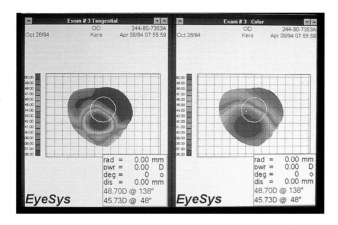

Figure 7.10 *Early keratoconus with maximal corneal power of 50.00 D and approximated keratometry readings of 45.73 D and 48.70 D. The tangential or corneal shape map on the left demonstrates a well-defined circular area greater than 47.00 D situated inferotemporal to the pupil, corresponding to the apex of the cone. In contrast the power map on the right suggests a larger area of increased power extending towards the limbus. (Scale: 36.00–50.00 D using 1.00 D incremental steps.) (Courtesy Eyesys Technologies.)*

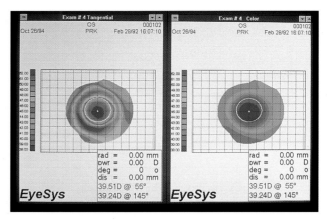

Figure 7.11 *These maps show a well-centred PRK procedure 18 months post-treatment. The tangential or true shape map, on the left, highlights a very sharp demarcation between the treated and untreated cornea. In the power map, shown on the right, a much more gradual transition in corneal power is evident and the effective PRK ablation zone appears larger than on the tangential map. (Scale: 38.00–52.00 D using 1.00 D incremental steps.) (Courtesy Eyesys Technology.)*

maps are derived by calculating a relative change in elevation by comparing the captured data to an ideal spherical or aspheric corneal model. These advances, while perhaps not quite the major step forward that manufacturers would have us believe, will certainly have applications in contact lens fitting, assessment of keratoconus and, perhaps, in the planning of keratorefractive retreatment cases.

SPECIALIZED CVK DISPLAY FORMATS

With a little computing assistance, and cooperation from manufacturers, practitioners should be able to customize CVK data displays to suit their practice; however, a brief outline of two commercially available displays, the Holladay Diagnostic Summary (HDS) and the Stars™ Display (pioneered by Daniel

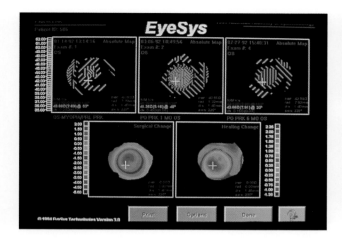

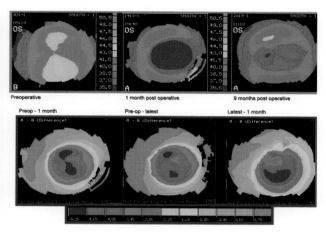

Figure 7.12 *An example of the STARS™ display, which generates two serial difference maps highlighting surgical change (bottom left) and the associated healing change (bottom right) in a post-PRK patient.*

Figure 7.13 *The McGhee–Orr Display (MOD), a simple research display developed by the authors, which highlights three chronological maps on an absolute scale of 1.50 D increments along the upper row (at pretreatment, 1 month and latest reviews), and three difference maps (pretreatment/1 month post-treatment, pretreatment/latest map and 1 month/latest map) along the lower row. These are combined with indices, including unaided vision, best spectacle corrected visual acuity and manifest refraction, to provide a single, one page, summary of the chronological topographic and refractive changes post-PRK.*

Durrie MD), (Fig. 7.12) and one example of a developing personalized display (Fig. 7.13), the McGhee–Orr Display (MOD), follows.

The Holladay Diagnostic Summary contains four colour maps and 15 itemized corneal parameters (Fig. 7.14). A standard scale refractive (power) map in 1 D increments from 37 to 51 D is provided, with the identical information displayed as an auto-scale, or normalized, refractive map in which the starting power and size of dioptric intervals are chosen to utilize the 15 colours for best visual display. A profile difference, or tangential, map is also highlighted and a relatively new concept, the distortion map, completes the four map display. This distortion map assumes that the best spherocylindrical lens is in place and maps distortion in terms of predicted Snellen acuity, ranging from blue (20/16) to red (20/200). It is suggested that by correlating optical irregularities of the cornea with visual performance this map is a useful addition in assessing quality of vision. Quantitative indices are highlighted below.

The Stars™ display, developed by Durrie and Spector, utilizes a five map display to highlight preoperative, 1 month postoperative and latest postoperative corneal power maps on a standardized, uniform dioptric scale, and two difference, or subtraction, map displays. The latter two displays firstly demonstrate the difference between the preoperative and 1 month post-PRK topographic maps – that is the surgical change – and, secondly, by producing a difference map between the 1 and 12 month (or latest) post-PRK maps, highlight the healing or regression in the ablation zone (Fig. 7.12).

The MOD display is simply a research display developed by the authors in 1994 and utilized to assess the usefulness of multiple data provision in the interpretation of outcome following PRK/PARK. Six maps and several indices, including unaided vision, best spectacle corrected acuity and manifest refraction are displayed to chronicle the postoperative course of PRK surgery and provide a one-sheet summary. The upper three topographic maps are

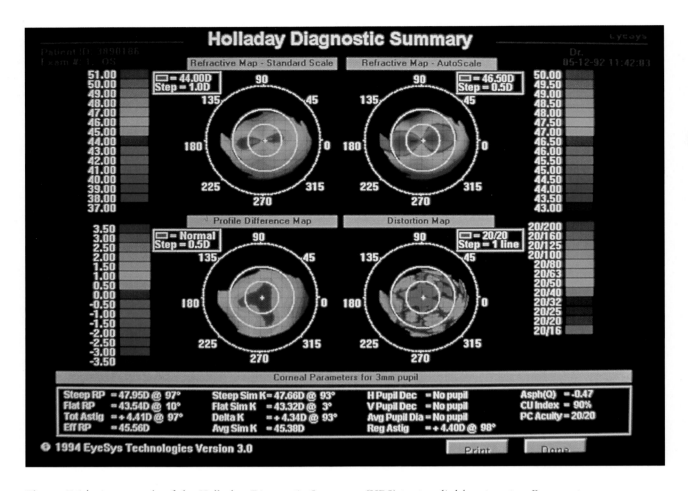

Figure 7.14 *An example of the Holladay Diagnostic Summary (HDS) post radial keratometry. Four maps are illustrated: the upper two show refractive power maps on standardized and autoscales; lower maps show a profile difference map and the distortion map. The scale on the last map highlights decreased visual potential to 20/80 in radial spokes (yellow) over the incision sites. Fifteen numerical indices are highlighted at the bottom of the display. (Courtesy Eyesys Technologies.)*

compiled on a uniform, absolute scale of 1.5 D increments, whereas the lower three represent three difference maps: pretreatment/1 month post-treatment, pretreatment/latest topographic map, and topographic map 1 month post-treatment/latest topographic map (Fig. 7.13). Such individualized displays are likely to become more common as surgeons refine the presentation of topographic data to provide an instant, easily interpretable, summary of the chronological changes in the post-PRK cornea.

QUANTITATIVE INDICES

The advantage of colour-coded topographic maps is the rapidity with which the information can be assimilated by the human eye and brain. However, although facilitating rapid pattern recognition has been one of the breakthroughs of these displays, the amount of quantitative data from these maps allows the formation of several useful numerical indices[14,15] (Fig. 7.15). Commonly used indices include

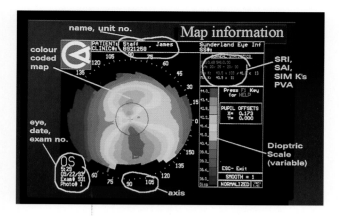

Figure 7.15 *A topographic map of a normal healthy cornea exhibiting with-the-rule astigmatism (WTR) with numeric data, including quantitative indices, highlighted.*

Table 7.2
Computerized videokeratography in clinical practice

1. Classification of normal topography
2. Identification of abnormal topography
3. Pre- and postoperative assessment in keratorefractive surgery
4. Management of astigmatism following intraocular surgery
5. Planning contact lens fit

Simulated Keratometry (Sim K), which approximates the equivalent readings of a mechanical keratometer, Surface Asymmetry Index (SAI), which increases with increasing asymmetry in the corneal power distribution, Surface Irregularity Index (SRI), which increases with increasing irregularity of the central cornea, and Potential Visual Acuity (PVA), which is an estimation of predicted visual acuity based upon the SRI.

The HDS display also contains a number of numeric indices including asphericity values (Q), regular astigmatism (Reg Astig), which is the amount and axis of regular astigmatism that can be neutralized by a spherocylindrical lens, the corneal uniformity index (CU), a measure of the uniformity of distortion over the pupillary area, and vertical and horizontal pupil decentration data.

COMPUTERIZED VIDEOKERATOGRAPHY IN CLINICAL PRACTICE

Computerized corneal videokeratography has proved most useful as a research tool but, in addition, has increasingly established its value in clinical ophthalmology and is essential in keratorefractive practice. The main clinical uses of CVK can be broadly divided into five categories, highlighted in Table 7.2. The

management of postsurgical astigmatism following intraocular surgery and the utilization of CVK data in the fitting of contact lenses are outside the scope of this chapter and will not be discussed further.

PRE-OPERATIVE CVK ANALYSIS

THE NORMAL CORNEA

When considering the topography of the cornea, it has to be remembered that there is a spectrum of 'normality' that blends continuously via a grey zone into frank abnormality. On the other hand, the exact morphology and topography of a given individual is unique.[16] The first widely recognized classification of computerized corneal topography illustrating the variation in a normal population was proposed by Bogan et al.[17] and described as five subgroups: round, oval, symmetric bow tie, asymmetric bow tie and irregular (Figs 7.16–7.19). It should be noted that some workers include oval with round in a combined category since neither is associated with significant corneal astigmatism.

The normal central cornea is approximately spherical (although the cornea as a whole is aspheric) and has an average radius of curvature of 7.8 mm, which equates to an average central power of 43.50 D.[18] The range of power found in the normal human cornea is 39–48 D, with highest power apically and lowest power peripherally; it should be noted, however, that a very small percentage of emmetropic subjects with normal corneas can have a central power of 50.00 D or more.[19] Interestingly, an individual's corneas are

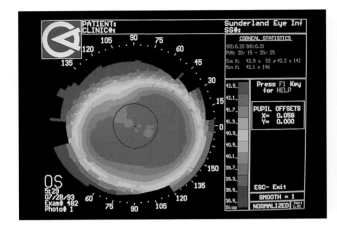

Figure 7.16 *A normal round or oval topographic appearance highlighted by a normalized scale in an almost spherical cornea. (Scale: 38.50–42.50 D using 0.40 D incremental steps.)*

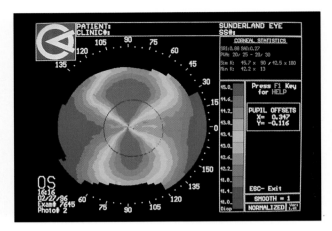

Figure 7.17 *A symmetric bow tie topographic appearance highlighted by a normalized scale in a cornea exhibiting +3.20 D of WTR astigmatism at 90°. (Scale: 41.00–45.00 D using 0.40 D incremental steps.)*

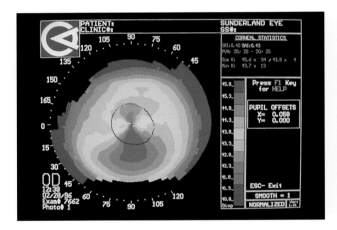

Figure 7.18 *An asymmetric bow tie topographic appearance highlighted by a normalized scale in a cornea exhibiting +1.80 D of WTR astigmatism at 94°. The cornea is more astigmatic inferiorly, thus producing the asymmetry in the bow tie pattern. (Scale: 40.80–45.80 D using 0.50 D incremental steps.)*

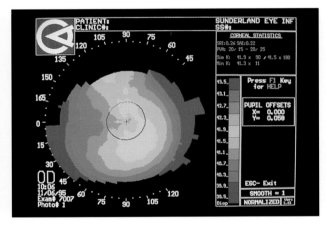

Figure 7.19 *An unclassifiable topographic appearance, highlighted by a normalized scale, that shows elements suggestive of both oval and asymmetric bow tie patterns, in an entirely healthy cornea. (Scale: 39.50–43.50 D using 0.40 D incremental steps.)*

often non-superimposable mirror images of each other (enantiomorphism)[6,16] and knowledge of this symmetry can be useful in deciding whether a cornea is normal or not, by comparison with topography of the contralateral eye (Fig. 7.20). As in any branch of medicine, a sound knowledge of the 'normal' must be appreciated before application of

new clinical tools, such as CVK, to common[19–24] and less common abnormalities.[25,26] The majority of corneas are toroidal aspheres and, therefore, it is unsurprising that the most common patterns identified are symmetric and asymmetric bow ties,[17] and that the prevalence of astigmatism increases with increasing ametropia.[27]

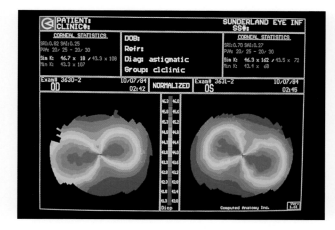

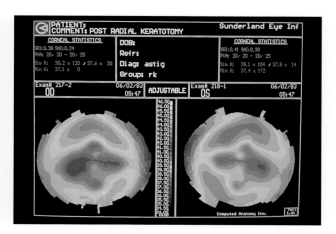

Figure 7.20 *Enantiomorphism, wherein an individual's CVK maps are non-superimposable mirror images of each other, can be useful in deciding whether a particular topography is abnormal or not, by comparison with the fellow eye. This case highlights oblique astigmatism of 3.40 D at 18° in the right eye, mirroring astigmatism of 2.80 D at 162° in the left eye in a patient who has been a long-term contact lens wearer. (Normalized scales: (right) 41.30–46.30 D using 0.50 D incremental steps; (left) 42.00–46.00 D using 0.40 D incremental steps.)*

Figure 7.21 *CVK maps of the right and left corneas of a patient 2 years after bilateral eight-incision radial keratotomy. The patient complained of fluctuating vision throughout the day in the left eye, which could only be fully corrected with a contact lens. Both topographic maps demonstrate a multifocal appearance to the central cornea, with 1.30 D of induced astigmatism in the left cornea. (Scale: 34.00–46.50 D using 0.50 D incremental steps.)*

THE ABNORMAL CORNEA

Because of dissatisfaction with spectacle or contact lens correction, subjects with irregular astigmatism or larger amounts of regular astigmatism frequently present to refractive surgery clinics. CVK is invaluable in screening potential candidates for refractive surgery. The role of CVK in the assessment of naturally occurring astigmatism preoperatively is discussed in Chapter 8 and this section will be restricted to the assessment of irregular astigmatism – specifically keratoconus and contact lens-related corneal warpage. However, the ophthalmologist must be aware of the potential for significantly altered topography, not only after refractive procedures such as radial keratotomy (RK) (Figs 7.21, 7.22), but also following keratitis, minor corneal trauma and corneal epithelial disturbance (Figs 7.23a,b).[25,26]

KERATOCONUS

The presence of visual symptoms or clinical signs (including retinoscopy and biomicroscopic examina-

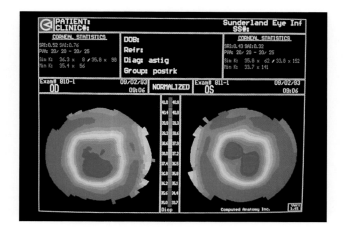

Figure 7.22 *CVK maps of the right and left corneas of a patient 3 years after bilateral eight-incision radial keratotomy. Both maps show a uniform reduction of central power over a wide area. The patient enjoyed 20/20 vision unaided right and left with no detracting visual symptoms. (Normalized scales: (right) 35.00–41.00 D using 0.60 D incremental steps; (left) 33.70–40.80 D using 0.70 D incremental steps.)*

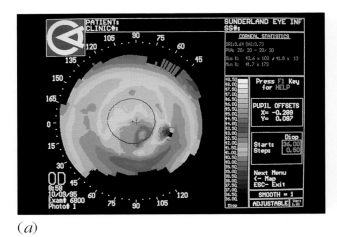

(*a*)

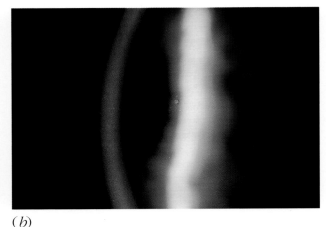

(*b*)

Figure 7.23 (*a*) *A corneal topographic lagoon: a focal, reproducible area of significantly reduced dioptric power more commonly found in post-traumatic recurrent corneal erosion syndrome.*[25] *The lagoon is highlighted as a small (1.0–1.5 mm diameter) blue green area of reduced dioptric power on the edge of the ablation zone (4 o'clock relative to pupil outline) in a patient complaining of transient recurrent corneal erosion symptoms in an eye following a −1.50 D PRK correction 2 years earlier. (Scale: 36.00–48.50 D using 0.50 D incremental steps.) (b) A slit-lamp biomicroscope photograph of the cornea illustrated in (a) highlighting a group of epithelial microcysts on the nasal border of the PRK ablation zone by retroillumination. These microcysts correspond to the region identified as a corneal topographic lagoon on the CVK map and may be the source of the patient's transient recurrent micro-erosion symptoms.*

tion) can be quite variable in this relatively common condition and in early cases may frequently be absent.[19] Therefore, the only means of making a diagnosis in the earliest subclinical cases is by CVK, which may also be useful for both monitoring and contact lens fitting in those with advancing disease. The prevalence of clinically significant keratoconus is 0.03–0.05%[20] but, in fact, may be as high as 6–12% in those presenting for refractive surgery. Topographical subtypes have been proposed[19,21,28] and include oval, with cone only involving one or two quadrants, usually inferiorly, with fairly normal appearance outside this area (Fig. 7.24); globus, in which the cone involves most of the cornea (Fig. 7.25); nipple, with cone involving less than 50% of the central cornea, surrounded by flatter normal cornea through 360° (Fig. 7.26); and astigmatic, where the cornea is characterized by an exaggerated bow tie astigmatism, often steeper above, involving less than 50% of the cornea but supported by clinical signs of keratoconus (Fig. 7.27).

Detection programs for screening and diagnosis of subclinical and clinical keratoconus have received much attention and may have value in the diagnosis of keratoconus by inexperienced observers, screening

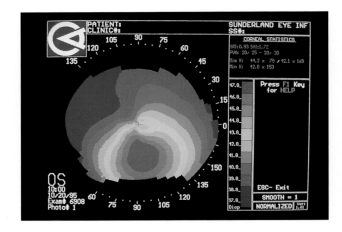

Figure 7.24 *Keratoconus of the oval topographic subtype, highlighted by a normalized scale. Because of increasing discomfort this patient presented for assessment for keratorefractive surgery with moderate corneal astigmatism (2.10 D) and no prior diagnosis of keratoconus. However, the pattern was noted to be keratoconic with an apical power of 47.8 D and careful slit-lamp examination demonstrated subtle early clinical signs of keratoconus. (Normalized scale: 37.80–47.80 D using 1.0 D incremental steps.)*

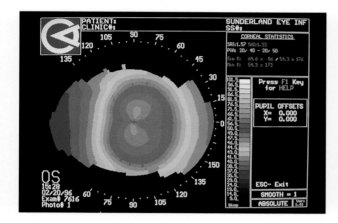

Figure 7.25 *Keratoconus of the globus topographic subtype using the Klyce absolute scale. More than 50% of the cornea demonstrates abnormal dioptric power (orange = 47.50 D) with an apical power of 71.50 D. (Klyce absolute scale: range 9.0–101.50 D in incremental steps of 1.50 D between 35.5 and 50.50 D, and in 5.00 D incremental steps outside this central range.)*

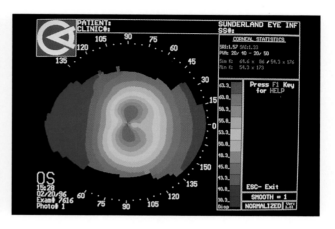

Figure 7.26 *Keratoconus of the nipple topographic subtype, highlighted by a normalized scale. The area of abnormally increased dioptric power represents less than 50% of the cornea, with normal topographic power throughout the periphery of the cornea (40.80–45.80 D) and an apical power of 63.30 D. (Normalized scale: 38.30–63.30 D using 2.50 D incremental steps.)*

of subjects presenting for refractive surgery, genetic (family) studies, and quantifying the progression of keratoconus. Subclinical topographic changes have been identified in a group of patients by Maguire,[22] and Rabinowitz and McDonnell,[23] who found central corneal power, difference in central corneal power between fellow eyes, and steepening of the inferior cornea compared with the superior cornea (I–S), to be significantly different in keratoconics compared to normal controls. Maeda et al.[24] used three quantitative approaches to identify keratoconus, simulated K values (Sim-K) >45.7 D, the modified Rabinowitz–McDonnell test (central corneal power greater than 47.2 D and/or inferosuperior asymmetry [I–S] value >1.4 D), and an expert system analyzer based upon eight topographic indices, including SAI. Sensitivity for the latter two tests was considerably better than simulated keratometry, being 96% for the modified Rabinowitz–McDonnell test and 98% for the expert system classifier. Therefore, for screening of refractive surgery patients for keratoconus, either of these tests, both exhibiting high sensitivity, is suitable. However, in terms of specificity, the expert classifier system (99%) is superior to the modified Rabinowitz–McDonnell test (85%) (p=0.001).

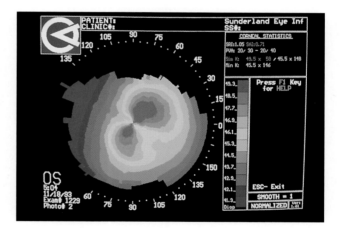

Figure 7.27 *Keratoconus of the astigmatic topographic subtype, highlighted by a normalized scale. This subtype is the one most likely to present to keratorefractive clinics having previously been undiagnosed. The appearance is of a symmetric or asymmetric bow tie astigmatism (often greater superiorly) supported by clinical signs of keratoconus on careful slit-lamp examination of the cornea. The cornea illustrated shows 4.00 D of astigmatism and an apical power of 49.30 D. (Normalized scale: 41.30–49.30 D using 0.80 D incremental steps.)*

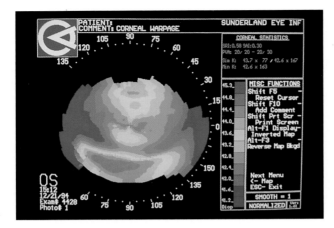

Figure 7.28a *Contact lens-related warpage in a PMMA lens wearer. Although Sim-K values only show 1.10 D of astigmatism and the SRI and SAI values are 0.58 and 0.30, respectively, the CVK map highlights central corneal warpage caused by a high-riding hard contact lens. (Normalized scale: 41.20–45.30 D using 0.40 D incremental steps.)*

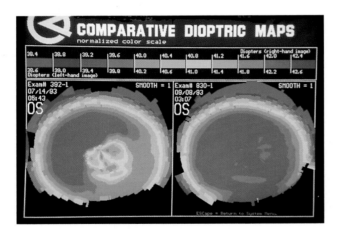

Figure 7.28b *CVK maps of the left eye of a patient presenting for PRK. The left map shows the topographic appearance 2 weeks after discontinuing PMMA contact lens wear, highlighting marked reduction in central power (flattening) due to corneal warpage. Interestingly, at this point the subject, who stated he had always had poor corrected visual acuity, was correctable to a BSCVA of 20/30 with a −5.50 D sphere. The patient was reviewed at fortnightly intervals and 2 months elapsed before the normal, round CVK appearance shown on the right returned, at which point the patient obtained a BSCVA of 20/15.*

CONTACT LENS-INDUCED CORNEAL WARPAGE

This has been defined as contact lens-induced changes in corneal topography, reversible or permanent, that are not associated with corneal oedema (to distinguish it from other pathologies).[29] Mechanical and/or metabolic factors are thought to be responsible. Warpage is more likely to occur in rigid (PMMA) lens wearers rather than rigid gas-permeable lens wearers (RGP) and clinically significant warpage is rare in soft contact lens wearers.[29] Rigid lens decentration is a known risk factor[29,30] while lenses must be worn for a minimum of 3 months to produce warpage.[31,32] Stable topography following discontinuation of lens wear may take as long as 8 months.[33] The importance of CVK screening to ensure stable corneal morphology prior to refractive procedures is obvious and the observation of a spherical refraction and reasonable corrected visual acuity (6/6–6/12) should not lull the ophthalmologist into a false sense of security (Figs 7.28a,b).

CVK FOLLOWING PHOTOREFRACTIVE SURGERY

GENERAL CONSIDERATIONS

It is difficult to generalize in respect of the frequency with which CVK analysis should be performed post-PRK/PARK. Whilst topographic maps can be obtained in many subjects by the 7th day postoperatively, a large number will exhibit artefact at this stage due to epithelial irregularities. However, in terms of avoiding failure to detect early phenomena, such as central topographic islands, or document the difference between true decentration and differential regression of the ablation zone, early rather than late CVK analysis is advisable. High quality, reproducible images should be obtainable from all eyes by 1 month post-treatment and, presuming no topographic abnormalities are identified, further images at 3, 6 and 12 months might represent reasonable topographic assessment.

Topographic images are a powerful educational tool and preoperative features, such as astigmatism, can be more readily explained to the patient. Similarly, postoperative features, such as central islands, regression, and the less common pupil/ablation zone disparity symptoms, such as night-time glare and halo, can be more readily comprehended by the patient when a graphical image is utilized in the education process.

Centration of ablation zone

Refractive surgery has been traditionally centred upon the geometric centre of the cornea, as defined by the first Purkinje–Sanson image of the operating microscope light. However, following the elegant exposition upon centring refractive procedures by Uozato and Guyton,[34] more recently surgeons have attempted to centre procedures on a point where the line of sight intersects the pupil, with the surgeon and patient coaxially fixating. Increasingly, there is general agreement that PRK/PARK procedures should be based on this point, which represents the centre of the virtual pupil, and therefore the biological pupil, with the patient fixating a co-axial target.[35] However, various methods have been described to centre PRK/PARK and only one large series reports a method of marking the pupil centre with both the surgeon and patient fixating coaxially.[36]

Decentration of ablation zone was particularly problematic with early excimer laser systems utilizing small ablation zones and non-coaxial microscopes. The mean magnitude of decentration has been noted to be in the range of 0.36–0.78 mm.[37,38,39,40,41,42] In a review of a personal series, the authors noted a mean decentration of 0.46 mm; however, in this, as in all series, it is the range of decentration that is important, with 96% being decentred less than 1 mm from the pupil centre and greatest decentration being 1.1 mm.[11]

Decentration of greater than 1 mm may be associated with troublesome night-time symptoms of glare and halo in younger subjects with large pupils, particularly if ablation zones of 5 mm diameter or less have been utilized (Figs 7.29a–c). However, ray-tracing and CVK analysis has demonstrated excellent visual acuity (20/40 or better unaided) even in the presence of moderate decentration (0.8–1.7 mm) of a 5 mm PRK ablation zone relative to the pupil centre. Indeed, in this small study, the patient with greatest decentration obtained 20/15 unaided vision and only one subject complained of troublesome visual symptoms.[43] In a larger study of 38 eyes, treated with a 5 mm ablation zone, multivariate analysis demonstrated that ablation zone decentrations of less than 0.89 mm from the pupil centre were not associated with untoward visual symptoms.[44] Nonetheless, major decentrations can be associated with persistent glare,

halo and induced astigmatism of up to 6.4 D[36] (Fig. 7.30) (see Chapter 23). Accurate centration of the ablation zone is particularly important when treating astigmatism with an elliptical ablation, since even in excimer lasers using a 6 mm diameter zone for spherical ablation, the short axis of the astigmatic ablation may be as little as 4.5–5.0 mm (Fig. 7.31).

Topography of ablation zones

Early studies demonstrated that post-PRK corneal topography patterns were variable and might change for up to 1 year post-treatment.[37] A variety of topographic patterns have been described post-PRK, including multifocal cornea;[45] however, two large series highlight most of the patterns.[46,47]

Using a VisX 20/20 laser, utilizing 5.0–6.0 mm ablation zones, Lin[46] classified 502 consecutive eyes at 1 month post-PRK into one of four ablation zone patterns: uniform (44%), keyhole (12%), semicircular (18%) and central island (26%). The latter group accounted for the majority of patients who exhibited lines of lost best spectacle corrected visual acuity (BSCVA); however, these central topographic features resolved spontaneously, with only 2% of eyes exhibiting central islands at 12 months post-PRK.

Hersh et al.[47] reporting CVK data on 181 eyes 1 year after PRK with a Summit Omnimed laser utilizing a 4.5–5.0 mm ablation zone, described seven topography patterns: homogenous (58.6%), keyhole, semicircular (2.8%), toric with axis (17.7%), toric against axis (2.8%), irregularly irregular (13.8%) and focal topographic variants (4.4%) (Figs 7.32, 7.33). No cases of central islands were identified. A chronological change in topographic appearance was identified in 41.1% of those eyes with topography available at 3 months and 1 year, with 54.3% demonstrating an evolution to a topographically better group, 17.4% remaining in an equivalent category and 28.2% changing to a poorer category.

Those with homogenous patterns obtained best uncorrected visual acuity (UCVA), whereas UCVA was worst in the toric against axis category, and approximately two lines poorer in the irregularly irregular group compared to the homogenous group. However, based upon topographic patterns, there was no statistical difference between groups in terms of BSCVA. The authors noted that estimations of change in refractive power, based upon topographic analysis, tended to underestimate for corrections less than −5.00 D and overestimate for corrections greater than −5.00 D.[47]

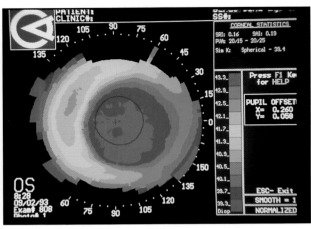

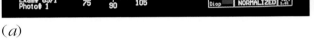

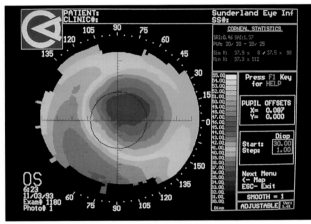

(a)

(b)

(c)

Figure 7.29 *(a) A well-centred 6 mm PRK ablation zone of uniform power is noted to have margins that are approximately equidistant from the pupil margin (highlighted in grey). (Normalized scale: 37.70–41.80 D using 0.40 D incremental steps.) (b) A 6.0 mm diameter PRK ablation zone of highly uniform power demonstrates approximately 1.0 mm decentration to the pupil. Because of the diameter of the ablation zone, and the limited excursion of the pupil in this 45-year-old subject, no adverse symptoms were experienced due to this decentration and the patient enjoyed unaided vision of 20/15. (c) A 5.0 mm diameter PRK ablation zone is decentred superotemporally by approximately 1.0 mm. The pupil is outlined in grey and a 10.0 mm scale, in 1.0 mm divisions, is centred upon the pupil centre. Despite a similar magnitude of decentration, due to the smaller ablation zone, unlike the case illustrated in Fig. 7.29b, this patient complained of secondary images and troublesome night-time visual symptoms. (Scale: 30.00–55.00 D using 1.00 D incremental steps.)*

Topographic central islands

Although PRK should preferably result in a fairly uniform area of decreased corneal power, caused by relative corneal 'flattening' over a wide central area[37,40,41] well-circumscribed central islands are not infrequently encountered.[46,48,49] Indeed, in the early postoperative period central islands may be the more common topographic pattern, with up to 67% of eyes demonstrating some degree of increased central power.[48] A 'central island' may be defined as a well-circumscribed, usually central, circular or oval area of relatively greater corneal topographic power (>3.00 D) within the region of reduced corneal topographic power created by excimer laser (PRK or PARK)[48,49] (Figs 7.34a,b, 7.35). These central island formations may contribute significantly to delayed visual rehabilitation and cause visual symptoms such as monocular diplopia and decreased best corrected visual acuity.[46] The origins of the central islands have been subject to much speculation.

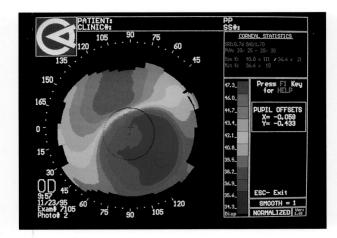

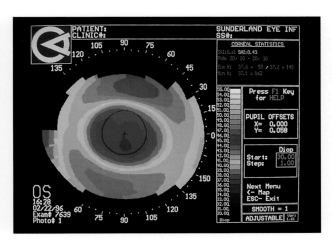

Figure 7.30 *This CVK map shows a 6.0 mm PRK ablation decentred inferonasally by approximately 1.50 mm relative to the pupil centre. It is notable that the pupil centre (grey dot) is offset by 0.433 mm inferior to the corneal vertex (grey cross) and, therefore, the ablation zone is actually decentred by almost 2.00 mm relative to the corneal vertex. An induced topographic astigmatism of approximately 3.40 D is present and SRI and SAI values are 0.76 and 1.70, respectively. Potential visual acuity (PVA) is 20/15 to 20/30 but the eye recorded a BSCVA of 20/20. Because of problematic daytime and low-light symptoms this patient requested retreatment. (Normalized scale: 34.3–47.3 D using 1.30 D incremental steps).*

Figure 7.31 *This CVK image demonstrates a well-centred, oval astigmatic PARK ablation zone of uniform power. However, it is noteworthy that although the zone is 6.0 mm in its long axis, it is only 4.5 mm in the short axis, therefore even relatively minor decentrations of such oval astigmatic PARK zones can lead to troublesome symptoms related to pupil/ablation zone mismatch. (Scale: 30.00–55.00 D using 1.00 D incremental steps.)*

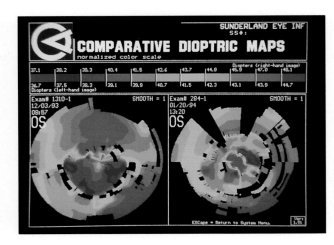

Figure 7.32 *Post-PRK topographic variants – irregular topography. CVK map appearance of the left eye 4 weeks (left) and 10 weeks (right) after a –6.50 D PRK correction using a 6.0 mm diameter ablation zone. Due to epithelial irregularity at 4 weeks the zone appears truncated superiorly (BSCVA 20/60). At 10 weeks the ablation zone looks more regular in the periphery but focal topographic anomalies persist centrally and at 5 o'clock relative to the zone (BSCVA 20/40). Six months post-PRK the zone had regularized and BSCVA improved to 20/20 with a residual refractive error of –1.50 D.*

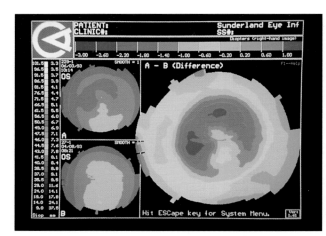

Figure 7.33 *Post-PRK topographic variants – semicircular ablation zone. A CVK subtraction map comparing preoperative topography (lower left) and 3 months post-PRK topography (upper left), clearly demonstrates a semicircular ablation zone following a –3.50 D PRK using a 6.0 mm ablation zone (right). Despite the appearance of this inferior peninsula of astigmatism the subject obtained 20/15 unaided vision and was entirely symptom free. (Scale: preoperative and postoperative maps on an absolute scale 9.00–101.50 D using 5.00 D increments, outside the central range 35.50–50.50 D that utilizes 1.50 D incremental steps, difference map scale is shown horizontally along the top of the figure).*

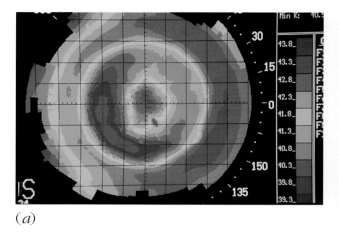

(*a*)

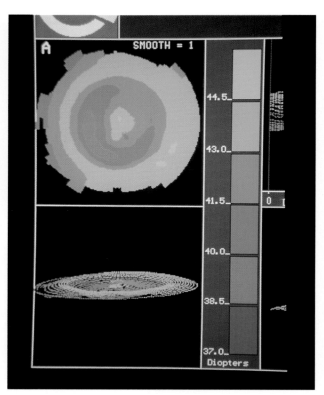

(*b*)

Figure 7.34 *Post-PRK topographic variants – central topographic island. (a) A central island of 5.00–6.00 D maximal power and approximately 2.5 mm diameter is clearly seen in the centre of a 6.0 mm PRK ablation zone 1 month after a –5.50 D correction. The patient complained of monocular secondary images but BSCVA was unaffected. This central island completely resolved without further treatment over the following 3 months. (Normalized scale: 38.80–43.80 D using 0.50 D incremental steps with a 1.0 mm grid overlay.) (b) The central island illustrated in Fig. 7.34a is shown here on an absolute scale of 1.50 D increments (upper image) and as a three-dimensional wire diagram (lower image).*

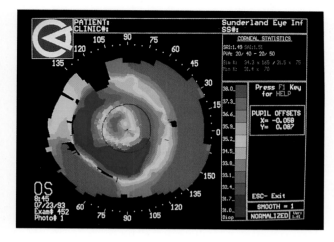

Figure 7.35 *A large central island, of approximately 7.00 D power and 3.0 mm diameter, 1 month after a PRK correction of −15.00 D utilizing a 6.0 mm diameter ablation zone. This island was associated with loss of three lines of BSCVA. The island fully resolved, without intervention, over a six month period and the patient regained preoperative BSCVA. Note extremely high SRI and SAI values of 1.49 and 1.51, respectively. (Normalized scale: 31.00–38.00 D using 0.70 D incremental steps.)*

Although many centres have recorded few or no instances of this complication,[47,50,51] others have recorded an incidence of 26–29% in the early postoperative period.[46,48,49] Theories regarding the origin of central islands are varied, and although no single explanation has yet gained universal acceptance, four possible explanations are commonly proposed:

- Firstly, there may be localized 'cold spots' within the laser beam, due to poor homogenization or because of imperfections or damage to laser optics. Subsequent regional differences in tissue ablation might, theoretically, lead to central islands; however, islands are not eliminated by frequent replacement of laser optics[48] and variable cold spots in the beam might reasonably be considered to be as likely to cause eccentric as central islands. Differences in laser beam profile, such as the top-hat configuration of the VisX laser compared to the more Gaussian distribution of the earlier Summit lasers, may also contribute to central island formation.

- Secondly, the plume of photoablative products rising from the corneal surface may partially absorb the laser energy centrally if the plume is not removed effectively, resulting in reduced laser energy reaching the central cornea and causing relative underablation of the underlying central stroma. Certainly, it has been noted that varying the position of the vacuum suction nozzle, which is designed to remove ablative products, may alter the incidence of central island formation.[48] This may occur as a result of eddy currents created by evacuation of the plume of ablation products or changes in hydration of the exposed corneal stroma.

- Thirdly, it has been proposed that there are regional differences in hydration of the cornea during photoablation, with fluid collection centripetally, which may result in 'masking' and undercorrection of the centre of the ablation zone. Indeed, central islands were initially described after discontinuation of the technique of blowing nitrogen over the cornea utilized in earlier excimer laser systems.[52] The use of nitrogen in this manner seemed to eliminate the occurrence of central islands and this may lend considerable support to the theory of local hydration excess.[41,53] Acoustic shock waves have been shown to occur as a result of the impact of excimer laser energy on the cornea[54] and, theoretically, these may displace surface fluid centripetally during ablation, resulting in overhydration centrally within the ablation zone.

- Finally, there may be increased stimulus to epithelial healing in the central, more deeply ablated, component of the ablation zone, leading to a focal increase in the degree of epithelial hypertrophy. Such hypertrophy, causing increased central epithelial thickness and the central steepening and increased dioptric power typical of central islands, may resolve with time due to epithelial remodelling to a uniform thickness. However, central islands have been demonstrated prior to re-epithelialization, which would support a stromal rather than epithelial origin.[55] Unfortunately, standard methods of pachymetry in general use cannot discriminate between the relative contribution of epithelium and corneal stroma to the increased central corneal thickness; therefore, it cannot be reliably demonstrated that the increased central thickness is due to epithelial hyperplasia rather than focal areas of lesser stromal ablation. However, studies of PRK in primates have shown markedly thicker epithelium over the ablation zone, with the epithelium being up to 12 cells deep (80 µm) compared to six cells deep (30 µm) in the periphery. This epithelial hyperplasia appears to regress with time and return to normal in 15–18 months.[56–58]

Central corneal topographic islands have most frequently been described in series utilizing a VisX excimer laser and corneal topographic analysis using the Topographic Modelling System (TMS-1) although, more recently, islands have been observed using other corneal topography systems.[59] The apparent preponderance of islands associated with this laser and CVK system has several possible explanations, excluding obvious features such as the greater central corneal coverage of the cornea by the TMS-1 compared to other CVK systems. In early series, using the Summit laser with 4.5–5.0 mm ablation zones, central areas of relatively higher power ('islands'), which may be 3 mm or more in diameter, may actually have occupied much of the ablation zone and, therefore, passed undetected by being misinterpreted as primary undercorrections; it has also been suggested that islands may only occur in larger diameter ablations, such as the 6 mm ablations pioneered by the VisX laser. Lastly, and perhaps most importantly, CVK has not been available in every centre performing excimer laser and, even in those centres that had access to CVK, topography was not always performed in the early postoperative period. Thus, although central topographic islands may have developed with equal frequency in other series, due to rapid resolution many may not have been documented. Indeed, in a study by the authors, had postoperative CVK analysis been

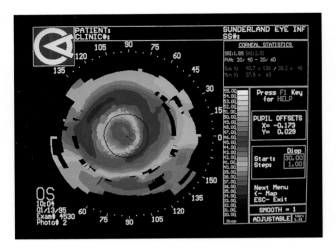

Figure 7.36 *A large central island, a little less than 3.5 mm diameter and 9.00 D power, 1 month after a transepithelial PRK of −9.50 D in a diabetic patient. Unless a central pretreatment, or modified anti-island algorithm is utilized, transepithelial ablation appears to produce central islands more commonly than PRK after manual epithelial debridement. Although this island decreased in power over a 6-month period, excimer PRK retreatment was required (see Fig. 7.43). (Scale: 30.00–55.00 D using 1.00 D incremental steps.)*

postponed to 6 months post-treatment rather than 1 month, only a 3% incidence of central islands, rather than the true incidence of 29%, would have been recorded![49]

Although anecdotal reports suggest some central islands persist for up to and beyond 1 year, little has been written regarding possible differences in the origin, morphology or treatment of persisting central corneal topographic islands. Fortunately, almost all central islands appear to resolve spontaneously within 6 months of the primary PRK procedure, without long-term detrimental effect on refractive outcome.[46,49] However, persisting central topographic islands have necessitated retreatment with excimer laser in some cases (Fig. 7.36).

Transient early postoperative visual problems induced by central topographic islands can be problematic, with up to 32% of eyes with central

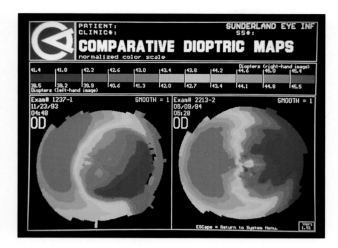

Figure 7.37 *Regression of effect in a PRK ablation zone is highlighted in these two CVK images of the right eye of a patient 3 months (left) and 9 months (right) after PRK. The CVK map on the left shows a degree of inferonasal decentration and a gradual increase in power across the zone from inferonasal (41.40 D) to superotemporal (43.00 D); nonetheless, the patient obtained 20/15 unaided vision with no visual symptoms at 3 months post-treatment. The CVK map on the right demonstrates extensive asymmetric regression of the temporal PRK zone (increased corneal power) and the patient exhibited loss of BSCVA, an unaided visual acuity of 20/120, and troublesome secondary images at this postoperative period. Three months later the patient underwent successful PARK retreatment. (Normalized scales: (left) 38.50–45.50 D using 0.70 D incremental steps; (right) 41.40–45.40 D using 0.40 D incremental steps.)*

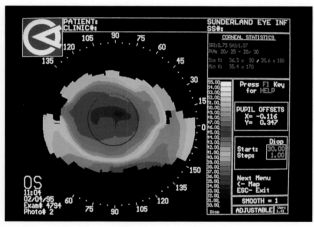

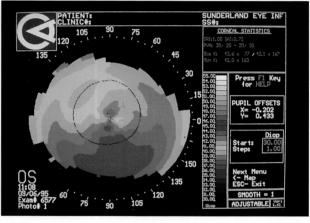

(a)   (b)

Figure 7.38 *Myopic regression with loss of myopic PRK correction can be dramatic, as illustrated by this sequence of CVK maps. (a) A 6.0 mm diameter, well-centred PARK ablation zone, of fairly uniform power, 2 months after a correction of −8.25 D spherical equivalent. At this juncture the patient achieved 20/20 unaided vision. However, progressive myopic regression, unresponsive to topical corticosteroids, commenced approximately 4 months after initial PARK treatment and resulted in widespread erosion of the induced myopic change in the lower half of the ablation zone (b) with regression of myopia to more than 50% of the pre-operative magnitude. A retreatment was performed 1 year after the primary PARK and, although initially very successful (20/15 unaided vision at 2 months post-retreatment), myopic regression occurred once more and the eye exhibited a final spherical equivalent of −2.50 D with BSCVA of 20/20. (Scales: 30.00–55.00 D using 1.00 D incremental steps.)*

islands losing two lines of BSCVA at 2 months post-PRK, compared to 8.7% loss of two lines in eyes not demonstrating islands at the same time point.[49] Therefore, although the natural history of such islands is spontaneous resolution, usually within 6 months, accompanied by recovery of lost lines of Snellen acuity, modifications have been incorporated to excimer laser treatment algorithms in order to reduce their occurrence and speed visual rehabilitation. This modification is usually in the form of additional laser treatment to the centre of the corneal ablation zone at some stage during the treatment.

Regression/healing

Corneal topography is vital in documenting the postoperative course of refractive surgery and provides myriad detail in comparison to the clinical brevity of refraction and unaided visual acuity as benchmarks of success or failure. Trends and subtle changes in corneal profile, immune to the probings of refraction, but often obvious to the patient, are readily exposed and highlighted. Whilst chronological topographic developments have certainly illuminated the healing process and enable appropriate patient education and counselling, unfortunately deleterious changes allow little room for intervention by the ophthalmologist (Figs

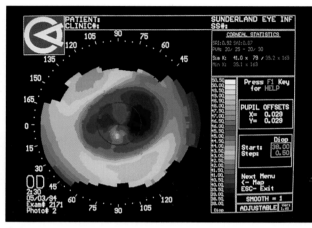

(a)

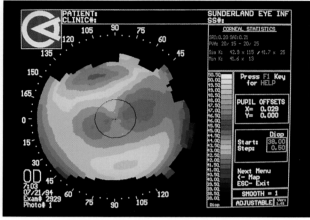

(b)

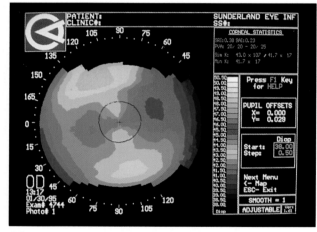

(c)

Figure 7.39 *This series of CVK maps demonstrates preferential regression of myopic cylindrical correction associated with myopic regression following PARK. (a) The CVK map of a right cornea 1 month after a PARK of −2.75/1.50 D at 30°. Although Sim-Ks suggest a topographic cylinder in the region of 1.80 D the patient enjoyed unaided vision of 20/15 with no manifest refractive error. (b) A CVK map of the same cornea 3 months post-PARK. The ablation zone is less well defined and a positive cylinder is evident at 115° on topography. The patient maintained a reasonable 20/20 unaided vision at this point, but corrected to 20/15 with −0.25/−0.50 D at 45°. (c) A considerable change from the 1 month post-PRK map, with poor definition of the ablation zone and the partial re-emergence of the preoperative symmetric bow tie appearance. The patient's unaided vision had reduced to 20/80 and a spectacle correction of −1.00/−1.00 D at 30° produced BSCVA of 20/15. It is notable that the astigmatic correction regressed by 66% in the original axis of the negative cylinder. The patient subsequently underwent a successful retreatment, which was also associated with a small degree of myopic astigmatic regression. (Scale: 38.00–50.50 D in 0.50 D incremental steps.)*

7.37, 7.38). Presently, in the face of myopic regression, over-exuberant healing or irregular astigmatism, the physician's armamentarium is largely limited to trial by corticosteroids (see Chapter 25), excimer laser retreatment (see Chapter 24) or the passage of time.

However, despite limited opportunity for intervention in the healing process, early and repeated topography from the first postoperative month is important if the practitioner is to avoid such common pitfalls as asymmetric healing being mistaken for decentration, or preferential healing of a cylindrical correction being presumed to be a primary undertreatment (Figs 7.39a–c, 7.40a–c). Such topographic information is vital in the planning of excimer laser retreatment.

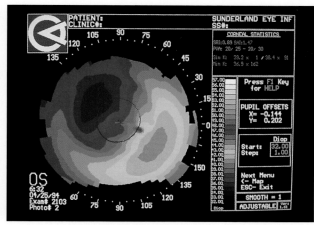

(a)

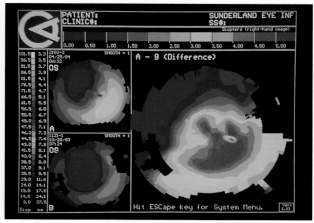

(b)

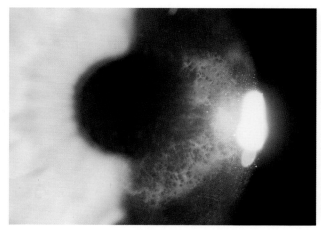

(c)

Figure 7.40 *Preferential healing and myopic regression of a PRK ablation zone can lead to a CVK map appearance suggestive of ablation zone decentration. (a) A CVK map of a left cornea 7 months after a PARK of −5.75/−0.50 D at 30°. The zone appears markedly decentred in a superonasal direction and the eye exhibits a refractive error of +0.25/−1.50 D at 15° with unaided visual acuity of 20/80 and BSCVA of 20/15. (Scale: 32.00–57.00 D in 1.00 D incremental steps.) (b) However, the subtraction or difference CVK map generated by comparing the well-centred ablation zone evident at 1 month post-PARK (B: bottom left) and the apparently decentred PARK zone observed at 7 months (A: top left), highlights that the change in the ablation zone appearance is due to preferential myopic regression (increasing power of up to +5.00 D) in the inferotemporal lower half of the ablation zone (A–B: right.) (Scale: difference scale i shown horizontally along the top of the image; 0.00–5.00 D using 0.50 D incremental steps.) (c) Examination of the cornea illustrated in (a) shows a focal area of grade II reticular haze in a crescentic shape occupying the lower half of the inferotemporal ablation zone. This area of increased haze corresponds closely to the area of focal myopic regression (increased power) shown by CVK analysis. This cornea subsequently underwent PARK retreatment and this is shown in Figs 7.42 a and b.*

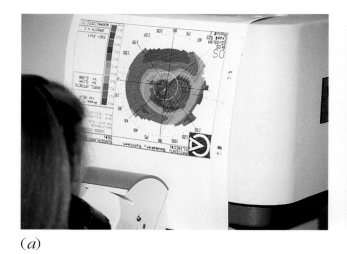

(a)

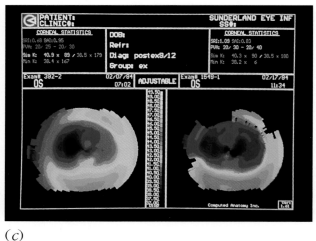

(c)

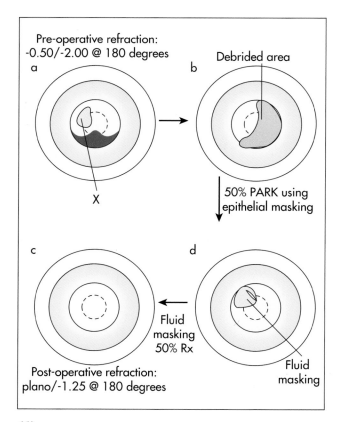

(b)

Figure 7.41 *The CVK map can be carefully annotated to delineate areas of treatment and masking (or focal epithelial debridement) and attached to the excimer laser, in an inverted orientation, to guide PRK retreatment (a). The cornea illustrated in (a) and (c) demonstrates the way in which CVK maps can be used to guide retreatment. (b) This eye suffered troublesome uniocular doubling of images when the pupil was mid-dilated due to an induced cylinder at 6 o'clock in the inferior ablation zone (20/40 unaided visual acuity; 20/15 BSCVA with −0.50/−2.00 D at 180°). However, the superonasal ablation zone demonstrated greater achieved correction than the temporal or inferior zone. Using the CVK map (divided into eight sectors) as a guide, an eight-blade RK marker was gently applied to the corneal epithelium and focal debridement was carried out over the undercorrected aspects of the zone (B). Thereafter, 50% of the −0.50/−2.00 D at 180° ablation was applied. The remainder of the epithelium was then removed (to allow a smooth transition between retreated and untreated areas) and the region of greatest initial correction (X) was masked by saline for the remaining 50% of the PARK ablation. (c) Preoperative (left) and 10 days post-PRK retreatment (right) CVK maps. Both maps are shown on the same scale (37.00–49.50 D in 0.50 D increments). The ablation zone is of more regular power following retreatment and has changed from a semicircular to a more even oval pattern, but it still exhibits a (more regular) degree of WTR cylinder. One year post-retreatment this patient was entirely free of any secondary images or glare and achieved 20/30 unaided visual acuity; however, a degree of cylindrical error had recurred during the first 6 months and final BSCVA was 20/15 with plano/−1.25 at 180°.*

Planning retreatment

Retreatment regimens are covered in detail elsewhere in this book (see Chapter 24); however, the value of CVK data in the planning of retreatment is briefly outlined below. It must be remembered when comparing preoperative corneal power with PRK-induced dioptric change, as evidenced on a difference or subtraction map, there may actually be a slight over- or underestimate of the refractive change deduced by subjective refraction and, in terms of corneal astigmatic power, CVK tends towards overestimation. Therefore, although the topographic map may be considered as a template for retreatment

planning, it must be guided and modified by the manifest refractive error.

Topographic maps are particularly valuable in the management of decentration or asymmetric healing of the ablation zone. Where it is intended to preferentially treat one area, to enlarge a zone or correct asymmetric astigmatism, it is useful to divide up the most recent topographic map into eight segments, akin to radial keratometry divisions, with a delimited central zone equivalent to 6.0–6.5 mm, depending on the diameter of the retreatment ablation zone. This map can then be positioned, in an inverted orientation, at eye level behind the oculars of the laser for reference during retreatment (Fig. 7.41a). Using an

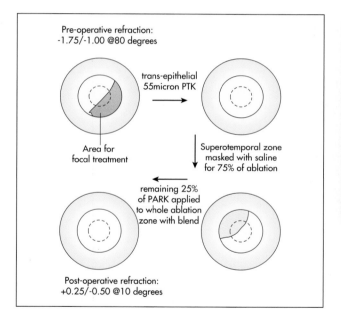

(a)

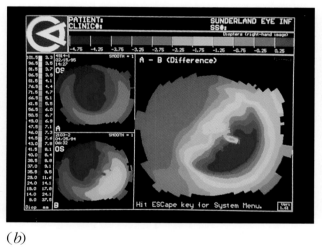

(b)

Figure 7.42 *The case of focal regression highlighted in Fig. 7.40 required PARK retreatment and this is outlined in (a). Because of the underlying focal reticular haze, a transepithelial PTK of 55 μm was performed to smooth the ablation surface, by using the epithelium as a masking agent, prior to the PARK stromal retreatment. Since only the inferotemporal zone required retreatment the superotemporal half of the ablation zone was masked with saline for the initial 75% of the −1.75/−1.00 D at 80° correction. The saline was then removed and the remaining 25% of the PARK ablation applied to the whole zone, utilizing small excursions of the head to blend the transition between maximally retreated and relatively untreated areas. (b) A difference map, created by utilizing the pre-retreatment CVK map (B bottom left) and the 9-month post-retreatment map (A top left), demonstrates that focal retreatment can be successfully guided by the CVK map and manifest refraction (A–B right) to produce, in this case, a myopic PARK correction localized to the inferotemporal zone, which had exhibited focal myopic regression. The patient recorded unaided visual acuity of 20/20 at 1 year post-retreatment and a BSCVA of 20/15 with +0.25 D/−0.50 D at 10°.*

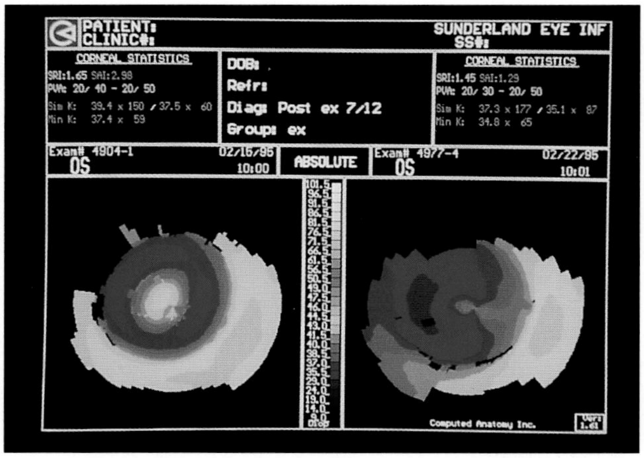

Figure 7.43 *The persisting central topographic island shown in Fig. 7.36 that demonstrated a topographic power of 9.00 D at 1 month, following a transepithelial PRK of −9.50 D, failed to resolve completely. This figure shows the same island prior to retreatment (left). With an apical power of 43.00–44.50 D and mean ablation zone power of 37.00 D, the central island had reduced in power to a maximum of approximately 6.00–7.50 D, with a diameter of 2.50 mm. Surprisingly, the subject obtained 20/60 unaided vision, but this could not be improved by refraction. Due to uncertainty as to the relative contributions of epithelium and stroma to this central island, a 55 µm transepithelial, 2.5 mm diameter, PTK was performed until stroma was uncovered. A conservative correction of the island power, in the form of a −5.00 D correction (diameter 2.5 mm) was then performed. The appearance following retreatment is shown on the right, with complete resolution of the island. As the eye settled over the next 2 months there was no recurrence of the island and 1 year postoperatively the patient achieved 20/40 unaided visual acuity and a regained BSCVA of 20/20 with +1.25/−2.50 D at 70°. (Klyce absolute scale: range 9.0–101.50 D in incremental steps of 1.50 D between 35.50 and 50.50 D, and in 5.00 D incremental steps outside this central range.)*

eight-blade RK marker and an appropriate optical zone marker the corneal epithelium is marked in an identical fashion to the guide marks upon the planning map (Figs 7.41b). By constant reference to the planning map the surgeon can accurately delineate areas to be treated and areas to be masked, either by preferential selective epithelial removal or by the application of a masking solution (Figs 7.42a,b, 7.43).

SUMMARY

Reawakened and wider interest in refractive surgery, highlighted by the precise nature of excimer laser PRK, may have been the wind that fanned the rapid developments in computerized corneal topography over the past decade. However, the original concept of unravelling the fuller nature of the cornea by examining its reflections rests in the renaissance of ophthalmology with such pioneers as Kepler and Scheiner. In everyday practice we are now much nearer to an understanding of the complexities and nuances of corneal power, with a precision and detail that the pioneers of corneal topography might only have dreamed of...

'...the keratoscopic image would furnish a complete record both of the corneal astigmatism and of the decentration of the visual axis. If only it were practical to fix them by instant photography and measure them under the microscope. Until this shall have been accomplished we must depend upon the ophthalmometer to obtain an approximate idea of the form of the anterior surface of the cornea.'

E Javal, System of Diseases of the Eye, 1888

REFERENCES

1. Duke-Elder S, The history of ophthalmic optics. In: Duke-Elder S, ed, *System of Ophthalmology Volume 5, Ophthalmic Optics and Refraction* (Henry Kimpton: London, 1970) 3–21.
2. Wilson SE, Klyce SD, Advances in the analysis of corneal topography, *Surv Ophthalmol* (1991) **35**:269–77.
3. Reynolds AE, Introduction: history of corneal measurement. In: Schanzlin DJ, Robin JB, eds, *Corneal topography: measuring and modifying the cornea* (Springer Verlag: New York, 1991) vii–x.
4. Bores LD, Corneal topography. In: Bores LD, ed, *Refractive*

eye surgery. (Blackwell Scientific: Oxford, 1993) 127–73.

5. Kraff CR, Robin JB, Topography of corneal disease processes. In: Schanzlin DJ, Robin JB, eds, *Corneal topography: measuring and modifying the cornea* (Springer Verlag: New York, 1991) 39–46.

6. Corbett MC, O'Brart DPS, Saunders DC, Rosen ES, The assessment of corneal topography, *Eur J Implant Ref Surg* (1994) **6**:98–105.

7. Wilson SE, Wang JY, Klyce SD, Quantification and mathematical analysis of photokeratoscopic images. In: Schanzlin DJ, Robin JB, eds, *Corneal topography: measuring and modifying the cornea* (Springer Verlag: New York, 1991) 1–9.

8. Maguire LJ, Corneal topography. In: Kaufman HE, Barron BA, McDonald MB, Waltman SR, eds, *The Cornea* (Churchill Livingstone: New York, 1988) 897–909.

9. Hannush SB, Crawford SL, Waring GO, Gemmill MC, Lynn MJ, Nizam A, Accuracy and precision of keratometry, photokeratoscopy and corneal modelling on calibrated steel balls, *Arch Ophthalmol* (1989) **107**:1235–9.

10. Hannush SB, Crawford SL, Waring GO, Gemmill MC, Lynn MJ, Nizam A, Reproducibility of normal corneal power measurements with a ketatometer, photokeratoscope and video imaging system, *Arch Ophthalmol* (1990) **108**:539–44.

11. Webber SK, McGhee CNJ, Bryce IG, Decentration of photorefractive keratectomy ablation zones after excimer laser surgery for myopia, *J Cataract Refract Surg* (1996) **22**:299–303.

12. Cohen KL, Tripoli NK, Holmgren DE, Coggins JM, Assessment of the power and height of radial aspheres reported by a computer-assisted keratoscope, *Am J Ophthalmol* (1995) **119**:723–32.

13. Eghbali F, Yeung KK, Maloney RK, Topographic determination of corneal asphericity and its lack of effect on the refractive outcome of radial keratotomy, *Am J Ophthalmol* (1995) **119**:285–80.

14. Dingledein SA, Klyce SA, Wilson SE, Quantitative descriptors of corneal shape derived from computer assisted analysis of photokeratographs, *Refract Corneal Surg* (1989) **5**: 372–8.

15. Wilson SE, Klyce SD, Quantitative descriptors of corneal topography. A clinical study, *Arch Ophthalmol* (1991) **109**:349–53.

16. Dingeldein SA, Klyce SD, The topography of normal corneas, *Arch Ophthalmol* (1989) **107**:512–18.

17. Bogan SJ, Waring GO, Ibrahim O, Drews C, Curtis L, Classification of normal corneal topography based on computer-assisted videokeratography, *Arch Ophthalmol* (1990) **108**:945–9.

18. Corbett MC, O'Brart DPS, Saunders DC, Rosen ES, The topography of the normal cornea, *Eur J Implant Ref Surg* (1994) **6**:286–97.

19. O'Brart DPS, Saunders DC, Corbett MC, Rosen ES, The topography of keratoconus, *Eur J Implant Ref Surg* (1994) **7**:20–30.

20. Kennedy RH, Bourne WM, Dyer JA, A 48-year clinical and epidemiological study of keratoconus, *Am J Ophthalmol* (1989) **101**:107–12.

21. Wilson SE, Lin DTC, Klyce SD, Corneal topography of keratoconus, *Cornea* (1991) **10**:2–8.

22. Maguire LJ, Bourne WM, Corneal topography of early keratoconus, *Am J Ophthalmol* (1989) **108**:107–12.

23. Rabinowitz YS, McDonnell PJ, Computer-assisted corneal topography in keratoconus, *Refract Corneal Surg* (1989) **5**:400–8.

24. Maeda N, Klyce SD, Smolek MK, Thompson HW, Automated keratoconus screening with corneal topography analysis, *Invest Ophthalmol Vis Sci* (1994) **35**:2749–57.

25. McGhee CNJ, Bryce IG, Anastas CN, et al, Corneal topographic lagoons: a potential new marker for post traumatic recurrent corneal erosion syndrome, *Australian NZ J Ophthalmol* (1996) **24**:27–31.

26. Anastas CN, McGhee CNJ, Bryce IG, Disciform keratitis causing severe irregular astigmatism, *Australian NZ J Ophthalmol* (1996) **24**:69–70.

27. Chitkara D, McGhee CNJ, Bryce IG, Corneal topographic analysis and classification of healthy ametropic and emmetriopic corneas. In: Proceedings of the Royal Australian College of Ophthalmologists, 26th Annual Scientific Conference (1994) (abst).

28. Bryce IG, Morgan SJ, McGhee CNJ, Anastas CN, A classification of keratoconus by computerized videokeratography. In: Proceedings of the 27th Annual Scientific Congress of the Australian College of Ophthalmologists (1995) 120 (abst).

29. Wilson SE, Lin DTC, Klyce SD, Reidy JJ, Insler MS, Topographic changes in contact lens-induced corneal warpage, *Ophthalmol* (1990) **97**:734–44.

30. Wilson SE, Lin DTC, Klyce SD, Reidy JJ, Insler MS, Rigid contact lens decentration: a risk factor for corneal warpage, *CLAO-J* (1990) **16**:177–82.

31. Levenson DS, Berry CV, Findings on follow-up of corneal warpage patients, CLAO-J, (1983) **9**:126–9.

32. Morgan JF, Induced corneal astigmatism and hydrophilic lenses, *Can J Ophthalmol* (1975) **10**:207–13.

33. Ruiz Montenegro J, Mafra CH, Wilson SE, Jumper JM, Klyce SD, Mendelson EN, Corneal topographic alterations in normal contact lens wearers, *Ophthalmol* (1993) **100**:128–34.

34. Uozata H, Guyton DL, Centering corneal surgical procedures, *Am J Ophthalmol* (1987) **103**:264–75.

35. Maloney RK, Corneal topography and optical zone location in photorefractive keratectomy, *Refract Corneal Surg* (1990) **6**:363–71.

36. Cantera E, Cantera I, Oliviera L, Corneal topographic analysis of photorefractive keratectomy in 175 myopic eyes, *Refract Corneal Surgery* (1993) **9(Suppl):**S19–S22.

37. Wilson SE, Klyce SD, McDonald MB, et al, Changes in corneal topography after excimer laser photorefractive keratectomy for myopia, *Ophthalmology* (1991) **98**:1338–47.

38. Cavanaugh TB, Durrie DS, Riedel SM, et al, Topographical analysis of the centration of excimer laser photorefractive keratectomy, *J Cataract Refract Surg* (1993) **19**:136–43.

39. Cavanaugh TB, Durrie DS, Riedel SM, et al, Centration of excimer laser photorefractive keratectomy relative to the pupil, *J Cataract Refract Surg* (1993) **19(Suppl):**144–8.

40. Klyce SD, Smolek MK, Corneal topography of excimer laser photorefractive keratectomy, *J Cataract Refract Surg* (1993) **19(Suppl):**122–30.

41. Lin DTC, Sutton HF, Berman M, Corneal topography following excimer laser photorefractive keratectomy for myopia, *J Cataract Refract Surg* (1993) **19(Suppl)**:149–54.

42. Schwartz-Goldstein BH, Hersh PS, The Summit Photorefractive Keratectomy Study Group. Corneal topography of phase III excimer laser photorefractive keratectomy; optical zone centration analysis, *Ophthalmology* (1995) **102**:951–62.

43. Maguire LJ, Zabel RW, Parker P, Lindstrom RL, Topography and raytracing analysis of patients with excellent visual acuity 3 months after excimer laser photorefractive keratectomy for myopia, *Refract Corneal Surg* (1991) **7**:122–8.

44. Doane JF, Cavanagh TB, Durrie DS, Hassanein KH, Relation of visual symptoms to topographic ablation zone decentration after excimer laser photorefractive keratectomy, *Ophthalmology* (1995) **102**:42–7.

45. Moreira H, Garbus JJ, Fasano A, et al, Multifocal corneal topographic changes with excimer laser photorefractive keratectomy, *Arch Ophthalmol* (1992) **110**:994–9.

46. Lin DTC, Corneal topographic analysis after excimer photorefractive keratectomy, *Ophthalmology* (1994) **101**:1432–9.

47. Hersh PS, Schwartz-Goldstein BH, Corneal topography of Phase III excimer laser photorefractive keratectomy, *Ophthalmology* (1995) **102**:963–78.

48. Levin S, Carson C, Garret SK, Taylor HR, Prevalence of central islands after excimer laser refractive surgery, *J Cataract Refract Surg* (1995) **21**:21–6.

49. McGhee CNJ, Bryce IG, The natural history of central topographic islands following excimer laser photorefractive keratectomy, *J Cataract Refract Surg* (1996) **22**:1151–58.

50. Salz JJ, Maguen E, Nesburn AB, et al, A two year experience with excimer laser photorefractive keratectomy for myopia, *Ophthalmology* (1993) **100**:873–82.

51. Dutt S, Steinert RF, Raizman MB, Puliafito CA, One year results of excimer laser photorefractive keratectomy for low to moderate myopia, *Arch Ophthalmol* (1994) **112**:1427–36.

52. Campos M, Cuevas K, Garbus J, et al, Corneal wound healing after excimer laser ablation: effects of a nitrogen gas blower, *Opthalmology* (1992) **99**:893–7.

53. Parker PJ, Klyce SD, Ryan BL, et al, Central topographic islands following photorefractive keratectomy, *Invest Ophthalmol Vis Sci* (1993) **34 (Suppl)**:803.

54. Bor ZS, Hopp B, Racz B, et al, Plume emission, shock wave and surface wave formation during excimer laser ablation of the cornea, *Refract Corneal Surg* (1993) **9(Suppl)**:S111–S115.

55. Colin J, Cochener B, Gallinaro C, Central steep islands immediately following excimer laser photorefractive keratectomy for myopia, *Refract Corneal Surg* (1993) **9**:395–6.

56. Hanna KD, Pouliquen YM, Savodelli M, et al, Corneal wound healing in monkeys 18 months after excimer laser photorefractive keratectomy, *Refract Corneal Surg* (1990) **6**:340–5.

57. Del Pero RA, Gogstad JE, Roberts AD, et al, A refractive and histopathological study of excimer laser keratectomy in primates, *Am J Ophthalmol* (1990) **109**:419–29.

58. Hanna KD, Pouliquen YM, Waring GO, et al, Corneal wound healing in monkeys after repeated excimer laser photorefractive keratectomy, *Arch Ophthalmol* (1992) **110**:1286–91.

59. Gangadhar DV, Talamo JH, The use of computerized videokeratography in keratorefractive surgery, *Semin Ophthalmol* (1994) **9(2)**:81–90.

Chapter 8 Patient assessment in photo-refractive surgery

Kathryn H Weed and Charles N J McGhee

INTRODUCTION

Comprehensive preoperative patient assessment is perhaps the pivotal element of excimer laser photo-refractive treatment, whereas the postoperative length of care and frequency of review is less defined for photorefractive keratectomy (PRK) or photoastigmatic refractive keratectomy (PARK) than for many other types of elective ophthalmic surgery. This chapter is divided into two sections, preoperative and postoperative assessment, and the important objective and subjective evaluations are illustrated at each stage.

PRE-OPERATIVE ASSESSMENT

FIRST CONTACT: THE BEGINNINGS OF PATIENT EDUCATION

As the frequently expressed maxim states 'first impressions count', and this opportunity normally presents itself at the first contact by telephone or letter communication. In the UK, which at one point in 1994 hosted no less than 55 active excimer laser sites (or approximately one per million of population), it became increasingly apparent to those active in the field that many prospective patients were 'shopping around' for the best service.

It became equally apparent that the patient's first contact would usually be by telephone and that this first call was not usually a casual enquiry for an information brochure, or more specifically for an appointment, but rather it usually involved a sequence of specific questions (presumably already asked of several other centers) that included: which surgeons were available; how long had the laser site been operational and how many patients had been treated

specifically by this technique; which laser was being utilized and was this a 'new' generation laser; what level of myopia was being treated; was astigmatism also being treated; was the procedure painful and how many days away from work might be anticipated postoperatively; would all necessary medications be included in the cost of treatment; and if enhancement or retreatment was required would there be an additional charge? Well-trained personnel can quite adequately answer all of these questions in general terms, although discussing an individual's refractive problem in specific terms is best avoided! Usually an informed approach to these frequently asked questions provides the patient with the positive feedback of a team approach to their future eyecare. Obviously the best individuals to answer many of these questions are those who have already undergone PRK treatment and many centers in the UK have successfully recruited individuals who had received treatment, or offered treatment to interested members of staff.

All enquiries, wherever possible, should be followed by the forwarding of an information package, which can set the tone of the patients' refractive surgery education, vital for the development of realistic expectations and knowledge of the relative benefits and risks of PRK/PARK surgery. Preferably patients should have read and studied carefully any such information guide prior to the initial assessment consultation. Obviously the detail included in such an information pack will vary from physician to physician and center to center. However, any clinician involved in keratorefractive activities must be fully aware of any patient education or promotional material that prospective patients are given. Even if such material, originating from the physician's clinic or laser center, does not actually identify the physician by name, any unsubstantiated or overly optimistic claims made in such literature, may later be construed as confusing or misleading informed consent in a legal setting.[1]

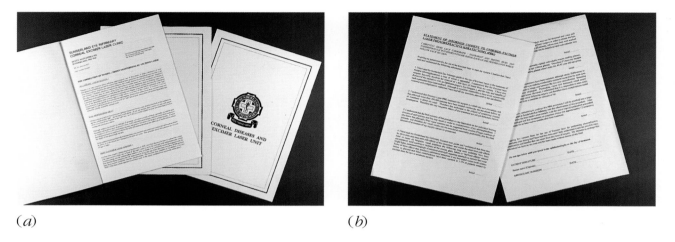

(a)   (b)

Figure 8.1 *Written information handout provided in the Sunderland Eye Infirmary (SEI) excimer laser study.*

WRITTEN PATIENT INFORMATION

The extent and content of patient information packs will not only vary depending upon the approach of the ophthalmologist involved, but is equally dependent upon the cultural and educational background of the patient base. Since commencing excimer laser activities in Sunderland Eye Infirmary (SEI), a UK National Health Service (NHS) Trust hospital, we have favored an extensive and comprehensive information pack consisting of six pages of single spaced typeface, about 2500 words, covering the following areas: explanations of myopia (near/short-sightedness), hyperopia (far/long-sightedness) and astigmatism; definitions of PRK, PARK, radial keratotomy (RK) and transverse astigmatic keratotomy (T-cuts); a brief explanation of the manner of excimer laser photoablation; a resumé of the results of recent representative large PRK/PARK studies in a text and tabulated form; a summary of the results for various refractive errors obtained in our unit; an extensive and explicit list of reported complications; reported complications from the SEI series; and answers to commonly asked questions (Fig. 8.1). Following approximately 2000 telephone requests and the forwarding of these comprehensive information packs, which some might suspect would tend to deter rather than encourage potential patients, this initial expression of interest was converted into a

Table 8.1
Satisfaction study results. Patient responses to information giving (n=90). From an anonymous questionnaire study following excimer laser PRK. (From McGhee et al.[2])

Sufficient written information	95.6%
Sufficient verbal information	94.5%
All questions adequately answered	95.6%
Further information readily available	100%
Operative procedure fully understood	98.9%
Discussion with patients who had already undergone PRK useful reassurance	84.1%

little under 600 procedures (without further patient follow-up by telephone or mail). An anonymous patient questionnaire was subsequently completed by 90 of the first 100 patients who proceeded to surgery, after having considered this patient information and undergone formal assessment (Table 8.1).[2]

PRE-ASSESSMENT INSTRUCTIONS

Current contact lens wearers should be advised to remove their lenses, for at least 7 days for soft hydrogel lenses and 2 weeks for rigid gas permeable or hard PMMA contact lenses, before attending for initial consultation. If the patient wears 'retainer lenses' for orthokeratology purposes then these lenses must be discontinued for a minimum of 6 months.[3] In the event, these recommendations for length of contact lens removal prior to review are rather arbitrary and patients should be informed that due to contact lens-related corneal warpage, a longer period of discontinued lens wear might be necessary for an accurate preoperative assessment.

Prospective patients should be requested to bring three or more copies of their refractive correction for the preceding 3–5 year period, if at all possible, in order to help establish the stability of refraction. A reminder should be provided that driving will not be possible following the assessment, due to pupil dilation for the purpose of thorough retinal examination, and that communication with their general medical practitioner or personal physician will be sought if they elect to proceed to surgery.

INITIAL APPOINTMENT

CLINIC ENVIRONMENT

The ambience of the waiting room dictates the physical comfort of the patient, necessary to help allay any misgivings or concerns of the unknown. It will also affect the initial professional image of the clinic, as does the reception area. Patient education can be continued with an information video on the PRK/PARK procedure running within the waiting room and by provision of additional information leaflets or posters. By establishing clinics that combine new patient assessments and review of patients who have already undergone PRK/PARK, new patients may be able to discuss 'real-life experiences' of the procedure with those who have previously been treated. In our experience this appears to be extremely beneficial in reassuring potential patients.[2] The need for realistic expectations of outcome cannot be stressed enough and this more than anything will color the level of subjective success. Therefore further copies of the patient information guides should be provided as leaflets and educational posters in the waiting area, such that reinforcement of this information can be made. Depending on the size and style of practice an ancillary health-care worker may be employed to cover salient points of the procedure with all new patients.

INITIAL ASSESSMENT

PATIENT HISTORY: REASONS FOR SEEKING TREATMENT

The prior knowledge the patient has assimilated through the popular media and the patient grapevine may have already accumulated into a preconceived, quite possibly erroneous, concept of what PRK can accomplish. This must be noted carefully and addressed. A unique visual analogue questionnaire was developed at SEI to determine the reasons why patients seek excimer laser treatment.[2] Improved unaided vision (85.6%), freedom from spectacles (83.3%), difficulties with the wearing of contact lenses (72.7%), and improved unaided vision enabling subjects to participate in sports (70%) were the most common reasons. In respect to those pursuing sporting activities, PRK should not predispose the globe to rupture in the event of blunt ocular trauma,[4] and Salz[5] observed corneal abrasions sustained during sport in the post-PRK cornea healed as would be expected in the normal untreated cornea. Improved cosmetic appearance was only considered important for 59.5%, but this was a higher figure than

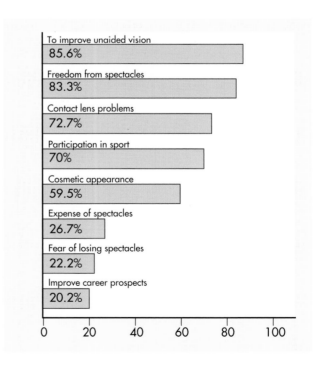

Figure 8.2 *Reasons for seeking excimer laser treatment of myopia. (From McGhee et al.[2])*

Kahle's study[6] where 'looking better' was considered of minor importance; unsurprisingly the highest-ranked motivation in this latter study was the desire to improve general vision. Interestingly, only 26.7% in the SEI series rated the expense of spectacles and contact lenses as reasons for interest in the procedure (Fig. 8.2).

OCULAR HISTORY

This should include previous ocular surgery, orthoptic treatment, and refractive history. In particular, an accurate contact lens history should be ascertained: when the lenses were last worn; the type of contact lens; the ongoing wearing success or not (e.g. wearing times past and present, dryness symptoms, whether tear supplements are being supplied, environmental and seasonal associations); and reasons for discontinuation of contact lens wear are equally essential points. In one questionnaire study the significant difference between those subjects who resumed contact lens wear after discontinuation, compared to those who did not, was found to be largely related to the 'inconvenience' of cleaning, inserting, and removing the contact lenses.[7] The ability to wear a contact lens in the non-operated eye is extremely helpful in highly myopic individuals to alleviate the anisometropia created following surgery to the first eye. Contact lens wear may be equally crucial to those in whom the final refractive outcome is not intended to be emmetropia, but rather a large reduction of the presenting myopia.

REFRACTIVE STABILITY

The stability of the patients' refractive status must be determined by previous copies of their refractive prescription. With regard to refractive stability, many practitioners arbitrarily suggest a lower age limit of 18 to 21 years of age for treatment. Girls antedate boys, in terms of refractive stabilization, by about 2 years and this pattern of myopia stability is true for some 87% females and 68% males. The majority of the remainder have a continuing myopic progression but at a much slower rate than during child and teenagehood, with only 6% of males showing an accelerated progression of myopia (see Chapter 5). Patients must be made aware of the possibility of such predetermined myopic progression in the future, which cannot be ascertained preoperatively, and that will not be ameliorated by photorefractive surgery.

Table 8.2
Relative ocular contraindications to excimer laser PRK.

Severe dry eye disease
Lagophthalmos
Severe atopic disease
Blepharitis
Past history of herpes simplex virus keratitis
Decreased corneal sensation/neurotrophic cornea
Keratoconus (with apical thinning)
Irregular astigmatism
Marked corneal vascularization

MEDICAL HISTORY: OCULAR AND SYSTEMIC CONTRAINDICATIONS

As with any new procedure the initial list of relative contraindications is inevitably extensive, but as greater clinical experience and knowledge of the technique is gained this list diminishes considerably. In respect to our present state of knowledge, relative ocular contraindications to PRK/PARK (Table 8.2) might include severe dry eye disease, lagophthalmos, severe atopic disease, blepharitis that has not been treated, history of herpes simplex virus keratitis, decreased corneal sensation/neurotrophic cornea, keratoconus (with apical thinning), irregular astigmatism, marked corneal neovascularization within 1 mm of the ablation zone,[8] and advanced glaucoma (see Chapter 23). Questions upon relevant family medical and ocular history, such as chronic open angle glaucoma, corneal dystrophies, etc. are pertinent.

Relative systemic contraindications (Table 8.3) that theoretically might affect healing and influence the refractive outcome include: pregnancy, diabetes

Table 8.3
Relative systemic contraindications to excimer laser PRK.

Pregnancy
Diabetes mellitus
Immunocompromise
Collagen disorders, e.g. SLE and rheumatoid arthritis
Systemic medication which affects healing, e.g. systemic steroids and HRT

First of all the spherical component of the objective refraction needs to be confirmed. This power is adjusted by requesting the patient to look at a letter on the last line of distinct vision and to reply if the letter improves in clarity or reduces with the addition of a powered lens. To ensure accommodation is not stimulated, demonstrate the addition of a positive lens first, using for example +0.25 DS. If there is no improvement in VA nor any deterioration, add the plus lens and repeat this addition until there is a deterioration of visual acuity. If there is initially a reduction in VA then add a –0.25 D lens and then add additional minus sphere as above, but be particularly careful there is no 'eating up' of the minus, which myopes tend to do, i.e. ensure that any increase in minus sphere correlates with improvement of VA.

To confirm that myopic overcorrection has not occurred, ask the patient to observe the duochrome (bichromatic test), which consists of letters or four black circles (each circle contains a smaller circle for definition). Two of the circles are on an illuminated green background, the other two are on an illuminated red background. The patient should be asked which circles look blacker or clearer, those on the red or the green background. The black circles should be just clearer on the green rather than the red; however, this should reverse to red on the addition of +0.25 D. If 'overminused', i.e. too much negative sphere has been added, the circles on the red will be blurred. Although previous ophthalmologic texts have suggested subjective refraction should remain on red just changing to green, it is the authors' opinion that in general the 'just green' is

more beneficial to the myopic patient, especially in poor illumination conditions. Research has established that night myopia can frequently induce an extra undercorrection of –0.25 DS;[10] if the patient has been left 'on the red' this could translate into a –0.50 DS undercorrection, which may have a noticeable impact, especially upon the ability to drive without refractive correction at night. The key principles to avoid overestimation of myopia are highlighted in Table 8.5.

DELINEATION OF CYLINDER MAGNITUDE AND AXIS

To refine the cylindrical component there are two widely used, and well-described methods utilizing either the Jackson cross-cylinder or the fan and block technique.[10,11] Both techniques can be utilized using a trial frame; however, if a phoropter unit is used the same principles apply. A cross-cylinder incorporates two lenses of equal power (usually 0.25 D) but opposite sign and therefore the mean spherical power is zero. It requires for the circle of least confusion to be on the retina as the cross-cylinder technique will alter the interval of Sturm (distance between the two focal lines) not the position of the circle relative to the retina (Fig. 8.4). Following further refinement of the magnitude of the cylindrical component of the refraction by one of the above methods, even if the cylinder is increased by a relatively small amount, then adjustment to the sphere component is also needed to keep the circle of least confusion on the retina, e.g. if cylinder power

Table 8.5
Key principles to avoid overestimation of myopia.

Fixate distant target
Contralateral eye blurred (6/12 or 20/40) during refraction
Neutralize 'with movement' first (with positive spheres, i.e. negative cylinders)
When adjusting spherical component use a positive sphere first
When adjusting cylinder power, adjust spherical component accordingly
Duochrome reversal with +0.25/–0.25 DS
+1.00 DS blur test
Binocular balancing with fogging technique

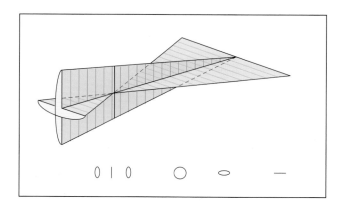

Figure 8.4 *Diagrammatic representation of the interval of Sturm and the circle of least confusion.*

is increased by −0.25 D then +0.12 D is added to the sphere component in the trial frame, to avoid inadvertent over- or undercorrection.

THE PENULTIMATE STAGE

At the endpoint of subjective refraction, place a +1.00 DS lens into the trial frame and record the VA obtained. This is called 'fogging' and the +1.00 DS lens is the 'fogging lens'. The VA should 'blur back', i.e. be reduced to approximately 6/12 (20/40) if the patient's correctable VA was approximately 6/5 (20/15). A point of note is that 6/12 (20/40) is the level of reasonably guaranteed unaided outcome postexcimer PRK for the majority of patients, and demonstration of this level of Snellen acuity on a chart, followed by encouraging the patient to look or walk around the clinic with the trial frame on, can be useful in appreciation of this level of unaided vision in a 'real-life' context. If the patient can still see the original line or that above with 'fogging', the patient has too much negative sphere incorporated into the subjective prescription and, therefore, if the duochrome is observed the black circles on the green background will be clear whilst the circles on the red will be blurred. Theoretically, if the patient's VA does 'blur back' by the 'fogging lens', if this fogging lens is removed and the duochrome is observed, the black circles will look equally clear on the red and the green. Sometimes this equal balance is not obtainable and in these circumstances it may be preferable, as previously stated, for the patient to be 'on the green', switching to red with an additional +0.25 DS to prevent undercorrection.

After both eyes have undergone this procedure, binocular balancing should always be performed. As the commonly employed 'Humphriss immediate contrast test'[10] requires a +1.00 DS blur to 6/12 (20/40), this balancing technique flows easily from the previous step. With the +1.00 DS lens placed in front of one eye the patient is asked to look at a letter on the 6/9 (20/30) line. A +0.25 DS then a −0.25 DS lens is placed in front of the 'non-fogged' eye and the patient asked which feels more comfortable. If he replies in the affirmative, and there is no deterioration of VA, then the appropriate lens is incorporated into the trial frame lenses and so forth until no subjective improvement is obtained. The +1.00 DS lens is then switched to the other eye and the procedure repeated. The fogging method relies on foveal vision in the 'fogged' eye being suspended but paracentral and peripheral vision being maintained.

This of course will not work in situations of compromised binocular vision such as amblyopia or alternating esotropia or exotropia. After binocular balancing carefully record the prescription and VA attained.

COMBINING DATA TO REFINE CYLINDRICAL CORRECTION

Occasionally one is fortunate enough to come across a patient with past refractive documentation of a cylindrical component that is virtually identical in both magnitude and axis to the preoperative astigmatism documented by the above techniques. Less frequently, this preoperative astigmatic magnitude and axis also corresponds exactly to the data obtained by computerized videokeratography (CVK), keratometry, and autorefraction. Videokeratography should also identify any asymmetric astigmatism and may assist in differentiating between astigmatism that is corneal or lenticular in origin. Lenticular astigmatism can be created by either or both lens surfaces or by decentration or tilting of the lens with respect to the cornea. It accounts for the difference between corneal astigmatism and total ocular astigmatism (spectacle lens), allowing for BVD. If the resultant ocular astigmatism axis is different to the corneal axis, then the former axis direction will have been created in accordance with the theory of obliquely crossed cylinders. Lenticular astigmatism has been found to have a narrow leptokurtic (peaked) distribution, the great majority of eyes falling between zero and 1.00 D against the rule.[12]

Some clinicians also take into account the astigmatic axis determined by autorefraction. However, although an autorefractor is a useful adjunct in the busy clinical setting, it cannot replace an experienced refraction utilizing retinoscopy, fogging, and binocular balancing techniques. Autorefractors are programmed to compute readings from the reflected reflex over the entire width of the pupil. Postoperative to PRK/PARK, especially in the first few months, one can frequently observe during retinoscopy the end point of a neutral reflex centrally whilst still maintaining an against movement in the periphery. These conflicting reflexes may adversely influence autorefractor accuracy, especially in patients with large pupils. Russell et al[13] found in patients with RK that although preoperatively the difference between mean sphere obtained by an autorefractor and subjective refraction was clinically acceptable at 0.25 D, postoperatively there was a statistically significant difference of 1.25 D, with the autorefractor detecting a more myopic refraction. Proximal myopia must also be considered, especially in younger patients. Although cycloplegic assessment does minimize this latter error, as previously noted, it compounds any associated considerations of pupil size and does not allow for subjective assessment. Autorefractors have been found to have excellent reproducibility in the healthy unoperated eye;[14] however, inaccuracies when measuring eyes with pathology, e.g. lens and corneal opacities, have been documented[15] and therefore their usefulness in the postoperative PRK eye is further compromised.

The possible errors of keratometry and CVK are described in detail elsewhere.[16,17] The crucial factors of position (centration, working distance) and fixation of the patient are relevant to avoiding error formation by clinician or equipment. Disregarding the possible errors, sensitivity of 0.25 D and reproducibility of 0.50 D, with the cylinder axis being within 10°, are tolerance figures to be expected from contemporary autorefractors. However, in contrast, formal refraction allows the facility to adapt, i.e. to concentrate only on the central part of the reflex, to cope with possible epithelial disturbance, which can vary throughout the ablation zone, and to manipulate accommodation without cycloplegia. Vital additional information such as reflex distortions due to keratoconus and contact lens warpage can also be detected by the retinoscopy reflex.

Therefore, some debate continues to surround which is the best method of ascertaining the correct cylindrical axis to use in programming excimer laser

PARK. Although some clinicians have suggested a mean of all three cylinder axes obtained in the preoperative work-up (i.e. definitive subjective axis, computerized corneal topographic axis, and autorefractive axis); if such a compromise axis is chosen, the subjective best-corrected VA with this axis should be compared to the definitive axis obtained by subjective refraction. Such a compromised axis should only be utilized if the VA is unchanged or improved by this change in axis and such a compromise axis probably only has a role in these occasional patients that exhibit a wide latitude (> ±5°) in preferred subjective axis. It should always be borne in mind that a 15° error in axis alignment can produce a 50% reduction in correction (Fig. 8.5).[18,19]

STANDARDIZING VISUAL ACUITY MEASUREMENT

As already mentioned, Snellen acuity distance test charts are the letter charts most frequently used and can be subject to variable illumination conditions that may obviously affect recorded VA. The minimum luminance for internally illuminated charts is 120 candelas/meter^2 (cd/m^2), (the minimum for new equipment being 150 cd/m^2) and for externally illuminated charts 480 lux (600 lux for new).[10] Regarding the evenness of the luminance or illumination, the minimum uniformity ratio should be 70%.[20] As one of the more common complications of PRK/PARK is that of loss of lines of best spectacle visual acuity (BSCVA), not only is a standard acuity chart set up important in terms of illumination, but ideally a more accountable method of recording visual acuity is needed. The Bailey–Lovie letter chart uses Log MAR acuity[21] whereby each letter correctly identified is credited.[22,23] There are high and low contrast, and near acuity versions of this chart.

NEAR VISION AND READING ACUITY

The residual, or induced, astigmatic error that can occur after PRK/PARK will affect near VA 'crispness' more so than general distance. This may cause possible symptoms of asthenopia especially with computer VDU work increasingly becoming an everyday visual task. Myopes presenting for PRK/PARK must also be made aware of the inherent advantages of lower levels of myopia with regard to presbyopia. Since many patients who seek this procedure are in the presbyopic age group, loss of this

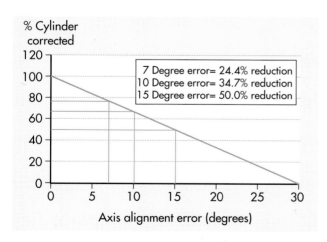

Figure 8.5 *Percentage cylinder correction versus error in cylinder axis alignment.*

unaided near vision facility can have an immediate effect. All patients must be made fully aware that if PRK/PARK results in emmetropia or low hypermetropia, reading glasses will be required as presbyopia develops.

Under these circumstances, some patients, already in the presbyopic age range, may elect for monovision, i.e. only one eye receiving PRK/PARK, or a deliberate undercorrection of one eye. However, such patients must be made aware that in this situation judgement of speed and depth of field will be affected due to the depreciation of the binocular status, especially so with night driving. The dominant eye should be used for distance and, therefore, is the eye of choice to undergo a fully correcting procedure. Ocular dominance can be assessed by using an alignment technique, whereby the patient is asked to point to a distance object with both hands held together. As both hands are held together hand dominance is eliminated and the fingers should instinctively line up with the dominant eye. If the patient closes each eye in turn, the 'line up' eye will become apparent. Similarly, a hole in a card can be used by asking the patient to look at a letter with the card extended in front of him/her, both eyes being open. The eye viewing the letter will be the dominant one. In contrast, where both eyes are to be treated, the authors' current practice is to treat the non-dominant eye first, in view of the small but appreciable risk of complications that might affect BSCVA.

ASSESSING SUBJECTIVE VISUAL SYMPTOMS PREOPERATIVELY

Subjective symptoms of glare, haloes, and ghosting are reported in various degrees after PRK/PARK;[24] however, it is important to realize that some subjects will have experienced these same symptoms prior to surgery[25] and these should be documented. This visual degradation can be measured by a low-contrast chart such as the Bailey–Lovie chart or by a contrast sensitivity test such as the Pelli–Robson chart.[26,27] Glare tests are also ways of quantifying possible subjective symptoms pre- and postoperatively[28] but must be evaluated prepachymetry and intraocular pressure (IOP) measurement. Glare testing has previously been found to be clinically useful in evaluating pseudophakes with posterior capsule opacification who complained of visual disability despite good Snellen VA under standard testing conditions.[29]

The pupil diameter may be difficult to measure but pupil size will have a bearing on all VA type measurements. Under the illumination conditions of the test, a pupil template is the easiest way to judge the pupil size. Hold the template half way over the patient's pupil, ask the patient to look at a distance object and match one of the pupils on the template to that of the patient's to form a complete pupil. To try and evaluate possible problems with pupil dilation at night time, one can use the pupil template in conjunction with just a Burton lamp, since under the cobalt blue light the fluorescence of the crystalline lens is seen and no room illumination is required.[30] Alternatively, using a slit lamp biomicroscope the slit height can be preset to the estimated pupil diameter and the biomicroscope is quickly turned on and off, with low room illumination. The slit height is then adjusted until coincident with the pupil diameter. Whichever method is employed, the dimensions of the pupil should be recorded under ambient and low-light conditions.

ASSESSMENT OF PHORIAS AND TROPIAS

To assess the muscle balance status pre- and postoperatively, at the very minimum, a cover test should be performed and any history of strabismus or amblyopia determined. It is possible that a near phoria may become decompensated after PRK due to the loss of the base in prism effect created by myopic spectacles, and esotropia subsequent to RK has previously been reported.[31] In eyes with gross myopic anisometropia, in which the more ametropic eye has not been routinely fully corrected, all reasonable attempts, e.g. by fitting temporary contact lenses and a full orthoptic assessment, must be made to exclude the possibility of postoperative diplopia.

COMPUTERIZED VIDEOKERATOGRAPHY

Undiagnosed keratoconics may, due to the visual dissatisfaction with spectacles or contact lenses, appear at excimer clinics in a greater percentage than expected from population studies.[32] Videokeratography can be a useful diagnostic aid and also part of the educational process. Measurement must be performed prior to IOP and pachymetry. Graphic representation of corneal power, in a readily comprehensible form, is empowering to the patients who often feel, after being shown such topographic maps with appropriate explanations, that they can relate to and understand more fully features such as astigmatism. Contact lens warpage is frequently identified, usually accompanying hard, and less frequently rigid gas permeable contact lens wear. On cessation there is progressive corneal flattening for the first 3 days, followed by corneal steepening usually leaving the cornea 0.50–0.75 D flatter[33] with associated increase in the 'with the rule' astigmatism.[34] Normal topography may not be achieved for several months following cessation of contact lens wear.[35] As these patients experience spectacle blur (in fact many will not have up to date spectacles), one eye will have to be chosen for cessation of contact lens wear and monitored with repeated CVK until the corneal shape has stabilized. Soft contact lens-induced warpage, although rarer, has been observed[36] and in such cases the corneal topography also needs to be monitored over time; however, resolution of corneal contact lens warpage with soft contact lenses is usually rapid and not under the same lengthy time constraints as hard contact lens warpage (see Chapter 7).

BIOMICROSCOPY

ASSESSMENT OF LIDS AND TEARFILM

Evaluation of the lid position and condition of lid margins is important. Blepharitis can be a potential cause of ocular infection and sterile corneal infiltrates postoperatively and should be treated by improved lid hygiene, with lid scrub and antibiotic cover if necessary. The tear quality can be quantified by the tear break up time (TBUT) using fluorescein (with local discontinuity in tear film translating to a discrete black area, and TBUT less than 10 seconds generally being considered abnormal),[37] phenol red thread test (thread changes from yellow to red due to pH of tears, normally between 9 and 20 mm in length in 15 seconds)[38] or by non-invasive techniques (NIBUT) such as the Tearscope (utilizing a cold light source) (Fig. 8.6),[39] stability of keratometer mires or by lactoferrin immunoassay testing (normal concentration 1.42 mg/mL).[37] Schirmer strips only provide quantitative information and the Schirmer test is considered normal when the filter paper strip wets more than 15 mm in 5 minutes,[38] but in practice an artificially increased reading may be produced by induced reflex tearing. Therefore non-invasive techniques, avoiding the addition of fluids such as fluorescein, which by lowering the surface tension destabilizes

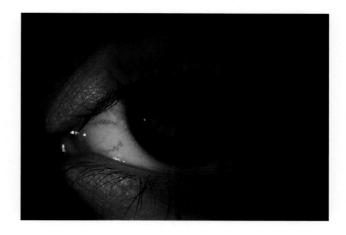

Figure 8.6 *Tearscope examination of tearfilm.*

the tear film, or obviating increased tear evaporation by biomicroscope illumination, are generally the more useful.

Documentation of tear film status can be important, as tear deficiency may delay or alter corneal epithelial healing post-PRK/PARK, in addition to the less dramatic, but frequently reported, subjective symptoms of variation in VA on blinking and the sensation of 'dryness' or grittiness postoperatively. Despite anecdotal reports, further investigation is still required to determine if there is a direct relationship between the quality of the precorneal tear film preoperatively and myopic regression and corneal haze. The presence of diffuse punctate epithelial erosions, or lower one-third corneal staining may be indicative of a clinically dry eye, or incomplete lid closure (lagophthalmus), both of which may compromise the healing response.

ASSESSMENT OF ANTERIOR SEGMENT

The cornea should be carefully assessed for any early signs of keratoconus such as Fleischer's ring, Vogt's striae, and differential thickness of the corneal optical section. The stroma must be thoroughly assessed in respect to preoperative evidence of focal haze or decrease in translucency, which may be related to age˙ (Fig. 8.7),[40] degenerative conditions, corneal dystrophies and long-term contact lens wear (Fig. 8.8).[41] Following biomicroscopic assessment of the corneal endothelium, if specular microscopy is

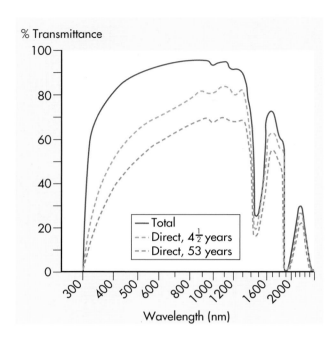

Figure 8.7 *Changes in corneal translucency with age. (Published in Boettner EA and Wolter JR,* Invest Ophthalmol *(1962)* **I**:776)

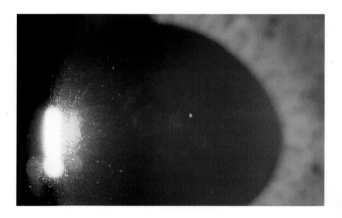

Figure 8.8 *Corneal stromal flecks related to long-term contact lens wear.*

unavailable, a careful slit lamp record of the appearance of the endothelial mosaic and the presence of any endothelial degenerative changes, including guttata, should be made. As patients within the presbyopic age group do present for PRK/PARK, careful evaluation of lenticular changes is required to exclude the possibility of cataract extraction, which

for high myopes might be a preferable refractive solution. One must also keep in mind the possibility of nuclear sclerosis inducing a myopic shift by lenticular refractive index changes. Other additional tests should include measurement of the IOP (with time of measurement), corneal thickness (pachymetry), corneal sensitivity (esthesiometry), endothelial specular photomicroscopy and corneal photography of any detected abnormalities (see Chapter 23).

ASSESSMENT OF THE OCULAR FUNDUS

A mydriatic fundus evaluation is essential. Of continued academic debate is the effect, if any, of the acoustic shock waves produced by excimer laser PRK upon asymptomatic peripheral retinal conditions, such as small holes and lattice degeneration. Nonetheless, any significant peripheral retinal degeneration should be referred for assessment, and possible prophylactic treatment, by a vitreoretinal colleague. In the first 100 consecutive patients reviewed in SEI, we identified 4% with asymptomatic peripheral retinal holes, including one large horseshoe tear in an eye with a refraction of –6.50 D (Fig. 8.9). The presence or absence of posterior vitreous detachment (PVD) should be established and we have personally encountered one case of sudden symptomatic PVD within 2 weeks of PRK. Whether this latter event represents coincidence or 'cause and effect' (as concluded by the patient) is obviously open to speculation.

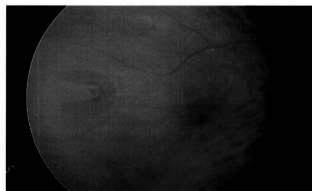

Figure 8.9 *Asymptomatic, horseshoe, retinal tear in a patient with moderate myopia presenting for myopic RK.*

Particular attention should be directed to examining and documenting the condition of the maculae, even in patients with good VA. Subtle changes may be more likely to provoke visual symptoms in the post-PRK eye with compromised transparency, and cystoid macular edema has been reported following PRK.[42]

FINAL PREOPERATIVE INTERVIEW

This is the time to address the patient expectations and provide a realistic probability of outcome following treatment. The individual clinic's results for unaided vision for a range of myopia or myopic astigmatism should be available for the patient to see. However, reinforcement of the fact that individual eyes will have different healing responses is vitally important. The distinct probability of occasional spectacle wear for demanding fine visual tasks such as night driving, theatre, cinema, reading, or VDU work should be emphasized. The relevant short-term and long-term effects of the PRK procedure should be discussed (see Chapter 23 for further information). All information discussed should be accurately documented in the patient file, this is important for future consultation and especially in consideration of the medicolegal climate in relation to refractive surgery. If the ophthalmologist relies only on signed consent forms and does not, in addition, document the consent discussion, the potential for patient allegations that he or she signed the forms without really understanding them is increased.[1]

During assessment and discussion time, the patient will have formed an opinion of the physician and the support staff and it is equally important for excimer laser providers to form a psychophysical profile of the patient. In a study carried out in SEI using the Hudson self-esteem questionnaire (1982) and the GHQ30 (Goldberg 1982) we identified 13% of potential laser candidates to have 'psychiatric' caseness (i.e. suffering from psychological stress) and 47% exhibited low self-esteem. The percentage 'caseness' is not statistically higher than is normally recorded in a general population; however, the number of patients presenting for excimer laser with low self-esteem is significantly higher. Postoperative trends might suggest that this low self-esteem improves with improvement in visual function post-PRK.[43] Further extensive studies are underway (see Chapter 10).

FULLY INFORMED CONSENT AND A 'COOLING-OFF' PERIOD

To ensure the patient has sufficient time to make an informed decision, a 'cooling off' period of 1–2 weeks is recommended. In our experience, of more than 600 procedures, this tends to reinforce to patients the importance of this decision and the significance of the operation and has only very rarely led to a change of mind. It is useful to provide the patient with the informed consent form to be read and considered carefully during this period. Consent forms will obviously vary from center to center but it is probably universally advisable that after each paragraph in the consent form that there should be a space allowing the patient to initial that they have both read and understood the particular implications of each paragraph in respect to the predictability and complications of PRK/PARK surgery. The 'bottom line' in any consent for PRK refractive surgery is that there can be no absolute guarantees and that it is impossible to state every conceivable complication that may occur following surgery.

On the day of treatment the informed consent form should be reviewed in the presence of the ophthalmologist, with each paragraph read and countersigned to acknowledge comprehension before being formally signed at the bottom by both parties. The patient should be encouraged and be given opportunities to discuss any last concerns or problems to ensure there are no more questions before progressing to the procedure (see Chapter 9). If the patient insists on expecting 'perfect' vision, it may be preferable to suggest that PRK surgery may not be suitable.[3]

POSTOPERATIVE ASSESSMENT

SCHEDULED REVIEWS

Review assessments will vary from physician to physician, but a reasonable postoperative protocol might include visits at day 1, day 3 (or until the epithelium has healed), 1 week, 1 month, 3 months, 6 months, and 12 months. Depending upon the political climate and professional relationships between ophthalmologists and optometrists, shared care may be appropriate in the postoperative care of PRK patients. Optometrists who take part in follow-up reviews must be aware of the time scale of potential

Table 8.6
Subjective ocular symptoms postoperatively.

Fluctuating acuity
Glare
Haloes/ghosting
Reduced night vision
Monocular diplopia/secondary images
Ocular discomfort

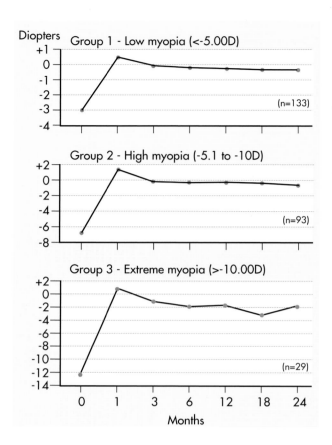

Figure 8.10 *Chronological changes in refraction following excimer laser PRK for myopia in the SEI study (the horizontal scale is non-linear.)*

minor complications and the symptoms they may give rise to. As in any shared-care arrangement, the patient care plan set and supervised by the physician, must be strictly adhered to with the ability to contact the physician immediately if necessary.

HISTORY AND SYMPTOMS

Specific questions on subjective symptoms need to be asked at each visit and can be tabulated in the form of a brief questionnaire for the clinician to complete in addition to the clinical details. An outline of important symptoms is illustrated in Table 8.6. It is very important that patients are aware of the individual variation in acuity post-treatment. It is not uncommon to find that two patients treated on the same day, with approximately identical refractions, will return for day 3 follow-up and whilst patient A might obtain 6/6 (20/20) unaided, patient B might struggle to see 6/60 (20/200). Since patients frequently discuss and compare outcomes in the waiting room, this might lead patient B to erroneously conclude that the surgical result has been poorer than for patient A. Therefore positive reinforcement of individual rate of recovery must be stressed again and again, particularly in the first week, and whilst most eyes with a preoperative myopia of less than −5.00 D might be anticipated to obtain 6/12 (20/40) or better by the seventh day postoperatively, surface irregularities can be such that even at 1 week, eyes that may ultimately obtain a good unaided VA, may nonetheless record a relatively poor unaided acuity. Reassurance and a discussion of the patient's perceived concerns at this early stage can pay substantial dividends in the longer term. The sequence of initial hyperopia followed by relative myopic regression and refractive stabilization (Fig. 8.10)[44] may mean that 6/6 is attained transiently for a few days or weeks (as refraction decays from early hyperopia to residual

myopia) and then lost. Patients' appreciation of these chronological changes in VA need to be reinforced.

ASSESSING REFRACTION POST-PRK

The extent of postoperative assessment will obviously vary from center to center and within the time course of follow-up. However, the basic minimum at any postoperative review must include: slit lamp biomicroscopy, assessment of IOP (especially if utilizing topical corticosteroids), unaided VA; objective and subjective refraction; and CVK. A comprehensive assessment might include all of the investigations listed in Table 8.7.

Unaided vision is recorded using the Snellen chart or, if available, high and low contrast vision is established with the Bailey–Lovie chart, followed by

Table 8.7

Comprehensive postoperative assessment (*these investigations might be regarded as optional).

Distance vision/near vision
Refraction
Contrast sensitivity/glare*
Computerized videokeratography
Tear evaluation/biomicroscopy
Esthesiometry*
Tonometry
Pachymetry
Specular microscopy*
Fundal examination

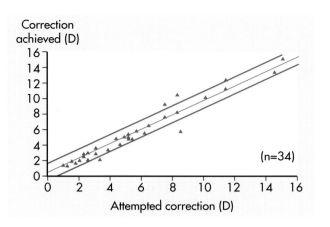

Figure 8.11 *Graph illustrating attempted correction (−1.75 to −15.00 D) and achieved correction at 8 weeks post-PRK/PARK, in the first 34 consecutive eyes treated by the authors using a 6 mm multizone algorithm. Although the majority of the eyes (84%) are within ±1.00 D of emmetropia, many continued to display a degree of myopic regression for up to 6 months or more. Beginning PRK surgeons should therefore view initial results conservatively.*

contrast sensitivity and glare measurement. After the refraction procedure, explained previously, VA measurements and subjective measurements are then recorded as per vision. Retinoscopy postoperatively generally provides a central 'with' movement surrounded by an annulus of 'against' movement. This differentiation diminishes with time postoperatively, as the 'elbow' of the junction between the ablation zone and the paracentral cornea reduces due to epithelial hyperplasia and stromal remodelling. The 'reflex' will also be affected by the presence of corneal haze, or any induced multifocal elements in the ablation zone. Interestingly, some patients can achieve an unaided vision of 6/6 yet still have an appreciable refractive element, frequently a residual cylinder, hence the need to refract all patients regardless of what the unaided vision may be. Patients with such minor residual refractive error may appreciate the provision of the refraction for occasional, demanding, visual tasks such as night driving and VDU work. Indeed, patients will often appreciate a surprisingly significant subjective improvement in VA from such minor prescriptions. If the expectations of the patient have been managed well, i.e. they have been appropriately advised of the possibility of occasional spectacle wear postoperatively, most will not consider the wearing of spectacles for fine visual tasks or reading an encumbrance, and will continue to relish their new unaided vision for general viewing.

When analyzing an individual laser unit's refractive outcome versus unaided vision results, the percentage of patients achieving a vision of 6/12, especially for the first 6 months postoperatively, can be higher than the percentage with a spherical equivalent

within ±1.00 DS of emmetropia.[45] Worthy of note in the early postoperative period, is that blinking, for some post PRK/PARK patients, has a quite dramatic effect upon improving unaided VA, presumably due to the tear film smoothing any microirregularities of the corneal surface.

The beginning PRK surgeon must be very aware of chronological refractive changes in order to avoid providing the patient with a too optimistic outlook early in the postoperative period. Indeed, the 1–3 month results are often highly successful, in refractive terms, regardless of preoperative myopia (Fig. 8.11); however, many patients with 5 D or greater myopia are likely to regress towards myopia until at least 6 months. Therefore, even 4–8 weeks post-PRK, a conservative approach on behalf of the surgeon, especially in expressing the likely final outcome to the patient, is to be encouraged. Complications encountered in the postoperative period are covered in Chapter 23.

ANISOMETROPIA POST-PRK

After the first eye has undergone PRK/PARK, if the patient is a current spectacle lens wearer, the spectacle lens for the treated eye may be replaced temporarily by a plano or appropriate myopic lens (for extreme myopes expected to have residual myopia). This can cause problems of anisometropia and, therefore, if the patient is able to wear a contact lens in the non-operated eye visual comfort will be greater, especially in cases of high myopia. A short period of time off work, usually 3–4 days, is advisable postoperatively, both to recover from the procedure and for the visual system to begin to adapt to the new transient hyperopic state of the operated eye, compared to the contralateral eye (particularly if presbyopia is present). As the degree of initial hyperopia diminishes unaided vision rapidly improves. If, as the eye settles, anisometropia is problematic and the operated eye has a minor residual prescription, the patient may cope better with this prescription incorporated into the spectacles and a plano lens in front of the non-operated myopic eye, if contact lens wear is not possible.

Depending on the unaided vision of the treated eye and the length of time required for refractive stability to be obtained, refitting of the contact lens in the non-operated eye will be necessary. A sizeable proportion of patients seeking PRK/PARK are contact lens wearers who have encountered problems of contact lens-related discomfort. Sometimes this is simply due to the need for an improved lens care regimen but, more frequently, a replacement contact lens is needed to maintain comfort and re-establish comfortable wear.

FITTING CONTACT LENSES IN THE PRK EYE

It may be desirable to fit an eye that has undergone PRK/PARK with a contact lens once the eye's refraction has stabilized, approximately 6 months postoperatively in medium to high myopia. In former contact lens wearers, a significant number have a history of contact lens intolerance, in which case contact lens fitting may not be possible. In non-contact lens wearers the ability to wear contact lenses will have to be ascertained. It is theoretically possible that tear film alterations following PRK, e.g. the reduced tear breakup time or the position where the tear film initially breaks up, may affect comfort of contact lens wear. There is of course a fundamental intrinsic difference to the corneal shape upon which the contact lens parameters will be based. Instead of a corneal model whereby the periphery is flatter in comparison to the central part of the cornea, the

periphery is now relatively steeper. As long as there is no appreciable corneal astigmatism, or induced irregular topography, hydrogel (soft) contact lenses can prove to be successful and are, most importantly, comfortable. These patients generally do not wish to return to, or begin with, contact lens wear and therefore contact lens fitting will no doubt be the last step in refractive management following PRK/PARK and careful counselling is needed for success.

As with soft contact lens fitting in the normal eye, one fits flatter than the flattest keratometry readings (K); however, remember this will be probably in the region of 9.00 mm rather than the normal corneal curvature of 7.8 mm.[46] The standard criteria of fitting soft lenses, i.e. lens centration, adequate movement, and lack of conjunctival indentation, pertain. If the soft lens follows the contour of the cornea the lens will flex and cause fluctuation in the visual acuity. If the lens 'vaults' over the ablation zone, although initial VA may be good, consideration must be made to the possible stagnation of tears centrally due to insufficient tear exchange. Rigid contact lenses in the form of rigid gas permeables are obviously able to compensate for irregularities of the cornea, unlike soft contact lenses. However, after PRK/PARK there is no longer a central corneal apex upon which the lens normally contours and, therefore, even weight distribution of the contact lens and thereby centration may prove difficult. Using a standard contact lens fit produces a pool of tears under the centre of the contact lens, causing a significant positive power 'tear lens', presuming normal lens movement and centration pertains (Fig. 8.12). The resultant contact lens power is in the region of the preoperative myopic

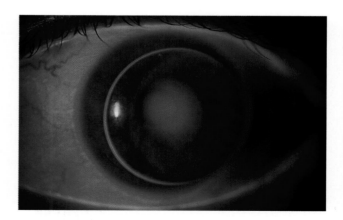

Figure 8.12 *Contact lens fit post-PRK.*

refraction, as extra negative power is required to compensate for this positive tear pool. Nonetheless, rigid contact lenses may enable eyes to regain preoperative BSCVA in cases of irregular topography. This can provide a useful demonstration to the patient that lines of VA can be restored, but it is unlikely that the comfort of the contact lens will be totally satisfactory to the patient who initially presented for surgery to obviate this mode of correction, and who might now have to slowly build up wearing time, especially if previously a soft contact lens wearer. Of course loss of BSCVA can be due to other factors, such as severe corneal haze, and in such cases there is no advantage in trying contact lenses. Counselling of loss of BSCVA is important since in most cases this complication is self-limiting. At present, contact lens manufacturers are designing rigid contact lenses with negative eccentricity that follow the flattened corneal apex to cope with the post-PRK fit.[47]

COMPUTERIZED VIDEOKERATOGRAPHY

Wherever possible, corneal topography should be performed at the earliest juncture postoperatively, i.e. 1 week or 1 month post-treatment. In addition to the important role of CVK in the clinical assessment of subjects postoperatively, topographic maps can continue to play an important part in the education of the patient by demonstrating complications such as irregular healing, central islands, irregular topography, induced astigmatism, decentration, and regression. Visual representation is often easier for the patient to comprehend, allows them to follow the corneal healing response at each stage, and enables appreciation of occasional symptoms, e.g. how decentration may cause subjective symptoms of haloes with a large pupil. Details of postoperative CVK analysis are covered more fully in Chapter 7.

ASPECTS OF BIOMICROSCOPY

Possible observations are delayed epithelial healing, mucous tags or plaques, epithelial inclusions, epithelial nodules, frank corneal erosions, corneal edema, allergic reactions to the prescribed drugs, ptosis, keratic precipitates, and corneal haze. The main distinguishing features of the above complications are covered in Chapter 23.

Several corneal haze grading scales are reported in the literature, including haze graded on a scale 0 to 4 (0 = no haze, 4 = severe haze),[48] a grading strategy of clear, trace, mild, moderate, and severe haze;[49,50] by separate subjective evaluations for the superficial and deep epithelium and the anterior and posterior stroma using a qualitative scale from 0 (no haze) to 5 (severe haze of the cornea which obscured the iris);[51] or grading according to the Food and Drug Administration (FDA) guidelines.[52-54] Lohmann et al[55] have developed a system for objective assessment of corneal clarity that enables one to differentiate between the back scattered light, which contributes to the clinician's view, and the forward scattered light that affects the quality of vision the patient experiences. Other examples of grading scales are shown in Table 8.8.[56-61] To monitor and document the development of corneal haze and to ensure consistency in magnitude for inter- or intraobservations, each excimer unit should implement a standard grading system. A selection of slides depicting varying degrees of haze relating to the particular classification of haze can be helpful. Obviously, too coarse a grading scale will needlessly reduce the clinician's ability to detect change in the parameter being assessed.[62] The question of whether the clinician should routinely grade severity of haze alone, or also indicate whether haze is homogeneous or heterogeneous and outline the relative position and percentage of ablation area involved, is important. The latter can be particularly important in distinguishing between asymmetric zone regression, with apparent zone decentration, and genuine zone decentration.

TREATMENT OF THE SECOND EYE

No arbitrary guidelines can be accurately established for the timing of treatment of the second eye. Indeed, some clinicians perform bilateral treatments at one session or with a time period of only 1 or 2 weeks in between each eye.[61] However, in the small percentage of patients who develop severe problems postoperatively, such an approach could, in a worst case scenario based upon results in individual eyes,[63-65] lead to bilateral best corrected visual acuities of 6/60 (20/200). In view of this relatively uncommon but devastating outcome, the authors suggest a 2–3 month delay between treatments in eyes with less than −5.00 D of myopia, and 3–6 months in eyes with greater than −5.00 D of preoperative myopia. These suggested intervals presume early stabilization of refraction and at least 1 month without topical corticosteroids. Where refraction continues to drift, especially in high myopia, a delay of up to 1 year is quite possible.

Table 8.8
Examples of corneal haze grading.

Grade	Kim et al[56]	McDonald et al[57]	Salz et al[58]	Ditzen et al[59]	Epstein et al[60]	Ehlers et al[61]
0	totally clear	clear possibly with faint haze	clear ablation not apparent	clear and slight reticular corneal haze but no light reflex from the corneal stroma seen at the slit lamp	completely clear	clear
trace	faint corneal haze seen by indirect broad tangential illumination					
0.5			barely visible			
1	mild seen easily with direct focal slit illumination	mild reticulated haze not affecting refraction	easily visible but does not interfere with refraction	traces of reticular or spot-like haze postoperatively VA=preoperative VA	faint haze detectable only with broad tangential illumination	minimal reticular opacification
2	moderate haze with dense opacity that partially obscures any iris detail	moderate haze refraction possible but difficult	easily visible but does not interfere with refraction	reticular or punctate subepithelial structures clearly visible at the slit lamp postoperative VA=preoperative VA	discrete haze visible with difficulty by focal illumination	distinct punctate or reticulate structures within ablated region
3	severely hazed with dense opacity that completely obscures the detail of the intra-ocular structure	opacity prevents refraction anterior chamber easily viewed	opacity easily visible and markedly interferes with refraction	confluent subepithelial structures causing haze-reduced VA	moderately dense opacity partially obscuring iris detail	confluent opacification in the central region
4		opacity impairs view of anterior chamber	opacity prevents view of anterior chamber details		severely dense opacity completely obscuring details of intraocular structures	
5		anterior chamber not visible				

CONCLUSIONS

The clinician should not underestimate the amount of personal research, both into the technique and in respect to available centers and lasers, that many potential patients will undertake prior to undergoing PRK surgery. Indeed, many patients will attend the first consultation armed with the brochures of other excimer centers, clippings from newspapers and magazines, and occasionally photocopies of scientific articles. Therefore, it is essential that whoever is delegated to take incoming enquiries from prospective PRK candidates is fully briefed on the basic answers to all of the above enquiries, and preferably will have attended a number of laser procedures and spoken to patients before and after the operative procedure. From experience, we have found that short training sessions for all practice staff who will come into contact with PRK patients is time well spent, both in terms of positive follow-up to initial enquiries and in reduced discussion time between the clinician and patient on basic questions.

Patients should be made aware, from the outset, of the expected level of success, the timescale of visual recovery, and possible complications that might occur. A stringent preoperative assessment, whilst time consuming, is likely to pay considerable dividends to both patient and practitioner in the long-term.

The length of time post-treatment to final refractive and visual stability is still under investigation, but appears to be very dependent on the individual healing response, the latter related, in large part, to the degree of refractive correction attempted. Therefore, a coherent strategy in respect to both the pre- and postoperative assessments, and the type and number of objective and subject evaluations needed at each visit, should be ascertained at the start of the clinic's development. In such a rapidly developing arena such assessment plans require regular re-evaluation if new technology becomes available, in light of published data, or in respect to patient demand. A postoperative follow up of 1 year might be considered the minimum reasonable length with respect to our present knowledge.

REFERENCES

1. Tiemeier CG, Abbott RL, Hauscheer Ellis J, Risk management issues in radial keratotomy surgery, *Surv Ophthalmology* (1994) **39**:52–56.
2. McGhee CNJ, Orr D, Kidd B, Stark C et al, Psychological aspects of excimer laser surgery for myopia: reasons for seeking treatment and patient satisfaction. *Br J Ophthalmol* (1996) **80**:874–79.
3. Bores LD, Patient Workup. In: Bores LD, ed, *Refractive Eye Surgery* (Blackwell Scientific: Oxford, 1993) 106–25.
4. Campos M, Lee M, McDonnell PJ, Ocular integrity after refractive surgery. Effects of photorefractive keratectomy, phototherapeutic keratectomy and radial keratotomy, *Ophthalmic Surg* (1982) **23**:598–602.
5. Salz JJ, Traumatic corneal abrasions following photorefractive keratectomy, *Refract Corneal Surg* (1994) **10**:36–37.
6. Kahle G, Seiler T, Wollensak J, Report on psychosocial findings and satisfaction among patients one year after excimer laser photorefractive keratectomy, *Refract Corneal Surg* (1992) **8**:286–9.
7. Weed KH, Fon D, Potvin R, Discontinuation of contact lens wear, *Optom Vis Sci* (1993) **70**:140.
8. McDonald MB, Leach DH, Myopic photorefractive keratectomy: U.S. Experience. In: Thompson FB, McDonnell PJ, eds, *Excimer Laser Surgery: The cornea* (Igaku-Shoin: New York, 1993) 37–51.
9. Emsley HH, *Visual Optics. Volume 1. Optics of Vision* (Butterworths: London, 1976).
10. Bennett AG, Rabbetts RB, *Clinical Visual Optics* (Butterworths: London, 1984).
11. Abrams D, *Duke Elder's Practice of Refraction* (Churchill Livingstone: Edinburgh, 1978).
12. Grosvenor T, Fitting the astigmatic patient with rigid contact lenses. In: Ruben M, Guillon M, eds, *Contact Lens Practice* (Chapman and Hall: London, 1994) 623–47.
13. Russell GE, Bergmanson JPG, Barbeito R, Gross WD, Differences between objective and subjective refractions after radial keratotomy, *Refract Corneal Surg* (1992) **8**:290–5.
14. Yeow EK, Taylor SP, Clinical evaluation of the Humphrey automatic refractor, *Ophthal Physiol Opt* (1989) **9**:171–5.
15. Hosaka N, The effect of various eye diseases on the measurement of refractive error using the Nikon autorefractometer. In: Brenin GM, Seigel IM, eds, *Advances in Diagnostic Visual Optics* (Springer-Verlag: Berlin, 1983) 75–83.
16. O'Brart DPS, Corbett MC, Sanders DC, Rosen ES, The topography of corneal astigmatism, *Eur J Implant Ref Surg* (1994) **6**:361–9.
17. Corbett MC, O'Brart DPS, Sanders DC, Rosen ES, The assessment of corneal topography, *Eur J Implant Ref Surg* (1994) **6**:98–105.
18. Pender PM, Photorefractive keratectomy for myopic astigmatism: Phase IIA of the Federal Drug Administrative study (12 to 18 months follow-up), *J Cataract Refract Surg* (1994) **20**:262–4.
19. Stevens JD, Astigmatic excimer laser treatment: Theoretical effects of axis misalignment, *Eur J Implant Ref Surg* (1994) **6**:310–18.

20. Specification for test charts for determining distance visual acuity. BS4274 (1968).

21. Bailey IL, Lovie JE, New design principles for visual acuity letter charts, *Am J Optom Physiol Opt* (1976) **53**:740–5.

22. Lovie-Kitchen JE, Validity and reliability of visual acuity measurements, *Ophthal Physiol Opt* (1988) **8**:363–70.

23. Reeves BC, Wood JM, Hill AR, Reliability of high and low contrast letter charts, *Ophthal Physiol Opt* (1993) **13**: 17–26.

24. Lohmann CP, Timberlake GT, Fitzke FW, et al, Corneal light scattering after excimer laser photorefractive keratectomy: the objective measurement of haze, *Refract Corneal Surg* (1992) **8**:114–21.

25. Lohmann CP, Fitzke FW, O'Brart D, et al, Halos—A problem for all myopes? A comparison between spectacles, contact lenses and photorefractive keratectomy, *Refract Corneal Surg* (1993) **9**:S73–S75.

26. Elliott DB, Bullimore MA, Bailey IL, Improving the reliability of the Pelli–Robson contrast sensitivity test, *Clin Vision Sci* (1991) **6**:471–5.

27. Rubin GS, Reliability and sensitivity of clinical contrast sensitivity tests, *Clin Vision Sci* (1988) **2**:169–77.

28. Butuner Z, Elliott DB, Gimbel HV, et al, Visual function one year after excimer laser surgery, *J Refract Corneal Surg* (1994) **10**:626–30.

29. Sunderaj P, Villada JR, Joyce PW, Watson A, Glare testing in pseudophakes with posterior capsule opacification, *Eye* (1992) **6**:411–13.

30. Phillips AJ, Stone J, *Contact Lenses* (Butterworths: London, 1984).

31. John ME, Howard C, Esotropia following radial keratotomy, *J Cataract Refract Surg* (1991) **17**:246–7.

32. Klyce SD, McDonald MD, Computerised corneal topography of surface ablations with the Tomey (TMS-1). In: Salz JJ, ed, *Corneal Laser Surgery* (CV Mosby: St Louis, 1995) 93–108.

33. Rengstorff RH, Variations in corneal curvature measurements: an after effect observed with habitual wearers of contact lenses, *Am J Optom* (1969) **46**:45–57.

34. Rengstorff RH, Astigmatism after contact lens wear, *Am J Optom Physiol Opt* (1977) **54**:787–91.

35. Corbett MC, O'Brart DPS, Sanders DC, Rosen E, The topography of the normal cornea, *Eur J Implant Ref Surg* (1994) **6**:286–97.

36. Morgan JF, Induced corneal astigmatism with hydrophilic lenses, *Can J Ophthalmol* (1975) **10**:207–13.

37. Vanley GT, Leopold IR, Gregg TH, Interpretation of tear film break up, *Arch Ophthalmol* (1977) **95**:445–48.

38. Silbert JA, *Anterior segment complications of contact lens wear* (Churchill Livingstone: Edinburgh, 1994).

39. Guillon JP, Guillon M, Tear film examination of the contact lens patient, *Contax* (1988) *May* 13–18.

40. Boettner TA, Wolter JR, Transmission of the ocular media, *Invest Ophthalmol* (1962) **1**:776–83.

41. Pimendies D, Steele CF, McGhee CNJ, Bryce IG, Deep corneal stromal opacities associated with long term contact lens wear, *Br J Ophthalmol* (1996) **80**:21–24.

42. Janknecht P, Soriano JM, Hansen LL, Cystoid macula oedema after excimer laser photorefractive keratectomy, *Br J Ophthalmol* (1993) **77**(10):681.

43. Kidd B, McGhee CNJ, Bryce I, Psychological assessment of patients undergoing excimer laser PRK for myopia, (*J Refract Surg*, in press).

44. Weed KH, McGhee CNJ, Bryce I, Hazy Days? The refractive outlook of photorefractive keratectomy (PRK) and photo-astigmatic keratectomy (PARK), *Ophthal Physiol Opt* (1995) **15**:367–9.

45. Gartry DS, Treatment of myopia with the excimer laser—is it really the bottom line? *Ophthal Physiol Opt* (1995) **15**:S2–S10.

46. Bennett ES, Basic Fitting. In: Bennett ES, Weissman BA, eds, *Clinical Contact Lens Practice* (JB Lippincott: Philadelphia, 1991) 1–20.

47. Kersley J, Edwards K, Hough DA, Contact lens management following photorefractive keratectomy, *J Br Contact Lens Assoc* (1995) **18**:S4.

48. Talley AR, Hardten DR, Sher NA, et al, Results one year after using the 193 nm excimer laser for photorefractive keratectomy in mild to moderate myopia, *Am J Ophthalmol* (1994) **118**:304-11.

49. Machat JJ, Tayfour F, Photorefractive keratectomy for myopia: Preliminary results in 147 eyes, *Refract Corneal Surg* (1993) **9**:S16–S19.

50. Ficker LA, Bates AK, Steele AD, et al, Excimer laser photorefractive keratectomy for myopia: 12 month follow-up, *Eye* (1993) **7**:617–24.

51. Leroux Les Jardins S, Auclin F, Roman S, et al, Results of photorefractive keratectomy on 63 myopic eyes with six months minimum follow-up, *J Cataract Refract Surg* (1994) **20**:223–8.

52. Tavola A, Brancato R, Galli L, et al, Photorefractive keratectomy for myopia: single vs double-zone treatment in 166 eyes, *Refract Corneal Surg* (1993) **9**:S48–S52.

53. Burratto L, Ferrari M, Photorefractive keratectomy for myopia from 6.00 D to 10.00 D, *Refract Corneal Surg* (1993) **9**: S34–S36.

54. Office of Device Evaluation Division of Ophthalmic Devices. Food and Drug Administration, Draft clinical guidance for the preparation and contents of an investigational device exemption (IDE). Application for excimer laser devices used in ophthalmic surgery for myopic photorefractive keratectomy (PRK), *Refract Corneal Surg* (1991) **6**: 265–69.

55. Lohmann CP, Gartry DS, Kerr Muir M, et al, Corneal haze after excimer laser refractive surgery: objective measurements and functional implications, *Eur J Ophthalmol* (1991) **1**:173–80.

56. Kim HJ, Hahn TW, Lee YC, et al, Photorefractive keratectomy in 202 myopic eyes: One year results, *Refract Corneal Surg* (1993) **9**:S11–S16.

57. McDonald MB, Frantz JM, Klyce SD, et al, Central photorefractive keratectomy for myopia, *Arch Ophthalmol* (1990) **108**:799–808.

58. Salz JJ, Maguen MD, Nesburn AB, et al, A two year experience with excimer photorefractive keratectomy for myopia, *Ophthalmology* (1993) **100**:873–82.

59. Ditzen K, Anschutz T, Schroder MD, Photorefractive keratectomy to treat low, medium, and high myopia: A multicenter study, *J Cataract Refract Surg* (1994) **20**: 234–8.

60. Epstein D, Fagerholm P, Hamberg-Nystrom H, Tengroth B, Twenty-four month follow-up of excimer laser photorefractive keratectomy for myopia, *Ophthalmology* (1994) **101**:1558–64.

61. Ehlers N, Hjortdal J, Excimer laser refractive keratectomy for high myopia, *Acta Ophthalmologica* (1992) **70**:578–86.

62. Bailey IL, Bullimore MA, Radsch TW, Taylor HR, Clinical grading and the effects of scaling, *Invest Ophthalmol Vis Sci* (1991) **32**:422–32.

63. Seiler T, Derse M, Pham T, Repeated excimer laser treatment after photorefractive keratectomy, *Arch Ophthalmol* (1992) **110**:1230–3.

64. Epstein D, Frueh BE, Indications, results and complications of refractive corneal surgery with lasers, *Curr Opin Ophthal* (1995) **6**:73–78.

65. Seiler T, Photorefractive keratectomy. European Experience. In: Thompson FB, McDonnell PJ, eds, *Excimer Laser Surgery: The cornea* (Igaku-Shoin: New York, 1993) 53–62.

Chapter 9 A very practical approach to excimer laser for myopia

Charles N J McGhee, Suzanne K Webber and Con N Anastas

INTRODUCTION

Despite extensive publications on the subject of excimer laser photorefractive keratectomy (PRK), most tend to skip many of the very practical points of the actual procedure and the essential interactions between surgeon and patients during treatment. Although PRK appears relatively straightforward compared to many ophthalmic procedures, there is undoubtedly a significant learning curve.[1,2] The purpose of this chapter is to outline in a *very practical* sense those aspects of the technique that occur recurrently and are not fully addressed elsewhere. No excuses are made by the authors for restating the apparently obvious at times, since the obvious only becomes so after it has been encountered in a large number of patients.

IMMEDIATE PREOPERATIVE REVIEW OF CONSENT

Fully informed consent and patient education should have been completed prior to the day of surgery; however, at this time it is worth reiterating in reasonable detail the risks and anticipated benefits of the planned surgery. Ideally the patient should also have been provided with an appropriate consent form, which they will have carefully studied at home prior to the day of surgery (Fig. 9.1). This consent form should be countersigned in the presence of the surgeon.

MAKING A PERSONAL NOTE OF INFORMED CONSENT

Regardless of the extensive nature of the consent form, it is also very useful to make a note in the

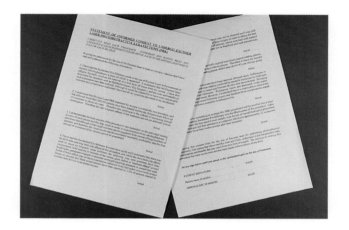

Figure 9.1 *Consent forms vary from center to center but should always include a reasonably comprehensive guide to possible complications. The consent form illustrated is divided into paragraphs followed by a space for patient signature to indicate that the relevant paragraph has been read and understood. A final section recording that the patient understood the consent and had all questions adequately answered preceeds final signature by the subject, which should be witnessed by the operating surgeon.*

surgeon's own handwriting[3] within the patient's notes of the final verbal consent provided to the patient. In the ideal circumstances this should include at least elements of the following statements:

- *The final refractive results of the procedure are not guaranteed* and depend on individual healing and, therefore, suggested acuity outcomes are only guidelines.
- *The approximate estimate of the anticipated final unaided visual acuity* suggested to the

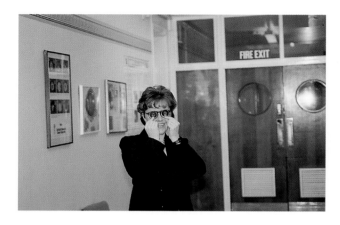

Figure 9.2 *Snellen acuity is an abstract concept to prospective patients and merely indicating 6/12 (20/40) on an acuity chart is of little value. A more appropriate impression of predicted unaided acuity can be obtained using an undercorrection in a trial frame, or by placing a +1.00 to +1.50 D addition in front of the patient's spectacles (to blur the patient to appropriate acuity) and allowing the patient to view everyday day objects at varying distances.*

patient, e.g. 80–90% prospect of 6/12 (20/40), 60–70% prospect of 6/6 (20/20). This estimation is most accurate if based upon the results of the clinic providing surgery, but if such data are unavailable appropriate data may be adapted from the scientific literature. However, it must always be remembered that a numerical value for predicted Snellen acuity, e.g. 6/12 (20/40), is an abstract concept as far as the patient is concerned. It is preferable to provide the patient with a real-life example of such acuity by under-correcting the trial frame prescription (or adding +1.00 to +1.50 D in front of existing spectacles) and allowing patients to view everyday near and distant objects at leisure (Fig. 9.2).

- *A statement of the nature of complications and their likely incidence* e.g. haze, scar, glare, halo, visual distortion, ghost images and decreased best spectacle corrected visual acuity (BSCVA). Although usually transient, these may all be permanent, and occur with an incidence of approximately 0–5% in the low-to-moderately myopic group (<–6.00 D), depending upon authors' classification of persisting significant

complications.[4-9] (High myopes should have a distinctly different statement of informed consent due to the greater risk of loss of BSCVA.)

- *Estimate of retreatment rate in cases of undercorrection or myopic regression*. The suggested approximate incidence in low myopia (<–6.00 D) is 1.4–5%, which may rise to 19.0% in extreme myopia (> –10.00 D).[10,11]
- *In a very small minority of cases, due to abnormal healing or complicating factors, treatment of the contralateral eye will not be recommended*. Unfortunately, a contemporary and exact estimate of the number of patients who remain uniocular, due to symptoms or complications associated with treatment of the first eye, is difficult to ascertain. Remaining untreated in the second eye has been noted to be as high as 10% in early series using small zone ablations,[12] but currently might be in the range of 1.0% or less for correction of low myopia.[13] Patients must be made aware of this discernible risk, which may create symptoms related to permanent anisometropia that will be particularly problematic if the individual cannot wear contact lenses.

DETAILED PREOPERATIVE DISCUSSION OF THE PROCEDURE

Although the procedure itself may seem very innocuous to the practitioner, there is no doubt that patients are very concerned and apprehensive on the day of the procedure even if they have received extensive counselling beforehand (Fig. 9.3).[14] Each relatively minor deviation from the patient's expectation of the procedure can be mistakenly perceived as an error or an unforeseen complication to which the patient may later attach inappropriate importance. Therefore, the surgeon should outline as exactly as possible, in a step-by-step explanation, the components of the treatment and what the patient should expect. This worthwhile explanation need not take more than 2–3 minutes and is likely to pay dividends both during treatment and in the postoperative period. Our personal guide to the patient is roughly as follows.

ANESTHESIA

Topical anesthetic (amethocaine) drops are applied to the eye three to four times in the 20 minutes prior

Question	% Positive response
Sufficient written information	95.2%
Sufficient verbal information	94.0%
All questions answered	95.2%
Fully understood PRK procedure	100%
Procedure performed professionally	98.9%
Operation as expected	83.2%
Operation distressing	23.9%

Figure 9.3 *Results of an anonymous questionnaire of 90 consecutive subjects who had undergone PRK at a single center. Although 100% of subjects felt that they understood the procedure preoperatively and 98.9% that the procedure was performed very professionally for a number of subjects the operation was not quite as expected and almost a quarter found it distressing. From these data it is obvious that despite maximum preoperative education patients do require further guidance and reassurance during the procedure. (McGhee et al, 1996[14].)*

to the procedure. The patient is informed that these drops will initially 'sting or smart' but become less uncomfortable with each additional drop. Patients are often concerned because they can still 'feel' the eye if they touch it through the closed lid. They are, therefore, reassured that these drops specifically affect the 'pain fibers' before the 'touch fibers' and, therefore, they should not seek to determine, nor cannot determine by themselves, that adequate anesthesia has occurred. This statement is made after having seen many patients in the waiting room tapping their eye with a finger through closed lid to determine if the anesthetic has really worked prior to treatment.

CONFIRMING PATIENT DETAILS AND MANAGEMENT OF CONTRALATERAL EYE

Patients are informed that they will be brought to the laser room, consent signature will be confirmed, they will be asked to confirm their name once more and requested to ***point to the eye*** to be treated (for medico-legal purposes). A less attractive alternative might be to mark above the eye to be treated and provide patient name tags. An eye shield will then be applied to the eye that is not being treated and it is

emphasized that this opaque shield is not to prevent all light, or any laser light from entering the eye, but rather to prevent visual distraction and cross-fixation. By using a shield rather than a patch the patient can keep this covered eye open, making contralateral eye opening easier and Bell's phenomenon less marked.

INSERTION OF LID SPECULUM

Details of the exact procedure must be given precisely. In the first instance patients are often gravely concerned about application of the lid speculum, which may have been likened, from discussion with other patients or from television/magazine articles, to some form of 'eye clamp'. It is always best to inform or demonstrate to patients that this is rather like a 'small wire clip' device which will painlessly hold the lids open. It is important to forewarn the patient that the reaction of the (unanesthetized) lids may be to blink and attempt closure, but that once the eyelids become accustomed to the speculum blepharospasm and associated Bell's phenomenon will settle.

EPITHELIAL DEBRIDEMENT

The second area that patients focus concern upon is that of epithelial debridement, the description of which often makes even the strong-willed queasy. When describing this it is always best to preface all descriptions with 'this is entirely painless' and that a simple blunt instrument, rather like a 'small windscreen wiper or hockey stick', will be used to 'rub off the surface cells that have been loosened by the anesthetic'. The term 'scrape' has connotations that upset many patients and is a term, therefore, best avoided!

OLFACTORY SENSATIONS

Patients may be aware of the 'smell of smoke'. Obviously, no smoke or significant thermal effect is generated by this procedure but the patient may be aware of their own photoablated carbon molecules passing their nostrils at the speed of sound. This may be simply explained by reminding patients that humans are essentially 70–80% water and the majority of the remaining 20% is carbon. Therefore, when the laser removes the thin corneal layer from the surface of the eye, the liberated carbon molecules

will pass the patient's nose and, if the patient becomes aware of this carbon smell then, due to pre-existing olfactory associations, they will associate this smell with smoke and, therefore, may believe tissue is burning.

It is vitally important to reassure patients on this matter preoperatively since, if they are not reassured specifically on this point, they may become rather distressed, not surprisingly, if aware of a 'burning smell' during the procedure. Some authors have suggested the use of colognes or perfumes to disguise this smell; however, such volatile agents interact with laser optics during laser action and may cause premature degradation of optics and a poor-quality laser beam.

AUDITORY AND TACTILE SENSATIONS

Patients should be made aware of the clapping sound generated by excimer laser pulses, which, due to proximity, sound louder to the patient than to observers. Occasionally patients describe the sensation of a gentle tapping on the eye with each pulse, which is presumably related to the acoustic shock wave generated by the photoablative process.

INTRAOPERATIVE TARGET FIXATION

Commonly, patients are rather concerned that they will be unable to fixate upon the laser target consistently throughout the procedure. It is worth reassuring maximally that the surgeon is able to stop and start the procedure to obtain refixation without any detrimental effect on the final outcome and it is worthwhile to suggest that one or two stops, in a procedure of greater than 30 seconds, is not uncommon. Patients should be warned about the brightness and intensity of the light before being positioned under the laser.

THE SURGICAL PROCEDURE

The procedure as outlined is the one that has been used by the authors over the last 3 years using a Visx 20/20B laser. Although some of the finer details will, therefore, differ from laser to laser, the basic techniques are applicable to all currently available excimer lasers.

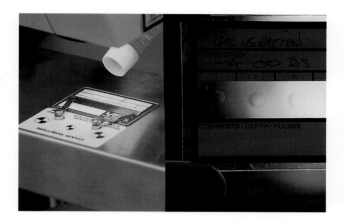

Figure 9.4 *Most laser systems now utilize a proprietary method to calibrate the excimer laser prior to treatment sessions. In the case of the Visx 20/20 B, plano, −4.00 D sphere and −4.00 D cylindrical ablations are performed onto a PMMA card before and during treatment sessions.*

EXCIMER LASER PREPARATION

The laser should be set up according to the manufacturer's instructions. Usually some form of objective calibration, often proprietary to the laser manufacturer, will be necessary before each laser session, or before each patient. In the case of the Visx 20/20B excimer laser used by the authors, this takes the form of lasering a PMMA card with a plano ablation, a −4.00 D spherical ablation and a −4.00 D cylindrical ablation (Fig. 9.4). The Poly-methyl methacrylate (PMMA) card is subsequently examined with a high power loupe to identify any inhomogeneities in the surface of the ablation zones and the dioptric power of the attempted correction checked with a focimeter. Achieved dioptric corrections on the PMMA card should be within ±5.0% of intended. The results are entered into the personal computer controlling the laser for final preoperative calibration.

Since there is no intraoperative indication to the surgeon, other than duration of treatment, of the magnitude of correction being achieved, accurate input of the desired correction is the fundamental step of the excimer laser procedure. The safest system probably requires the data to be input and then checked on the computer screen by both surgeon and assistant, comparing the programmed

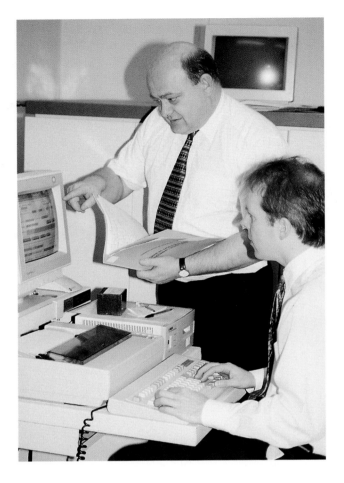

Figure 9.5 *A final check of intended refractive correction, comparing patient notes and input computer display data, should be made by both surgeon and laser operator prior to commencing photorefractive surgery.*

correction directly with the refraction in the patient's notes (Fig. 9.5).

SURGEON PREPARATION

Most excimer laser procedures take place in a clean office environment rather than a surgical theatre. Since the procedure is entirely extraocular, formal surgical gowning is seldom employed. Hands should be washed before each case but the adoption of gloves, surgical scrubs, masks or theatre hats is entirely an individual physician preference (Figs 9.6a–c).

TOPICAL ANESTHESIA

Photorefractive keratectomy may be adequately performed under simple topical anesthesia. However, the anesthetic agents and regimens in which they are used vary immensely, from topical cocaine to its synthetic analogues and from a few drops of topical agent to a full regimen including intravenous sedation and analgesia.

Topical anesthetics work by a reversible blockade of the sensory nerve endings in the cornea. Cocaine was the first acknowledged and widely used topical anesthetic for ophthalmic use. However, it may cause epithelial erosions, edema, cloudiness and even desquamation of the corneal epithelium which, despite its effectiveness, renders it less commonly used nowadays.

Proxymetacaine hydrochloride (Ophthaine, proparacaine), amethocaine (tetracaine), benoxinate (oxybuprocaine) and lignocaine (lidocaine) all have similar modes of action. They are low in toxicity and although minor differences have been reported in their potency, time of onset and length of action, there is clinically little significant difference between them.[15,16] Although low in toxic side effects, there are reports demonstrating various changes in epithelial cell metabolism and ultrastructure, including changes to the epithelial oxygen uptake, inhibition of cell migration, decreased mitosis and loss of microvilli. In view of these potential inhibitors of epithelial healing it would seem prudent to use the minimum of the least toxic anesthetic required to achieve sufficient anesthesia.

For routine PRKs the authors use two to four drops of amethocaine 1% (tetracaine) to the operative eye in the 20 minutes prior to treatment. If desired, a drop of anesthetic may be applied to the fellow eye as this may have the additional benefit of decreasing the patient's blink rate and allow a more steady fixation during the operative procedure. Some clinicians use a fixation device, such as the Thornton fixation ring, to hold the eye in a stable position during surgery (Fig. 9.7). In such circumstances, drops of topical anesthetic may occasionally provide insufficient anesthesia. If required, a pledget or limbus–sized sponge ring, soaked in anesthetic, may

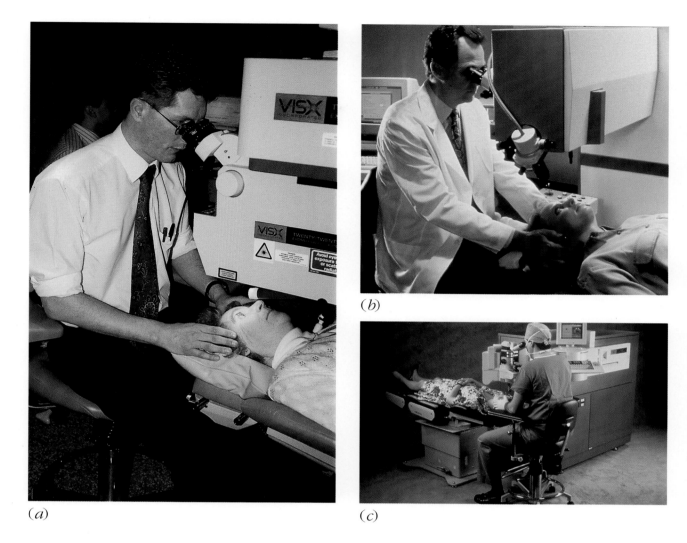

(a) *(b)* *(c)*

Figure 9.6 *The PRK/PARK procedure is usually performed in an office rather than operating room environment. Many practitioners merely wash hands thoroughly prior to treatment without adverse affect on the surgical outcome (a). However, white coats (b) or surgical scrubs (c) and gloves may be worn depending on the preference of the ophthalmologist.. Note the use of both hands by the surgeon to steady the patient's head, which not only allows minor head adjustments to maximise centration, but also provides the patient with an added sense of security and confidence. ((b) Courtesy of Coherent–Schwind; (c) Courtesy of Visx).*

be applied to the eye for a few minutes to increase the depth of anesthesia. The routine use of fixation devices has been shown to provide slightly inferior centration to unaided patient self-fixation.[17]

The use of oral or intravenous premedication is optional and is seldom used in the UK. Nonetheless, some clinicians have advocated the use of two paracetamol (acetaminophen) or codeine tablets and 10–15 mg diazepam with, in some instances, dramamine.[18] Rarely, it may be considered necessary to administer intravenous agents during the surgery.

POSITIONING THE PATIENT

The patient should have undergone formal assessment as highlighted in Chapter 8 prior to completing formal written consent as previously outlined. After ascertaining the patient's name and the eye to be treated an opaque shield is placed over the eye that is not being treated, the patient is reclined and the head adjusted comfortably within the conforming cushion (Fig. 9.8).

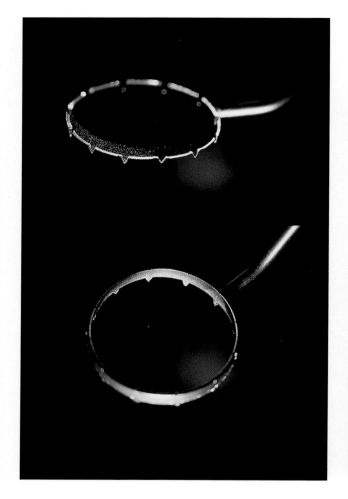

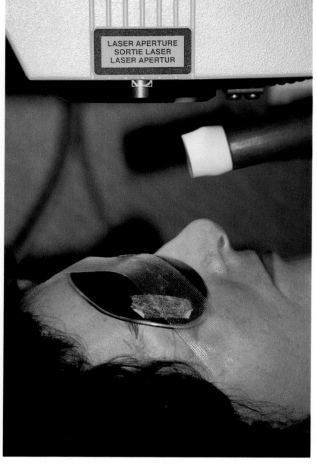

Figure 9.7 *A fixation device should always be available during PRK procedures to augment centration if self-fixation is inadequate. Although fixation devices such as the Thornton ring (illustrated) may require the practitioner to refocus due to a degree of retropulsion of the globe, if used carefully, torsional effects should be less than those produced by forceps. Torsion of the globe during PARK can lead to undercorrection of cylinder by creating axis malalignment.*

Figure 9.8 *Covering the contralateral eye with an opaque shield prevents crossfixation during the PRK procedure. Using a shield rather than a patch allows the patient to keep both eyes open, which diminishes the Bell's phenomenon and improves fixation.*

A wire-lid speculum is gently inserted to separate the lids and prevent any eyelashes becoming interposed between the laser beam and the cornea. The surgeon should always have a pediatric lid speculum available for any profound blepharospasm in patients with narrow interpalpebral fissures. An adjustable/ lockable lid speculum should also be available for subjects with very pronounced orbicularis spasm. Fortunately, in more than 600 consecutive cases we have only had to use a local anesthetic lid block on one occasion. Marked blepharospasm is often exacerbated by the photophobia associated with the microscope illumination and can be significantly reduced by turning down the light intensity.

If blepharospasm is associated with the superior drift of the cornea due to Bell's phenomenon the patient should be encouraged to keep the contralateral eye open under the opaque shield. If this proves difficult, a single drop of topical anesthetic to this contralateral eye can occasionally remedy the situation.

ALIGNING THE ASTIGMATIC AXIS

Obviously, several crucial factors may result in inaccurate photoastigmatic refractive keratectomy (PARK) ablation, including preoperative considerations (such as inaccuracy in measuring the axis and magnitude of the astigmatism), laser axis alignment and effectiveness of treatment algorithms (see Chapter 14). Cyclotorsion is another potential source of axis error. Although it is acknowledged that some axis error may be introduced in this physiological sense, recent publications show no significant predictable positional effect on eye torsion, with a recorded mean rotation of astigmatic axis between the seated and supine positions of 2.3 ± 1.9° (mean ± standard deviation).[19,20] This mean difference in astigmatic axis between the seated and supine positions was not statistically significant, although the authors noted that eyes of a subset of patients might undergo a higher degree of cyclotorsion. However, this is unpredictable in both magnitude and direction.

Head tilt, and the associated tilt of corneal axes, is an operative factor that has previously received little attention. An assumption is made that head tilt translates to an equal degree of ablation axis malalignment, although compensatory incyclotorsion or excyclotorsion might theoretically be considered to partially reduce this malalignment. The authors have documented a range of head tilt, or malalignment of 0–7° with a mean of 2.1° and 3.0° tilt when patients were aligned by an experienced and less experienced PRK surgeon, respectively.[21] It is the range of error, however, that is more important, as the upper range of deviation could potentially produce significant cylindrical undercorrection (see Chapter 8). Malalignment of intended corneal cylindrical axis and ablation axis, even by relatively small amounts, will result in a reduced effective correction of astigmatism. For the maximum alignment error of 7° observed in this study a theoretical reduction in effective cylinder treatment of 24.4% occurs and, for an error of 10°, a 34.7% reduction in effective cylinder correction would occur. Therefore, improved head,

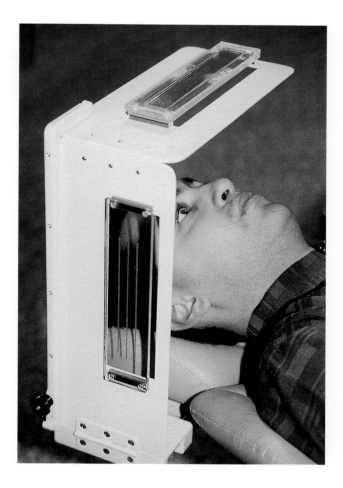

Figure 9.9 *The APAD device designed by the authors to prevent head and corneal axis malalignment by accurately aligning the eyes in the Z axis and the head in the X and Y axes. (Patent pending McGhee/Anastas).*

and thereby corneal axis, alignment should result in a significant improvement in cylindrical correction. Great care should, therefore, be exercised when aligning patients on the surgical couch to ensure that their head position is not tilted or laterally flexed relative to the principal horizontal axes of the laser beam (Fig. 9.9).

Although malalignment of corneal axis has not previously been extensively documented, axis alignment is currently being addressed in several clinical studies. Techniques that are currently on trial include limbal marking of the axis at a slit-lamp followed by narrow slit transepithelial test pulses to confirm

correct axis,[22] and devices combining a potential acuity meter with a lensometer, allowing a patient to 'rock the cylinder' and hence permit a subjective best axis to be achieved by patient focusing.[23] A variant of the latter is the Visx subjective alignment device, which incorporates parallel lines that the reclining patient rotates into sharpest focus as per the sharpest axis on an astigmatic fan, the axis of the parallel lines denoting the axis of the subjective minus cylinder. (Professor Hugh Taylor MD, personal communication). Other axis alignment techniques have also been described in the popular medical press, such as the device recently outlined by Dr Neal Sher MD. The clinical effectiveness of any one device awaits the results of current clinical trials. This area of clinical refinement in the accurate alignment of corneal and laser axes is likely to be the next big hurdle to be conquered in the treatment of astigmatism by PARK.

MARKING THE CORNEA AND CENTERING THE ABLATION ZONE

Once fully reclined and comfortable, the patient is encouraged to identify and look directly at the fixation target, which should be coaxial with the laser beam. Once the patient's eye is lined up in the center of the microscope field, using the XY shift of the couch, the center of the ablation zone can be determined.

Traditionally, refractive surgery has been centered upon the apparent geometric center of the cornea, i.e. the first Purkinje–Sanson image, or reflection of the operating light. This corneal light reflex is a virtual image of the light source created by reflection from the anterior surface of the cornea and lies approximately 3.9–4.0 mm behind the anterior surface of the cornea. This image is, therefore, subject to parallax and its exact position depends on the correct positioning of the examiner's eye directly behind the fixation light and correct fixation of the target by the patient. Uozato and Guyton[24] have elegantly analyzed errors associated with the various methods of determining centration in refractive surgery and concluded that best results would be obtained by centering upon the center of the patient's entrance pupil, ignoring the corneal reflex.

Therefore, the Purkinje–Sanson images or corneal reflexes to the target light should NOT be used for centration. The center of the (virtual) entrance pupil should be identified with the patient and the surgeon fixating coaxially. The imaginary line that connects the center of the entrance pupil and the fixation

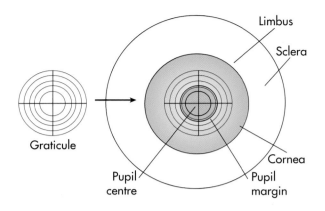

Figure 9.10 *If a graticule resides in the coaxial ocular used by the surgeon to visualize the (virtual) pupil whilst the patient is viewing the fixation target, by using the X–Y shift to superimpose a ring of the graticule concentrically with the pupil edge the surgeon can identify the center of the entrance pupil. This should be the center of the debridement and ablation zones. The position of the graticule relative to the pupil margin can be utilized to aid centration during the PRK procedure.*

object, is the line of sight, and the intersection of this line with the cornea should be used for centering refractive corneal procedures.[24,25] Pilocarpine should not be used since this may cause a pharmacologically induced shift of the pupil. Although many surgeons feel the best way to mark the pupil center is with binocular stereoscopic visualization, it has been demonstrated that only about half of those surgeons asked to sight centration upon a cornea binocularly actually do so.[24] Further aspects of centration are discussed in Chapter 23.

The authors suggest sighting monocularly via the eyepiece, which is coaxial with the fixation target. The eyepiece graticule should also reside in this eyepiece. With the patient viewing the fixation target, and surgeon and patient coaxial, the pupil center can be determined in a simple visual estimation manner, or the X–Y shift used until one of the center circles of the graticule superimposes the outline of the pupil. At this point the center of the graticule represents the centre of the entrance pupil and the cornea can be marked (Fig. 9.10) with a blunt ended instrument such as an intraocular lens (IOL) dialling hook

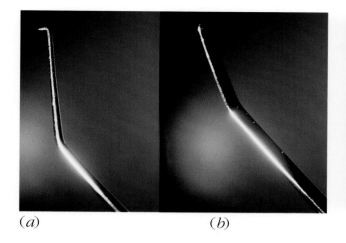

(a)   (b)

Figure 9.11 *The center of the entrance pupil can be marked upon the corneal epithelium using an IOL dialling hook (a) providing a ready reference for centration of the optical zone marker (Fig. 9.12a). The authors utilize a custom modified iris repositor to perform epithelial debridement (b).*

(Fig. 9.11a). The peripheral limits of the debridement zone can then be superimposed on this central mark by using a 'cross hair' 6.5 or 7 mm optical zone marker (Figs 9.12a,b).

AUGMENTING ANESTHESIA AND FINAL REMARKS

Depending upon the amount of topical anesthetic applied prior to this stage, the surgeon may choose to soak the corneal epithelium for another 30–60 seconds with a 6 mm diameter cellulose sponge soaked in amethocaine (tetracaine) (Figs 9.13a,b), which facilitates both anesthesia and a loosening of the central corneal epithelium. During this short period it is worth reminding the patient of the various events that will occur in the ensuing few minutes and remarks might include:

- The surface cells will be rubbed off, which will not be painful; however, the patient may notice the eye moving a little and associated flashing or distorted lights as the instrument moves across and distorts the cornea.

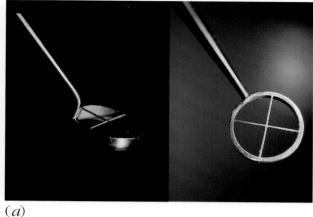

(a)

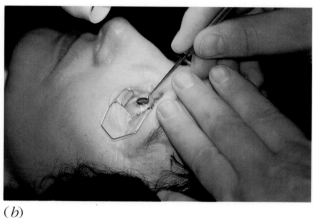

(b)

Figure 9.12 *(a) Optical zone markers are a matter for personal preference but the authors believe cross hair markers provide more ready centration than gunsight markers. Ultra-low profile markers should be avoided as the cross hairs may indent the epithelium centrally and this indentation may be reproduced on the stroma if a laser transepithelial technique is utilized. (b) The marker should be applied with sufficient compression, without a rotational movement, to produce a lasting epithelial indentation, which will not only delimit the epithelial debridement zone but, if placed concentrically with the pupil, provide a second landmark to assist ablation zone centration.*

- As the laser fires, the patient will be aware of a loud 'clap' which may cause the patient to be startled initially and at the same time they might feel, or have the impression, that a gentle tapping is occurring on the front of the eye.

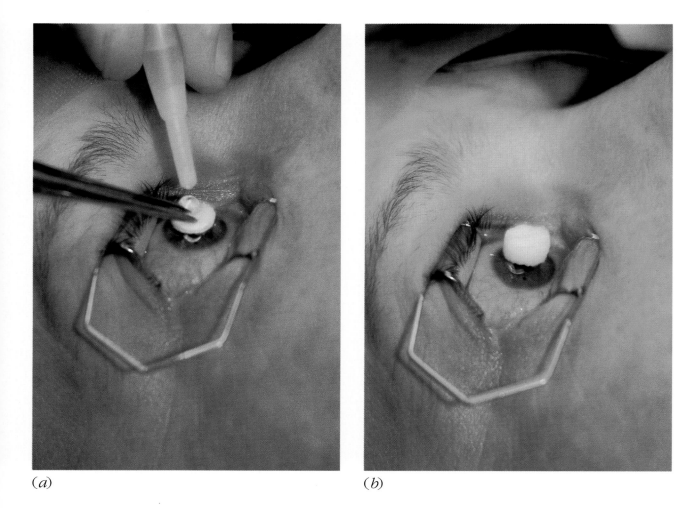

(*a*)   (*b*)

Figure 9.13 *A fiber-free circular cellulose sponge can be utilized to apply preservative-free topical anesthetic to the cornea just prior to epithelial debridement (a). By keeping the sponge moist, anesthetic can be applied directly to the central 6–7 mm of the corneal epithelium whilst sparing the peripheral cornea from additional anesthetic (b).*

- It is worth reminding the patient that during the procedure a carbon or smoke smell may occur but that no burning or thermal damage is occurring.
- Reassure the patient that the target light does not move and, therefore, they should not seek to look around if it should 'disappear'. The patient must be instructed that the target light will apparently 'come and go' during the procedure, depending on dehydration and stage of the ablation procedure. Notably, in extreme myopia, patients often remark that the target light has 'disappeared' entirely.

EPITHELIAL DEBRIDEMENT

There are three methods of epithelial removal: mechanical debridement, alcohol augmented debridement and laser removal.

MECHANICAL EPITHELIAL REMOVAL

Mechanical removal is the most commonly used method and is the method routinely recommended by both Visx and Summit. This should be accom-

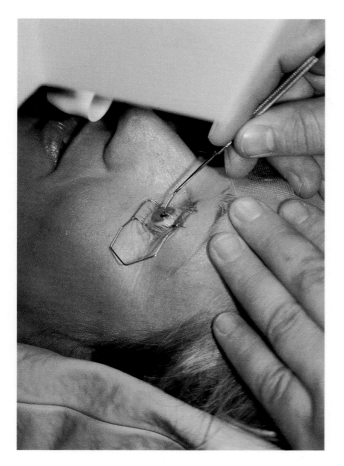

Figure 9.14 *Debridement should be performed in an efficient manner from periphery to center of the debridement zone. Central epithelium should not be left to last, nor should debrided epithelium be heaped in the center of the zone, since both actions might lead to a relatively greater central stromal hydration. A hand resting upon the patient's forehead helps to stabilize the eye and the surgeon's hands during this stage of the procedure.*

plished as quickly and as safely as possible. To this end it is probably best to time the duration of the procedure and aim, as far as possible, to complete debridement within a maximum of 2 minutes from its start.

There are several different techniques,[18] although debriding from the outer marker towards the center is probably the safest (since large strips of epithelium may be loosened beyond the demarcation zone if debridement is carried out from center to periphery).

The choice of instrument is up to the individual surgeon (Figs 9.11b and 9.14); we use a blunt instrument that avoids damage to Bowman's layer but this means that debridement takes 60–120 seconds. Care should be taken not to deform the underlying stroma with undue downward pressure since this might create focal areas of lesser hydration.

Although it is believed that little of the laser energy is consumed in the vaporization of water, decreased corneal hydration is associated with increased stromal ablation, and increased corneal stromal hydration with reduced effect of the ablation.[26] For this reason, fluid should not be added to the corneal surface during or after epithelial removal since it will be rapidly imbibed by the corneal stroma in the absence of epithelium. Strips of epithelium should be debrided in a motion that crosses the zone center, and central epithelium should not be left to the last, nor should debrided epithelium be allowed to accumulate in the center of the zone. By preferentially protecting the central debridement zone from dehydration, by either of the latter two methods, the practitioner is likely to produce relatively higher central hydration compared to the mid and peripheral area of corneal epithelial debridement, increasing the potential for central island formation.

Obviously, debridement can be accomplished more quickly with sharper instruments but with the possible risk of damage to Bowman's layer, thus creating small irregularities in the surface to be ablated. The area debrided of epithelium should be approximately 1.0 mm greater in diameter than the intended ablation zone. Once the epithelium has been removed a quick wipe with a dry or minimally dampened cellulose sponge can be employed if any small areas of cellular debris are identified.

Pallikaris has developed a rotating, circular, nylon brush to remove the surface epithelium. Apparently, this technique is fast and leaves a very neat border to the area of debridement. However, at the time of writing this device has yet to become widely available.

ALCOHOL AUGMENTED MECHANICAL DEBRIDEMENT

Application of alcohol can be used to make epithelial removal easier. A round sponge, soaked in 18% alcohol, is placed on the cornea for 10–20 seconds. This loosens the epithelium, making removal quicker

and easier. Refractive outcome and complication rates utilizing this method appear to be little different from manual debridement techniques.[27] However, this practice is not recommended because alcohol is likely to affect the hydration of the cornea, which in turn will affect the ablation rate. In addition, there is experimental evidence that demonstrates toxic effects of alcohol on the corneal epithelium, stroma and endothelium, albeit in concentrations and doses different to those likely to be used in clinical practice.[28,29]

REMOVAL OF THE EPITHELIUM BY EXCIMER LASER

Laser removal of the epithelium is rapid and provides a smooth surface from which to start the PRK. The central corneal epithelium is approximately 50 μm thick and an ablation arbitrarily set to this depth can be performed prior to commencing the PRK; however, if the epithelium is thinner, stromal ablation will occur, and if the epithelium is thicker refractive undercorrection is likely.

Alternatively, ablation depth can be set to 60 μm or greater and, by monitoring the cornea during ablation, the end-point of epithelial removal is determined by a change in epithelial fluorescence to a dark background, as the epithelium is removed and Bowman's layer exposed. However, in practice the end-point is often difficult to determine visually and may lead to under- or overablation of the epithelium. Some workers compromise by deliberately underablating the epithelium with a 40 μm depth ablation followed by mechanical debridement of the thin layer of basal epithelium remaining.

Laser ablation of the epithelium is not widely used in the UK, except in cases of retreatment, where epithelial thickness is variable and the stromal surface irregular. However, some Canadian practitioners, especially those performing bilateral surgery, have modified the laser algorithm appropriately and utilize transepithelial PRK with success. Transepithelial ablation does not produce a statistically significant difference in refractive outcome when compared to manual epithelial removal; however, there is a tendency towards greater refractive correction, which might lead to overcorrection.[30] Although no published data are available, theoretically, transepithelial ablation may also be associated with a higher incidence of persisting central corneal islands. (Stephen Trokel MD, personal communication).

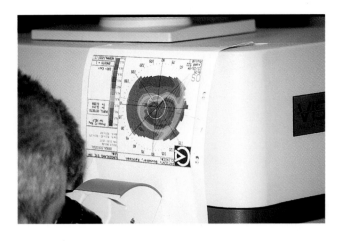

Figure 9.15 *In cases of retreatment, focal debridement and ablation can be guided by an inverted and appropriately annotated computerized corneal topographic map in the surgeon's field of vision.*

It has been suggested that laser removal of the epithelium helps with the problem of decentration, since off-center treatments may be detected prior to any refractive effect being reached at the stroma. Yet, conversely, it has been noted that once the stroma has been reached it is less easy, with laser epithelial removal, to make the small centration corrective adjustments that are possible with the wider mechanical debridement. Because the area of de-epithelialization with laser removal is slightly smaller than with mechanical removal, it is likely that postoperative pain is reduced since epithelial healing time will be reduced. Laser has also been suggested to be preferable when treating astigmatism in penetrating keratoplasty since no mechanical pressure is applied directly to the graft.

In cases of PRK retreatment in which Grade II or greater haze is present, by using a transepithelial ablation the epithelium can be utilized as a 'masking agent' to smooth the underlying irregular stromal surface. In retreatment cases where only selective areas of epithelium will be removed, e.g. to treat central islands or improve decentration, the appropriately annotated corneal topographic map can be attached to the laser, in ready view of the surgeon, to assist in delineating areas of debridement and retreatment upon the cornea (Fig. 9.15) (see Chapters 7 and 24).

SURGEON–PATIENT INTERACTION DURING THE LASER PROCEDURE

Delay should be avoided between completion of epithelial debridement and commencing the actual laser procedure. Any final alignment should be made and it should be rechecked that the patient has identified the correct fixation target. One final warning with regard to the 'clapping and tapping' effects should be made. The surgeon's hands should be placed on both the left and right forehead and temples of the patient (Fig. 9.16). This allows the surgeon to move the head, and thereby the eye, to maintain perfect centration.

IT MUST ALWAYS BE REMEMBERED THAT STOPPING THE PROCEDURE EITHER TEMPORARILY OR ALTOGETHER IS PREFERABLE TO PROCEEDING WITH THE ABLATION IF POOR CENTRATION HAS OCCURRED AND ADEQUATE FIXATION CANNOT BE RE-ESTABLISHED.

If patients have more than 4.00–5.00 D of myopia it is quite common to have to stop at least once, or as often as two to three times, in any procedure to realign the patient and allow them to refixate to obtain the best centration. As long as the delay is no more than 10–20 seconds at each interval it probably has little effect on the outcome, other than to improve centration. It must be remembered that the patient's view of the fixation target is compromised by myopia, epithelial debridement and the ablation process (Fig. 9.17). Thus, the target is likely to appear blurred, rather than a point focus. Due to this blurred view of the target, gentle pressure on either side of the patient's head allows minor movement of the head and eye to maintain perfect centration, whereas, if the subject were able to identify the target clearly, one would anticipate compensatory eye movement to take up original (decentered) fixation, which would negate the effect of movement of the head by the surgeon.

During the initial procedure the surgeon has two anatomical landmarks to maintain the ablation centration; firstly, the pupil, which will be obvious during the early part of the procedure whilst the ablation zone expands (Fig. 9.10) and, secondly, the edge of the debridement zone. However, the pupil becomes much less readily visible (and, therefore, a less useful landmark) as the procedure advances. However, during debridement the surgeon should attempt to maintain the epithelial removal just within the 6.5 or 7 mm mark, leaving an intact circular zone mark on the remaining epithelium. Prior to firing the laser it is

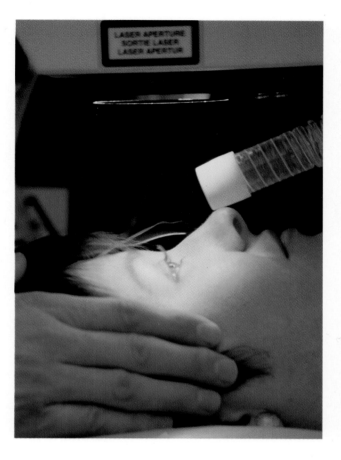

Figure 9.16 *By placing hands on either side of the subject's head the surgeon simultaneously reassures the patient and can make minor corrective movements of the head to improve ablation zone centration.*

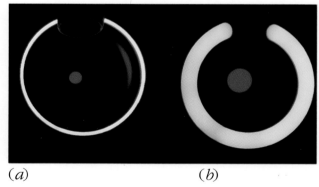

(a)   *(b)*

Figure 9.17 *A patient's eye view of the fixation target (red) as seen by an emmetropic or corrected eye (a), becomes a rather more blurred and less discrete target to a simulated uncorrected 5.00 D myopic error (b), a phenomenon that will be compounded by epithelial debridement and stromal ablation.*

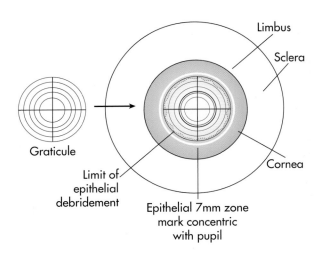

Figure 9.18 *As the PRK ablation progresses, the pupillary margin may become more difficult to discern; however, if the optical zone mark has been made concentric with the pupil and epithelial debridement contained within this mark, the graticule in the sighting, coaxial microscope optic can be aligned with this mark to maintain centration.*

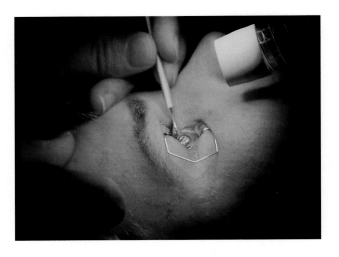

Figure 9.19 *Fixation of the globe in normally sighted eyes is seldom required, whereas in PTK of eyes with compromised visual acuity, globe fixation, in this case with a Thornton ring, is frequently necessary.*

useful to assess the exact position of the epithelial mark, relative to the alignment graticule' when the patient is properly viewing the fixation target (presuming this mark is concentric to the pupil). Thus, in the latter part of the procedure (when the pupil may no longer be a useful reference landmark) this demarcation zone can be appropriately aligned with the graticule to maintain accurate ablation centration (Fig. 9.18). Ultimately, centration is both surgeon and patient dependent and improves with surgical experience.

A fixation device should always be available for those patients who become unable to hold steady fixation. Whilst this might be accomplished by a pair of forceps, these will occupy both of the surgeon's hands, preventing minor corrective movements of the patient's head by the surgeon. These may also induce a torsional element, which is undesirable if a PARK is being performed. The authors use a Thornton fixation ring or similar but have found this necessary in less than 2% of sighted eyes, although fixation may be necessary in partially sighted eyes (Figs 9.7 and 9.19).

VERBAL REASSURANCE DURING THE PROCEDURE

During the procedure it is vitally important to continually reassure the patient and, whilst it may sound 'corny', encouraging phrases such as 'it's going well', 'try to concentrate harder on the target', 'we're half way there', 'only 10 seconds to go', etc, are most useful. Inform the patient throughout the procedure approximately how far into the treatment they have progressed. Whilst verbal reassurance may seem common sense and stating the obvious, having seen many ophthalmic surgeons perform this procedure, it is surprising how many, perhaps concentrating upon the procedure, remain very quiet, if not totally silent, during this vital 1–2 minutes.

POSTOPERATIVE CARE

At the end of the procedure the surgeon's choice of medication should be given to the patient; the regime used in the Sunderland Eye Infirmary series comprised: single application guttae diclofenac, guttae

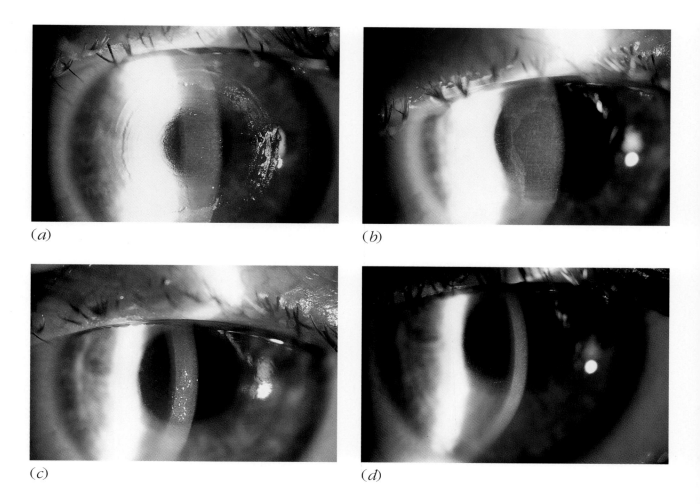

Figure 9.20 *Normal post–operative epithelial healing. (a) Appearance immediately after a –10.00 D correction with manual epithelial debridement. (b) Twenty–four hours post-PRK epithelial closure is already almost 50% advanced. (c) Forty–eight hours post-PRK only a minor epithelial defect remains. (d) Seventy–two hours post-PRK, epithelial closure is complete with a BSCVA of 6/12 (20/40).*

homatropine, an antibiotic ointment and application of a pad (patch) for 24 hours. A mild-to-moderate oral analgesic was provided, such as a paraceta-mol–codeine preparation, and guttae diclofenac drops, one drop to be taken 4–6 hourly for ocular pain, if required.

Fortunately, only about 10% of patients experience pain following the procedure but this pain may be severe. Therefore, it is prudent to warn all patients they should go home, sit in a slightly darkened room if possible, sit or sleep with their eyes closed, and generally be supported by their partner or friends in the 48 hour postoperative period. The worst pain is

usually felt by those who go home, feel the eye is well and continue as if they have not undergone an operation. It must be re-emphasized 'ad nauseum' that this is an operative procedure and the patient should relax and take things very easy for the immediate 2–3 days post-treatment. Within the UK, the use of bandage contact lenses has been very limited; however, they have been widely utilized post-PRK in North America.

At the end of the procedure the patient should be reassured about how well the procedure has gone and that their best vision may not return for several days or even several weeks. Since patients treated on

the same day may well come back for review on similar days, the patient with −2.00 D who obtains 6/6 (20/20) unaided on day 3 may well worry the patient with −8.00 D who does not obtain this unaided visual acuity for 3–4 weeks. Similarly, due to variations in healing, patients with identical refractions can see as well as 6/5 (20/15) or as poorly as 6/60 (20/200) on day 3. This individual variation in healing and variable rate of visual recovery must be re-emphasized and patients should not feel, since others have regained their best acuity earlier, some error or catastrophe has actually occurred in their own treatment.

Generally, epithelial closure occurs within 2–4 days (Figs 9.20a–d) and a significant improvement in unaided visual acuity should be noted within 7 days. However, due to transient induced hyperopia, older subjects with higher attempted corrections may have relatively poor unaided visual acuity for a few weeks. In the immediate postoperative period poor visual acuity may also be due to central corneal islands or irregular epithelial healing, which may be highlighted by computerized corneal topography. Postoperative follow-up is discussed in Chapter 8, the use of corticosteroids is discussed in Chapter 25, and postoperative complications, including decentration, are outlined in Chapter 23.

INTRAOPERATIVE LASER FAILURE

Fortunately, intraoperative machine or computer failure is extremely uncommon with modern excimer lasers if they are properly serviced and operated; however, contingency plans should always be made for the unexpected. If the excimer laser failure occurs due to a computer malfunction, rather than an intrinsic laser malfunction (which should lead to immediate cancellation) before epithelial debridement, the procedure can simply be abandoned or postponed. However, if failure to fire occurs after epithelial debridement is complete four options are available:

- Abandon the procedure immediately and allow the epithelium to heal with a view to treatment at a later date when the epithelium and cornea have returned to the pre-debridement state.
- If the fault can be corrected within 2–3 minutes, shield the eye to prevent dehydration and proceed as planned.
- If a 4–6 minute delay is encountered, wet the corneal surface evenly with saline and gently wipe off with a cellulose sponge to compensate for the inevitable corneal dehydration that will have occurred during the delay. This is likely to produce a relative overhydration of the stroma as the saline is imbibed by the bare Bowman's surface, possibly leading to a slight underablation. The patient should be made aware of this. Nonetheless, a primary underablation will be more susceptible to retreatment than hypermetropia produced by overablation of dehydrated stroma.
- If the laser cannot be brought safely back on line in a maximum of 5–6 minutes, the treatment should be abandoned in view of potential regional variations in corneal hydration secondary to prolonged exposure of bare Bowman's membrane after epithelial debridement.

REFERENCES

1. Krueger RR, Excimer laser: a step up in complexity and responsibility for the ophthalmic laser surgeon? *J Refract Corneal Surg* (1994) **10**(2);83–86 (edit).
2. Tavola A, Carones F, Galli L, Fontanella G, Brancato R, The learning curve in myopic photorefractive keratectomy, *J Refract Corneal Surg* (1994) **10**:S188–S193.
3. Tiemeier CG, Abbot RL, Ellis JH, Risk management issues in radial keratotomy surgery, *Surv Ophthalmol* (1994) **39**:52–6.
4. Talley R, Hardten D, Sher NA *et al.* Results one year after using the 193 nm excimer laser for photorefractive keratectomy in mild to moderate myopia, *Am J Ophthalmol* (1994) **118**:304–11.
5. Salz JJ, Maguen E, Macy JI *et al.* One year results of excimer laser photorefractive keratectomy for myopia, *Refract Corneal Surg* (1992) **8**:269–73.
6. Schallhorn SC, Blanton CL, Kaupp SE, Sutphin J *et al.* Preliminary results of photorefractive keratectomy in active–duty United States Navy personnel, *Ophthalmology* (1996) **103**:5–22.
7. Kim JH, Hahn TW, Lee YC, Sah WJ, Excimer laser photorefractive keratectomy for myopia: Two year follow–up, *J Cataract Refract Surg* (1994) **20**:S229–S233.
8. Salz JJ, Maguen E, Nesburn AB, Warren C *et al.* A two year experience with excimer laser photorefractive keratectomy for myopia, *Ophthalmology* (1993) **100**:873–82.

9. Dutt S, Steinert RF, Raizman MB, Puliafito CA, One year results of excimer laser photorefractive keratectomy for low to moderate myopia, *Arch Ophthalmol* (1994) **112**:1427–36.

10. Sutton G, Kalski RS, Lawless MA, Rogers C. Excimer retreatments for scarring and regression after photorefractive keratectomy for myopia, *Br J Ophthalmol* (1995) **79**:756–9.

11. Snibson GR, McCarthy CA, Aldred GF, Levin S, Taylor HR, Retreatment after excimer laser photorefractive keratectomy, *Am J Ophthalmol* (1996) **121**(3):250–7.

12. Gartry DS, Kerr–Muir MG, Marshall J, Excimer laser photorefractive keratectomy: 18 month follow–up, *Ophthalmology* (1992) **99**:1209–19.

13. McGhee CNJ, Weed KH, Bryce IG, Anastas CN, Webber SK, Assessment and management of complications following PRK/PARK. In: Proceedings of the Third Annual UK International Ophthalmic Excimer Laser Congress. *Eye News* (1996) **3**(2):Suppl 5–6.

14. Orr D, McGhee CNJ, Stark C, Kidd B *et al.* Psychological aspects of excimer laser surgery for myopia: reasons for seeking treatment and patient satisfaction, *Br J Ophthalmol* (1996) **80**:874–79.

15. Catterall W, Mackie K. Local Anaesthetics. In: Hardam JG, Goodman, Gillman A, Linbird LE, eds, *Goodman and Gillman's The Pharmacological Basis of Therapeutics*. 9th edn. (McGraw Hill: 1996) 331–40.

16. Craig EL, Anaesthesia. In: Mauger TF, Craig EL, eds, *Havener's ocular pharmacology*, 6th edn. (Mosby: St Louis, 1994) 201–12.

17. Maguen E, Salz JJ, Nesburn AB *et al.* Results of excimer laser photorefractive keratectomy for the correction of myopia, *Ophthalmology* (1994) **101**:1548–57.

18. McDonald M, Leach DH, Myopic photorefractive keratectomy: US experience. In: Thompson FB, McDonnell PJ, eds, *Colour atlas/text of excimer laser surgery of the cornea*. (Igaku–Shoin Medical Publishers: New York, 1993) 41–5.

19. Smith EM, Talamo JH, Assil KK, Petashnik DE, Comparison of astigmatic axis in the seated and supine positions, *J Ref Corn Surg* (1994) **10**: 615–20.

20. Smith EM, Talamo JH. Cyclotorsion in the seated and supine patient, *J Cataract Refract Surg* (1995) **21**:402–3.

21. McGhee NJ, Anastas CN, Bryce IG, The influence of head tilt and corneal axis malalignment on the success of PARK surgery. *Proceedings of the Second Annual UK International Ophthalmic Excimer Laser Congress* (1995) **2**:28 [abst].

22. Campos M, Hertzog L, Garbus J, Lee M, McDonnell PJ, Photorefractive keratectomy for severe postkeratoplasty astigmatism, *Am J Ophthalmol* (1992) **114**:429–36.

23. Pender PM, Photorefractive keratectomy for myopic astigmatism: phase IIA of the Federal Drug Administration study (12 to 18 months follow–up), *J Cataract Refract Surg* (1994) **20**(Suppl): 262–4.

24. Uozato H, Guyton DL, Centering Corneal surgical procedures, *Am J Ophthalmol* (1987) **103**:264–75.

25. Maloney RK, Corneal topography and optical zone location in photorefractive keratectomy, *Refract Corneal Surg* (1990) **6**:363–71.

26. Dougherty PJ, Wellish KL, Maloney RK, Excimer laser ablation rate and corneal hydration, *Am J Ophthalmology* (1994) **118**:169–76.

27. Jenkins L, A comparison between the use of 18% alcohol and simple scraping for epithelial debridement, Proceedings of the Third Annual UK International Ophthalmic Excimer Laser Congress. *Eye News* (1996) **3**(2): Suppl 7–8.

28. MacRae SM, Brown B, Edelhauser HF, The corneal toxicity of pre-surgical skin antiseptics, *Am J Ophthalmol* (1984) **97**:221–32.

29. Soukiasian SH, Asdourian GK, A complication from alcohol swabbed tonometer tips, *Arch Ophthalmol* (1988) **105**:424 [lett].

30. Gimbel HV, DeBroff BM, Beldavs RA, van Westenbrugge JA, Ferensowicz M, Comparison of laser and manual removal of corneal epithelium for photorefractive keratectomy, *J Refract Surg* (1995) **11**(1):36–41.

Chapter 10 Psychological associations of myopia in relation to excimer laser photorefractive surgery

Brian A Kidd and Cameron Stark

INTRODUCTION

Excimer laser photorefractive keratectomy (PRK) is a novel surgical treatment for myopia which may ultimately replace the technique of radial keratotomy, due to its higher success rate and improved predictability of outcome. Despite the risks of corrective eye surgery, patients have been shown to prefer radial keratotomy to an external form of optical correction such as contact lenses or spectacles.[1] Numerous studies have shown that spectacle wearers tend to see themselves as unattractive[2] and, when contact lenses have been worn successfully, their replacement with spectacles has been shown to induce considerable anxiety.[3] However, the long-term wear of contact lenses is inevitably time limited, and even amongst those who successfully tolerate them, the majority will eventually have to consider alternative forms of optical correction either due to ocular discomfort or drastically reduced wearing time. It is in this setting that excimer laser photofractive surgery for myopia has flourished and the patient demand for a safe and effective surgical correction of myopia has driven the rapid expansion in the provision of this service within the UK.

It is well established that there is a relationship between visual acuity and psychological profile.[4] However, psychological explanations for myopia have often been influenced by the fashionable theory of the day. For example, Freud described the visual loss of myopia as a castration symbol![5] Modern day research into the etiology and modification of myopia has often involved psychological assessments of myopic individuals, with the 'focus' being on aspects of personality and intelligence.[6,7] Behavioral psychological treatments for myopia have been shown to have some success, adding yet another confounding variable to the apparently straightforward science of light refraction and the amelioration of refractive error.[7,8] When a new treatment such as Excimer laser PRK/PARK for myopia is introduced and evaluated it is essential that we acknowledge the importance of psychological factors in the development of myopia and patient perception of their myopia in order to properly explore the possible impact of such factors on presentation for treatment, objective outcomes (treatment success or failure) and subjective outcomes (patient satisfaction).

PSYCHOLOGICAL INFLUENCES ON MYOPIA

ETIOLOGY OF MYOPIA

In order to understand the possible influence of psychological factors on myopia, a brief review of the demographics and etiological theories is required. Myopia is not unique to man, with some species such as horses and cattle, showing a prevalence of up to 30%.[9] There are also considerable racial differences.[10–14] The higher prevalence of myopia in Europeans compared to Eskimos or Negroes has been explained, by some authors, as the result of the longer history of European civilization, with the subsequent reduction in the importance of natural selection within the population, a process which would normally reduce the number of myopes in a society.[15] Notably, the prevalence of myopia is actually increasing in industrial countries[16] and myopia has consistently been shown to be more prevalent in those who are successful academically or perform clerical work.[17]

The only consistent physical finding in myopic individuals is an increased axial length of the eyeball.[18] The cause of this phenomenon is still under debate, though increased intraocular pressure resulting from squinting[19] or overuse[20] and increased tension of the extraocular muscles[21] are some of the etiologies which have previously been indicated in acquired myopia. Alterations of accommodation are also found in myopia and abolition of accommodation may prevent development of myopia in animals.[22–24]

The influences on myopia development can be classed as either genetic or environmental. The ethnic differences would appear to support the case for a genetic cause though research into family histories has shown that only individuals developing myopia in early life have a greater prevalence of myopia in their parents.[25] Twin studies have also suggested a genetic link[26] but no studies of adopted away twins have been performed to remove the influence of environment – a likely confounding variable. The case for environmental influence is strong and is based on Young's finding of a massive change in the prevalence of myopia in an Eskimo community after the introduction of compulsory schooling.[27] This near work hypothesis which suggests that myopia results from excess reading or close-work, has gained considerable support. It is, however, known that in animals growth of the visual pathways is positively related to use, with a lack of use in early life leading to underdevelopment.[28,29] In humans, underuse due to astigmatism might possibly lead to myopia[30] whilst optical correction appears to slow its development.[31,32] This is the argument many use to support the early correction of myopia in children. Unfortunately no randomized controlled trials have been performed to support this preventive approach.[33]

In summary, the only physiological or anatomical factor consistently associated with myopia is the increased axial length of the eyeball. It seems likely that a multifactorial etiology exists for this phenomenon, involving genetic and environmental influences which may act through a number of processes possibly involving the autonomic nervous system and/or mechanical forces (see Chapter 5). Using this model, the research linking psychological factors with the development or modification of myopia will now be examined. Previous studies have mainly looked at the myopic personality, intelligence and achievement of myopes, and possible behavioral modification/treatment of myopia. Descriptive studies of personality and intelligence will be described first,

followed by work addressing the question of any etiological relationship. Evidence for behavioral treatments of myopia will also be outlined.

THE MYOPIC PERSONALITY – DESCRIPTIVE STUDIES

Many studies have examined the myopic personality.[7,11] Initially descriptions were based on clinical experience, describing 'myopes' as 'bookish', introspective, introverted characters preferring sedentary activities'.[34,35] Other more unpleasant personality characteristics have also been described, including introjective, demanding, defensive and perseverative.[36] Therman B Rice's 1930 articles on *Physical defects in character* echoed these classical stereotypes, describing the myope as a character who is 'not dependent on others for entertainment and is liable to grow rather contemptuous of the abilities of others. He does not adapt himself to the surroundings and is not willing to make compromises. He is often severe in his rightness and may become a disagreeable personage.'[37]

It was not until 1948 that Mull objectively examined the myopic personality using a standardized personality inventory.[38] This work confirmed the myopic individual to be introverted, a finding which has been consistently repeated.[39,40] Other recurring observations are a disinclination for motor activity and a tendency for social leadership,[41] a greater tolerance for anxiety and passivity towards stress[39]. Some workers, in stark contradiction, have failed to demonstrate any significant relationship between refractive error and personality.[42,6] Therefore the apparent associations of personality and myopia which have been repeated to date are confusing. However, on balance, it does seem likely that, at the very least, the stereotypical picture of the 'introverted myope' is supported in fact.

INTELLIGENCE AND ACADEMIC ACHIEVEMENT – DESCRIPTIVE STUDIES

Research has shown there to be a definite relationship between academic achievement and myopia.[43,44] Indeed, myopic individuals have consistently been shown to gain higher grades in examinations,[17,40] to be represented in greater numbers in honors programs,[36] and to complete more educational grades[6] than emmetropic or hypermetropic subjects. Myopes have also been shown to spend more time reading on average, than other members of the population.[45] However, these parameters do not measure intelligence. Studies examining Intelligence Quotient (IQ) and refractive error have revealed confounding results: Young[45] and Nadell[46] initially found no correlation between IQ and refractive error while Hirsch[47] concluded from his work that 'hypermetropes have an average IQ below the mean of 113, while the myopes have an average value considerably above this.' Myopes have been shown to be better at certain intelligence tests[48] and it may be that this apparent discrepancy in IQ relates to the actual tests used. In a repeat study, Young[43] once more found no significant differences in IQ but a weak correlation on the California Test of Mental Maturity – a test requiring greater reading proficiency. When the test was repeated using a test in which reading was less important this difference was eliminated; notably, the myopes were significantly better at reading than the other group. This seemed to support the notion that reading ability could explain the myope's 'superior IQ'. In contrast, when tests requiring no reading skills were utilized by Grosvenor,[49] the myopic group still had a higher mean IQ, though small groups precluded the demonstration of statistical significance. This latter finding would appear to refute the suggestion that greater reading skills alone are the basis of higher IQ scores in studies of myopic groups. In order to fully test this premise an oral IQ test would be required, and once again, as in the case of myopic personality, there is a decided need for definitive studies.

PSYCHOLOGICAL INFLUENCES ON MYOPIA – CAUSE OR EFFECT?

Many potential relationships between psychological factors and myopia have been proposed.[4,11] Three theories will be addressed: a) psychological characteristics are the direct result of myopia, b) myopia results from a particular psychological type, c) a common causal factor results in myopia and certain psychological features.

Myopia affects personality/intelligence

This theory echoes the early work of Thorington[34] and Rice[37] and suggests that, as a result of an inability to see in the distance, the myope develops a rather introverted and self-sufficient personality. (S)he takes to non-physical pursuits, such as reading,

resulting in greater intelligence and poorer physical fitness, and thus will perform better academically and be more likely to have a successful career. The descriptive studies described above have done little to clarify this cause or effect debate.

Psychological factors affect myopia

This second hypothesis suggests that aspects of a person's personality can cause the development of myopia. Recent research has refuted the importance of personality profile and psychosocial stress as etiological factors for myopia.[4] Workers have, however, been able to demonstrate manipulation of myopia using psychological techniques.[7] Bates claimed to improve visual acuity in myopes using modified behavioral therapy methods[50] whilst Bell demonstrated improvements only in low-anxiety myopes[51] using a tone to condition the patients. Visual training methods[52] have shown improvement in visual acuity but not refractive error (only in motivated subjects), suggesting to Sells and Fixott that a perceptual rather than physiological change was taking place.[53] However, they failed to consider the possibility that autonomic conditioning, a phenomenon well recognized in other clinical areas such as blood pressure control, might influence myopia, despite the fact that operant methods were used. Studies employing hypnotism have shown an average improvement of 20/50 to 20/20 in visual acuity.[54,55] Similar results were achieved when a haploscope was used, implying that lens or eyeball shape changes had resulted from the treatment. However, use of a cycloplegic confirmed that no alteration in the lens shape was responsible and Kelley therefore hypothesized alterations in eyeball length, perhaps mediated through some effect on the external musculature.

Common etiological factors

It has been shown that eyes with a longer axial length are more likely to be myopic and that larger brains tend to be more intelligent.[56] In his review of the existing literature Miller hypothesizes that the pleiotropic relationship between myopia and intelligence could arise with a single genetically controlled mechanism affecting both brain and eye size.[56] Such a theory has yet to be tested or confirmed. The effect of the autonomic balance of an individual on both personality and refractive error has been investigated, however, and may have a part to play.[24] Personality traits have been linked to parasympathetic (PNS) or sympathetic (SNS) dominance within the autonomic system, with PNS dominance being related to introversion and SNS dominance to extraversion.[57,58] Since accommodation is facilitated by a PNS-mediated contraction of the ciliary muscle, with consequent thickening of the lens and near focusing[59] it has been hypothesized by some that this may be the common path leading to the associations of personality and myopia.[24]

CONCLUSIONS

Myopia is associated with certain psychological characteristics, though the nature of this relationship remains unclear. The consistent findings of an introverted myopic personality and a greater likelihood of higher IQ with better academic achievement in myopes are valid, but with our existing level of knowledge we cannot clarify the question of etiology.

PSYCHIATRIC MORBIDITY AND SELF-ESTEEM IN PATIENTS PRESENTING FOR EXCIMER LASER CORRECTION OF MYOPIA

We can now acknowledge that certain psychological findings are linked with, and may influence, myopia while myopia itself may affect the development of these psychological characteristics. Research has already shown that stress may influence the degree of myopia in an individual.[4] Behavioral processes can be used to improve visual acuity, at least subjectively[7] and it seems likely that autonomic nervous systems play a role in such a process.[24]

During assessment prior to excimer laser PRK, a detailed measurement of refractive error is undertaken. Minor errors in this assessment will affect the treatment settings and could have significant implications regarding the likelihood of success of the procedure. If the role of a patient's psychological state can influence the apparent degree of myopia, it would seem remiss of the physician to omit an assessment of psychological stress preoperatively. The laser procedure is also generally requested by the patient, perhaps in a situation where the ophthalmologist would not necessarily recommend this course of

action. Although there are many clear clinical indications for excimer laser PRK, it may be requested simply for reasons of vanity. Addressing aspects of the patient's self-image and self-esteem may help clarify if the patient is actually making an informed choice and help the physician to fully counsel them. This may help to avoid possible dissatisfaction after the procedure. Finally, among ophthalmologists, there has been anecdotal concern that a significant number of those patients self-presenting for PRK would be defined as unusual characters. Despite the potential effects on treatment outcome and patient satisfaction it would seem that little research has addressed any of these issues in the group of patients receiving PRK.

THE SUNDERLAND EYE INFIRMARY STUDY

In 1993 a large prospective study was commenced in the Corneal Diseases and Excimer Laser Unit of Sunderland Eye Infirmary, in order to determine the degree of psychological stress and self-esteem problems in those presenting for excimer laser PRK.[60] A cohort of 90 consecutive PRK patients (subjects) were assessed pre-operatively using the GHQ30 version of the General Health Questionnaire[61] and the Hudson Self-esteem Questionnaire.[62] Normal ophthalmic examination was undertaken and a control group of 50 consecutive myopes presenting for contact lens assessment to a local optometrist (controls) were similarly assessed. The questionnaires were relatively short, taking only a few minutes to complete while the patients sat in the waiting room prior to their appointments.

Results

A satisfactory response rate was achieved for both subjects (90% for both questionnaires) and controls (98% for the GHQ30 and 100% for the Hudson). Demographic data showed the subject group to be significantly older (p=<0.001) though no significant differences were demonstrated with regard to gender. The subject group were more myopic as measured by sphere equivalent (p=0.01) while the controls had a poorer best spectacle visual acuity (p=0.001).

Of the subjects, 14% were shown to be psychiatric cases as defined by the GHQ30[61] while 41% showed evidence of low self-esteem on the Hudson Questionnaire. Of the controls, 31% were cases while

34% showed low self-esteem. No significant differences could be demonstrated regarding the absolute scores on the GHQ30 (p=0.07), incidence of caseness on the GHQ30 (p=0.10), absolute scores (p=0.69) or normal/low self-esteem scores on the Hudson Questionnaire (p=0.29).

Discussion

It was felt that the age difference may reflect the fact that excimer laser PRK is an expensive, private procedure available only to more established individuals who are more financially stable. It may, however, be that this older group has a longer history of optical correction with an associated increase in contact lens tolerance problems. The subject group was more myopic but had a superior corrected visual acuity. It was felt that this illustrated that excimer PRK patients needed stronger optical correction (spectacles or contact lenses) which would probably be worn more often, which would again increase the chance of lens intolerance and corneal problems, a possible indication for seeking PRK. However, the results of the GHQ30 and Hudson Self-Esteem Questionnaire suggest that patients presenting for excimer laser PRK are no more likely to have self-esteem problems or to be under abnormal psychological stress than other myopes.

Conclusion

Some form of psychological examination should be a standard part of the preoperative assessment of excimer laser PRK patients. This can easily be achieved in an outpatient setting if short, simple questionnaires are used. The GHQ30 is known to be a good gauge of psychological stress[61] while the Hudson Self-esteem Questionnaire adequately measures low self-esteem.[62] Both instruments can readily be used in an outpatient setting and could constitute an adequate basic battery of tests for this group. Other instruments, assessing such areas as personality, need to be evaluated in the field.

While differences exist between the PRK patients and myopic controls with regard to age, refractive error and best spectacle visual acuity, no significant differences have been demonstrated with regard to the psychological tests used. This implies that, contrary to the concerns of ophthalmologists, patients presenting for excimer laser PRK are no different from other myopic individuals.

PATIENT SATISFACTION WITH EXCIMER LASER PRK

A discussion of patient satisfaction with excimer laser PRK has to be considered in the context of previous work on satisfaction with medical care in general. This section reviews the reasons why patient satisfaction is important, discusses dimensions of satisfaction and describes ways of measuring it, before going on to review previous work in ophthalmology. The final section discusses ways of making use of information gathered by these methods, and of building on this previous research work.

THE IMPORTANCE OF PATIENT SATISFACTION

Patient satisfaction is important for three main reasons:[63]

It is an outcome measure

Satisfaction with treatment has long been regarded as an end in itself[64] and as a measure of the quality of treatment. It also has importance because dissatisfaction with treatment may affect patient compliance.[65,66] Roghmann et al found a relationship between patient satisfaction and service utilization.[67] When they compared different providers, differences in patient satisfaction improved the performance of models designed to predict frequency of clinic attendance, with greater satisfaction being associated with increased attendance. Work in Health Maintenance Organizations in the United States also indicates that dissatisfied patients move to other healthcare providers.[68]

It provides information on communication

Satisfaction with information giving is one of the most commonly examined types of satisfaction.[69] Patients' views can be used to improve the communication processes within a particular healthcare service.

It allows services to choose between different forms of treatment delivery

Where there are alternative ways of delivering a service, with no clear difference in clinical outcomes, patients' satisfaction with the competing strategies can be used to choose between them.[70]

COMPONENTS OF SATISFACTION

Many studies examining consumer satisfaction ask about overall satisfaction . This may be a useful short-hand for a service to use, but there are difficulties associated with its interpretation. Experience indicates that a high proportion of patients always indicate that they are either satisfied or very satisfied with a service, although this effect may be less pronounced in younger people. This is comforting for the provider, but gains them little useful information. How should such results be interpreted, and do they mean that there is little scope for improvement to the service examined?

Although professional healthcare staff often fear that patients' judgments will be arbitrary and influenced more by personal liking for a particular professional than by any real measure of the technical quality of a service,[63] there is evidence that patients may dislike components of a service without allowing it to unduly influence their overall satisfaction. Fitzpatrick and Hopkins found that, while patients attending a neurology clinic formed judgements on doctors' communication and caring abilities, these were of secondary importance compared to their ability to relieve the presenting symptoms.[70] Similarly, Stark found that while women attending for mammography expressed considerable dissatisfaction, both about pain during the procedure and a perceived lack of support from radiographers, they were still satisfied with the treatment overall and intended to re-attend.[71] Questions about overall satisfaction may, therefore, tell services something about patients' views of service outcomes, but if the greatest possible information is to be obtained, it will be necessary to focus on more clearly demarcated aspects of the service.

In 1975, a detailed review of patients attending a Health Maintenance Organization suggested that there were at least four components of satisfaction which could be distinguished using factor analysis:[72] the qualities of the physician (such as humaneness), availability of services (presence of hospitals, specialists etc.), continuity and convenience of care, and access mechanisms (such as cost and payment methods, as well as availability of emergency care). Since then, surveys have reviewed many dimensions of patient satisfaction and Hall and Dornan, after reviewing the literature, listed 12 dimensions which have been used in previous studies (Fig. 10.1).

Dimensions of Patient Satisfaction	
Overall Satisfaction	Access
Cost	Overall Quality
Humaneness	Competence
Information Supplied	Administrative Arrangements
Physical Facilities	Attention to psychosocial problems
Continuity of care	Outcome of care

Figure 10.1 *Dimensions of patient satisfaction.*

Measures of overall quality tended to be less comprehensive than overall satisfaction, and to include measures such as the time spent with the patient. Physical facilities included the appearance of the facility, parking, adequacy of equipment etc. The most surprising measure to professional eyes may be competence. Many healthcare providers believe that patients are not generally capable of forming an opinion on the technical quality of care, and that such a judgement can only be made by professional colleagues. There is, however, some evidence that patients can form reasonable judgements of aspects of technical quality which correlate with professional judgements of technical quality.[73–75] It may prove to be the case that ocular laser surgery is too technical an area to allow patients to make any valid judgement of professional ability, but this will require further exploration before it can be confidently assumed.

MEASURING PATIENT SATISFACTION

Deciding on the components to measure

Hall and Dornan examined the frequency with which the components listed above were measured in published studies of patient satisfaction, and the overall ranking of each aspect across studies.[69] They found that the items given the highest satisfaction ranking by patients were overall quality, humaneness, competence, outcome, and facilities. Those ranked lowest were information giving, cost, administrative arrangements and, ranked lowest of all, attention to psychosocial problems. The most commonly reported measures were humaneness, information giving, overall quality, competence, and overall satisfaction, while the least reported measures were cost, facilities, outcome, continuity and, again lowest of all, attention to psychosocial problems. Interestingly, there was a moderate positive correlation between the two measures, with items with the highest patient satisfaction tending to be asked most often.

This work suggests that, if service providers follow the lead of previous studies, they will be unlikely to ask about the components of satisfaction which have been associated with the highest levels of reported patient dissatisfaction in other areas of medicine. Most services will, nevertheless, want to ask about overall satisfaction, humaneness, and information giving. If they also wish to identify areas likely to cause problems, they should consider extending their information gathering to other, additional areas of patient satisfaction.

Questionnaire development

The structure and content of a questionnaire depends on the method of administration. Fitzpatrick provides a useful summary of the competing advantages on self-administered and interviewer-based questionnaires, and discusses design.[63,76] In general, self-administered questionnaires are cheaper to use and, if anonymous, are less likely to result in patients feeling obliged to praise their treatment than in a face-to-face interview. Their main disadvantages are the problems associated with literacy, language barriers and the loss of qualitative information which could be obtained by an experienced interviewer. Interviewer-based systems lose some of the advantages of self-completion questionnaires, but tend to produce higher response rates.

Satisfaction questionnaires vary in the type of question asked. They are, like any survey, susceptible to biases from question phrasing and choice of sample. Individual questions can be of the yes/no type, but these almost inevitably produce positive responses.[76] As a service will wish to gain as much information as possible, scales with more than two responses are normally used. These can be visual analogue scales—a line of fixed length with a word anchor at each end, e.g. not satisfied at all, extremely satisfied,[77] or scales such as Likert scales, which are similar to visual analogue scales but are on an agree, disagree continuum. A variant of this provides an adjectival scale where the respondent chooses between descriptions, such as disagree

strongly, disagree, neither agree nor disagree etc. Other variations include the use of smiley faces, but the use of such variations seems to be limited by the age and cultural make up of the subject group. The statistical analysis varies according to the type of scale used.

Most patient satisfaction scales are developed by the workers who use them. It is uncommon for the scales themselves to be subjected to analysis of their face and content validity, and even less common for measures of reliability such as test-retest and split half reliability to be undertaken. This necessarily limits the uses to which questionnaires can be applied. The lack of standard measures makes it difficult to draw broad conclusions across studies using different measures, and examining different components, of patient satisfaction.

SATISFACTION WITH EXCIMER LASER PRK

Haverbeke reviewed patient satisfaction following radial keratotomy, and their preference compared to contact lens wearing.[1] The sample included consecutive attenders at the author's office, with some attending 13 years after their surgery. Although not discussed in the paper, this may have had the effect of over-representing those with adverse effects from their surgery. Haverbeke found that, although 50% experienced impaired night vision following the procedure, and other individual adverse effects were experienced by up to 10% of the sample, all patients were at least rather satisfied. Of these individuals, 93% stated that they would undergo the operation again, and only one individual declined a procedure on the second eye because of dissatisfaction with the technique. These results are in keeping with work in other areas suggesting that patients are able to make judgements about overall outcome despite experiencing adverse effects. Although a self-completion questionnaire was used, clinical details were also recorded, so it is possible that patients were not responding anonymously. This may have had the effect of decreasing adverse comment.

Studies of excimer laser treatments that include measures of satisfaction are listed in Figure 10.2. Some authors include measures which would not, in other fields, be regarded as patient satisfaction measures (e.g. halo and glare), as these are adverse effects of PRK which may influence satisfaction but are not, of themselves, satisfaction measures. In the

Study	Subject	Measures of Satisfaction	Findings
Heitzman et al (1991) (Ref 79)	18 patients (23 eyes)	Overall Outcome No specific measure: implied from their continuation of treatment	No patient refused treatment for second eye
Kahle et al (1992) (Ref 80)	26 patients	Change to Quality of Life (3 point scale) Satisfied with results of myopia correction (3 point scale)	Quality of life: 75% improved, 21% no change, 4% worse Satisfaction: 84% satisfied, 4% indifferent, 12% dissatisfied
Gimbel et al (1993) (Ref 78)	52 patients (104 eyes)	Overall rating of vision (good to excellent/fair) Overall rating of refractive results (satisfied to very satisfied/dissatisfied)	Vision: good to excellent 88.1%, fair 11.9% Refractive results: Satisfied to very satisfied 90.5%, dissatisfied 9.5%
Fichte and Bell (1994) (Ref 81)	74 patients (104 eyes)	Overall Satisfaction (5 point scale) Quality of vision (6 choices, not mutually exclusive) Intent to have second eye treated (Yes/No) Benefits in work, home or social life (Yes/No) Recommend to a friend (Yes/No)	Overall Satisfaction: 92% very satisfied, 8% neutral or rather dissatisfied 93% intended to have second eye treated Benefits: 89% yes, 11% no Recommend: 96% yes, 4% no
McGhee et al (1996) (Ref 82)	100 patients	38 item visual analogue scale Quality of life Sight as good as expected Pleased they had surgery Understood operation Operation distressing Post-op pain relief	85.5% improved quality 82% sight as good 95.5% pleased 98.9% understood 23.9% distressed 15.7% insufficient

Figure 10.2 *Studies of patient satisfaction in excimer laser patients.*

area of PRK, no authors have yet reported characteristics of questionnaires, such as reliability and validity, far less undertaken a factor analysis to identify related factors. This may be a reflection of the comparatively small number of patients treated with PRK, which makes such measures difficult to address at present. These questionnaire qualities are likely to be tested as numbers increase.

The findings to date show high overall satisfaction with the procedure in several different sites. Gimbel et al have begun the process of examining influences on satisfaction.[78] Using simple correlations, they demonstrated associations between overall patient satisfaction and night-driving problems: uncorrected visual acuity and residual myopia; having to continue to wear glasses; problems in dim or artificial light; and experiencing adverse effects of the procedure, such as ring and halo effects. This is a valuable first attempt to establish the contribution of different factors to overall satisfaction.

PRACTICAL APPLICATIONS

Researchers have undertaken patient satisfaction research on PRK largely because it is a new technique. As discussed above, there are high overall satisfaction levels across studies, but this is similar to

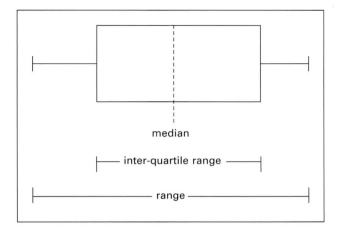

Figure 10.3 *A 'box and whiskers' graph allows median, range and inter-quartile range to be presented in a form which allows comparison through time/among differing services.*

results for most health care procedures. One of the major challenges for ophthalmic surgeons and researchers involved with PRK is to develop more sophisticated measures that are capable of providing information on more subtle details than overall satisfaction. This information can provide physicians with feedback on their own services and so enable them to identify aspects of their service which can be improved, as well as providing them with reassurance about components of their service which are functioning well. Researchers will have an important role in helping to develop questionnaires with carefully reviewed characteristics which can be applied across different services. This will allow all participating laser centers to participate in audit with other providers and to obtain comparative data on their own performance.

For this to become a reality, information will also have to be provided in a user-friendly format that provides helpful information for clinicians. The authors are presently developing a graphic presentation for patient satisfaction results which will allow ready assimilation and easy comparison (Fig. 10.3). The information will be presented in a 'box and whiskers' format, with the box showing the median and interquartiles of responses on a 10-point scale, and the whiskers showing the range. The findings for each item can be scrutinized by the clinical team regularly, allowing them a visual measure of compo-

nents of patient satisfaction. Similar presentations could be made of summed data when reliable subcomponents of satisfaction are developed.

IDENTIFICATION OF THE POTENTIAL PROBLEM PATIENT OR TREATMENT FAILURE

Treatments can fail in terms of objective outcomes (such as failure to attain the expected/desired refractive error or visual acuity postoperatively) or subjective outcomes (such as experience of pain and satisfaction with the procedure and result). Objective outcomes are largely precise measurements made by the physician and are likely to be related to characteristics of the surgical technique (method of epithelial removal used, alignment, etc.), the laser system used, and the degree of residual myopia or associated visual problems (such as induced astigmatism or myopic regression) occurring in any individual case. It may well transpire, however, that softer variables such as psychological state, self-esteem or personality of the patient may impact on these objective measures of success. Research is currently underway to explore this relationship.

Subjective measures have been extensively discussed in the previous section. There is clearly a need to develop an effective and reproducible measure of satisfaction for use with PRK patients. In recent years, PRK has been given considerable positive publicity and has been perceived as a safe and simple alternative to spectacles by the general public.[81] This has been in spite of ophthalmologists' attempts to promote a more cautious approach—at least until the procedure is adequately researched. In 1994–96 however, increasingly negative responses to the procedure surfaced and were widely covered by the UK media, simply fuelling the need for good quality objective evaluation of the treatment and its objective and subjective outcomes.

One important area of development will be the exploration of links between satisfaction and both pre- and postoperative factors including psychological profile, clinical characteristics, expectations and adverse effects. The development of pre-operative predictors of satisfaction may allow surgeons to advise patients on their suitability for surgery for other reasons than the purely clinical, and to minimize the risk of dissatisfied patients.

REFERENCES

1. Haverbeke L, Patient preference – contact lens or Radial Keratotomy? *Refractive and Corneal Surgery* (1992) **8**:315–18.
2. Knoll HA, Eyeglasses and contact lenses: What people think about them. *J Am Optom Assoc* (1978) **49**:861–66
3. Terry RL, Zimmerman DJ, Anxiety induced by contact lenses and framed spectacles. *J Am Optom Assoc* (1970) **41**:257–59.
4. Angi M, Giampietro R, De Bertolini C, Bisantis C, Personality, psychophysical stress and myopia progression. *Graefe's Arch Clin Exp Ophthalmol* (1993) **231**:136–40.
5. Freud S, Psychogenic visual disturbances according to psychoanalytic conceptions, In Freud S., *Collected Papers II*, (Hogarth Press and the Institute of Psychoanalysis: London, 1948).
6. Gawron VJ, Differences among myopes, emmetropes and hyperopes. *Am J Optom Physiol* (1981) **58**:753–60.
7. Lanyon RI, Giddings JW, Psychological approaches to myopia: a review. *Am J Optom Physiol* (1974) **51**:271–81.
8. Giddings JW, Lanyon RI, Modification of refractive error through conditioning: an exploratory study. *Behavioural Therapy* (1971) **2**:538–42.
9. Foster J, Curiosa Ophthalmica. *Transcripts of the Ophthalmological Society of Australia* (1953) **12**:28.
10. Rasmussen OD, Incidence of myopia in China. *Br J Ophthalmol* (1936) **20**:350–60.
11. Baldwin WR, A review of statistical studies of relations between myopia and ethnic, behavioural and physiological characteristics. *Am J Optom Physiol* (1981) **58**:516–27.
12. Jackson E, Norms of refraction. *JAMA* (1932) **98**:132–37.
13. Jones CP, A study of one hundred refraction cases in Indians fresh from the plains. *JAMA* (1908) **51**:308–12.
14. Scott JG, The Eye of the West African Negro. *Br J Ophthalmol* (1945) **291**:12–19.
15. Post RH, Population differences in vision acuity. *Eugenics Quarterly* (1962) **9**:189.
16. Sperduto RD, Seigel D, Roberts J, Rowland M, Prevalence of myopia in United States. *Arch Ophthalmol* (1983) **101**:405–7.
17. Young FA, Singer RM, Foster D, The psychological differentiation of male myopes and non-myopes. *Am J Optom Physiol* (1975) **52**:679–86.
18. Baldwin WR, The relationship between axial length of the eye and certain other anthropomorphic measures of myopes. *Am J Optom and Arch Am Acad Optom* (1964) **41**:513–22.
19. Coleman DJ, Trokel S, Direct-recorded intra-ocular pressure variations in a human subject. *Arch Ophthalmol* (1969) **82**:637–40.
20. Collins CC, Evoked pressure responses in the rabbit. *Science* (1967) **155**:106–8.
21. Bach-Y-Rita P, Collins CC, Tengroth BM, Influence of extra-ocular muscle co-contracture on globe length. *Am J Ophthalmol* (1968) **66**:906–908.
22. Young FA, The etiology of myopia. *Optom Weekly* (1965) **56**:17–24.
23. Rasmussen OD, (1951) *Thesis on the Cause of Myopia* (Tonbridge Free Press: Tonbridge).
24. Gawron VJ, Ocular accommodation, personality and autonomic balance. *Am J Optom Physiol* (1983) **60**:630–39.
25. Bullimore MA, Myopia in optometry students: family history, age of onset and personality. *Ophthalmol Physiol Opt* (1989) **9**:284–88.
26. Sorsby A, Leary GA, Fraser GR, Family studies on ocular refraction and its components. *J Med Genet* (1966) **3**:219–73.
27. Young FA et al, The transmission of refractive errors within Eskimo families. *Am J Optom and Arch Acad Optom* (1969) **46**:676–85.
28. Wiesel TN, Raviola E, Myopia and eye enlargement after neonatal lid fusion in monkeys. *Nature* (1977) **266**:66–68.
29. Troilo D, Wallman J, The regulation of eye growth and refractive state: an experimental study of emmetropization. *Vision Res* (1991) **31**:1237–50.
30. Fulton AB, Hansen RM, Petersen RA, The relation of myopia and astigmatism in developing eyes. *Ophthalmology* (1982) **89**:298–302.
31. Angi MR, Pucci V, Forattini F, Formentin PA, Results of photorefractometric screening for amblyogenic defects in children aged 20 months. *Behav Brain Res* (1992) **49**:91–7.
32. Parssinen O, Hemminki E, Klemetti A, Effect of spectacle use and accommodation on myopic progression: final result of a three year randomised clinical trial among school children. *Br J Ophthalmol* (1989) **73**: 547–51.
33. Birnbaum MH, Undercorrection and myopia development. *Am J Optom Physiol* (1988) **65**:974–5.
34. Thorington RN, *Refraction and How to Refract* 2nd Edition (P. Blakiston & Son, Philadelphia, 1900).
35. Gould GM, Diagnoses, diseases and therapeutics of ametropia. *Br J Ophthalmol* (1918) **2**:305–8.
36. Young FA, Myopia and personality. *Am J Optom and Arch Am Acad Optom* (1967) **44**:192–201.
37. Rice TB, Physical defects in character II Nearsightedness *Hygiea* (1930) **8**:644–6.
38. Mull HK, Myopia and introversion. *Am J Psychol* (1948) **61**:575–6.
39. Van Alphen GWHM, On emmetropia and ametropia. *Ophthalmologica Supplement* (1961) **142**:1–92.
40. Beedle SL, Young FA, Values, personality, physical characteristics and refractive error. *Am J Optom* (1976) **53**:735–9.
41. Schapero M, Hirsch MJ, The relationship of refractive error and Guildford-Martin Temperament Test scores. *Am J Optom and Arch Am Acad Optom* (1952) **29**:32–5.
42. Brown B, Stewart J, Moo G, LaRocca R, Are myopic children more anxious than their non-myopic peers? *Clin Exp Optom* (1987) **70**:46–52.
43. Young FA, Reading, measures of intelligence and refractive errors. *Am J Optom and Arch Am Acad Optom* (1963) **40**:257–64.
44. Tay MT, Au Eong KG, Ng CY, Lim MK, Myopia and educational attainment in 421,116 young Singaporean males. *Annals of the Academy of Medicine, Singapore* **21**:785–91.
45. Young FA, Myopes versus non-myopes – a comparison. *Am J Optom and Arch Am Acad Optom* (1955) **32**:180–91.
46. Nadell MC, Socio-cultural factors related to the incidence of refractive errors. *Am J Optom and Arch Am Acad Optom* (1987) 34:523–36.
47. Hirsch MJ, The relationship between refractive state of the eye and intelligence test scores. *Am J Optom and Arch Am Acad Optom* (1959) **36**:12–21.

48. Parssinen O, Era P, Leskinen AL, Some physiological and psychological characteristics of myopic and non-myopic young men. *Acta Ophthalmol* (1985) **63 Suppl. 173**:85–7.

49. Grosvenor T, Refractive state, intelligence test scores and academic ability. *Am J Optom and Arch Am Acad Optom* (1970) **47**:355–61.

50. Bates WH, The cause of myopia. *N Y Med J* (1912) **95**:529–32.

51. Bell GK, Conditioning visual acuity: increased perceptual responses as a function of myopia and manifest anxiety. Doctoral dissertation, University of Tennessee, 1956.

52. Berens C, Girard LJ, Fonda G, Sells SB, Effects of tachistoscopic training on visual functions in myopic patients. *Am J Ophthalmol* (1957) **44**:25–48.

53. Sells SB, Fixott RS, Evaluation of research on effects of visual training on visual functions. *Am J Ophthalmol* (1957) **44**:230–6.

54. Kelley CR, Psychological factors in myopia. Doctoral dissertation, New School for Social Research, New York, 1958.

55. Kelley CR, Psychological factors in myopia. *J Am Optom Assoc* (1962) **33**:833–7.

56. Miller EM, On the correlation of myopia and intelligence. *Genet Soc Gen Psychol Monogr* (1992) **118**:361–83.

57. Wenger MA, Preliminary study of the significance of measures of autonomic balance. *Psychosom Med* (1947) **9**:301–9.

58. Eppinger H, Hess L, Vagotonia: A clinical study in vegetative neurology. In Porges SW, Coles MGH, eds. *Psychophysiology* (Dowden Hutchinson & Ross, Stroudsburg, 1976).

59. Hurwitz BS, Davidowitz J, Chin NB, Breinin GM, The effects of the sympathetic nervous system on accommodation. 1. Beta sympathetic nervous system. *Arch Ophthalmol* (1979) 87:668–74.

60. Kidd B, Stark C, McGhee CNJ, Anxiety and self-esteem in patients presenting for excimer laser surgery for myopia. *J Refract Surg* (1997) **13**:40–44.

61. Goldberg D, Williams P, *A User's Guide to The General Health Questionnaire* (NFER Nelson, Basingstoke, 1988).

62. Hudson WW, *The clinical measurement package: A field manual* (Dorsey Press, Chicago, 1982).

63. Fitzpatrick R, Surveys of patient satisfaction: I – Important general considerations. *Br Med J* (1991) **302**:887–9.

64. Koos EL, *The Health of Regionville* (Hafner, New York, 1954).

65. Kirscht JP, Becker MH, Eveland JP, Psychological and social factors as predictors of medical behaviour. *Med Care* (1976) **14(5)**:422–31 .

66. Kincey J, Bradshaw P, Ley P, Patients' satisfaction and reported acceptance of advice in general practice. *J R Coll Gen Pract* (1975) **25**:558–76.

67. Roghmann KJ, Hengst A, Zastowny TR, Satisfaction with medical care: its measurement and relation to utilization. *Med Care* (1979) **17**:461–77.

68. Weiss B, Senf J, Patient satisfaction survey instrument for use in Health Maintenance Organisations. *Med Care* (1990) **28**:434–45.

69. Hall JA, Dornan MC, What patients like about their medical care and how often they are asked: a meta-analysis of the satisfaction literature. *Soc Sci Med* (1988) **27**:935–9.

70. Fitzpatrick R, Hopkins J, Problems in the conceptual framework of patient satisfaction research: an empirical exploration. *Sociology of Health and Illness* (1983) **5**:297–311.

71. Stark C, Factors affecting attendance and consumer satisfaction with breast screening. MPH Thesis. University of Glasgow, 1992.

72. Ware JE, Snyder MK, Dimensions of patient attitude regarding doctors and medical care services. *Med Care* (1975) **13**:669–82.

73. Linn BS, Burn patients' evaluation of emergency department care. *Ann Emerg Med* (1982) **11**:255–9.

74. Wilson P, McNamara JR, How perceptions of a simulated physician-patient interaction influence intended satisfaction and compliance. *Soc Sci Med* (1982) **16**:1699–1705.

75. Roter D, Hall JA, Katz NR, Relations of physicians' behaviour to analogue patients' satisfaction, recall and impressions. *Med Care* (1987) **25**:437–51.

76. Fitzpatrick R, Surveys of patient satisfaction: II – Designing a questionnaire and conducting a survey. *Br Med J* (1991) **302**:1129–32.

77. Streiner DL, Norman GR, *Health measurement scales: a practical guide to their development and use.* (Oxford Medical Publications. London, 1989).

78. Gimbel HV, Van Westenbrugge JA, Johnson WH, Willerscheidt AB, Sun R, Ferensowicz M, Visual, refractive, and patient satisfaction results following bilateral photorefractive keratectomy for myopia. *Refractive and Corneal Surgery* (Supplement) **(1993)** 9:S5–S11.

79. Heitzmann J, Binder PS, Kassar BS, Nordan LT, The correction of high myopia using the excimer laser. *Arch Ophthalmol* (1991) **3**:1627–33.

80. Kahle G, Seiler T, Wollensak J, Report on psychosocial findings and satisfaction among patients 1 year after excimer laser photprefractive keratectomy. *Refractive and Corneal Surgery* (1992) **8**:286–9.

81. Fichte CM, Bell AM, Ongoing results of excimer laser photorefractive keratectomy for myopia: subjective patient impressions. *J Cataract Refract Surg* (1994) **20** (Supplement):268–70.

82. Orr D., McGhee CNJ, Bryce IG, Stark C., Kidd BA, Patient satisfaction following excimer laser treatment for myopia and astigmatism. *Br J Ophthalmol* (1996) **80**:874–79.

Chapter 11 USA: Summit and Visx FDA studies

Marguerite B McDonald and Deepak Chitkara

INTRODUCTION

Excimer laser was first used to ablate corneal tissue by Stephen Trokel and co-workers and reported in their landmark paper published in 1983.[1] In this paper they reported that the excimer laser photoablative technique could be used for corneal surgery and for correction of refractive errors in particular. Subsequently, many studies attempted to use the excimer laser to perform radial keratotomy.[2–5] This effort failed to consistently improve the predictability of the refractive outcome compared to conventional incisional surgery. Wide area superficial ablation was therefore developed to correct refractive error, thereafter known as photorefractive keratectomy (PRK).

In 1988, Munnerlyn, Koons and Marshall published a computer-generated algorithm relating diameter and depth of the ablation to the required dioptric change.[6] Using these calculations, non-human primate studies confirmed the effectiveness of the excimer laser in inducing predictable refractive change in the eye. These wide area superficial lamellar keratectomies in primates subsequently provided corneal tissue samples for light and electron microscopy. Histopathological examination of recently operated eyes showed that the epithelium was slightly hyperplastic but surprisingly there was no evidence of inflammation or abnormal keratocyte activity.[7] Following these early experiments, the Food and Drug Administration (FDA) issued stringent guidelines for the clinical evaluation of this new technique in the United States. After completion of a large series of primate eyes, Taunton Technologies was issued the first investigational device exemption (IDE) from the FDA. This allowed the establishment of clinical trials in the Phase I (blind eyes) PRK study.

INITIAL HUMAN STUDIES

In February 1987, the first human eyes to have superficial keratectomies were three blind eyes, or eyes destined for enucleation, in a series of 11 patients. The surgeries were performed by L'Esperance and colleagues at Columbia University.[8] The first excimer PRK for myopia on a 'normally sighted' human eye was performed by McDonald and colleagues later that same year in July 1987 at the Louisiana State University (LSU) Eye Center. In the Visx FDA phase I study, nine legally blind eyes underwent PRK for myopia. Favourable results in this blind eye study encouraged the FDA to allow 10 partially sighted (20/50 or worse best corrected) to have excimer PRK, still under the phase I protocol at the LSU Eye Center.

PHASE II FDA STUDIES

Further favorable results were followed by phase IIA and IIB of the PRK study. In phase IIA beginning June 1989, 40 patients who were considered 'normally sighted', i.e. correctable to 20/50 or better, were treated at two sites, LSU Eye Center and University of Missouri at Kansas City. Phase IIB followed, in which 80 fully sighted patients were treated. Both phase II studies showed excellent visual results with no sight-threatening complications. Concurrent with these PRK studies, several other studies on the use of excimer laser for removal of superficial corneal scars and irregularities were also being investigated in the phototherapeutic (or PTK) protocols.

PHASE III FDA STUDIES: SUMMIT AND VISX LASERS

In Spring 1991, the final component of FDA refractive studies for mild to moderate myopia, PRK III, were commenced. Two laser manufacturers, Summit Technology of Waltham, Massachusetts and Visx (by now merged with Taunton Technology) of Santa Clara, California were allowed to begin these studies. Seven hundred patients at a maximum of 10 laser sites were enrolled throughout the country for each of these two laser companies. Both study protocols were authorized by the FDA under protocol requirements for evaluating the laser treatment, which were both extremely rigorous and laid down in great detail. The progress of the trials were closely monitored, and the Summit and Visx results from all the sites were collated and presented to the FDA with full approval for 6 mm zone PRK treatment for up to −7.00 D of myopia being granted to Summit in December 1995, at which time conditional approval was also recommended for treatment using the Visx laser, with full FDA approval in March 1996.

A minimum of 2 years follow-up was required for the patients enrolled in these Phase III studies and this chapter examines the results of the patients treated with the Visx and Summit lasers as presented to the FDA.

MYOPIC PRK WITH THE VISX EXCIMER LASER

The Visx PRK III study started in the Spring of 1991, with a protocol that required 500 or more cases to be followed for 2 years. The primary aim of the FDA Phase III study was to document the clinical safety and effectiveness of the excimer laser device. The effectiveness can be expressed in terms of the efficacy, predictability, and stability of the planned treatment. The safety assessments are considered in terms of the rate of adverse reactions, loss of vision or visual potential, retreatments, and the rates of less severe non-vision-threatening complications.

PATIENT SELECTION: FDA PHASE III TRIALS

Patient selection was critical because the excimer laser is considered an investigational device. The inclusion criteria for this study were that patients must be at least 18 years old, with −1.00 D to −6.00 D spherical equivalent at the corneal plane. All patients required best corrected visual acuity (BCVA) of 20/40 or better in both eyes. In addition the astigmatic component of the manifest refraction was limited to <1.00 D. Contact lens wearers removed their contact lenses at least 2 weeks prior to baseline measurements. Patients were advised that any retreatments, if required, could only be performed more than 6 months after the initial treatment.

PREOPERATIVE EXAMINATIONS

Preoperative examinations were performed within 45 days of the scheduled surgery and the preoperative examination included a complete ophthalmic examination of both eyes. Uncorrected visual acuity (VA) measurements were taken along with both manifest and cycloplegic refractions. The PRK III study also required other measurements including: computerized videokeratography (CVK), pachymetry, glare testing, evaluation of visual fields, contrast sensitivity measurement (performed using the Vector Vision CSV 1000, studying four spatial frequencies). Glare testing was performed with the Brightness Acuity Test (BAT) and CSV contrast sensitivity devices.

SURGICAL TECHNIQUE

The surgical technique included the use of topical anesthesia, manual removal of a 7 mm diameter disc of epithelium, and patient self-fixation. The early Visx cases utilized a fixation hand piece with nitrogen gas blown across the corneal surface in addition to aspiration of the debris. Other studies by non-US surgeons indicated that this technique resulted in excessive drying of the cornea, with increased corneal haze (see Chapter 23). This technique was therefore replaced with self-fixation on the part of the patient, with aspiration of the debris only (no-gas blowing). At the completion of the procedure, topical antibiotics[5] and a topical non-steroidal anti-inflammatory drug (NSAID) were applied, and a pressure patch or a bandage contact lens was applied to the eye. A tapered steroid regimen was used for the first 4 months post-operatively. The patients were examined daily until the cornea was fully epithelialized. Subsequent follow-up examinations were carried out at 1, 3, 6, 12, 18, and 24 months. Subepithelial haze was graded clinically on a scale of

Figure 11.1(a) *Clinical investigators enrolled for Visx Phase III FDA protocol*

Investigators	Location	No. of eyes
1. Tennant	Dallas Eye Institute, Dallas	142
2. Dello Russo	New Jersey Eye Center, Berengfield	128
3. Salz	Cedars-Sinai Medical Center, Los Angeles	105
4. Peibenga	Eye Foundation of Kansas City, Kansas City	87
5. McDonald	Louisiana State University, New Orleans	59
6. Haight	Manhattan EET Hospital, New York	41
7. Kasear	Mericos Eye Center, San Diego	40
8. Kraff	Kraff Eye Institute, Chicago	32
9. O'Donnell	O'Donnell Eye Foundation, St. Louis	32
10. Aquavella	Rochester Eye Foundation, Rochester	25

Figure 11.1(b) *Clinical investigators enrolled for Summit Phase III FDA protocol*

Investigators	Location	No. of eyes
1. Brint	New Orleans	104
2. Durrie, Hunkeler, Cavanaugh	Kansas City	136
3. Galusha	Tulsa	54
4. Repose	St. Louis	36
5. Gold, Milstein	Galveston	68
6. Gordon	San Diego	89
7. Michelson, Owen	Birmingham	58
8. Steinert, Puliafito	Boston	39
9. Wright	Colorado Springs	67
10. Waring, Stulting, Thompson	Atlanta	50

Figure 11.1 *Investigators and sites for (a) Visx and (b) Summit FDA studies.*

clear, trace, mild, moderate, or marked, as described elsewhere.[9–11]

ONE YEAR RESULTS WITH VISX LASER

At the time of the most recent FDA presentation, 521 Visx cases from a study population of 691 had completed the 1 year visit.[12] Data was collected from 10 sites as shown in Figure 11.1a. The study population consisted of 60% males and 40% females, with an average age of 38 years. The mean preoperative spherical equivalent was –3.8 D.

At 1 year, 48% of the PRK patients were ±0.5 D, 78% were ±1 D and 95% were ±2 D of the intended refraction. Fifty per cent of the patients had 20/20 or better uncorrected visual acuity and 88% were 20/40 or better at 1 year. Only 1.5% of patients suffered a loss of 1.6 lines or greater BCVA and 3.5% gained greater than or equal to 1.6 lines of acuity. This loss of BCVA was not as dramatic as it first appears: two patients fell from 20/12.5 to 20/20, three regained the loss by 18 months, two lost eight letters of vision and one lost nine letters of vision. All these patients who lost some degree of corrected acuity had undergone ablation with the nitrogen blow technique. The surgical technique was changed midway through the study and, using the revised no-blow technique, no further cases lost best corrected acuity.

Of the 691 patients in the study, 72 (10.4%) required retreatment with PRK for undercorrection, and two for corneal haze associated with undercorrection. One case was retreated twice, with a final outcome of 20/20 uncorrected visual acuity.

At 1 year, 2% of the eyes were assigned a haze score greater than 1 and none of the eyes scored higher than 2 (Fig. 11.7). The postoperative change in keratometric cylinder at 12 months was within 1 D of preoperative cylinder in 91.5% of patients (Fig. 11.8). Corneal endothelial cell loss was of the order of 4.5% at 1 year; this level of loss is within measurement

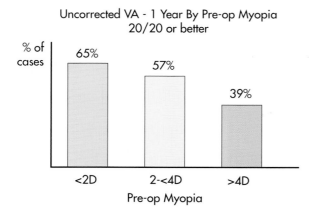

Figure 11.2 *Visx: Uncorrected visual acuity of 20/20 or better at 1 year post-PRK classified by preoperative myopia.*

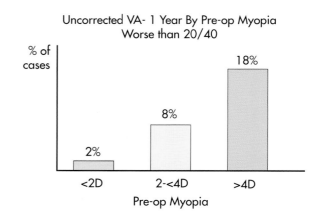

Figure 11.3 *Visx: Uncorrected visual acuity worse than 20/40 at 1 year post-PRK classified by preoperative myopia.*

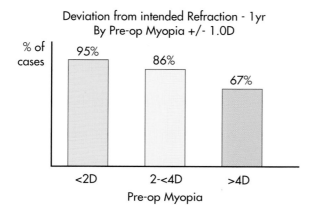

Figure 11.4 *Visx: Deviation from intended refraction at 1 year classified by preoperative myopia.*

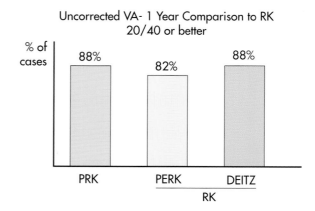

Figure 11.5 *Visx: Uncorrected visual acuity of 20/40 or better at 1 year compared to the PERK and Deitz radial keratotomy studies.*

error for this technique and probably is not clinically significant.

Contrast sensitivity was performed on 100 cases preoperatively and at 12 months postoperatively. There was a 0.1 log unit decrease in postoperative values at 12 and 18 cycles per degree but the values were still within the normal range. This change is not thought to be clinically significant. Similarly, glare testing was abnormal in only 1% of patients at 12 months. Corneal topography on 100 cases showed central islands in 13% of cases at 1 month. This resolved in all but one case by the 12-month period.

MODERATE MYOPIA STUDY

In the Moderate Myopia Study, 89 eyes of 80 patients with moderate myopia (between 6 D and 8 D, with a

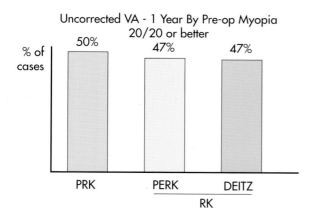

Figure 11.6 *Visx: Uncorrected visual acuity of 20/20 or better at 1 year compared to the PERK and Deitz radial keratotomy studies.*

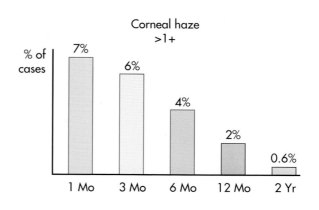

Figure 11.7 *Visx: Prevalence of corneal haze greater than 1+ over a 24 month follow-up period demonstrating a maximum involvement of 7% of eyes at 1 month and 0.6% of eyes at 2 years.*

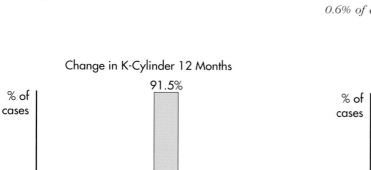

Figure 11.8 *Visx: Change in keratometric cylinder at 12 months post-PRK.*

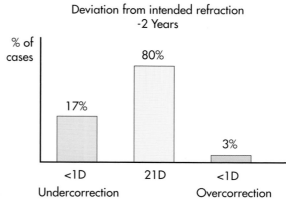

Figure 11.9 *Visx: Deviation from intended refraction 2 years post-PRK.*

mean preoperative spherical equivalent of −6.98 ±0.90 D) underwent PRK at nine investigational sites. Sixty eyes received single-zone 6.0 mm ablations and 29 eyes received two-zone ablations; all patients were treated with the Visx laser using standard settings.

At 1 year, 71% were ±1 D of intended correction for the single-zone technique and 50% for two-zone technique. With the two-zone technique, 29% and 21% were undercorrected by 1–2 D and >2 D, respec-

tively. However, corneal haze was greater in the single-zone as compared to two-zone technique at 1 year; 14% in the single-zone and 4% in the two-zone had greater than grade 1 haze at 12 months.

TWO-YEAR FOLLOW-UP DATA

Two-year data supports the safety and predictability of this procedure, with 80% of eyes being within

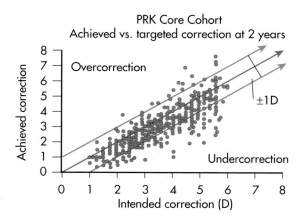

Figure 11.10 *Visx: Scattergram of PRK core cohort achieved versus targeted refractive correction at 2 years.*

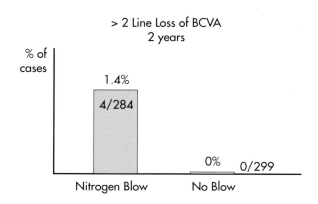

Figure 11.11 *Visx: Eyes losing two lines or more of best corrected visual acuity at 2 years post-PRK.*

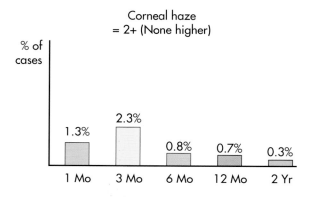

Figure 11.12 *Visx: Prevalence of moderate corneal haze (grade 2+) at intervals during a 24 month follow-up period.*

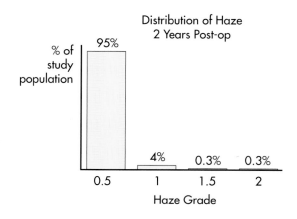

Figure 11.13 *Visx: Distribution of corneal haze 2 years postoperatively.*

±1.00 D of intended refraction (Figs 11.9 and 11.10) and only four eyes (0.7%) from 583 cases losing two or more lines of visual acuity (Fig. 11.11). Grade 2 corneal haze peaked at 3 months, affecting 2.3% of eyes, and progressively resolved thereafter, and although significant corneal haze was more evident in the nitrogen blow group, no eyes developed greater than grade 2 haze (Fig. 11.12). At 2 years only 0.6% of eyes demonstrated greater than grade 1 haze

(Fig. 11.13). The overall retreatment rate was 14% following PRK (Fig. 11.14).

These results suggest that Visx laser for treatment of low myopia appears to be a safe and effective procedure. Early results from further protocols such as the Visx Moderate Myopia Study Group are also encouraging. PRK for moderate myopia is safe and reproducible with large diameter ablation zones.

Phase III- Post second eye treatment

- n=289 at 1 year
- 88.6% 20/20 or better in at least one eye
- 83.4% 20/20 or better and within 0.5 diopters

Figure 11.14 *Summit: Unaided visual acuity and refractive results at 1 year in 289 eyes. FDA Phase III post second eye treatment.*

Phase III- First eyes
Patient survey
Reliance on corrective wear

Use of corrective eye wear for near or distance vision dramatically reduced

% of patients wearing corrective eyewear 1 year after PRK on both eyes

Preop prior to first eye treatment (n=701 89.8%)

1 year after fellow eye treatment (n=310 10.1%)

Figure 11.15 *Summit: Phase III—first eyes. Patient survey; reliance on corrective eyewear.*

MYOPIC PRK WITH THE SUMMIT EXCIMER LASER

The FDA issued stringent guidelines for the clinical evaluation of PRK with the Summit Excimed UV200 LA excimer laser in the same way as the Visx laser system. The phase III study protocol for this laser was approved in June 1991. Patient enrolment has been completed and both 1 year and 2 year follow-up results are now available.[13]

Seven-hundred-and-one treated eyes of 701 patients were entered into the study at the sites shown in Fig. 11.1b. The attempted corrections ranged from –1.5 D to –6.0 D spherical equivalent myopia with a mean of –4.07 D.

SURGICAL TECHNIQUE

A standard surgical procedure was used throughout. All surgeries were done under local anesthetic using 1% proparacaine or tetracaine. Patient fixation was demonstrated by delivering several laser pulses on the cornea protected by 1% methylcellulose. This was later removed with a sponge. The epithelium was debrided manually and 1% methylcellulose was again applied to the cornea. The laser energy at the corneal surface was 180 mJ/cm^2, with a repetition rate of 10 Hz. In the early phase III, all patients received 4.5 mm optical zone treatment. This later expanded to 5.0 mm and 58% of patients received a 5.00 mm ablation zone treatment.

Postoperatively dexamethasone–tobramycin ointment and an eye patch were used overnight with oral analgesics as required. Dexamethasone–tobramycin ointment and optional patching were continued until the corneal epithelium healed. Patients were then placed on fluoromethalone alcohol 2.5% drops five times daily for 1 month, fluorometholone 1% four times daily for the second month, three times daily for the third, and then tapered at the surgeon's discretion.

ONE YEAR RESULTS WITH THE SUMMIT LASER

In October 1993, the 1 year data on 585 eyes were submitted to the FDA (Figs 11.14 and 11.15). Corneal re-epithelialization of the ablated area was complete in all eyes at 1 week and within 72 hours in 91% of eyes. The uncorrected VA at 1 year was 20/40 or better in 90.7% of patients and 20/20 or better in 66.4% of patients. The refractive predictability at 1 year to within 1.00 D was obtained in 77.7% of patients and within 0.5 D in 58.0% of patients.

Eighteen eyes (3%) lost ≥ two lines of BCVA at 1 year. Most of these patients had preoperative VA better than 20/20 and postoperative VA 20/30 or 20/25. One patient with 20/80 postoperative VA had received an eccentric ablation. Retreatment in this patient improved VA to 20/25. Mild haze was present in 12.2% of patients and moderate haze in 2.6% of patients.

COMPARISON OF VISX AND SUMMIT ONE YEAR RESULTS

It is of interest to compare the two largest series, the USA, i.e. Visx and Summit, to presently submit data to the FDA. As noted earlier, both series had follow-up of more than 500 cases each (Visx = 555 and Summit = 585) with between 1 and 6 D of preoperative myopia. Both groups averaged approximately −4.00 D of myopia preoperatively. At 1 month postoperatively, the mean refraction was in the hyperopic range for both groups, both regressed with time and their regression curves look remarkably similar. However, at 1 year the Summit group final refraction averaged a small hyperopic correction, whereas Visx cases demonstrated a mean refractive error of −0.25 D myopia.

Presumably this difference in mean refractive error between the two groups of data means that a greater proportion of Summit cases were slightly overcorrected (hyperopic) and (taking into consideration the age of the patient groups) this could account for a greater proportion of Summit cases (50%) obtaining 20/20 uncorrected vision compared to the Visx group (16%). The proportion seeing 20/40 or better was similar, at about 90%. Fifty-eight percent of Summit cases were within ±0.5 D of intended correction, whereas only 48% of Visx cases were in this group. Accuracy to within ±1 D was similar, being approximately 77% and 78% respectively.

The major difference between the two series was in the reported incidence of corneal haze. Mild haze was reported in 0.7% (Visx) and 12.2.% (Summit). Visx only reported a 0.4% incidence of moderate haze while Summit reported 2.6% incidence. Loss of BCVA of two lines was also greater for Summit as compared to Visx (3.1% compared with 0.7%, respectively). This difference is even more marked when comparing Summit results with the present Visx technique of nitrogen no-blow. In this latter series there were no reported cases of moderate haze in the Visx group, compared to a 2.6% incidence in the Summit group. The difference in loss of BCVA of more than two lines in the two groups demonstrated a similar pattern, with 0% in the Visx series compared to 3.1% in the Summit series.

Although Visx and Summit have similar chronological refractive curves, the Summit cases demonstrate more hyperopia early on and final mean refractive error closer to emmetropia. Correspondingly, the incidence of uncorrected VA of 20/20 or better is also higher in the Summit study and results were also slightly better with regard to predictability in the ±0.5 D range. In contrast, the incidence of haze and, possibly related to this phenomenon, the loss of BCVA is much lower in the Visx study group.

SUMMIT—2 YEAR RESULTS

In June 1994, the 2 year data on Summit treated patients were submitted to the FDA and in October 1994 the data was discussed by the FDA panel meeting. The pertinent results presented at this review are summarized below. The compliance rate for follow-up was 82% at 2 years and 'the lost to follow-up' occurred primarily in young male subjects due to relocation. The mean age of the chart populations was 37 years and the preoperative mean myopia was −4.2 D.

At 2 years, 77.8% of patients were within 1.00 D of attempted correction, 12.2% were overcorrected, and 10.0% were undercorrected (Fig. 11.16). If success is defined as ±0.5 D of intended correction, only 59% were successful, 17.9% were hyperopic 'failures', and 21.6% were myopic 'failures'. However, 92% of patients obtained an uncorrected VA of 20/40 or better. If the criteria of success is defined as 20/20 in one eye uncorrected and within ±0.50 D of intended correction, only 52.1% were successful. Nonetheless, this may be an underestimation since only one eye was involved in the above equation of success; indeed, for bilateral PRK, if both eyes are considered, then using the above definition of success, 77% of cases would be considered successful (Fig. 11.17).

The BCVA of two lines or more was assessed at two separate pupil sizes: 2–4 mm and 6–8 mm. For the 2–4 mm pupil diameter the loss of BCVA of more than two lines was 6.9% at 24 months, whereas for the 6–8 mm diameter, pupil loss was 9.3% (Figs 11.18 and 11.19).

Phase III-First eye Two year predictability	
• ± 0.5 D336 eyes	54.9%
• ± 1.0 D 476 eyes	77.8%
• ± 2.0 D 579 eyes	94.6%

Figure 11.16 *Summit: Phase III—first eyes. Two year postoperative refractive predictability.*

Phase III-First eyes Uncorrected visual acuity			
	Preop	1yr	2yr
• 20/20 or better	0.0%	66.7%	66.4%
• 20/40 or better	0.01%	91.0%	92.1%
• 20/200 or worse	81.0%	1.0%	1.6%

Figure 11.17 *Summit: Phase III—first eyes. Uncorrected visual acuity at years 1 and 2.*

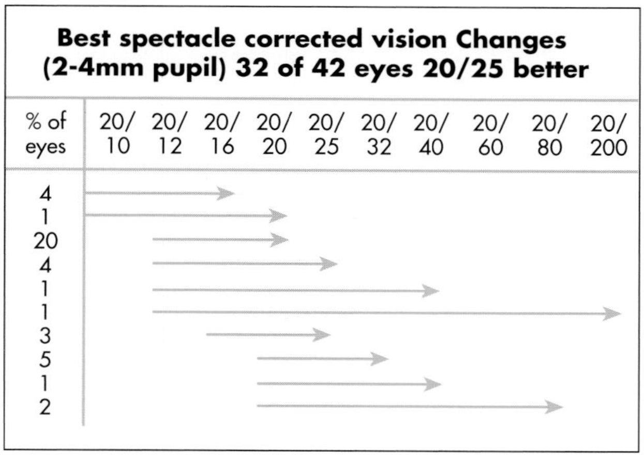

% of eyes	20/ 10	20/ 12	20/ 16	20/ 20	20/ 25	20/ 32	20/ 40	20/ 60	20/ 80	20/ 200
4										
1										
20										
4										
1										
1										
3										
5										
1										
2										

Best spectacle corrected vision Changes (2-4mm pupil) 32 of 42 eyes 20/25 better

Figure 11.18 *Summit: Best spectacle corrected vision changes with a 2–4 mm pupil (32 of 42 eyes 20/25 or better).*

Phase III- First eye Change in BSCVA (2-4mm pupil)@ 2 years (n=611)		
	% of eyes	%
Decrease of 12 lines	1	0.2%
Decrease of 6 lines	2	0.3%
Decrease of 5 lines	1	0.2%
Decrease of 4 lines	0	0.0%
Decrease of 3 lines	6	1.0%
Decrease of 2 lines	32	5.2%
No change	455	74.4%
Increase of 2 lines	77	12.6%
Increase of 3 lines	86	5.9%
Increase of 4 lines	0	0.0%
Increase of 5 lines	1	0.2%

Figure 11.19 *Summit: Phase III—first eyes. Changes in BSCVA (2–4 mm pupil) at 2 years post-PRK (n=611).*

Failure can be defined as: spectacle dependence, two lines of BCVA loss, or >1 D of overcorrection. Based on these criteria, the subjects have a 47.9% chance of reading glasses after the procedure, 12.2% chance of having significant hyperopia, and 7.9% chance of losing more than two lines of BCVA. There was no significant difference in incidence of BCVA loss at 2–4 mm and 6–8 mm pupil diameter (Fig. 11.20).

The loss of BCVA is the key safety issue. However, it must be remembered that in the ETDRS chart there are four lines better than 20/20. Therefore a two line loss could be from 20/10 to 20/16 and not readily noticeable by the patient. Of the 42 patients who lost more than two lines of BCVA, 32 had a final VA of 20/25 or a better BCVA. It was also noted that patient dissatisfaction was highly correlated with loss of more than four lines of BCVA. Between 12 and 24 months, 89% of refractions were stable as defined by ±1.0 D. The mean change in uncorrected VA between 12 and 24 months was a loss of 0.6 D or one-tenth of a line.

Phase III- First eyes
Best spectacle corrected vision changes

At two years postop, there were a total of 6 eyes with a loss of 4 or more lines of best corrected vision with a 6.8mm pupil. These patients were as follows:

Patient	Preop BCVA	2 yr BCVA	Comment
C.I.	20/16	20/200	Cornea abraded with applanation toxometer during 1 month follow-up exam (L.O. 20/32)
C.W.	20/16	20/80	Bilateral macular cyst
J.B.	20/20	20/80	Moderate haze/irreg astigmatism(L.O.20/20)
S.B.	20/12	20/40	Regression w/PRK retreatment
C.C.	20/20	20/50	Irregular astigmatism (L.O.20/32)
V.E.	20/16	20/40	Mild epithelialdefect and resolved keratitisdue to soft contact lens UCVA 20/32

Figure 11.20 *Summit: Phase III—first eyes. Best spectacle corrected vision changes.*

Endothelial cell loss was correlated with higher degrees of correction. There was no significant cell loss in the low myopes, whereas in the 5–6 D range, the eyes had 4.8% cell loss at 24 months.

The largest loss of contrast sensitivity was seen in the population that had the 4.5 mm ablation zone, with undilated pupils, i.e. 28% loss at 24 months. In the 5 mm ablation group, the loss was 19% at 24 months.

The rates of other adverse reactions were minimal: rate of cataract formation was 0.3% at 12 months, the incidence of corneal scarring was 0.2% at 24 months, and the incidence of ulceration was 0.2% at 12 months.

FDA APPROVAL FOR SUMMIT

Based on these presentations, the FDA panel agreed to grant 'conditional approval' status to the Summit laser. The FDA required the Summit laser company to meet over a dozen stringent conditions for approval, many of which required Summit to bring back many patients for additional examinations.

The most important of these approval conditions were:

- reliability and quality issues to be fully addressed
- reporting of adverse reactions in more detail
- repeat corneal endothelial cell evaluation exams on at least 150 patients
- BCVA to be repeated on 500 patients with a requirement that no more than 5% lose two or more lines of BCVA
- presentation of detailed data on patients' VA and refraction based on an end point of 20/20 or better and ±0.5 D of intended refraction
- baseline deviations in halo, glare, and VA to be presented
- postoperative surveillance required annually on 500 eyes for an additional 2 years
- in eyes that were 20/20 BCVA preoperatively, 75% must achieve 20/25 uncorrected VA, and cycloplegic refraction between −1.00 and +0.50 D
- approval would then be restricted to treatment of myopia between 1.5–6.0 D and for patients with cylinder less than 1.5 D
- treatment must also be limited to a 5.00 mm optical zone as the data presented for larger zone ablation at that time was considered 'inadequate'.

Although FDA phase II trials had commenced upon sighted eyes in 1989, the earliest possible timescale for this final FDA approval was mid-1995. The FDA granted final approval to Summit Technology in December 1995.

APPROVAL FOR VISX AND EXPANSION OF EXCIMER LASER PROVISION

Rapidly following Summit approval by the FDA, Visx received approval for treatment of myopia in March 1996. However, the expected rapid expansion of excimer laser provision, and public demand for PRK within the USA, has been much slower than anticipated and RK retains a substantial proportion of the refractive market. Whilst a large number of ophthalmologists have added PRK to their repertoire, estimates vary wildly in respect to the total number of operational excimer lasers installed by December 1996, but it is probably in the region of 250–300 lasers.

PHOTOTHERAPEUTIC KERATECTOMY—VISX EXPERIENCE

Phototherapeutic keratectomy (PTK), like PRK, has undergone FDA-sponsored multicenter trials to assess its safety and therapeutic effectiveness in humans. All patients entering the FDA-sponsored PTK trials had significant functional impairment and are candidates for conventional invasive surgery. In accordance with FDA regulations, these patients met the appropriate eligibility criteria as defined by the Visx protocol.

The primary aim of the study was to significantly improve best corrected acuity and decrease corneal opacity. The reduction of patient comfort and ocular symptoms from the corneal surface disorders was a secondary aim. For the study it was assumed that these aims could be adequately tested by 3 months post-treatment, although patients were followed up for 2 years. Two-hundred-and-sixty-nine patients were enrolled in the study from 17 different US centers. Of these, 77% have been examined at 1 year or more postoperatively. Patient selection and exclusion criteria are described in detail in Chapter 22.

The average improvement in BCVA was 1.8 lines. Eight per cent of patients lost two or more lines of BCVA, while 53% gained two or more lines at 1 year. Six percent of patients lost three or more lines, while 41% gained three or more lines at 1 year. The decrease in BCVA was due to corneal surface irregularity induced by PTK.

The patients were divided into quartiles based on the date of treatment. The first quarter had an average 5.5 D of hyperopic effect and the last had less than 2.0 D of hyperopia. This demonstrates that marked hyperopic shifts are becoming a much less significant problem. At 1 year, 83% of patients had an improvement in the density of epithelial opacity and 17% remained the same. For anterior stromal opacities, 65% of cases showed an improvement. All cases reported a reduction in ocular discomfort or pain, 94% showed an improvement in tear film, 82% reported less photophobia and all cases had an improvement in the foreign body sensation. One of the objectives of PTK is to delay or postpone penetrating kerato-plasty in patients with severe, chronic, debilitating corneal diseases that are often associated with systemic diseases. The penetrating keratoplasty rate at 1 year in this study population was 4.8%.

The success rate in treating recurrent granular or lattice dystrophy in a graft appears to be very high and is similar to that for primary Reis–Buckler's dystrophy in which the deposits are limited to Bowman's layer.[14] There is evidence of minimal corneal haze following PTK, but the principal undesired effect is the central flattening of the cornea. In the Visx PTK study, PTK significantly improved the BCVA and decreased the corneal opacities. Phototherapeutic keratectomy also improves

patient comfort and reduces ocular symptoms related to the surface corneal disorders treated.

PHOTOTHERAPEUTIC KERATECTOMY – SUMMIT EXPERIENCE

The phase II and phase III Summit Excimed laser clinical trials for PTK were performed on 67 eyes.[15] The eye disorders treated were grouped into those with corneal opacity (lattice dystrophy, corneal scar, band keratopathy, Schnyder's crystalline dystrophy, and Reis–Buckler's dystrophy, postpterygium removal scars, and other corneal scars), and those with epithelial breakdowns (recurrent erosion and band keratopathy).

The surgical technique involved the use of methyl-cellulose as a 'polishing' agent. The PTK was performed using a 'polish technique', where the surgeon moves the patient's head in a brisk controlled circular manner while the laser treatment is performed. This allows the beam to 'polish' the corneal surface and prevents the ablation from producing an abrupt transition to the untreated cornea (also see Chapters 21 and 22).

Of the 67 eyes treated, 22 were in the corneal opacity group, 27 eyes were in the irregular surface group, and 11 eyes were in the recurrent epithelial breakdown group. The average length of follow-up was 8.2 months (range 3–21 months).

Uncorrected VA improved in 64–69% of cases in the three treatment groups. Best corrected visual acuity improved in 77% of the corneal opacity group, in 70% of the irregular surface group, and in 36% of the recurrent erosion group. Between 18 and 22% of eyes lost at least one line of BCVA in the three groups.

The change in patients' spherical equivalent was variable. In the corneal opacity group there was an average myopic shift from +0.75 D preoperatively to −0.92 D postoperatively, with a range of −10.25 to +3.00 D. In the irregular surface group, the average change was not significant (preoperative +0.37 D to +0.39 D postoperatively but, again with a range of −5.75 to +5.00 D). In the recurrent epithelial break-down group only minimal hyperopic refractive change was observed from −1.59 D preoperatively to −0.94 D postoperatively.

Phototherapeutic keratectomy with the Summit Excimed excimer laser system appears to be an effective treatment for superficial corneal disease. It has the potential to decrease morbidity as well as being cost-effective in the long run by avoiding the need for lamellar or penetrating keratoplasty. In October 1994, the FDA panel recommended approval of excimer laser PTK with the Summit laser.

PHOTOREFRACTIVE KERATECTOMY FOR ASTIGMATISM

Smooth ablation of the cornea using the 193 nm excimer laser promises to be a more predictable and efficacious approach to correct astigmatism. This procedure to correct astigmatism is still under study and phase IIa and IIb of the FDA-sponsored clinical trials have been completed. The study was carried out at five investigative sites and 90 procedures carried out on 66 patients have been fully evaluated.

The Visx 20/20 system for correcting astigmatism incorporates modifications of their hardware and software to produce toric ablations. The hardware consists of a dual operative system: an iris diaphragm, which can expand or constrict (circular aperture), and a pair of parallel adjustable blades (rectangular aperture) that can rotate 180°. The blade separation and the circular aperture size are controlled by the computer software. Two programs are combined to create the toric (elliptical) ablation for correction of compound myopic astigmatism. The idea is to create an elliptically shaped toric ablation by simultaneously opening the rectangular aperture while opening the circular aperture. This creates a smooth ablation with no transition zones. This program cannot be used if the refractive error is only cylindrical or if the spherical component is not at least as large as the cylindrical component (also see Chapter 15).

Patients were enrolled with more than 0.75 D, but not more than 4.5 D of refractive cylinder. The preoperative spherical equivalent was 1.0–6.0 D and the spherical component was at least as large as the cylindrical component. The vision had to be 20/40 or better in both eyes. The mean age was 39.5 years with a range of 24 to 71 years. Sixty-three per cent of patients were male and available data is on 72% of patients with at least 6 months' follow-up.

At 6 months no patient had more than 1+ haze. The mean preoperative cylinder was 1.49 D, which was reduced to a mean of 0.44 D at the 1 month visit. This mean refractive cylinder remained stable over 1 year of follow-up. The mean targeted increase in spherical equivalent in the compound myopic astig-

matism cases was 4.0 D and the mean deviation from targeted correction, a measure of predictability, was −0.13 D at 6 months.

At 12 months, all cases were 20/25 or better except one case, which was 20/30. Three cases lost two or three lines of BCVA. Preoperatively, 94% of cases had uncorrected vision 20/80 or worse and 55% were worse than 20/200. At 12 months, 67% had uncorrected vision 20/25 or better and 28% saw 20/30 or 20/40. One case lost a significant level of uncorrected vision, associated with a regression of effect.

The treatment of astigmatism with photoastigmatic refractive keratectomy (PARK) can be successfully performed, with good stability of effect. There is marked improvement in uncorrected VA and no significant loss of best corrected vision. Currently studies are underway to evaluate the ability of the Visx 20/20 laser to steepen the cornea and correct hyperopia. If successful, this approach should allow for steepening of the flat corneal meridian, thereby providing a treatment for hyperopic astigmatism.

PRK FOR HYPEROPIA WITH THE VISX LASER

Correction of hyperopia is much more difficult to accomplish than correction of myopia. Surgical options are limited to procedures that remain controversial at best. Hexagonal keratotomy, an incisional procedure, is associated with poor predictability, limited range of correction, and induction of irregular astigmatism that adversely affects best corrected vision. Holmium:YAG thermokeratoplasty is another procedure under investigation. In this technique a laser system is used to apply heat to the stromal collagen, causing shrinkage and central corneal steepening.

The Visx and Summit excimer laser systems for correction of hyperopia are currently under study. The Visx laser system projects the laser beam through a spinning, off-set slit, which creates a ring-shaped beam that spares the central 1 mm of the cornea (see Chapter 17 for initial Summit data).

FDA Phase I clinical trials utilizing the Visx 20/20 laser were conducted on a group of 10 legally blind eyes.[16] In all the patients the target correction was 4.00 D in the corneal plane. The treatment zone ranged from 8 to 9 mm. The mean change at 1 month was a −3.21 D decrease in spherical equivalent. This showed some regression of effect at 6 months to −2.64 D. Similarly, the mean keratometry regressed over 6 months by an average of 40%. Thus, at 6 months the patients retained an average of 2.6 D of refractive change. All the corneas healed well and re-epithelialized within 1–5 days with minimal haze. These phase I patients are the first clinical cases.

Further refinements in the nomograms to improve target strategies are forthcoming. This approach to correction of hyperopia looks promising.

REFERENCES

1. Trokel SL, Srinivasan R, Braren B, Excimer laser surgery of the cornea, *Am J Ophthalmol* (1983) **96**: 710–15.

2. Marshall J, Trokel S, Rothery S, et al, An ultrastructural study of corneal incisions induced by an excimer laser at 193 nm, *Ophthalmology* (1985) **92**: 749–58.

3. Puliafito CA, Steinert RF, Deutsch TF, et al, Excimer laser radial keratotomy, *Ophthalmology* (1985) **92**: 741–8.

4. Cotliar AM, Schubery HO, Madel ER, et al, Excimer laser radial keratotomy, *Ophthalmology* (1985) **92**: 206–8.

5. Marshall J, Trokel S, Rothery S, et al, A comparative study of corneal incisions induced by diamond and steel knives and two ultraviolet radiations from an excimer laser, *Br J Ophthalmol* (1985) **70**: 482–501.

6. Munnerlyn CR, Koons SJ, Marshall J, Photorefractive keratectomy: a technique for laser refractive surgery, *J Cataract Refract Surg* (1988) **14**: 46–52.

7. Beuerman RW, McDonald MB, Shofner RS, et al, Quantitative histological studies of primate corneas after excimer laser photorefractive keratectomies, *Arch Ophthalmol* (1994) **112**: 1103–10.

8. L'Esperance FA Jr, Taylor DM, Warner JW, Human excimer laser keratectomy: short-term histopathology, *J Refract Surg* (1988) **4**: 118–24.

9. Anrade HA, McDonald MB, Liu JC, et al, Evaluation of an opacity lensometer for determining corneal clarity following excimer laser photoablation, *Refract Corneal Surg* (1990) **6**: 346–51.

10. Lohmann C, Fitzke F, Timberlake G, et al, Corneal transparency after excimer laser photorefractive keratectomy: a new technique for objective measurement of haze, *Refract Corneal Surg* (1992) **8**: 15–2.

11. Lohmann C, Gartry D, Kerr-Muir M, et al Haze in photorefractive keratectomy: its origins and consequences, *Lasers Light Ophthalmol* (1991) **4**: 15–34.

12. Riberio JC, Ancel JM, McDonald MB, et al, A comparison of clinical results of photorefractive keratectomy for mild to moderate myopia with the VISX and Summit excimer lasers: A retrospective study, ARVO abstract, *Invest Ophthalmol Vis Sci* (1994) **35(Suppl)**: 2017.

13. Thompson KP, Waring GO III, Steinert R, et al, Excimer laser photorefractive keratectomy for myopia: Preliminary results at one year, *SPIE Proc Ophthalmic Tech II* (1992) **1644**: 20–31.

14. Stark WJ, Chamon W, Kamp MT, et al, Clinical follow-up of 192 nm ArF excimer laser photokeratectomy, *Ophthalmology* (1992) **99**: 805–11.

15. Maloney RK, Ghiselli G, Thompson V, et al, A multicenter trial of excimer laser phototherapeutic keratectomy for coneal opacities and irregularities.ARVO abstract, *Invest Ophthalmol Vis Sci* (1994) **25(Suppl)**: 1488.

16. McDonald MB, Telfair WB, Nesburn AB, et al, Excimer laser hyperopia PRK Phase I: The blind eye study, ARVO abstract, *Invest Ophthalmol Vis Sci* (1994) **35(Suppl)**: 1488.

Chapter 12 European experience with excimer PRK/PARK

Jerry Jayamanne and Charles N J McGhee

European clinical experience with the Summit, Visx and Meditec laser systems

INTRODUCTION

Most ophthalmologists in the USA have been severely restricted, under FDA regulations, in their ability to utilize excimer laser as a refractive tool. European ophthalmologists have been under considerably less constraint. This has enabled clinicians in Europe to build up a considerable long-term experience in a variety of excimer laser systems, notably Summit, Visx, Meditech, and Technolas, with Schwind and Nidek lasers becoming more widely available recently. This section will largely deal with the first three systems, with clinical data on Technolas systems being covered in Chapter 13.

Although a great many clinical teams, indeed too many to name individually, have contributed to the wealth of knowledge accrued from the many European studies, three groups have been pre-eminent in pushing back the boundaries, both in the laboratory and the clinical setting. No discussion of excimer laser photorefractive keratectomy (PRK) would be complete without identifying the pioneering work by Professor Theo Seiler and his co-workers in Berlin. At about the same time, Professor John Marshall was assembling a team in London, which included David Gartry and Malcolm Kerr Muir, whilst in Stockholm, Sweden, a third research team, which included Professor Bjorn Tengroth and his colleagues Drs Epstein, Fagerholm and Hamberg-Nystrom, started out upon clinical trials using the Summit laser, but later became one of the few large groups in Europe to also gain invaluable experience with a second laser system (Visx). Between 1989 and 1993, together these three groups produced more than 50% of the ophthalmic excimer literature published from European sites, thus producing a firm core foundation upon which to develop excimer laser in Europe.

BACKGROUND

Numerous studies have been published on the results of excimer laser PRK and, by convention, data concerning efficacy of refractive correction following PRK generally report two overall measures: the percentage of eyes that achieve a postoperative refraction within one diopter (D) of intended correction or emmetropia; and the percentage of eyes that achieve 20/40 (6/12) or better uncorrected visual acuity. It is important to remember that, although the above measures are helpful in assessing predictability of the procedure, these are not absolute measures of refractive success; for example, a residual myopia of −1.5 D in an eye which was highly myopic prior to surgery (> −10.0 D) might quite rightly be considered a successful result. On the other hand, complications such as loss of contrast sensitivity, which might significantly affect night vision, may not be detected under conditions used for measuring visual acuity.

A major parameter cited as a measure of the safety of PRK is loss of best spectacle corrected visual acuity (BSCVA). Visual loss of two or more lines of best corrected visual acuity is reported by most studies and is a useful measure of clinically significant visual deterioration. Although some studies also report on the postoperative period required for stabilization of refraction, due to the relatively short follow up frequently reported (6–12 months), this has yet to be exhaustively established.

EUROPEAN EXPERIENCE WITH SUMMIT EXCIMER LASER SYSTEM

SUMMIT: THE BERLIN STUDIES

The first clinical application of the excimer laser to a human cornea for the correction of astigmatism was performed in 1985 by Professor Theo Seiler and his associates.[1] Since that time numerous European studies have been published on the results of excimer laser PRK. In 1991, Seiler[2] reported the results of PRK on an initial series of 26 sighted eyes with preoperative refractive errors ranging from –1.4 to –9.25 D. Ablation zones were 3.5 mm in diameter and 92% of the eyes were within ±1.0 D of intended final refraction at 1 year, with stability of refraction (±0.25 D) in 58% of the eyes between 6 and 12 months. Uncorrected visual acuity had improved to 20/40 or better in 96% of the eyes and to 20/20 or better in 48% of the eyes. None of the patients had lost or gained more than one line of best corrected visual acuity 1 year after surgery and these excellent early results were associated with a low incidence of complication.

Subsequently, Seiler and co-authors[3] reported the results of a prospective study in 193 eyes of 146 patients using a small ablation zone diameter of 3.5 mm. Twelve months after surgery, the percentage of eyes showing refraction within ±1.0 D of attempted correction was noted to be dependent upon the intended refractive change, with 97% of eyes in the lower myopia group (≤ –3.0 D), 91.8% in the middle myopia group (–3.1 to –6 D), 44.4% in the higher myopia group (–6.1 to –9 D) and 25% in the highest myopia group (more than –9 D) being within ±1.0 D of attempted refraction. Undercorrections of greater than 1.0 D occurred in only 2.4% of the eyes in the lower myopia group, compared to 50% of eyes in the highest myopia group. This trend to undercorrection in higher myopia was to be echoed by many other studies in Europe using a variety of lasers. Changes in refractive astigmatism were considered to be significant if the cylinder power increased or decreased by more than 0.5 D. At 2 years, surgically induced increase in astigmatism was reported in 1.7% of the eyes and a decrease in 0.6% of the eyes.

None of the eyes examined at the 2 year follow-up showed a refraction that was more than 0.75 D hyperopic than at the 1 year examination. Regression during the second year after surgery, of 1.0 D or more, was not detected in eyes with baseline refractions of ≤ –3 D; however, 8.6% of the eyes with

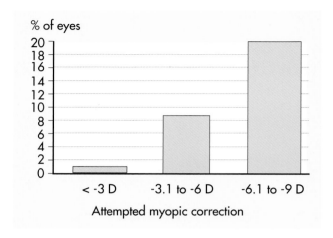

Figure 12.1 *Regression during the second year after photorefractive keratectomy of –1.0 D or greater. (Seiler et al, 1994[3].)*

baseline refractions between –3.1 and –6.0 D, and 20% of the eyes with baseline refractions between –6.1 and –9.0 D did demonstrate regression during the second year of 1 D or more (Fig. 12.1). Based upon 126 eyes, with 2 year follow-up, the refractive change between 1 and 2 years after surgery was statistically significant only in the group with a preoperative refraction of –6.1 to –9.0 D.

Change in BSCVA at 1 year after PRK showed that loss of more than two lines of visual acuity was not detected at 1 year in the group with corrections up to –3.0 D; however, 5% of the eyes with corrections between –3.0 and –6.0 D, 19% of the eyes with corrections between –6.0 and –9.0 D and 43% of the eyes with corrections of more than 9.0 D had lost more than two lines of visual acuity at 1 year. Manifest scars occurred in 10 eyes appearing between 1 and 3 months after surgery in six eyes, between 3 and 6 months after surgery in three eyes, and after 12 months in one eye. The incidence of scarring was greater if the attempted correction was greater than –6.0 D. All 10 eyes were reoperated and no recurrence of the scars were manifest at 2 years (Table 12.1). At 1 year, a total of 15 eyes were reablated and a further 12 eyes required reoperation at 2 years. Of these 27 eyes, 17 eyes required reablation for undercorrection without scars and 10 eyes due to undercorrection with scars. The distribution of reoperations, according to attempted correction, revealed increasing incidence with greater attempted correction being 0% in the myopia group > –3.0 D,

Table 12.1

Outcome of excimer laser PRK for myopia related to attempted correction. (Seiler et al, 1994[3].)

Number of patients	Myopia treatment range (D)	Loss of three lines of BSCVA (% of eyes)	Gain of three lines of BSCVA (% of eyes)	Incidence of manifest scars after PRK (%)	Reoperations within 2 years after PRK (%)
48	≤ −3.0	0	2.4	0	0
93	−3.1 to −6.0	5	2.3	1.1	6.5
40	−6.1 to −9.0	19	3.7	17.5	40
12	≥ −9.1	43	0	16.7	41.6

compared to 6.5%, 40% and 41.6%, respectively, in each of the increasingly myopic groups previously defined. None of the reoperated eyes lost one line of BSCVA compared with baseline. The authors concluded that PRK showed good refractive results for corrections up to −6.0 D with tolerable regression during the first 2 years after surgery.

Complications such as loss of visual acuity under glare conditions may be secondary to increased spherical abberation of the cornea after excimer laser PRK. Seiler and colleagues, have recently addressed this problem by performing PRK for myopia using a new aspherical algorithm.[4] Although there appeared to be a statistically significant subjective reduction in halos reported in the aspherically corrected eyes, because of the small number of eyes in the study the results should be interpreted cautiously.

SUMMIT: THE EARLY LONDON STUDIES

Gartry et al initially reported on excimer laser PRK treatment of cadaver eyes and 25 eyes with anterior corneal disease in 1991.[5] Later that same year, Gartry and co-workers reported the results of PRK using Summit technology.[6] The refractive results were presented for a total of 136 patients (16 blind and 120 sighted eyes), with a range of preoperative myopia from −1.5 to −17.5 D, followed up for at least 1 year. The authors reported that 90% of the eyes undergoing −2.0 D correction and 75% of the eyes undergoing −3.0 D corrections were within ±1.0 D of attempted correction; however, this figure fell to 40% and 20% for the groups undergoing −6.0 and −7.0 D corrections, respectively.

Best corrected visual acuity was reported as greater than, or equal to, preoperative acuity in 93% of the patients and no eyes lost more than two lines of

BSCVA; however, six patients lost one line of Snellen acuity at 6 months and a further three were reported to have lost two lines of best corrected acuity. These latter three patients were in the group with the highest attempted correction of myopia. The authors noted that 78% of the patients identified halo around lights at night, more markedly so in the early postoperative period.

In a subsequent article (1992), Gartry and co-workers presented their 18 month results of PRK for −2.0 to −7.0 D attempted correction in 120 eyes of 120 patients[7] utilizing a 4 mm diameter ablation zone. Ninety-five per cent of eyes undergoing −2.0 D, 70% of eyes undergoing −3.0 D, 40% of the eyes undergoing −6.0 D and 20% of the eyes undergoing −7.0 D corrections, respectively, were within ±1.0 D of attempted correction. Refractions were stable by 3–6 months.

Overall, 11% of the eyes had lost one or two lines of best spectacle corrected Snellen visual acuity. Anterior stromal haze, detected in 92% of patients, was reported to be maximum at 6 months. Halation, due to the relatively small 4 mm diameter ablation zone, was reported by 78% of the patients in the early postoperative period; however, only 10% of the patients declined treatment of the other eye because of the persistence of this problem.

SUMMIT: THE STOCKHOLM GROUP

Tengroth and co-workers[8] used a Summit laser to perform PRK on 420 sighted eyes with a minimum of 1 year follow-up. Ablation zones of 4.3–4.5 mm were used and preoperative refraction ranged from −1.25 to −7.5 D. Twelve months postoperatively, 86% of the eyes were within 1.0 D of emmetropia and 91% of eyes achieved an uncorrected visual acuity of at least

20/40. At 3 months postoperatively, a myopic shift in refraction, greater than or equal to −0.5 D, appeared to be associated with increasing magnitude of attempted myopic correction. Regression, when it occurred, was usually noted between 3 and 6 months postoperatively and was more frequently identified in eyes that had received topical steroids for only 5 weeks postoperatively than in those eyes treated for 3 months. Tengroth concluded that argon fluoride excimer laser can correct myopia with good predictability, that higher preoperative myopia is associated with greater incidence of regression, and topical steroids postoperatively seem to play a crucial role in refractive outcome. The latter deduction has subsequently been widely questioned (see Chapter 25).

Epstein and co-workers (1994), using a Summit laser to perform PRK, reported on the 24 month refractive outcome[9] of 495 sighted myopic eyes which were entered into the study with preoperative refractive errors ranging from −1.25 to −7.5 D. Once more, ablation zone diameters of 4.3 and 4.5 mm were used. Interestingly, mean refraction at 12 months was statistically different from the mean at 18 months, and there was also a significant difference between 12 and 24 month mean refractions; however, there was no significant difference between the means at 18 and 24 months, suggesting that stabilization of refractive error has probably occurred by 18 months post-PRK.

On subgroup analysis, patients with low to moderate myopia (up to −3.9 D) had significantly better refractive outcomes than those with higher myopia. At 24 months, it was noted that 91% of the eyes had an uncorrected visual acuity of at least 20/40 and 81.5% had an uncorrected visual acuity of at least 20/30, whilst 87% and 71.7% of the eyes, respectively, were within 1.0 and 0.5 D of emmetropia (Table 12.2).

Only 0.4% of eyes lost one line of BSCVA and none lost two lines or more. The authors concluded, after analyzing outcomes 24 months post-PRK, that the procedure was safe, with reasonably predictable and effective results, although refraction after PRK was slow to stabilize, and only appeared to reach stability by 18–24 months after surgery.

SUMMIT: OTHER LARGE EUROPEAN STUDIES

An 81 patient study of PRK with a 12 month follow-up was reported by Ficker and colleagues in 1993.[10] PRK was performed with the aim of correcting a range of myopic errors between −1.0 and −10.0 D. At 1 year, 81% of the patients were within ±1.0 D of emmetropia, with unaided vision of 6/12. Fifteen per cent of the eyes lost a single line of best corrected Snellen acuity. Contrast sensitivity dropped immediately from a mean value of 1.8 to a value of 1.51 in the first week; thereafter gradual recovery occurred over 12 months to a mean value of 1.6; no correlation between loss of contrast sensitivity and intended correction was identified. Regression of myopia was more commonly seen among moderate and high myopes (greater than −4 D). Steroids were commenced in 37 patients with regression ranging from −0.25 to −3.5 D and this myopic regression was reported to be reversed in 82% of the eyes, for the duration of steroid therapy.

Brancato and co-workers[11] reported the results of PRK conducted in Italy to evaluate the efficacy, safety, predictability and complications of the technique. In an extensive series of 1236 myopic sighted eyes from 16 centers, the attempted correction ranged from −0.8 to −25.0 D, and 12 month follow-up was available for 330 eyes. Twelve months after surgery, 71.2% of the patients with attempted

Table 12.2

Postoperative corneal haze and loss of best spectacle corrected visual acuity (BSCVA) following excimer laser PRK in eyes with attempted corrections between −1.25 and −7.5. (Epstein et al, 1994[9].)

Number of patients	Myopia treatment range (D)	Lines of BSCVA lost (%)			Postoperative corneal haze (%)		
		1	*2*	*3*	*1+*	*2+*	*3+*
495	−1.25 to −7.5	0.4	0	0	16	2–4	1

correction of –0.8 to –6.0 D were within ±1.0 D of attempted correction, whereas only 34.5% of the patients with attempted corrections of –6.1 to –9.9 D were within ±1.0 D of attempted correction. In eyes with attempted correction of greater than –10.0 D, only 28.2% were within ±1.0 D of attempted correction. Interestingly, despite the attempted correction of high levels of myopia, only 2.4% of the patients had lost two or more Snellen lines of BSCVA.

Specifically looking at the ability to correct low to moderate myopia, Tutton and co-workers (1993)[12] reported results of PRK with a 5 mm diameter ablation zone in 95 eyes with myopia from –1.0 to –6.0 D. Six months post surgery, 70% of the eyes were within ±0.5 D, 88% were within ±1.0 D, and 99% were within ±2.0 D of attempted correction. However, 5% of the eyes had lost one line and 2% of the eyes had lost two lines of best corrected visual acuity. A degree of corneal haze was noted in 72% of the treated eyes and the authors reported more haze in those eyes that had undergone larger corrections. Overall, there appeared to be no relationship between corneal haze and BSCVA.

Salorio and colleagues[13] used a Summit laser with a 5 mm ablation zone to treat 178 myopic eyes. Ninety of these eyes had attempted treatment of more than –6.0 D, the remaining 88 eyes had attempted correction of –6.0 D or less. Although 95% of the eyes with initial refraction of less than –6.0 D were within ±1.0 D of attempted correction, eyes with greater initial refraction were more frequently over- or undercorrected. No eyes in this series lost BSCVA.

Orssaud and co-workers[14] reported on excimer laser PRK in 176 eyes of 176 patients. Preoperative refractions ranged from –1.0 to –8.5 D and the procedures were performed with a 4 mm ablation zone. Six months after PRK, 100% of the eyes in the group with intended correction of less than –2.9 D and 86% of the eyes in the group with intended correction between –3.0 D and –5.9 D were within ±1.0 D of emmetropia. Over the same period of time, only 43% of the eyes with intended correction of –6.0 D or more had a refraction within ±1 D of emmetropia, and results were reported to be similar at 1 year. Six months after PRK, 58% of the eyes in the low myopia group, 45% of the eyes in the medium myopia group and 18% of the eyes in the high myopia group had uncorrected visual acuity of 20/20 or better (Fig. 12.2). The average best corrected visual acuity was 20/20 in the eyes where the intended correction was less than –5.9 D; this compared to the average best corrected visual acuity of 20/25 in the eyes where intended correction was greater than –6.0 D. At 1 year post surgery, 8% of

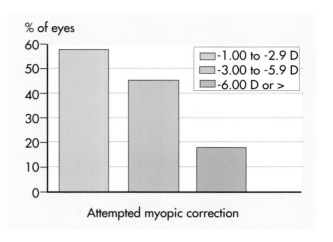

Figure 12.2 *Percentage of eyes with uncorrected visual acuity (UCVA) of 20/20 6 months after PRK. Total number of patients 176. (Orssaud et al, 1994[14].)*

the eyes in the group where intended correction was less than –2.9 D, and 9% of eyes where the intended correction was less than –5.9 D had lost two or more lines of best corrected visual acuity. This was in stark contrast to 38% of the eyes with an attempted correction greater than –6.0 D which had lost two or more lines of BSCVA at the same time point.

Murta and co-workers reported on PRK in 98 consecutive normal myopic eyes[15] with 31 eyes followed-up for 6 months. Preoperative myopia ranged from –1.25 to –12.00 D. A 5 mm ablation zone was used in eyes with up to –6.0 D of preoperative myopia, a 4.9–4.6 mm optical zone in eyes with preoperative myopia of –6.12 to –9.0 D, and a 4.5 mm ablation zone to correct more than –9.0 D of myopia. All of the eyes which had attempted correction of between –1.25 and –3.0 D were within 0.5 D of desired refraction at 6 months and 100% of the eyes in the group with attempted correction between –3.12 and –6.0 D were within ±1.0 D of attempted correction. Results for higher myopia were also encouraging, with 89.9% of the eyes with attempted correction of between –6.12 and –9.00 D within ±1.0 D of desired refractive correction. However, as always, the reporting of 6 month data in high myopia can be misleading since there may be a continual myopic drift for up to 1 year or more.[16]

Other studies with longer follow-up have reported the results of excimer laser PRK using Summit technology in high myopia. Buratto and Ferrari (1993) described the results of surgery in 40 eyes

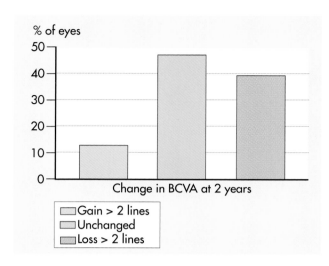

Figure 12.3 *Change in best spectacle corrected visual acuity (BSCVA) at 2 years post-PRK in eyes with attempted correction of –6.0 to –10.0 D (Buratto and Ferrari, 1993[16].)*

with between –6.0 and –10.0 D of myopia, with a follow-up of at least 24 months.[16] At the end of the follow-up period, only 35% of the eyes were within ±1.0 D of desired correction and 65% of the eyes had undercorrection of more than 1.0 D from the desired result. The uncorrected visual acuity was 20/100 or better in 60% of the eyes and BSCVA declined two or more lines in 40% of the eyes (Fig. 12.3). In 65% of the eyes, the authors observed a regression of the refractive effect after 6 months and 85% of the eyes had persisting corneal haze at the end of the follow-up period. The authors concluded that there appeared to be poor predictability and significant refractive regression in this series.

SUMMIT: MULTIZONE TECHNIQUES

Multizone PRK has been suggested to increase the predictability of higher myopic correction. The technique essentially consists of dividing the intended correction between two or three different concentric ablation zones, which require a less deep ablation and, theoretically, produce a smoother transition ablation profile, than a single zone ablation for an equivalent attempted correction (Table 12.3).

In a large series, Lavery[17] reviewed the results of PRK for refractions ranging between –1.25 and –9.6 D (with less than 1.25 D of astigmatism). In this series of 472 myopic eyes, refractive errors up to –6.0 D were treated with a single zone spherical ablation, whilst eyes with greater than –6.0 D of myopia were treated with a dual zone procedure. Six months after surgery, 92% of the eyes in the group with refractive errors up to –6.0 D had a refraction within ±1.0 D of intended correction. In eyes with corrections between –6.0 and –9.6 D, at 6 months, 45% of the eyes exhibited a refraction within ±1.0 D of emmetropia and 84% were within ±2.0 D of emmetropia. Overall, at 1 year post surgery, 94% of all eyes achieved uncorrected visual acuity of 20/40 or better.

Tavola and associates[18] reported PRK results with Summit technology for correction of myopia ranging between –6.5 and –10.00 D using multizone PRK. Fifty-eight eyes were treated with a single zone, and 58 eyes with a double zone ablation. Regression of refractive effect was more pronounced in the single zone group; however, at 6 months, a greater number of eyes in the single zone treatment group had achieved correction within ±2.0 D of attempted correction. The authors concluded that eyes treated with a double zone procedure had less corneal haze and less regression than the single zone group,

Table 12.3

Results from two studies of excimer laser PRK for moderate-to-high myopia using Summit laser dual zone technique.

Group (year) reference	Follow-up (months)	Pre-PRK myopia (D)	Within ± 1 D of emmetropia	Within ± 2 D of emmetropia	Within ± 3 D of emmetropia
Lavery (1993)[17]	6	> –6.0	45%	84%	NR
Tavola et al. (1993)[18]	6	–6.5 to –10.00	50%	70%	75%

probably because the depth of ablation in the first group was less than in the second group; nonetheless, there was no statistically significant difference in refractive predictability between the groups.

Scialdone and co-workers[19] also reported on multizone PRK for eyes with refractions between –6.0 and –9.0 D over a follow-up period of 1 year. Once more the authors reported that there was no statistically significant difference in refraction of the single zone group as compared to double zone PRK.

SUMMIT: EFFECT OF INCREASING ABLATION ZONE DIAMETER

During the evolution of PRK, ablation zone diameters have progressively increased from 3.5 to 6.0 mm or greater. Major reasons for this increase in diameter are: the high incidence of symptomatic halos during night driving conditions with small ablation zones;[2] a reduction in the initial hyperopic shift with lasers that employ beam diameters greater than 5 mm;[20] and greater predictability in the treatment of higher myopia (see Chapter 16).

To determine the effects of ablation zone diameter on the outcome of PRK, O'Brart et al[21] conducted a study on 33 patients undergoing bilateral PRK with identical dioptric corrections in both eyes, except that first eyes received 4 mm and second eyes received 5 mm ablation zones. Identical postoperative medication regimes were used in both eyes of each subject. The authors reported that there was no statistically significant difference in preoperative refraction between the first and the second eyes; however, mean reductions in myopia, up to 1 year post surgery, were significantly greater in eyes treated with 5 mm ablation diameters. None of the eyes treated with 4 mm zones were overcorrected at 12 months postoperatively, whereas 15% of the eyes treated with 5 mm beams had a refraction greater than +1.0 D. No statistically significant difference in the amount of anterior stromal haze between the two groups was reported at any stage despite greater depths of stromal ablation with 5 mm zones. Subjective and objective improvement of night halos was reported by patients in respect to eyes treated with 5 mm zones.

Pursuing this line of investigation, O'Brart and colleagues[22] also reported on the effects of ablation diameter on the outcome of PRK in 80 patients treated with either a 5 or 6 mm zone. All eyes in this study underwent either a –3.0 or –6.0 D correction based on preoperative refraction. Eyes treated with a 6 mm diameter ablation zone showed reduction in hyperopic shift for both treatment groups (–3.0 and –6.0 D corrections) and at 6 months the induced refractive change was closer to that intended with 6 mm, rather than 5 mm, diameter ablation. Five eyes treated with a 5 mm zone experienced a regression of the correction and a reduction of three or more lines of best corrected visual acuity over 6 months. None of the eyes treated with 6 mm zones were similarly affected. Night halo problems were significantly less in the 6 mm treatment groups in both the –3.0 and –6.0 D corrections 1 month postoperatively. The authors concluded that treatment with 6 mm ablation diameters precipitated less initial overcorrection and greatly improved the predictability of PRK and was associated with reduction in complications that impaired postoperative visual rehabilitation.

In the most recent study reported by this group (1996),[23] 100 eyes were prospectively randomized to receive –3.00 D corrections in a 5 or 6 mm single zone ablation (n=40) or –6.00 D corrections utilizing a 5 mm, 6 mm or tapered dual zone ablation (n=60). In a carefully constructed experimental protocol, the –6.00 D multizone 6 mm ablation was restricted to the same depth as the 5 mm –6.00 D correction, by restricting the initial 5.00 D to a 4.6 mm diameter zone and then overlaying this, following a variable delay of up to 2 minutes, with a 1.00 D 6 mm diameter ablation. Although technically a multizone procedure, the use of a central 4.6 mm zone for 83% of the ablation in the latter subgroup might, rather predictably, lead to results and visual symptoms more akin to 5 mm ablations than 6 mm ablations.

At 1 year postoperatively in the group receiving –3.00 D corrections, 100% of 6 mm diameter zone eyes but only 71% of 5 mm zone eyes achieved a refractive outcome ±1.00 D of intended. The differences were even more marked in the group receiving a –6.00 D correction, with 67% of the 6 mm ablation group achieving ±1.00 D of intended refraction, compared to 20% in the 5 mm zone and 26% in the multizone group. Interestingly, no eyes in either the –3.00 or –6.00 D group treated with a 6 mm ablation zone exhibited loss of two or more lines of BSCVA, whereas the 5 mm and multizone groups demonstrated 10–21% of eyes with two lines or more of lost BSCVA. Overall, the authors concluded that the 6 mm ablation zone was superior to 5 mm zones in terms of smaller hyperopic shift, more predictable and stable refractive outcome and smaller halos. This improved outcome was attributed, by the authors, largely to the decreased rate of change of slope over the entire ablation zone in the 6 mm ablations.

SUMMIT: ASSESSING AND MINIMIZING COMPLICATIONS

The St Thomas' group[24] have also investigated disturbances in night vision after excimer laser PRK using Summit technology. The phenomenon of significant postoperative halos around light sources at night, which prevent patients from driving comfortably, was noted in early clinical trials in which small ablation zone diameters were used. The authors reported on PRK with 5 mm ablation zone diameter[2], and at 3 months postoperatively 45% of the patients complained of disturbances in night vision compared with 25% preoperatively. At 12 months, 38% of patients were aware of night halos; however, only 5% of the patients reported significant problems. In their most recent study, using a 6 mm diameter ablation zone, no severe subjective night vision problems were recorded in subjects receiving −3.00 or −6.00 D corrections, whereas these were still reported in 5% of those receiving a −6.00 D 5 mm ablation.[23]

Many investigators using Summit technology have utilized corticosteroids postoperatively to improve refractive outcome or reverse myopic regression. Great debate in respect to the efficacy, or otherwise, of using corticosteroids in the post-PRK eye continues[8,25–30] (see Chapter 25). O'Brart and co-workers[30] reported on a prospective study of 86 patients randomized to fluorometholone, plasmin inhibitor (aprotinin) or placebo following PRK. The authors reported that the steroid-treated eyes had greater refractive changes at 3 and 6 months but the difference became non-significant 3 months after steroids were discontinued. Aprotinin did not affect refractive error but was associated with greater haze at 12 months post surgery. However, there were only 13 eyes treated with steroids and 14 controls in eyes with attempted correction of -6.0 D; therefore the narrow margin by which statistical analysis failed to prove significance in the steroid-treated group must be interpreted with caution.

Summit lasers have also been used for retreatment of regression following PRK. Epstein and co-workers[31] reported results from 17 eyes retreated with excimer PRK. At 6 months after retreatment, 67.7% of the eyes had an uncorrected visual acuity greater than or equal to 20/40 and 58.8% were within 1 D of emmetropia; however, two eyes showed a loss of one or two lines of BSCVA. Seiler[32] performed repeat PRK on 30 eyes of 30 patients at least 6 months after initial PRK, with indications for retreatment being undercorrection and corneal scaring. Sixty-three per cent of eyes achieved a refraction within 1 D of

attempted correction and only one eye demonstrated scar formation after the second treatment during the period of follow-up (see Chapter 24).

Radial keratotomy (RK) undercorrections have also been treated with Summit laser technology, with results in small studies suggesting that PRK can correct small degrees of residual myopia post RK effectively and safely.[33,34]

SUMMIT: SUMMARY OF EUROPEAN EXPERIENCE

Summit laser systems have been used in much of the pioneering work in Europe over the last 10 years. Although the 3.5–4.0 mm diameter ablation zone was associated with significant regression and a degree of unpredictability, it resulted in up to 92% of eyes in the moderate myopia group (−3.00 to −6.00 D) achieving ±1.00 D of intended refraction.[3,6,7] Later studies using 4.3 and 4.5 mm ablation zones demonstrated improved predictability up to −7.5 D, with 91% of eyes obtaining 6/12 unaided and being within ±1.0 D of intended correction.[8,9] Further increases in ablation diameter to 5 mm[12,13,15] and more recently 6 mm[23] have also been associated with increased predictability, decrease in lost lines of BSCVA, and virtual elimination of significant night time visual disturbance in corrections up to −6.00 D. However, results for attempted corrections of extreme myopia greater than −10.0 D have generally been poor in terms of predictability and outcome and only moderate success (40–45% ±1.00 D) has been encountered in attempted corrections between −6.00 and −9.00 D.[16–19] The treatment of astigmatism by ablatable or erodible masks within Europe has been rather limited but is discussed later in this chapter and more fully in Chapter 15. Selected representative studies using Summit laser technology are summarized in Table 12.4.

EUROPEAN EXPERIENCE WITH VISX EXCIMER LASER SYSTEMS

Many of the European mainland sites, and almost all of the excimer lasers installed in the UK prior to 1992 were Summit laser systems, and most of these data have previously been discussed. However, developments within the UK in the period 1992–1996 are worth relating as a salutory experience to those in presently undersubscribed refractive laser markets.

Table 12.4

Summary results of large representative European studies using Summit laser technology to perform myopic photorefractive keratectomy.

Group (year) reference	Number of eyes	Follow-up (months)	Pre-PRK myopia (D)	Within ± 1 D emmetropia	20/40 + UVA	Eyes losing 2 or more lines of BSCVA
Gartry et al (1991)[6]	176	8-18	−1.5 to −7	50%	61%	NR
Tengroth et al (1993)[8]	420	12	−1.5 to −7.5	86%	91%	NR
Ficker et al (1993)[10]	81	12	−1 to −10.00	81%	NR	NR
Brancato et al (1993)[11]	146	12	−0.8 to −6	71%	NR	1.4%
	145	12	−6.1 to −9.9	35%	NR	2.1%
	39	12	−10 to −25	28%	NR	7.7%
Tutton et al (1993)[12]	91	6	−1 to −6.0	88%	NR	2%
Lavery (1993)[17]	99	12	−1.2 to −9.6	93%	84%	1%
Epstein et al (1994)[9]	495	24	−1.5 to −7.5	87.5%	91%	0%
Seiler et al (1994)[3]	193	12	up to −3	97%	NR	0%
		12	−3.1 to −6	91.8%	NR	5%
		12	−6.1 to −9	44.4%	NR	19%
		12	> −9	25%	NR	43%

Within the UK, a very rapid expansion occurred between 1992 and late 1994, with the number of excimer laser units multiplying from less than 10 to an estimated 55 fully operational systems. With the UK population of 58 million at the peak of this expansion, this represented almost one system per million of the populus. For a variety of reasons, including an overestimation of demand for PRK in a traditionally cautious population, an oversupply in geographic terms with the majority of systems within a 150 mile radius of London and, not least, a recurring backlash in the popular press after initial media enthusiasm for the 'miracle treatment', the number of patients seeking excimer laser PRK began to fall and by August 1996 the number of operational laser systems had fallen by more than one-third. The majority of the remaining 30 UK systems are Summit lasers, with a handful of Technolas and Nidek excimer lasers complemented by 10 Visx installations. Two of these latter systems are in academic refractive research units, namely Moorfields Eye Hospital,

London and the Corneal Diseases and Excimer Laser Unit, Sunderland Eye Infirmary (SEI), Sunderland, and data from these two centers will be discussed later.

Not unsurprisingly, due to widespread early footholds gained by Summit within Europe, the volume of literature available upon Visx systems is much less than Summit, although the Visx experience with wider ablation zones, multizone treatment in high myopia and photoastigmatic refractive keratectomy (PARK) is much greater.

VISX: THE STOCKHOLM GROUP

Hamberg-Nystrom and co-workers,[35] being one of the few teams using both Summit and Visx lasers, reviewed the results of PRK comparing Summit and Visx systems. Visual outcome in terms of unaided visual acuity, contrast sensitivity, residual refractive error and centration of the surgically ablated area were assessed. Forty eyes of 40 consecutive patients undergoing PRK to correct myopia (range −2.0 to −5.0 D, with less than 0.75 D of astigmatism) were enrolled. Ablation zone diameter was 5 mm in all cases. A mean refraction of ±0.0 D in the Summit group and −0.5 D in the Visx group was reported 12 months postoperatively. The uncorrected visual acuity was 20/40 or better in 100% of the Summit-treated eyes, whereas only 85% of the Visx-treated eyes achieved 20/40 or better (it should be noted that at this time the Visx algorithm was deliberately programmed to produce a residual refractive error of −0.5 D). Contrast sensitivity and dark vision were the same in both groups, as was centration of ablation zones. The slightly more myopic outcome of the Visx laser explained the poorer uncorrected visual acuity outcome in this group.

VISX: THE FRENCH EXPERIENCE

Professor Danielle Aron-Rosa and co-workers have been involved in European excimer laser research since 1986[36] and recently this group presented a multicenter study[37] using Visx 20/20B laser technology to perform PRK/PARK on 265 eyes at two centers—Paris and Brest. Preoperative refractive errors range from −0.7 to −19.4 D. The results from 124 eyes with 6 months follow-up were reported. The outcomes were assessed according to preoperative refractive error: mild myopia group (spherical equivalent (SE) −3.0 D or better), moderate myopia group (SE −3.1 to −7.0 D), and severe myopia group (SE greater than −7.0 D).

The results in the mild-to-moderate myopia groups were significantly better than those in the severe myopia group. In eyes with mild myopia (n=35), the mean deviation from intended correction was less than −0.5 D at 6 months with 83% ±1.0 D, whereas in moderate myopia (n=52), the mean deviation from intended correction was less than −0.6 D with 79% of the eyes being within ±1.0 D of intended refraction. However, in the group with severe myopia greater than −7.0 D (n=37), the mean deviation from the intended correction was almost −2.0 D, with only 43% of the eyes ±1.0 D of intended. Eyes with mild and moderate myopia stabilized between 2 and 4 months postoperatively, whereas eyes with severe myopia stabilized between 4 and 6 months. Overall, 63% of the patients obtained uncorrected visual acuity of 20/40 or better at 6 months; unfortunately the authors do not provide a breakdown of unaided visual acuity by severity of myopia but, based on the preceding

figures, 20/40 uncorrected vision must have been much more frequent in those with less than −7.00 D corrections. The authors reported no statistically significant difference among the groups in the intensity or evolution of haze related to the degree of myopia. Unfortunately, no comment on lines of lost BSCVA, a good pointer to safety of technique, is made, although it is notable that one eye had regressed to 20/200 unaided acuity, associated with corneal haze, and one eye developed a contact lens-related infection. Decentration of ablation zones greater than 1 mm was not noted in any patient 6 months after PRK. Myopic regression after excimer laser PRK appeared to be related to the depths of ablation performed, and neither patient age nor sex influenced the process.

VISX: UK STUDIES

The largest UK prospective study using the Visx 20/20B laser commenced at Moorfields Eye Hospital, London, under the supervision of Mr Arthur Steele in 1992. This group have previously reported on their PRK studies with a Summit[10] laser and although they have yet to publish a comprehensive account of their Visx 20/20B results, some of this information is available from scientific abstracts and conference reports in the popular ophthalmic press.

Comparing the outcome of a prospective randomized steroid regime in 214 patients, Stevens et al,[38] used a 20/20B with 6 mm diameter treatment zone to treat myopia of −2.00 to −12.00 D with associated astigmatism of 0.0 to 2.0 D. Six months post-treatment, the group randomized to 3 weeks treatment with dexamethasone (n=103) exhibited a refraction of −1.03 ± 1.38 D (mean ± standard deviation), whereas the group randomized to 6 months topical dexamethasone had a mean refraction of −0.91 ± 1.31 D. No statistical difference was observed between the groups, suggesting that prolonged topical corticosteroid treatment was of no refractive benefit.

Stevens,[39] in an early comparison of PRK and PARK, demonstrated, in a study of 116 eyes treated for spherical myopia, compared to 50 eyes tested by PARK for myopia associated with up to 2.0 D of astigmatism, no statistical difference in uncorrected visual acuity or residual myopic error. In those eyes that underwent astigmatic correction, the mean preoperative cylinder was reduced from 1.34 to 0.67 D at 6 months.

Stevens[40] further reported that approximately 20% of patients experienced regression of more than 1.5 D

3 months postoperatively. During the same period post-PRK, 32% of the eyes had regressed between 0.5 and 1.5 D. Interestingly, however, the author reported that 11% of the eyes had moved in a hyperopic direction at 3 months, and between 3 and 6 months 7% moved in this 'plus' direction. The author advised that due to the variability in refractive changes for 1 year post surgery, PRK retreatments should be delayed until at least 1 year postoperatively.

In respect to retreatment of myopic regression, Gartry et al working within the Moorfields group conducted a prospective randomized trial of 106 eyes that exhibited significant regression.[41] The eyes were initially divided into two subgroups—those with mild haze and those with severe haze (2+) and these were then randomized to two treatment protocols:

1) with exact correction of refractive error or
2) correction plus 50% deliberate overcorrection.

The mean time between primary PRK and retreatment was 11.6 months (range 6–23 months) and mean follow-up post retreatment was 12 months. The two subgroups with 50% deliberate overcorrection achieved a statistically better refractive outcome than those with exact correction and the single most important predictor of poor outcome post retreatment was the development of significant corneal haze after the primary treatment. The authors suggested that highly myopic eyes that had regressed beyond (approximately) −3.00 D and demonstrated more than 2+ haze should be retreated with caution, if at all, in view of the risk of further loss of BSCVA.

The SEI prospective study of PRK/PARK commenced in May 1993 with a 3 year protocol to enrol 500 eyes to be treated with a Visx 20/20B using a single pass multizone 'keycard' controlled technique. All eyes were treated with a 6 mm diameter ablation zone, with low myopia (< −5.00 D) being treated in a single 6 mm zone, high myopia (−5.1 to −10.0 D) treated in two zones, −5.0 D in the 6 mm zone and the remaining refraction in a 5.5 mm zone, and extreme myopia (−10.1 to −15.0 D) treated in three zones, 5.0 D in at 6 mm, 5.0 D at 5.5 mm and the remaining refraction greater than −10.00 in a 5 mm zone.

Early results were encouraging[42] and 6 month results in a series of 120 consecutive eyes with a mean error of −5.33 D (range −0.87 to −16.5), divided into low (≤ −5.00), high (−5.1 to −10.0 D) and extreme myopia (> 10.1 D), demonstrated unaided

visual acuity of 6/12 or better in 100%, 78% and 33% of eyes in each myopia group, respectively. Empirical astigmatism was reduced by a mean of 64.3% in the low myopia group, although this was less well corrected (38.6%) in the high myopia group. Overall, three eyes (2.5%) lost two lines or more of BSCVA, all having undergone attempted corrections of greater than −6.00 D.

In an in-depth prospective analysis of complications and refractive outcome, the same authors reported on 100 consecutive myopic eyes that had undergone excimer laser PRK with the Visx laser system,[43] using the previous definitions of low, high and extreme myopia. In terms of spherical reduction, the mean myopia SEs reduced from −2.88 to −0.22 D in low myopia, −5.94 to −0.43 D in high myopia and −12.61 to −1.83 D in the group that underwent greater than −10.0 D correction. The overall cylindrical reduction appeared to decrease with increasing associated myopia, being 53% in the low myopia group, 29% in the moderate myopia correction and 23% in extreme myopia.

Overall 66% of all eyes were reported to have been within ±1.0 D of attempted correction and 80% achieved a vision of 6/12 or better; however, the authors reported that the percentage of eyes achieving 6/12 vision decreased from 93% to 76% in the low-to-high myopia groups and only 40% of eyes treated for greater than −10.0 D achieved 6/12 unaided. At 6 months, six eyes (6%) had lost two or more lines of BSCVA and in four eyes this was associated with significant corneal haze. Myopic regression (defined as at least 0.75 D of residual myopia or an undercorrection representing 25% of the preoperative SE) was reported in seven eyes at 6 months postoperatively. In two cases the regression was halted or reversed with the use of topical steroids and 6 months post surgery only one eye required retreatment.

Decentration of ablation zones, even one as large as 6 mm, can result in unwanted visual symptoms and theoretically produce induced astigmatism and reduction in BSCVA. Specifically addressing this point, the Sunderland group analyzed 53 eyes of 53 consecutive patients undergoing purely spherical corrections with a 6 mm zone.[44] Mean decentration of the ablation zone was 0.46 mm from the pupil center, with only two cases decentered by more than 1 mm. Within this small range of decentration, no association between magnitude of decentration and unaided visual acuity was identified.

Phelan and colleagues (1995)[45] reported the preliminary results of excimer laser PRK for high and

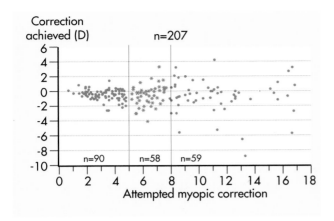

Figure 12.4 *Scattergram of refractive correction achieved compared to attempted myopic correction at 6 months post PRK/PARK in 207 consecutive eyes treated in the Sunderland series. Tight clustering around emmetropia is obvious for corrections up to –8.00 D, higher attempted corrections are associated with greater scatter of refractive outcome.*

extreme myopia in 21 eyes ranging from –6.5 to –17.5 D with astigmatism of up to –5.0 D.

At a mean follow-up time of 8.05 months (range 6–22 months), the mean refractive error had reduced from –10.9 to +0.25 D (range –2.25 to +4.0 D). Unaided visual acuity of 6/18 or better was reported in 90.5% and 6/9(20/30) or better in 57%. One eye lost two lines and another lost one line of BSCVA.

In the latest update on the Sunderland series, McGhee et al (1995)[46] reviewed results of PRK using Visx laser technology in the first 226 consecutive eyes. Preoperative myopic SE ranged from –0.88 to –22.00 D, with a mean of –5.80 ± 3.5 D, associated with a mean myopic astigmatism of –0.98 ± 0.83 D. For analysis purposes, eyes were divided into three groups of low, high, and extreme myopia, as previously noted. Mean follow-up was 12.2 months and data on the 176 eyes that had reached 9 months postoperatively was available. In the low myopia group (mean –3.31 ± 1.09 D) the postoperative mean SE was –0.27 ± 0.68 D and 84% of eyes were within ±1.00 D of emmetropia. In the high myopia group (mean –6.71 ± 1.2 D), the mean postoperative SE was –0.42 ± 1.48 D, with 58% of the eyes within ±1.00 D of emmetropia. In the extreme myopia group (mean preoperative SE –13.39 ± 3.2 D), the mean post-treatment refractive error was –1.91 ± 3.22 D and only 28% of the eyes were within 1.00 D of intended

correction (Fig. 12.4). Unaided visual acuity was 20/40 (6/12) or better in 94%, 83% and 32% of eyes in the low, high and extreme myopia groups, respectively. Only 2% of the eyes that had reached 1 year post treatment lost two or more lines of BSCVA and the overall retreatment rate was 13%.

In respect to those eyes retreated, of 32 eyes with a mean follow-up of 7 months, all cases that had reached 6 months post retreatment achieved 6/12 unaided, with 75% achieving 6/6 unaided.[47] However, although the majority of eyes regained lines of BSCVA and only one eye lost two lines of BSCVA following retreatment, at latest follow-up, seven of the 32 eyes (22%) had lost two lines of BSCVA compared to preoperative acuity prior to initial PRK. This suggests that retreated eyes, although often achieving 6/12 unaided acuity, are unlikely, as a group, to enjoy as favorable visual outcomes as those eyes that require only one treatment. The authors noted that the visual recovery period after retreatment might be as long as 12 months.

Williams[48] reported the results of Visx multizone PRK using the Visx laser system in 88 highly myopic eyes, ranging from –6.0 to –20.0 D, with astigmatism of up to 5.5 D. Ablation zones were 5–6 mm. At 12 months postoperatively, 63.6% of the eyes were within ±1.0 D of attempted correction and 85% were within ±2.0 D. However, 14% of eyes had lost two lines of best corrected visual acuity at 1 year. In the group with lower myopic errors (–6.0 to –10.0 D), the regression rate was 14%, compared to 20% for corrections from –10.0 to –15.0 D and 33.3% for corrections over –15.0 D. Interestingly, 83% of the eyes had residual astigmatism of 1.0 D or less. All eyes had corneal haze of grade 1 or less at 6 months. The author concluded that high myopia can be treated with reasonable success using excimer laser and a multizone technique. Predictability was greater in the group with myopia ranging from –6.0 to –10.0 D.

VISX: SUMMARY OF EUROPEAN STUDIES

Excimer laser PRK/PARK using a Visx 20/20B with 6 mm multizone algorithm appears to be highly successful for treating myopia up to –10.00 D. European results have demonstrated that in low myopia of up to 5.0 or 6.0 D, approximately 85–94% of eyes will obtain 6/12 unaided acuity and more than 80% will be ±1.0 D of intended correction,[35,36,42,43,46] whereas in high myopia of –6.00 to –10.00 D, although more than 75% of eyes may achieve 6/12 unaided,[42,43,46] less than two-thirds

Table 12.5

Summary results of large representative European studies utilizing Visx* or Meditec† laser technology to perform myopic photorefractive keratectomy.

Group (year) reference	Number of eyes	Follow-up (months)	Pre-PRK myopia (D)	Within ± 1 D emmetropia	20/40 + UCVA	Eyes losing 2 or more lines of BSCVA
McGhee et al* (1995)[46]	176	9	≤ –5	84%	94%	0%
			–5.1 to –10	58%	83%	0%
			–10.1 to –15	28%	32%	2%
Aron-Rosa et al* (1995)[37]	124	6	–0.7 to > –19	NR	63%	NR
Williams* (1994)[48]	88	6–12	–6 to –20.00	63.6%	NR	14%
Les Jardins et al† (1994)[52]	63	> 6	≤ –3	91%	NR	NR
			> –3 to < –6	62%	NR	NR
			> –6.01	41%	NR	14%

will be ±1.0 D of intended correction.[46,48] Although results for treatment greater than –10.0 D look promising, insufficient long-term data on a large number of patients are available in this extremely myopic group, and due to the increased risk of loss of BSCVA at this level and the increasing availability of LASIK, many practitioners are currently placing a voluntary upper limit of –8.00 to –10.0 D for surface-based PRK. Successful retreatment of myopic regression looks feasible if patients are selected carefully and sufficient time is allowed between initial PRK and retreatment; however, despite improved visual results following retreatment, many of these eyes will still lose significant lines of BSCVA. Results of Visx laser PRK are summarized in Table 12.5.

MEDITEC: THE EUROPEAN EXPERIENCE

The scanning slit technique of PRK was developed by Meditec/Aesculap in Germany and the photoablation pattern for myopic or hyperopic correction is achieved by (non-erodible) masks mounted on suction rings that have to be adjusted and fixed to the subject's eye (Fig. 12.5).

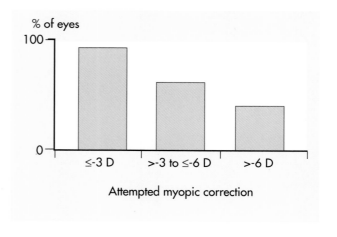

Figure 12.5 *Percentage of eyes within ±1.0 D of emmetropia after PRK related to attempted myopic correction. (Leroux les Jardins et al, 1994[52].)*

Dausch and co-authors conducted a retrospective study on 134 sighted eyes treated by a Meditec laser system.[49] The attempted correction ranged from –3.0 to –15.0 D, using an optical zone diameter of 5 mm. Postoperatively, the authors reported a reduction in myopia by 10.6 D in a group with high myopia (–10.0

to –20.0 D), and this compared with a mean correction of 13.4 D in a group with extreme myopia (over –20.0 D). In eyes with myopia of less than –6.00 D, 88% of the eyes achieved a refraction within ±1.0 D of desired correction 3 months postoperatively. Regression was reported by the authors to have occurred in all patients during the first 6 months post surgery (range 2.0–5.0 D) but only 2% of the patients were reported to have had clinically significant corneal haze at 6 months.

Ehlers and co-workers[50] reported results of excimer laser PRK using the Meditec system in 40 eyes of 20 patients, again using a 5 mm diameter ablation zone. At 6 months, the eyes with an attempted refractive change of –5.0 to –8.0 D, were undercorrected by 2.5 D in 10% of the cases and in the higher treatment group, with attempted refractive change of between –9.0 and –12.0 D, 50% of the eyes were undercorrected by more than 2.5 D. At 6 months follow-up, 72% of the eyes with an attempted refractive change of between –5.0 and –8.0 D had an unchanged or improved best corrected visual acuity; however, in eyes with attempted refractive correction of between –9.0 and –12.0 D, BSCVA had actually decreased in 56% of eyes. Corneal haze was more severe in eyes with 9.0 to 12.0 D of attempted refraction change.

In a larger study of excimer laser PRK using Meditec laser technology in 325 myopic eyes, Ditzen et al[51] reported higher attempted corrections were associated with greater myopic regression. Indeed, in eyes with the least myopia (≤ –6.0 D), mean regression after 12 months was 1.0 D, whereas, in corrections of between –6.25 and –15.0 D, the mean regression was approximately 2.0 D and, in eyes with extreme myopia (greater than –15.5 D), up to 5.0 D of regression was reported. At 6 months, 83% of the eyes had regained preoperative BSCVA, increasing to 99% after 12 months. Subepithelial corneal haze occurred in nearly all the patients after PRK and the risk of a confluent scar increased with ablation depth in excess of 100 μm. Interestingly, the haze appeared less intense in female patients. The authors concluded that corrections for extremely high myopia were not as stable as in the eyes with less myopia and that ablation depth is the main factor in regression after PRK for myopia.

Leroux les Jardins and colleagues reviewed the result of PRK with a 5 mm ablation zone in 73 myopic eyes of 54 patients[52] with preoperative myopia of –1.25 to –9.0 D. Mean preoperative myopia for all eyes was reported as –3.8 D and mean postoperative myopia was –0.6 D after 6 months, with an associated mean unaided visual acuity of

20/30. Six months after PRK, 91% of the eyes with preoperative refractions of less than –3.0 D, 52% of the eyes with preoperative refraction between –3.1 and –6.0 D, and 41% of the eyes with preoperative refractions of greater than –6 D were within 1 D of emmetropia (Fig. 12.5).

These authors reported significant loss of best corrected visual acuity with 8% of the eyes losing one line and 15% of the eyes losing two lines or more of BSCVA at 6 months. Notably, at 1 year, 4% had lost one line whilst 20% had lost two or more lines of BSCVA. The mean regression from 1 month to 6 months was reported to be 0.38 D in the low myopia group, 1.00 D in the medium myopia group, and 1.7 D in the high myopia group (Fig. 12.6). The authors concluded that the main complication in this study was undercorrection rather than overcorrection.

To improve the stability of refraction after PRK attempting to correct higher degrees of myopia, Dausch and co-authors[53] developed a new ablation profile with a 1.5 mm wide tapered transition zone bordering the refractive zone. The diameter of the refractive zone was 4 mm, whilst the total area of treatment was 7 mm. With attempted corrections between –10.0 to –13.0 D, the results of six eyes of

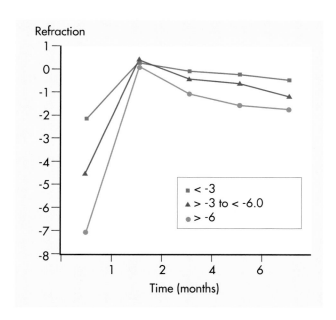

Figure 12.6 *Evolution of mean refraction, preoperative to postoperative, related to attempted myopic correction. (Leroux les Jardins, 1994[52].)*

six patients were reported. In contrast to the regression noted in previous studies,[49–52] the change in refraction in five eyes, 12 months after surgery, was less than or equal to 1.0 D as compared with the first month postoperatively.[53] The authors concluded that a tapered transition zone for high myopia produced less regression after PRK when compared with a conventional ablation profile.

Wetterwald,[54] reporting results of PRK in 30 myopic eyes between –4.0 and –16.0 D, noted a tendency to overcorrection in higher myopia and undercorrection in low myopia. Regression of up to 3.0 D was common in high myopia and no regression was reported in low myopia.

In a recent series reporting 1 year follow-up on 100 myopic eyes treated by a Meditec laser,[55] 88% of the patients with –6.0 D or less attempted correction achieved a refraction within ±1.0 D of emmetropia and 50% of eyes in the group with myopic correction between –6.1 and –10.1 D achieved a refraction within ±1.0 D of emmetropia. However, only 33% of the patients with myopia over –10 D achieved a refraction within ±1 D of emmetropia.

From the published data it is evident that early Meditec series demonstrate a high level of myopic regression and a surprisingly high level of eyes demonstrate loss of BSCVA. In later studies, refractive predictability appears to approach that of Summit and Visx in corrections of up to –6.00 D. Further data are required to assess the efficacy of the Meditec system in high or extreme myopia.

NIDEK AND COHERENT SCHWIND EXCIMER LASERS

Although many Schwind and Nidek units are presently operating in Europe, no publications on the results of PRK with these machines have yet reached the scientific press.

A preliminary report on the results of a single-center study from Bratislava, Slovakia, documents first-year data with the Coherent Schwind excimer laser.[56] One-hundred-and-seventy-five eyes of 97 patients with myopia between –1.00 and –7.50 D were evaluated between 3 months and 1 year post PRK. At latest follow-up, in eyes treated for low myopia (< –3.00 D), 98% were ±1.00 D of intended, whilst in moderate myopia (–3.25 to –7.50 D), 83% of eyes were within ±1.00 D of emmetropia. Overall, 98% of eyes obtained 20/40 or better unaided acuity

and loss of two lines of BSCVA occurred in 0.6%. These are very promising results but represent very short-term follow-up. Further data are eagerly awaited.

Short-term data on the Nidek EC-5000 also show promise. Flayeh reported 90% of eyes within ±1.00 D and 98% 6/12 or better 3 months post PRK, in a group of 162 eyes with attempted corrections of –1.0 to –11.0 D.[57] Lavery noted similar results with 96% predictability within ±1.00 D up to –6.00 D, and 65% predictability between –6.10 and –12.50 D.[58]

ASTIGMATISM RESULTS WITH SUMMIT, VISX AND MEDITEC LASERS

A fuller discussion of excimer laser photoastigmatic refractive keratectomy is covered in Chapter 15 and, therefore, only a few salient features of the European experience will be covered in this section.

Lipshitz and colleagues[59] performed combined astigmatic keratotomy and PRK for compound myopic astigmatism. Eleven eyes underwent astigmatic keratotomy 1 month prior to PRK. In nine eyes arcuate incisions were performed, in one eye a modified Ruiz procedure was performed and in one eye radial T-cuts were done. The mean SE was –8.26 ±2.51 D after the astigmatic keratotomy but before PRK, and this was reduced to an SE of –0.36 ± 0.93 D after PRK. The mean cylinder of –3.11 ± 1.16 D prior to PRK was reduced to 0.13 ± 0.9 D following PRK. The authors concluded that combined astigmatic keratotomy and PRK are effective treatments for compound myopic astigmatism (Fig. 12.7).

Seiler and colleagues (1988)[60] initially corrected astigmatism with the excimer laser by creating linear corneal T excisions in 13 eyes of 12 patients. Although induced refractive changes of up to 4.6 D were obtained, this technique was abandoned due to unpredictability of result and cylindrical regression. Schipper and colleagues,[61] revisiting this technique (1994), reported results on transverse keratectomies with excimer laser on seven eyes of four patients with a range of astigmatism from 4.25 to 7.0 D. Mean astigmatism prior to laser surgery was 5.32 D and 1 year post excimer laser this had reduced by only 12% to 4.68 D.

Another early method employed for toric ablations involved the use of an ablatable mask.[62,63] The mask was placed on the cornea and the beam applied to the surface of the mask. The surgeon had to

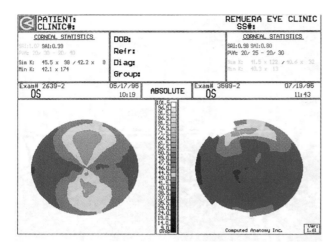

Figure 12.7 *Preoperative corneal topography of a left eye with a refraction of −0.75/−3.25 at 180° (left image). Following transverse astigmatic keratotomy combined with a spherical PRK the patient obtained 6/6 vision without correction and corneal astigmatism was reduced from 3.3 D at 8° to 0.9 D at 32° (right image). (Courtesy of Dr Peter Ring MD.)*

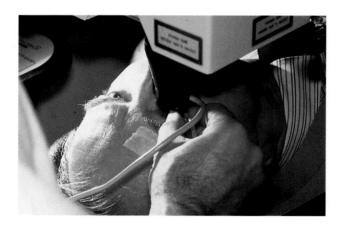

Figure 12.8 *Meditec astigmatism mask in situ during treatment of myopic astigmatism. (Courtesy of Meditec.)*

manually hold the eye-cup and center the mask along the laser axis. A mask is moulded so that the superficial surface represents the desired final contour of the cornea. This superficial surface contour is then transposed to the cornea by mask ablation. Despite early promise[64,65] of the technique and variations in the method of fixating the mask,[66]

the technique has never been widely utilized, and is presently being supplanted by the newer 'mask in rail' apogee system, in which the mask is placed in the path of the beam, within the excimer laser, rather than held in front of the cornea.

Dausch and colleagues[67] reported on a technique of toric ablation to correct astigmatism using the Meditech excimer laser and a non-ablatable mask with an hour glass-shaped opening. The mask rotates variably over 360° and by varying the angular distances the surgeon can increase ablation depth in any desired meridian (Fig. 12.8). A total of 73 eyes with simple, myopic, mixed or irregular astigmatism were treated. In the group with simple astigmatism, preoperative refractive cylinder ranged from −1.0 to −11.0 D (mean refractive cylinder −3.3 ± 2.4 D) and in 19 eyes, with follow-up of 12 months, the refractive cylinder was reduced to −0.3 ± 0.58 D (mean ± standard deviation). (See Chapter 15 for further discussion of this technique.)

MISCELLANEOUS CLINICAL POINTERS

Tavola and colleagues[68] evaluated the results of 160 consecutive unilateral PRKs to assess the role of surgeons' skill on the final results of the surgery. At 1 year follow-up, uncorrected visual acuity and refractive errors were used as parameters of efficacy and predictability, and BSCVA loss and corneal clarity as safety parameters. In order to draw up a learning curve, the mean values for each parameter were calculated by arbitrarily grouping the first 10 cases of each surgeon (n=4) in the first group, and the second 10 cases in the second group and so forth. The authors concluded an increase in uncorrected visual acuity, smaller residual refractive error and corneal clarity appeared to improve as the surgeon became more experienced, while the loss of BCSVA was not significantly influenced by increased surgical experience. Data from this study suggest that the surgeons' skill does, indeed, play a part in the final results of PRK in the correction of myopia.

A common complication of radial keratotomy, diurnal fluctuation of vision, is not common following PRK. Seiler and colleagues[69] reported on morning and evening visual acuity measurements, refractions, autorefractor and autokeratometry readings on 10 patients who complained of diurnal fluctuations in vision after PRK. The authors noted that post-PRK eyes demonstrated a mild hyperopic shift as the day progressed, but no change in autorefraction or autokeratometry were measured. Although the mechanism for this phenomenon is unknown, the authors concluded that the refractive shift may be due to a reduced accommodation in the evening.

Environmental factors may play a role in PRK outcomes.[70] Stevens et al noted that patients who underwent PRK during the summer months were significantly more undercorrected at 1 month than patients who had the procedure during winter. The difference of 0.5 D was maintained at the 3 and 6 month assessment. The authors concluded that temperature or humidity levels may interfere with the preoperative calibration of the laser, or absorption of laser energy. The authors also noted that anecdotal reports abound of patients who develop severe post-PRK haze shortly after an episode of sunbathing or skiing, and a possible role of increased sun or ultraviolet light in the summer as a causal agent in regression in these eyes remains to be ascertained, although it must always be noted that strong sunlight in the UK is uncommon, even in the 'summer'.

Intraocular pressure (IOP) increases have been reported in clinical series of excimer laser PRK, and appear to be related to prolonged therapy with topical corticosteroids. Studies have demonstrated a rise in IOP following prolonged administration of topical steroids in 30% or more of 'normal' eyes.[71] However, Gartry and colleagues[7] noted a significant rise in IOP in only 12% of eyes following PRK.

It has been confirmed that there is a positive correlation of measured IOP using applanation tonometry with increasing corneal curvature.[72] Possible inaccuracies of the Goldmann applanation tonometry technique following PRK, due to relative flattening and thinning of the central cornea, which may result in falsely low IOP measurement, were first highlighted by Phelan and colleagues.[73] These authors concluded that until definitive studies have been completed, glaucoma and ocular hypertension are relative contraindications to PRK.

REFERENCES

1. Seiler T, Wollensak J, In vivo experiments with the excimer laser—technical parameters and healing processes, *Ophthalmologica* (1986) **192**:65–70.
2. Seiler T, Wollensak J, Myopic photorefractive keratectomy with the excimer laser. One year follow-up, *Ophthalmology* (1991) **98**(8):1156–63.
3. Seiler T, Holschbach A, Derse M, Jean B, Genth U, Complications of myopic photorefractive keratectomy with the excimer laser, *Ophthalmology* (1994) **101**(1):153–60.
4. Seiler T, Genth U, Holschbach A, Derse M, Aspheric photorefractive keratectomy with excimer laser, *Refract Corneal Surg* (1993) **9**(3):166–72.
5. Gartry D, Kerr Muir M, Marshall J, Excimer laser treatment of corneal surface pathology: a laboratory and clinical study, *Br J Ophthalmol* (1991) **75**(5):258–69.
6. Gartry DS, Kerr Muir MG, Marshall J, Photorefractive keratectomy with an argon fluoride excimer laser: a clinical study, *Refract Corneal Surg* (1991) **7**(6):420–35.
7. Gartry DS, Kerr Muir MG, Marshall J, Excimer laser photorefractive keratectomy. 18 month follow-up, *Ophthalmology* (1992) **99**(8):1209–19.
8. Tengroth B, Epstein D, Fagerholm P, Hamberg-Nystrom H, Fitzsimmons TD, Excimer laser photorefractive keratectomy for myopia. Clinical results in sighted eyes, *Ophthalmology* (1993) **100**(5):739–45.
9. Epstein D, Fagerholm P, Hamberg-Nystrom H, Tengroth B, Twenty-four month follow-up of excimer laser photorefractive keratectomy for myopia. Refractive and visual acuity results, *Ophthalmology* (1994) **101**(9):1558–63.
10. Ficker LA, Bates AK, Steele AD, et al, Excimer laser photorefractive keratectomy for myopia: 12 month follow-up, *Eye* (1993) **7**:617–24.
11. Brancato R, Tavola A, Carones F, et al, Excimer laser photorefractive keratectomy for myopia: results in 1165 eyes. Italian study group, *Refract Corneal Surg* (1993) **9**(2):95–104.
12. Tutton MK, Ramsell TG, Garston JB, et al, Photorefractive keratectomy for myopia: 6-month results in 95 eyes, *Refract Corneal Surg* (1993) **9**(Suppl):S103–S104.
13. Salorio DP, Costa J, Larena C, et al, Photorefractive keratectomy for myopia: 18-month results in 178 eyes, *Refract Corneal Surg* (1993) **2**(Suppl):S108–S110.
14. Orssaud C, Ganem S, Binaghi M, et al, Photorefractive keratectomy in 176 eyes: one year follow-up, *Refract Corneal Surg* (1994) **10**(Suppl):S199–S205.
15. Murta JN, Proenca R, Van Velze RA, Travasso A, Photorefractive keratectomy for myopia in 98 eyes, *Refract Corneal Surg* (1994) **10**(Suppl):S231–S234.
16. Buratto L, Ferrari M, Photorefractive keratectomy for myopia from 6.00 D to 10.00 D, *Refract corneal surg* (1993) **9**(Suppl):S34–S36.
17. Lavery FL, Photorefractive keratectomy in 472 eyes, *Refract Corneal Surg* (1993) **9**(Suppl):S98–S100.
18. Tavola A, Brancato R, Galli L, Carones F, Esente S, Photorefractive keratectomy for myopia: single vs double-zone treatment in 166 eyes, *Refract Corneal Surg* (1993) **9**(Suppl):S48–S52.
19. Scialdone A, Carones F, Bertuzzi A, Brancato R, Randomized study of single vs double exposure in myopic PRK, *Refract Corneal Surg* (1993) **9**(Suppl):S41–S43.
20. Salz JJ, Maguen E, Nesburn AB, et al, A two year experience with excimer laser photorefractive keratectomy for myopia, *Ophthalmology* (1993) **100**:873–82.

21. O'Brart DP, Gartry DS, Lohmann CP, Muir MG, Marshall J, Excimer laser photorefractive keratectomy for myopia: comparison of 4.00 and 5.00 millimeter ablation zones, *J Refract Corneal Surg* (1994) **10**(2):87–94.

22. O'Brart DP, Corbett MC, Lohnmann CP, Kerr Muir MG, Marshall J, The effects of ablation diameter on the outcome of excimer laser photorefractive keratectomy. A prospective, randomized, double-blind study, *Arch Ophthalmol* (1995) **113**(4):438–43.

23. Corbett MC, Verma S, O'Brart DP, Oliver KO, Heacock G, Marshall J, Effect of ablation profile on wound healing and visual performance 1 year after excimer laser photorefractive keratectomy, *Br J Ophthalmol* (1996) **80**:224–34.

24. O'Brart DP, Lohmann CP, Fitzke FW, et al, Disturbances in night vision after excimer laser photorefractive keratectomy, *Eye* (1994) **8**:46–51.

25. Gartry DS, Muir MGK, Lohmann CP, Marshall J, The effect of topical corticosteroids on refractive outcome and corneal haze after photorefractive keratectomy: a prospective, randomized, double-blind trial, *Arch Ophthalmol* (1992) **110**:944–52.

26. Fagerholm P, Hamberg-Nystrom H, Tengroth B, Epstein D, Effect of postoperative steroids on the refractive outcome of photorefractive keratectomy for myopia with the Summit excimer laser, *J Cataract Refract Surg* (1994) **20**(Suppl):212–5.

27. Carones F, Brancato R, Venturi E, Scialdone A, Bertuzzi A, Tavola A, Efficacy of corticosteroids in reversing regression after myopic photorefractive keratectomy, *Refract Corneal Surg* (1993) **9**(Suppl):S52–S56.

28. Gartry DS, Kerr Muir M, Marshall J, The effect of topical corticosteroids on refraction and corneal haze following excimer laser treatment of myopia: an update. A prospective, randomised, double-masked study, *Eye* (1993) **7**:584–90.

29. Tengroth B, Fagerholm P, Soderberg P, et al, Effect of corticosteroids in postoperative care following photorefractive keratectomies, *Refract Corneal Surg* (1993) **9**(Suppl):61–64.

30. O'Brart DPS, Lohmann CP, Klonos G, et al, The effects of topical corticosteroids and plasmin inhibitors on refractive outcome, haze, and visual performance after photorefractive keratectomy. A prospective, randomised observer-masked study, *Ophthalmology* (1994) **101**:1565–74.

31. Epstein D, Tengroth B, Fagerholm P, Hamberg-Nystrom H, Excimer retreatment of regression after photorefractive keratectomy, *Am J Ophthalmol* (1994) **117**(4):456–61.

32. Seiler T, Derse M, Pham T, Repeated excimer laser treatment after photorefractive keratectomy, *Arch Ophthalmol* (1992) **110**:1230–3.

33. Seiler T, Jean B, Photorefractive keratectomy as a second attempt to correct myopia after radial keratotomy, *Refract Corneal Surg* (1992) **8**(3):211–4.

34. Meza J, Perez-Santonja JJ, Moreno E, Zato MA, Photorefractive keratectomy after radial keratotomy, *J Cataract Refract Surg* (1994) **20**(5):485–9.

35. Hamberg-Nystrom H, Fagerholm P, Tengroth B, Epstein D, Photorefractive keratectomy for low myopia at 5 mm treatment diameter. A comparison of two excimer lasers, *Acta Ophthalmologica* (1994) **72**(4):453–6.

36. Aron-Rosa D, Gross M, Boulnoy JL, et al, Excimer laser of the cornea: qualitative and quantitative aspects of photoablation according to the energy density, *J Cataract Refract Surg* (1986) **12**:27–33.

37. Aron-Rosa DS, Colin J, Aron B, et al, Clinical results of excimer laser photorefractive keratectomy: a multicentre study of 265 eyes, *J Cataract Refract Surg* (1995) **21**:644–52.

38. Stevens JD, Steele AD McG, Ficker LA, et al, Prospective randomized study of two topical steroid regimes after excimer laser PRK, *Invest Ophthalmol Vis Sci* (1994) **35**(4):1839 (abst).

39. Stevens JD, Ficker LA, Steele AD McG, et al, Excimer laser treatment of myopia with primary astigmatism, *Invest Ophthalmol Vis Sci* (1993) **34**:799 (abst).

40. Stevens JD, One year wait urged for photorefractive keratectomy retreatment, *Ocular Surgery News* (1995) **13**(15):24.

41. Gartry DS, Larkin DFP, Hill AR, Ficker LA, Steele AD McG, Retreatment for significant regression following excimer laser photorefractive keratectomy (PRK): a prospective, randomised, masked trial, *Proceedings of the 2nd Annual Scientific meeting of MCLOSA* (abstract) (1995).

42. Bryce IG, McGhee CNJ, Weed KH, Anastas CN, Excimer laser surgery for myopia and astigmatism with the VisX 20/20B, *Proceedings of the second annual United Kingdom International Ophthalmic Excimer Laser Congress* (1995) **2**:21 (abst).

43. Weed KH, McGhee CNJ, Bryce IG, Hazy days? The refractive outlook of photorefractive keratectomy/photo-astigmatic keratectomy, *Ophthalmic Physiological Optics* (1995) **15**:367–9.

44. Webber SK, McGhee CNJ, Bryce IG, Decentration of photorefractive keratectomy ablation zones after excimer laser surgery for myopia, *J Cataract Refract Surg* (1996) **22**:299–303.

45. Phelan PS, Bryce IG, McGhee CNJ, The successful treatment of high and extreme myopia by excimer laser, *Proceedings of the second annual United Kingdom International Ophthalmic Excimer laser congress* (1995) **2**:49 (abst).

46. McGhee CNJ, Bryce IG, Anastas CN, Weed KH, Two year follow-up of photorefractive keratectomy and photo-astigmatic keratectomy, *Proceedings of the Royal Australian College of Ophthalmologists 27th Annual Scientific Congress*, (1995) **S14**:69 (abst).

47. McGhee CNJ, Webber SK, Bryce IG, Anastas CN, Weed KH, Individualizing retreatment by excimer laser, *Proceedings of the International Society of Refractive Surgery 1995 Mid-Summer Symposium* (1995) 92–93 (abst).

48. Williams DK, Excimer laser photorefractive keratectomy for extreme myopia, *J Cataract Refract Surg* (1996) **22**:910–14.

49. Dausch D, Klein R, Schroder E, Photoablative, refractive keratectomy in treatment of myopia. A case study of 134 myopic eyes with 6-months follow-up, *Fortschritte der Ophthalmologie* (1991) **88**(6):770–6.

50. Ehlers N, Hjortal JO, Excimer laser refractive keratectomy for high myopia. 6-month follow-up of patients treated bilaterally, *Acta Ophthalmologica* (1992) **70**:578–86.

51. Ditzen K, Anschutz T, Schroder E, Photorefractive keratectomy to treat low, medium and high myopia: a multicentre study, *J Cataract Refract Surg* (1994) **20** (Suppl):234–8.

52. Leroux les Jardins S, Auclin F, Roman S, Burtschy B, Leroux les Jardins J, Results of photorefractive keratectomy

on 63 myopic eyes with six months minimum follow-up, *J Cataract Refract Surg* (1994) **20**(Suppl):223–8.

53. Dausch D, Klein R, Schroder E, Dausch B, Excimer laser photorefractive keratectomy with tapered transition zone for high myopia. A preliminary report of six cases, *J Cataract Refract Surg* (1993) **19**(5):590–4.

54. Wetterwald N, 2 years experience in the treatment of myopia with photokeratectomy, *Klinische Monatblatter fur Augenheilkunde* (1994) **204**:416–7.

55. Benjamin L, Cox SN, Jenkins LM, One year results of myopia treatment with the Meditech excimer laser, *Proceedings of the first annual United Kingdom excimer laser congress 1994* (Abst).

56. Krueger RR, Cernak A, Marcellino G, Singer V, Assil K, Schanzlin D, Photorefractive keratectomy for low and medium myopia with the Coherent Schwind excimer laser, *Proceedings of the International Society of Refractive Surgery 1995 Mid-Summer Symposium* (1995) **39** (abst).

57. Flayeh H, Photorefractive keratectomy for myopia and myopic astigmatism using the Nidek EC-5000 excimer laser, *Proceedings of the second annual United Kingdom International Ophthalmic Excimer Laser Congress* (1995) **2**:20 (abst).

58. Lavery FL, Twelve months follow-up using the Nidek EC5000 excimer laser, *Proceedings of the International Society of Refractive Surgery 1995 Mid-Summer Symposium* (1995) **37** (abst).

59. Lipshitz I, Loewenstein A, Lazar M, Astigmatic keratotomy followed by photorefractive keratectomy in the treatment of compound myopic astigmatism, *Refract Corneal Surg* (1994) **10**(Suppl):S282–S284.

60. Seiler T, Bende T, Wollensak J, Trokel S, Excimer laser keratectomy for correction of astigmatism, *Am J Ophthalmol* (1988) **105**:117–24.

61. Schipper I, Suppelt C, Senn P, Correction of astigmatism with excimer laser transverse keratectomy, *Acta Ophthalmologica* (1994) **72**(1):39–42.

62. Gordon M, Brint SF, Durrie DS, Photorefractive keratectomy at 193 nm using an erodible mask, *Ophthalmic Technologies II Proc SPIE* (1992) **1644**:11–19.

63. Muller D, Laser reprofiling system and methods, U.S. Patent Number 4: 856, 513.

64. Brancato R, Carones F, Trabucchi G, Scialdone A, Tavola A, The erodible mask in photorefractive keratectomy for myopia and astigmatism, *Refract Corneal Surg* (1993) **9**(Suppl):S125–S130.

65. Cherry PM, Tutton MK, Bell A, Neave C, Fichte C, Treatment of myopic astigmatism with photorefractive keratectomy using an erodible mask, *Refract Corneal Surg* (1994) **10**(Suppl):S239–S245.

66. Gobbi PG, Carones F, Scagliotti F, Venturi E, Brancato R, A simplified method to perform photorefractive keratectomy using an erodible mask, *Refract Corneal Surg* (1994) **10**(Suppl):S246–S249.

67. Dausch D, Klein R, Landesz M, Schroder E, Photorefractive keratectomy to correct astigmatism with myopia or hyperopia, *J Cataract Refractive Surg* (1994) **20**(Suppl):252–7.

68. Tavola A, Carones F, Galli L, Fontanella G, Brancato R, The learning curve in myopic photorefractive keratectomy, *Refract Corneal Surg* (1994) **10**(Suppl):S188–S193.

69. Seiler T, Hell K, Wollensak J, Diurnal variation in refraction after excimer laser photorefractive keratectomy, *Ger J Ophthalmol* (1992) **1**:19–21.

70. Stevens JD, Seasonal variation seen in photorefractive keratectomy results, *Ocular Surgery News* (1995) **13**(15): 24.

71. Becker B, Hahn KA, Topical corticosteroids and heredity in primary open-angle glaucoma, *Am J Ophthalmol* (1964) **57**:543–51.

72. Mark HH, Corneal curvature in applanation tonometry, *Am J Ophthalmology* (1973) **76**:223–4.

73. Phelan PS, McGhee CNJ, Bryce IG, Excimer laser PRK and corticosteroid induced intraocular pressure elevation: the tip of an emerging iceberg? *Br J Ophthalmol* (1994) **78**:802–3.

Chapter 13 Photorefractive keratectomy and LASIK with the Chiron–Technolas Keracor 116 excimer laser: the European experience

Chris P Lohmann, Jose L Guell, Helmut Sachs and Johannes Junger

THE KERACOR 116 EXCIMER LASER

The Chiron–Technolas Keracor 116 excimer laser (Fig. 13.1) is a 'new generation laser', which has the capability of two approaches to photorefractive keratectomy (PRK), both the large area technique and the scanning technique.

Basically, the laser consists of a laser chamber, a gaseous mixture tank, a condenser for electric charge emission, an optical arm for transmission of the laser beam, a coaxial microscope, an alignment system consisting of both a green helium neon laser and a red diode laser, and a computer. The computer software controls the laser action, the mechanical iris diaphragm, and the scanning mirror. The laser medium of this excimer laser is argon fluoride (ArF) with an emission wavelength of 193 nm, a switchable pulse repetition rate of either 2, 5, or 10 Hz and a fixed radiant exposure of 120 mJ/cm² at the cornea.

The optical ray consists of seven optical elements (Fig. 13.2). The excimer laser tube has a maximum energy of approximately 500 mJ per pulse, and in order to keep the energy density at the following optical elements as low as possible, the electrodes within the laser tube have a very gentle curvature. A beam homogenizing system converts the laser beam profile from a Gaussian profile to a linear profile at the center of the beam. The laser beam then passes through a mechanical iris diaphragm, placed concentric to the laser beam. This motorized iris diaphragm progressively opens with a given number of laser pulses being directed through the aperture in the diaphragm at each aperture size, resulting in an ablation pattern with concentric circular steps. The maximum diameter of the iris diaphragm is 14 mm. The following projecting lens system reduces the size of the laser beam by half such that the maximum available beam size at the cornea is 7 mm in diameter.

The 'scanning mirror' consists of two mirrors, which direct the laser beam on the corneal surface within an area of 15 × 15 mm². This mirror system allows the circular laser beam to be placed accurately anywhere upon the corneal surface within this area. For refractive surgery, the iris diaphragm and the position of the scanning mirrors are under control of the computer software according to certain nomograms, which allow the treatment of myopia, astigmatism, and hyperopia.

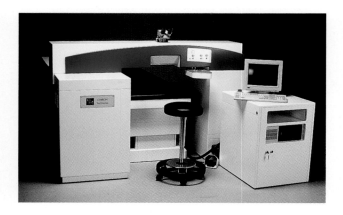

Figure 13.1 *The Chiron–Technolas Keracor 116 excimer laser.*

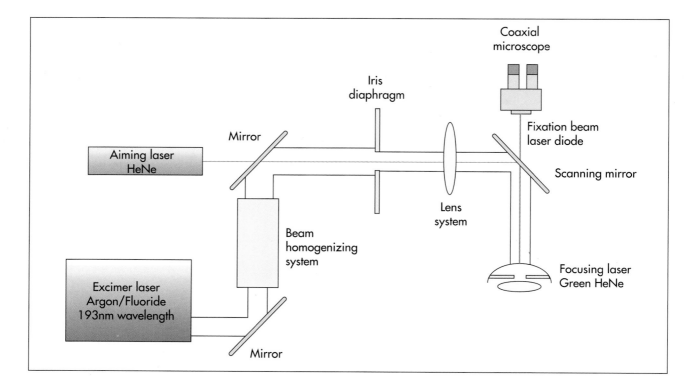

Figure 13.2 *Schematic diagram of the various optical elements of the Keracor 116 excimer laser.*

EYE TRACKING

A feature of the Keracor 116 excimer laser is the use of an automatic eye tracker. This eye tracker consists of an infrared lighting system, which does not interfere with the surgical illumination, and a high resolution S-VHS camera. The eye tracker uses the entrance pupil as the reference marker for the position of the cornea. The camera is able to detect 50 frames per second with the output signal of the camera being analyzed in real time at a spatial resolution of 25 μm/pixel. The pupil edge is recognized at the beginning of the procedure and the computer calculates the co-ordinates of its center. Pupil identification takes place every 20 ms during ablation and the position of the pupil edge is compared to the initially evaluated image. If a displacement is detected the laser beam is realigned in the direction of the pupil displacement. The correction time for the whole procedure is 40 ms; however, if the eye moves more than 2.5 mm in the vertical or horizontal axis, the camera will lose the image of the pupil and the laser is automatically turned off.

PHOTOREFRACTIVE KERATECTOMY

The Chiron–Technolas Keracor 116 excimer laser was first introduced into European clinical trials in July 1992. Since then, more than 14 000 myopic eyes, with or without astigmatism, have been treated with this excimer laser at 40 clinics in Europe.

ALGORITHMS FOR MYOPIA

For myopia two software versions are available, the 'transition zone software', and the 'multizone software'. The difference between both software versions are highlighted in Figure 13.3. In respect to the following data analysis (n=1369), 986 eyes were treated with the transition zone software, and 383 procedures were performed with the multizone software.

PATIENT SELECTION

Careful patient selection and appropriate counselling are essential before refractive surgery is performed. Patients consenting to undertake excimer laser PRK should understand the nature of the treatment and have detailed information. It is most important that prospective patients have realistic expectations in relation to the outcome of the procedure (see Chapter 8). The phenomenon of presbyopia and the possible need for reading glasses must be explained prior to surgery.

The current inclusion criteria for PRK were based on the results of various clinical studies, which predicted that treatment to within ±1.00 D of intended correction may be achieved in eyes with a preoperative myopic refraction of up to 8.00 D.[1–12] Patients were over the age of 18 and demonstrated stable refractions for at least two years.

Any patient with a history of eye disease, in particular keratoconus, herpes keratitis, glaucoma or macular diseases was excluded. Patients with systemic disorders such as diabetes, autoimmune or collagen vascular diseases, were also excluded because of the potentially serious problems of delayed or abnormal postoperative wound healing.

Patients were informed that treatment would be performed to one eye in advance of the other, with an interval of at least four months being advisable before treatment of the second eye. Between the two PRK procedures either a contact lens was worn in the untreated eye, or, if spectacles were used, a balance lens was worn for the treated eye.

PATIENT PREPARATION

Ophthalmic examination included uncorrected and corrected visual acuity, refraction, routine detailed anterior and posterior segment examination, and intraocular pressure measurement. Corneal topography was assessed with computerized videokeratography (CVK) to exclude patients with undiagnosed corneal disorders. Patients were asked to remove hard contact lenses for a minimum of four weeks and soft contact lenses for two weeks prior to surgery.

THE PRK PROCEDURE

The photorefractive keratectomy only required topical anesthetics. The eye to be treated was aligned beneath the laser aperture, and the other non-treated eye was taped shut to facilitate fixation. The patients practised fixating on a red target light until this could be sustained for the predicted duration of the procedure. The patient was informed of the noise and 'burn-like' smell associated with the procedure. The

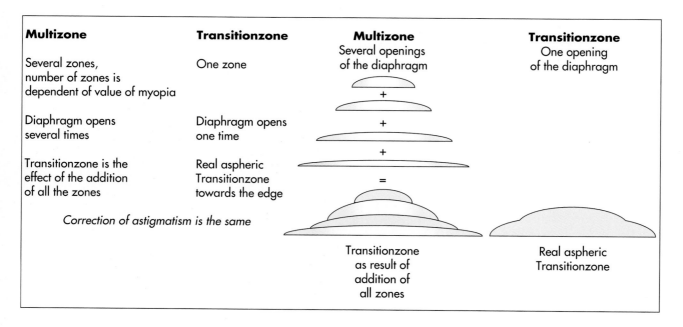

Figure 13.3 *The two software versions available for the treatment of myopia and astigmatism.*

Table 13.1.

Pre- and postoperative refraction for four discrete treatment groups at 1 year after PRK using the Keracor 116 excimer laser.

Preoperative refraction (D)	No. of eyes	Postoperative refraction (D) (mean ± standard deviation)	
up to −2.00	358	−0.25	±0.38
−2.25 to −4.00	472	−0.61	±0.23
−4.25 to −6.00	331	−0.97	±1.16
−6.25 to −8.00	208	−0.65	±0.96

whole PRK procedure took about 15 minutes, which included informing and training the patient, manual debridement of the corneal epithelium, and the surgery. The actual laser beam exposure lasted on average 30 seconds, depending on the amount of myopia to be treated.

POSTOPERATIVE PHARMACEUTICAL TREATMENT

Immediately after the treatment mydriatic drops were instilled. In some clinics a soft contact lens, together with non-steroidal anti-inflammatory drops were used, and in others antibiotic ointment was instilled, and the eye padded until re-epithelialization had occurred.

All study centers used topically applied corticosteroids, mainly fluoromethalone, after re-epithelialization. Unfortunately, since use and duration of topical steroid was physician-preference dependent, there was a large variation in the length of this postoperative treatment, ranging from 1 to 3 months.

CLINICAL RESULTS WITH THE TECHNOLAS-KERACOR 116

In all eyes (n=1369) re-epithelialization took between 48 and 72 hours and no epithelial disorders persisting longer than 4 days were observed.

After a period of hypermetropic overcorrection, of about 2–4 weeks, the refraction tended to stabilize between 1 and 3 months postsurgery, depending upon the degree of myopia corrected. The overall success rate for refractive correction, defined as the percentage of treated eyes in the range of ±1.00 D from the intended final refraction was approximately 91% for corrections up to 8.00 D at 1 year postsurgery. In summary, the mean postoperative

refraction for eyes in this study group was: eyes up to −2.00 D preoperative refraction achieved −0.25 ± 0.38 D (mean ± SD); eyes between −2.00 and −4.00 D achieved −0.61 ± 0.23 D; preoperative refraction between −4.00 and −6.00 D achieved −0.97 ± 1.16 D and refraction between −6.00 and −8.00 D achieved −0.65 ± 0.96 D (Table 13.1).

Uncorrected visual acuity improved postoperatively in all treated eyes. At 12 months 93% of the patients had an unaided Snellen visual acuity (VA) of 6/12 or better, and about 80% of eyes achieved 6/6 or better. Significant changes in best corrected visual acuity (BCVA) have not been observed so far.

A marginal loss of corneal transparency ('haze') could be detected in virtually all patients during the early postoperative period. A faint diffuse subepithelial haze was first apparent after about 4 weeks, increased in intensity to a maximum at about 3 months, and then decreased gradually. After 1 year almost all corneas were clear. None of the treated eyes showed a manifest

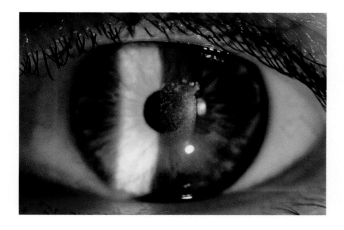

Figure 13.4 *Representative photograph of maximum haze after −5.00 D PRK procedure.*

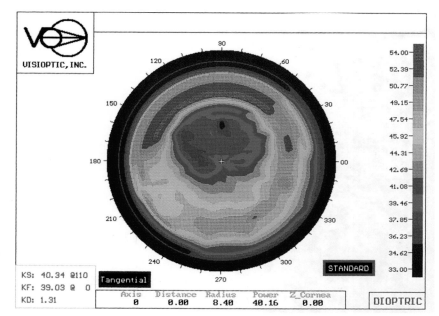

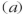
(a)

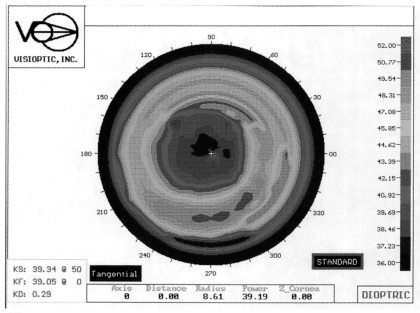

(b)

Figure 13.5 *Corneal topography maps of corneas after myopic PRK treatment. (a) Without the use of the eyetracker. (b) With the use of the eyetracker.*

scar. A typical sample of maximum haze obtained 3 months after PRK is shown in Figure 13.4.

Grossly decentered ablation zones in relation to the pupillary center have not been reported. However, centration was better with the use of the eye tracker (Fig. 13.5). Without the use of the eye tracker (n=988), mean decentration was 0.4 mm, with a range of 0.3–1.1 mm horizontally and 0.3–1.0 mm vertically. In contrast, with the eye tracking system, (n=381) mean decentration was reduced to 0.15 mm, with a range of 0.0–0.2 mm horizontally and 0.0–1.0 mm vertically.

A mild postoperative blepharoptosis was observed in three eyes during the first two postoperative months. This phenomenon may have been related to the use of a lid speculum during surgery.

Approximately 10% of the patients had a measurable rise in intraocular pressure (IOP) of more than 5 mm/Hg detected at 1 month due to topical corticosteroid medication. A change of the steroid type (from dexamethasone to fluorometholone where dexamethasone had been employed) and the application of beta-blockers returned the IOP to within normal limits within 2 weeks.

CONCLUSIONS

Photorefractive keratectomy using the Chiron–Technolas Keracor 116 excimer laser seems to be a safe and effective procedure for the correction of low and moderate degrees of myopia. The patient satisfaction is very high, with around 89% of the patients pleased that they underwent PRK. Even patients with higher degrees of myopia, in whom emmetropia was not achieved, benefited from this surgery by having their myopia significantly reduced. These patients with partial correction were usually pleased, as they benefit from considerable improvement in their unaided vision and less absolute dependence on spectacles or contact lenses. Although not observed in our present patient cohort, potential complications such as loss of BCVA or corneal haze must always be taken into account.

A main advantage of the Chiron–Technolas Keracor 116 excimer laser compared to other commercially available excimer laser systems is the possibility of using a single large ablation zone of up to 7.0 mm. Initial studies in animal models suggested the need to minimize the depth of stromal ablation to avoid detrimental effects of the healing process such as regression of the intended correction and loss of corneal transparency ('haze').[13–16] As small diameter ablation zones result in high dioptric corrections with limited ablation depths,[17] the concept of conservation of stroma resulted in most early clinical trials being conducted with ablation diameters of 4.00 mm or less.[1–3] However, in these early clinical studies it became apparent that the use of such small-sized ablation diameters resulted in visual disturbances associated with pupillary excursions. The combination of large pupillary excursions with small ablation diameters results in the generation of myopic blur

circles.[18] These are apparent to the patient as haloes around point sources of light at night and may cause significant and persistent impairment of night vision.[19,20] In fact, the appearance of haloes around point sources of light at night was one of the most reported complaints in these initial series. This phenomenon resulted in a number of dissatisfied patients who declined treatment of their second eye despite good refractive outcomes. With a 7.00 mm ablation zone, as obtained with the Keracor 116 excimer laser, patients rarely experience the phenomenon of haloes.

Large diameter ablation zones also seem to have a positive effect on the refractive outcome of PRK. In a recent clinical study it was obvious that an ablation zone diameter of 6.00 mm gave a more predictable refractive outcome compared to former trials with small ablation zones by the same investigators.[21]

In conclusion, an improvement in predictability and stability of the refractive change and a reduction in complications impairing performance is found in eyes treated with ablation zone diameters of 6.00 mm or more. In our study using a 7.00 mm ablation zone, the predictability of PRK, in respect to achieving 6/12 unaided VA and refractions within ±1.00 D of intended, is high in procedures up to −10.00 D. Therefore, we suggest that excimer laser myopic PRK should be performed with large ablation zones.

CORRECTION OF ASTIGMATISM

Astigmatism occurs when the refractive elements of the eye are not spherical. It can be defined as that type of refractive anomaly in which no single point focus is formed owing to the unequal refraction of the incident light by the dioptric system of the eye in different meridians.[22,23] Astigmatism can be regular, where the refractive power changes gradually from one meridian to the next by uniform increments, or irregular where the irregularities in the curvature of the meridians conform to no geometrical pattern.[24] The corneal surface is responsible primarily for any astigmatic error and the average difference between the refractive powers of the major and minor corneal meridians is usually between 0.50 and 1.00 D. Such small degrees of ocular astigmatism are of little visual effect; however, astigmatism is a major problem in limiting visual recovery after ocular surgery.[25]

Two experimental approaches have been investigated for excimer laser PRK in the treatment of astig-

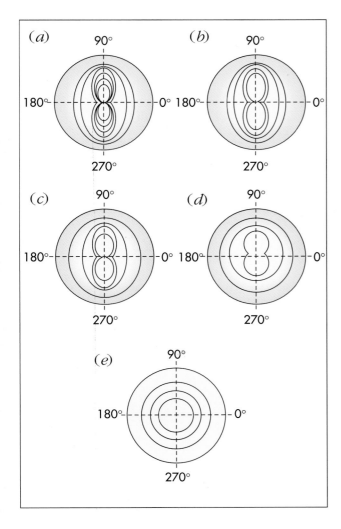

Figure 13.6 *Correction of astigmatism. (a–d) The corneal tissue is removed by the scanning mechanism with increasing beam diameter along the negative cylinder. (e) The result is a spherical cornea.*

directly a new refractive surface. A number of techniques have been developed to create such toric ablations.[27–29]

The Chiron–Technolas Keracor 116 excimer laser creates such a toric photoablation by removing corneal tissue by a scanning mechanism, with increasing beam diameters along the cylindrical axis. The computer orientates the long axis of the slit parallel to the axis of the refractive cylinder expressed in minus cylinder form (flatter meridian). Subsequently, the steeper areas of the cornea are differentially ablated, resulting in a change in the refractive power, while the flatter meridian, which lies along the long axis of the slit, is therefore uniformly ablated, resulting in no change in the refractive power (Fig. 13.6).

TREATING ASTIGMATISM: PATIENT SELECTION AND PREPARATION

This study presents the results of 98 eyes. In all eyes astigmatism was naturally occurring and there was no history of previous surgical procedures or ocular disorders other than the refractive error. All patients underwent a detailed ophthalmic examination as described for the treatment of myopia. Mean pre-operative astigmatism was –3.25 D (range –1.50 to –5.50 D). Mean spherical refractive error was –4.50 D (range –2.00 to –7.50 D).

THE SURGICAL PROCEDURE

The surgical technique is basically similar to that for ablations to correct spherical myopia. The axis of the astigmatism should be marked at the slit lamp preoperatively in order to allow a proper alignment of the excimer laser. This is of critical importance because it has been shown that an axial error of 10° can result in an astigmatic undercorrection of 40%.[30]

POSTOPERATIVE PHARMACEUTICAL TREATMENT

The postoperative pharmaceutical regimens are similar to the regimens after myopic PRK. Immediately after the treatment mydriatic drops were instilled. In some clinics, a soft contact lens together with non-steroidal anti-inflammatory drops were used, and in others antibiotic ointment was instilled, and the eye was padded until re-epithelialization had

matism. In early studies, the laser was used to create precise linear or arcuate incisions into peripheral corneal tissue, similar to conventional techniques such as radial keratotomy. In the untouched central cornea, a new stress equilibrium is established producing a new optical zone.[26] The current approach to astigmatic correction using the excimer laser involves ablating tissue from the anterior central cornea in a cylindrical fashion in order to define occurred. All clinics used topical applied cortico-steroids, mainly fluorometholone, after re-epithelialization. Unfortunately, once more, there was a variation in the length of this postoperative treatment, ranging from 1 to 3 months, depending upon physician preference.

RESULTS OF PHOTOASTIGMATIC REFRACTIVE KERATECTOMY

The refraction tended to stabilize at around 3 months after the surgery. The mean preoperative astigmatism of –3.25 D was reduced to –0.56 D (range, plano to –1.25 D) 1 year after photoastigmatic refractive keratectomy (PARK). In general, the amount of empirical astigmatism (non-vector corrected) was reduced by about 80% postoperatively. The residual astigmatism showed an axis within ±5° compared to preoperatively. The mean preoperative spherical correction of –4.50 D was changed to a mean figure of –0.50 D (range +0.5 D to –1.00 D).

Uncorrected VA improved in all treated eyes. At 1 year, all patients had an uncorrected Snellen VA of 6/12 or better, and 85% of eyes achieved 6/6 or better. Significant changes in BCVA have not been observed; indeed, 97% of the treated eyes did not lose or gain a line. However, 3% of the treated eyes actually gained one or two lines of Snellen VA.

TREATMENT OF ASTIGMATISM: CONCLUSIONS

In our early experience the data indicate that myopic astigmatism can be treated with the Chiron–Technolas excimer laser. Overall, the postoperative results and resultant uncorrected VA are encouraging. However, it is of interest that the amount of cylinder as determined by manifest refraction was only around 80% corrected, and the associated spherical component was slightly overcorrected.

TREATMENT OF HYPEROPIA

In the treatment of hyperopia, the central 4.5–5.0 mm of the cornea is ablated with an associated large transition zone extending to a 10 mm diameter.

Clinical trials for the treatment of hyperopia have just commenced and therefore no clinical data are currently available for the Chiron–Technolas laser.

LASER-ASSISTED IN SITU KERATOMILEUSIS

The technique of keratomileusis was initially proposed by Jose Barraquer in 1949.[31] Keratomileusis is indicated for higher degrees of myopia, particularly when other surgical techniques are considered to be insufficient to achieve the desired results. In this procedure, a disc of anterior cornea, usually 9 mm in diameter and 300 μm thick, is removed with a microkeratome. The stromal side of this corneal button is reshaped either by cryolathing,[32] or by cutting a mould,[33] and then sutured back to its original position. After the surgery, it may take several months for the refraction to stabilize.[34] However, most published studies indicated that the refractive results of keratomileusis are unpredictable, with 26–87% of treated eyes having final postoperative refractions within ± 2.00 D of the intended correction.[35–38]

The development and application of the 193 nm ArF excimer laser in corneal surgery has permitted further advances in keratomileusis. A major advantage of excimer laser photoablation is the ability to reshape the anterior corneal surface with a submicron accuracy of approximately 0.25 μm per pulse, without causing any significant damage to adjacent structures.[39] However, several experimental and clinical studies have shown that there is a progressive filling in of epithelium, newly synthesized collagen, and glycosaminoglycans into the surgical site during the first 3–6 weeks, resulting in a loss of the initially intended dioptric correction.[40] It has been suggested that some form of cellular and extracellular communication between the epithelium and the stroma exists, in that keratocyte activity, and subsequently collagen synthesis, is not initiated before the epithelium has completely re-covered the wound bed. Keratomileusis has the advantage of maintaining the intregrity of the anterior corneal layers and, therefore, theoretically might not initiate such a strong wound healing response as seen in high myopic corrections after surface-based photorefractive keratectomy.

Basically, two surgical procedures can be discriminated: laser in situ keratomileusis (LASIK) and excimer laser intrastromal keratomileusis (ELISK).

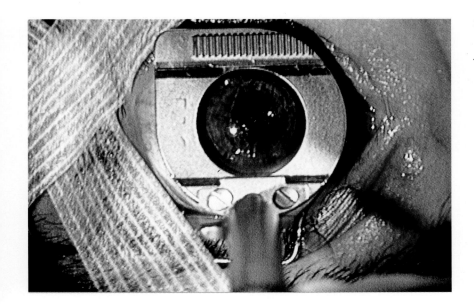

Figure 13.7 *Photograph to show the position of the microkeratome fixation ring on the sclerocorneal limbus and centered on the pupil center.*

Both techniques employ a microkeratome that produces a corneal flap. In LASIK, which was first described by Pallikaris and co-workers,[40,41] the flap is turned back and corneal tissue is removed from the central surface of the stromal bed. In contrast, in ELISK, first described by Burrato and co-workers,[42] the microkeratome cuts across the whole cornea producing a free corneal disc. This disc is then placed under an excimer laser with the stromal side up and a refractive lenticule is removed by the laser. The disc is then repositioned on to the cornea. Although both techniques seem to produce comparable postoperative refractive results, LASIK requires less surgical time and no suturing of the corneal flap. In the following section we only report our results of LASIK.

PATIENT SELECTION AND PATIENT PREPARATION

The criteria for selecting patients for LASIK and the preoperative evaluation were basically the same as for PRK. However, the refractive range was extended, in that highly myopic eyes (above −10.00 D) were also treated with this technique.

SURGICAL TECHNIQUE

A stringent and standardized surgical technique, including both correct handling and maintenance of the keratome and the excimer laser, are essential to achieve good refractive results and to avoid most of the complications associated with this procedure.

LASIK was performed as an outpatient procedure. The patient was instructed to have a light meal on the day of surgery, and was administered a 5 mg tablet of diazepam 30 minutes before the procedure. Prior to surgery, corneal topography was repeated along with ultrasonic central pachymetry. Topical oxybuprocaine and tetracaine were instilled in the eye to be treated. The contralateral eye was occluded. The cornea was marked with a four incision RK-marker. After adequate preparation of the surgical area, the adjustable suction ring of the microkeratome (Automated Corneal Shaper, Chiron Vision) was carefully placed on the sclerocorneal limbus and centered upon the pupil centre (Fig. 13.7). The suction ring induced an intraocular hypertension with an IOP between 65 and 80 mm/Hg. The suction ring was set at its lowest height in order to obtain the largest possible resection diameter, which can be between 7.2 and 8.5 mm. In practice we have used

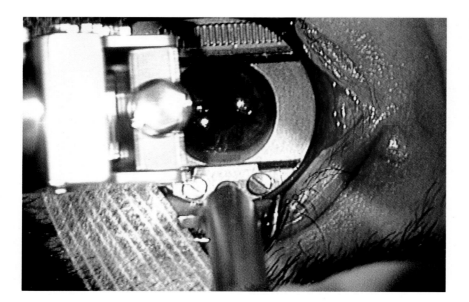

Figure 13.8 *Photograph demonstrating insertion of the microkeratome into the fixation ring. The microkeratome advances across the suction ring from temporal to nasal to produce the corneal flap.*

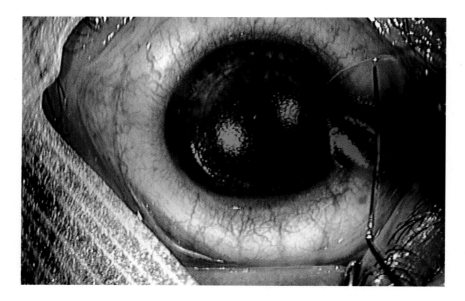

Figure 13.9 *The 160 micron flap is elevated and laid flat nasally utilizing a cyclodialysis spatula. Note the straight edge where the flap remains hinged to the underlying cornea.*

the maximum diameter of 8.5 mm. After placement of the suction ring, the IOP was checked using a Barraquer applanation tonometer, an 8.5 mm diameter contact lens was positioned and the suction ring adjusted such that the diameter of the applanated cornea coincided with the 8.5 mm diameter circle on the contact lens. Up to this stage of the surgery the cornea was kept completely dry. With the automatic

microkeratome, a corneal disc was cut up to the edge, leaving it still joined to the cornea as a flap ('hinge technique') (Fig. 13.8). We utilized a corneal disc of 160 μm thickness and 8.5 mm diameter. In order to avoid problems during the resection of the lenticule, a new blade must be used for each procedure and the guides of the microkeratome always kept moistened. After the lamellar resection, the

Table 13.2
Pre- and postoperative refraction for four discrete treatment groups at 1 year after LASIK using the Keracor 116 excimer laser.

Preoperative refraction (D)	No. of eyes	Postoperative refraction (D) (mean ± standard deviation)	
−3.00 to −6.00	18	−0.34	±0.34
−6.25 to −10.00	35	−1.03	±1.04
−10.25 to −15.00	32	−1.96	±1.30
−15.25 to −21.00	14	−2.04	±1.49

microkeratome and the suction ring were removed and the lenticule turned down using a modified iridodialysis spatula (Fig. 13.9). The excimer laser ablation was performed on a completely dry stromal bed. The laser beam was focused on the center of the pupil and both myopia and astigmatism were corrected using the 'multizone mode' with a maximum diameter of 7.0 mm. After the ablation, the stromal surface was washed with balanced salt solution (BSS) in order to remove all tissue debris. The flap was replaced on to a wet stromal bed and the resection border was carefully dried (Fig. 13.10). No sutures were necessary and eyes were not occluded after the surgery. Topical antibiotics were prescribed for the first week and artificial tear substitutes continued for the first 4 weeks.

LASIK RESULTS

Data was collected from 81 myopic eyes, treated by one surgeon (JLG), with a follow-up for 1 year. Based on their pre-operative refraction, patients were allocated to one of three groups as follows:

- Group I—between −6.00 and −10.00 D (35 eyes)
- Group II—between −10.12 and −15.00 D (32 eyes)
- Group III—between −15.12 and −21.00 D (14 eyes).

The mean postoperative refraction at 1 year in Group I was -1.03 D (SD ± 1.04 D), in Group II it was −1.96 D (SD ± 1.30 D), and in Group III it was −2.04 D (SD

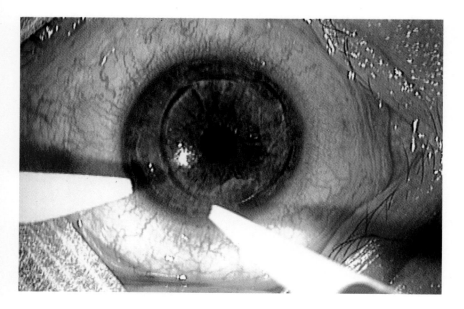

Figure 13.10 *Replacement of the corneal flap after excimer laser photoablation. The flap is allowed to dry into position for 2–5 minutes and integrity checked by striae and blink tests. The central epithelium should be kept moist during this period.*

± 1.49 D) (Table 13.2). Stabilization of the refraction occurred after 3 weeks. No hypermetropic overcorrections were observed.

COMPLICATIONS OF LASIK

No significant changes in BCVA were observed, with only one eye losing one line of Snellen acuity. Night vision ('starburst-effect') was reported in 60% of the treated eyes during the first postoperative month; however, none of the patients reported night vision problems after 6 months. None of the patients showed a decentration of the ablation zone of more than 1.0 mm. In nine cases (10%) an epithelial ingrowth was observed, and in two of these eyes (2.5%) the epithelial cells had to be removed surgically.

LASIK: CONCLUSIONS

Although the results of LASIK seem to be very promising, more prospective studies have to be undertaken with larger patient numbers and longer follow-up time in order to show the possibilities and limitations of this procedure. The main advantages of LASIK are: minimal postoperative pain, rapid recovery of useful visual acuity, wide range of myopic corrections, and the (apparently) minimal effect of epithelial and stromal healing on refractive outcome. However, the main disadvantages are: the expensive and complex equipment needed, the handling of the interface (deposits, epithelial ingrowth), the possibility of inducing irregular astigmatism, the partial absence of intraoperative surgical monitoring as the keratome creates the flap, and a very long surgical 'learning-curve'. Currently, LASIK does not appear sufficiently advanced to treat accurately astigmatism or hyperopia.

REFERENCES

1. McDonald MB, Miu JC, Byrd TJ, et al, Central photorefractive keratectomy for myopia: partially sighted and normal sighted eyes, *Ophthalmology* (1991) **98**: 1327–37.
2. Gartry D, Kerr Muir M, Marshall J, Photorefractive keratectomy with an argon fluoride excimer laser: a clinical study, *Refr Corneal Surg* (1991) **7**: 420–35.
3. Seiler   ensak J, Myopic photorefractive keratectomy with t   .mer laser: one year follow-up, *Ophthalmology* (1991) **18**: 1156–63.
4. Tengroth B, Epstein D, Fagerholm P, et al, Excimer laser photorefractive keratectomy for myopia: clinical results in sighted eyes, *Ophthalmology* (1993) **100**: 739–45.
5. Salz JJ, Maguen E, Nesburn AB, et al, A two year experience with excimer laser photorefractive keratectomy for myopia, *Ophthalmology* (1993) **100**: 873–82.
6. Kim JH, Hahn TW, Lee YC, et al, Photorefractive keratectomy in 202 myopic eyes: one year follow-up, *Refract Corneal Surg* (1993) **9**: S11–S16.
7. Brancato R, Tavola A, Carones F, et al, Excimer laser photorefractive keratectomy for myopia: results in 1165 eyes, *Refract Corneal Surg* (1993) **9**: S95–S104.
8. Seiler T, Wollensak J, Results of a prospective evaluation of photorefractive keratectomy at one year after surgery, *Ger J Ophthalmol* (1993) **2**: 135–42.
9. Lavery FL, Photorefractive keratectomy in 472 eyes, *Refract Corneal Surg* (1993) **9**: 98–100.
10. Gimbel HV, Van Westenbrugge JA, Johnson WAS, et al, Visual, refractive and patient satisfaction results following bilateral photorefractive keratectomy for myopia, *Refract Corneal Surg* (1993) **9**: S5–S10.
11. Talley AR, Hardten DR, Sher NA, et al, Results one year after using the 193 nm excimer laser for photorefractive keratectomy in mild to moderate myopia, *Am J Ophthalmol* (1994) **118**: 304–11.
12. Dutt S, Steinert RF, Raizman MB, et al, One year results of excimer laser photorefractive keratectomy for low to moderate myopia, *Arch Ophthalmol* (1994) **112**: 1427–36.
13. Lohmann C, Gartry D, Kerr Muir M, et al, Haze after photorefractive keratectomy: its origins and consequences, *Laser and Light in Ophthalmology* (1991) **4**: 15–34.
14. Marshall J, Trokel S, Rothery S, et al, Long-term healing of the central cornea after photorefractive keratectomy using an excimer laser, *Ophthalmology* (1988) **95**: 1411–21.
15. Tuft S, Zabel RW, Marshall J, Corneal repair following keratectomy: a comparison between conventional surgery and laser photoablation, *Invest Ophthalmol Vis Sci* (1989) **30**: 1769–77.
16. Goodman GL, Trokel S, Stark WJ, et al, Corneal healing following laser refractive keratectomy, *Arch Ophthalmol* (1989) **107**: 1799–1803.
17. Munnerlyn CR, Koons SJ, Marshall J, Photorefractive keratectomy: a technique for laser refractive surgery, *J Cataract Refract Surg* (1988) **14**: 46–52.
18. Lohmann C, Fitzke F, O'Brart D, et al, Halos—a problem for all myopes? *Refract Corneal Surg* (1993) **9**: S72–S75.
19. O'Brart D, Lohmann C, Fitzke F, et al, Night vision after excimer laser photorefractive keratectomy: haze and halos, *Eur J Ophthalmol* (1994) **4**: 43–51.
20. O'Brart D, Lohmann C, Fitzke F, et al, Disturbances in night vision after excimer laser photorefractive keratectomy, *Eye* (1994) **8**: 46–51.
21. O'Brart D, Corbett M, Lohmann C, et al, The effects of ablation diameter on the outcome of excimer laser photorefractive keratectomy (PRK): a prospective randomised, double blind study, *Arch Ophthalmol* (1995) **113**: 438–43.
22. Young T, The mechanisms of the eye, *Phil Trans* (1801) **91**: 23.

23. Duke Elder S, System of Ophthalmology, Vol 5 (Kimpton: London, 1970) 274.

24. Donders F, On the anomalies of refraction and accommodation of the eye, London (1864).

25. Swinger CA, Post operative astigmatism, *Surv Ophthalmol* (1987) **31**: 219–48.

26. Seiler T, Bende T, Wollensak J, et al, Excimer laser keratectomy for correction of astigmatism, *Am J Ophthalmol* (1988) **105**: 117–24.

27. McDonnell PJ, Moreira H, Garbus J, et al, Photorefractive keratectomy to create toric ablations for correction of astigmatism, *Arch Ophthalmol* (1991) **109**: 710–13.

28. Spigelman AV, Albert WC, Cozean CH, et al, Treatment of myopic astigmatism with the 193 nm excimer laser utilising aperture elements, *J Cataract Refract Surg* (1994) **20**: 258–60.

29. Gordon M, Brint SF, Durrie DS, et al, *Photorefractive keratectomy at 193 nm using an erodible mask*, In: Parel JM ed. *Ophthalmic Technologies II. Proc SPIE (1992)* **1644**: 11–19.

30. Campos M, McDonnell PJ, Photorefractive keratectomy: astigmatism. In: Thompson FB, McDonnell PJ eds. *Colour Atlas/Text of Excimer Laser Surgery. The Cornea.* Igaku-Shoin: New York (1993) 93–103.

31. Barraquer JI, Queratoplastica refractiva est, *Inform Oftal (Inst Barraquer)* (1949) **2**: 10.

32. Barraquer JI, Keratomileusis for myopia and aphakia, *Ophthalmology* (1953) 701–708.

33. Krumeich JH, Swinger CA, Non-freeze epikeratophakia for the correction of myopia, *Am J Ophthalmol* (1987) **103**: 397–403.

34. Swinger CA, Barker BA, Prospective evaluation of myopic keratomileusis, *Ophthalmology* (1984) **91**: 785–92.

35. Swinger CA, Barraquer JI, Keratophakia and keratomileusis—clinical results, *Ophthalmology* (1981) **88**: 709–15.

36. Nordon LT, Fallor MK, Myopic keratomileusis: 74 non-amblyopic cases with one year follow-up, *J Refract Surg* (1986) **2**: 124–8.

37. Dossi F, Bosio P, Myopic keratomileusis: results with a follow-up over one year, *J Cataract Refract Surg* (1987) **13**: 417–20.

38. Arenas-Archila E, Sanchez-Thorin JC, Noranjo-Urtibe JP, Hernandez IA, Myopic keratomileusis in situ: a preliminary report, *J Cataract Refract Surg* (1991) **17**: 424–31.

39. Krauss JM, Puliafito CA, Steinert RF, Laser interactions with the cornea, *Surv Ophthalmol* (1986) **1**: 37–53.

40. Pallikaris IG, Papatzanaki ME, Stathi E, et al, Laser in situ keratomileusis, *Laser Surg Med* (1990) **10**: 463–8.

41. Pallikaris IG, Papatzanaki ME, Siganos DS, et al, A corneal flap technique for laser in situ keratomileusis, *Arch Ophthalmol* (1991) **145**: 1699–1702.

42. Burrato L, Ferrari M, Rama P, Excimer laser intrastromal keratomileusis, *Am J Ophthalmol* (1992) **113**: 291–5.

Chapter 14 Photorefractive surgery in Australia and Asia Pacific

David B Cano and Hugh R Taylor

EXCIMER LASER USE IN AUSTRALIA AND ASIA

Ophthalmic excimer laser use in Australia and Asia Pacific region is fairly widespread. In fact, there are currently more than 65 excimer lasers in use within South Korea alone; more than any other country. From a survey of the current excimer laser manufacturers, we have determined that there are over 150 excimer lasers in Asia and over a dozen in Australia and New Zealand being used for ophthalmic treatments.

From a survey of about 20 ophthalmologists with excimer lasers in Australia and Asia in January 1995, we estimated that between 100 and in excess of 1000 cases were likely to be treated annually by each machine and that more than 100 000 eyes had already been treated in Asia and Australia.

The current distribution of the different commercially available excimer lasers varies in each country, but currently the Summit and Visx lasers are the most commonly used excimer lasers and most of the currently published clinical research from Australia and Asia is based on these two lasers (Table 14.1).

Table 14.1

Excimer laser use and distribution in Australia and Asia as of January 1995

COUNTRY	Summit	Visx	Laser-sight	LASER Nidek	Schwind	Medi-tech	Chiron	LEI	Nova-tech	TOTAL
South Korea	25	30			9	2	1			67
China	5	4	17	3	2		3			34
Japan	5	3	5	7		3				23
Australia	7	1			1			1		10
Thailand	4					1				5
India	2			1		2				5
Singapore	3			1						4
Taiwan	2			1						3
Hong Kong	2	1								3
New Zealand	1	1						1		3
Malaysia	2			1						3
Indonesia			1	1				1		3
Philippines	1									1
Total	59	40	23	15	12	8	4	3	0	164

LOCAL HISTORY OF EXCIMER LASER USE

The first excimer laser to be used in Australia was developed in Perth in 1987 and the first human therapeutic keratectomy trial started at the Lions Eye Institute in February 1991.[1] It was not until 1991 that the first commercially available lasers were used in Australia. They were a Summit Med UV200 used by the Sydney Refractive Surgery Centre and a Visx 20/20 used by the Melbourne Excimer Laser and Research Group.[2,3] In Japan the first excimer laser was used at the Department of Ophthalmology, Musashino Red Cross Hospital in Tokyo in 1990.[4] JH Kim's group began the first reported Korean PRK clinical study in 1991.[5] MacRobert and Ho reported using the first excimer laser in Hong Kong in late 1991.[6]

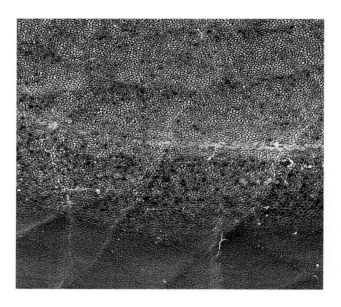

Figure 14.1 *Scanning electron microscopy of rabbit endothelium 24 hours after excimer laser photorefractive keratectomy showing reversible endothelial changes.*

EXPERIMENTAL EXCIMER LASER TRIALS AND RESEARCH STUDIES

Since the late 1980s the excimer laser has been used experimentally in Australia. In 1990, van Saarloos and Constable published their initial studies of the effect of beam homogeneity and ablation rate on bovine corneal stroma with the Lions' Eye Institute (LEI) laser that they had developed.[7] Recently, this group has reported on a spatial filtering system and an image rotator for beam smoothing, which appears to be effective in reducing regression following corrections of myopia with the excimer laser.[8] Morlet et al in Sydney reported the effect of topical interferon-alpha-2b on corneal haze after excimer laser surgery in rabbits.[9] Interferon-alpha-2b inhibits glycosaminoglycan production, but increases collagenase production. They demonstrated a decrease of corneal haze with interferon-alpha-2b and that dexamethasone had an additive effect, but they also noted that when higher doses of interferon were used there was reduced effect. Gillies et al in Melbourne have found similar results in a small clinical trial with interferon-alpha-2b on the reduction of corneal haze[10] and further investigation is warranted.

Using the excimer laser for glaucoma surgery has been one topic of research interest. Allan et al in Perth used the excimer laser for glaucoma surgery for open-angle glaucoma using an ab externo, modified open-mask system.[11] An air jet was incorporated to dry the target area during the ablation and a conjunctival plication method to create a sclerostomy in porcine cadaver eyes and in rhesus monkeys with experimental glaucoma.[12] They created a sclerostomy in nine pseudophakic patients with advanced open-angle glaucoma and had good intraocular pressure control in eight.[13] Complications included temporary fibrinous sclerostomy occlusion and profound early hypotony including one case with suprachoroidal hemorrhage. Brooks et al in Melbourne performed excimer laser filtration surgery in human and pig cadaver eyes as well as in seven patients with severe glaucoma.[14] Precise ablation of Schlemm's canal was confirmed by scanning electron microscopy, and this ab externo technique allowed for the formation of a bleb external to the trabecular tissue. Either intraoperative mitomycin C or postoperative 5-fluorouracil was used as adjunctive treatment in some patients. There was no report of fibrinous sclerostomy occlusion, hypotony or suprachoroidal hemorrhage with this procedure. The overall success rate was 71% without significant complications.

Because of the interest in postoperative corneal haze, Cherny et al used Scheimpflug densitometry as a measure of corneal opacification following excimer laser surgery.[15] A Nidek EAS 1000 Anterior Segment Analysis System with a Scheimpflug slit was utilized

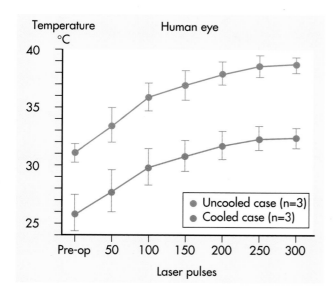

Figure 14.2 *Thermal change on living human corneas after 300 shots with a 193 nm excimer laser. (Reproduced with permission of the American Society of Cataract and Refractive Surgery,* J Refract and Corn Surg, *Niizuma et al. 1994;10:SS264[19]).*

to measure corneal opacity and Cherny et al consequently developed an index of corneal opacity which was found to be superior to subjective assessment.

A rabbit model for lamellar keratoplasty using the excimer laser to create the bed and the donor button has been reported by Cano et al from Melbourne.[16] They demonstrated little interface opacity or long-term damage to the endothelium (Fig. 14.1), but significant postoperative astigmatism was noted. A related study of wide-zone ablation (6 mm) in human and porcine cadaver eyes noted that the endothelium demonstrated damage immediately after ablation to a depth of 65%, but these effects moderated after 24 hours in organ culture.[17]

Another study of endothelial changes was reported by Sano et al in Tokyo. It was found that a vibration of 120 Hz with an amplitude of 2 mm for 3 minutes on the central cornea of rabbits caused changes in both Descemet's membrane and in the endothelium. These findings were similar to those previously seen following excimer laser ablations of rabbit corneas.[18]

Several experimental studies of the untoward effects related to the keratorefractive use of the excimer have been reported from Japan. Niizuma et al in Japan investigated cooling of the cornea to prevent the side effects of PRK.[19] They noted in pig eyes that

1000 laser pulses increased the temperature by 10–12°C; in rabbit eyes 500 laser pulses resulted in a rise of 9–10°C; and in human eyes increases of 6–7°C with 300 pulses. Cooling the cornea with balanced salt solution apparently resulted in less damage to collagen fibrils, and less reduction in normal distribution of proteoglycans (Fig. 14.2). Patients experienced less pain, subepithelial corneal haze and damage to corneal endothelium with cooling.

Tsubota et al in Tokyo made a similar observation in three highly myopic patients undergoing PRK in which the ocular surface was cooled with balanced salt solution prior to treatment.[20] Their patients had less pain and corneal haze. This group also reported on one patient who underwent PRK with endothelial changes noted on specular microscopy four days after treatment.[21]

Amano et al in Tokyo, Japan performed a specular microscopic evaluation of the corneal epithelium after PRK in 19 patients.[22] They noted a normal epithelial pattern in 18 eyes at 1 and 3 months and in all eyes at 6 months.

This group recently reported on a study of optical performance of the cornea following excimer laser myopic photorefractive keratectomy using a ray-tracing technique and weighted focal distribution in 35 eyes one year after PRK with uncorrected visual acuity of 20/20 or better for attempted correction of −5.00 D or less. They noted that the optical performance of the cornea after PRK can be improved by decreasing the decentration, but the optical performance of a successful PRK is inferior to that of the normal cornea.[23] They also noted in a previous study that downward displacement of the ablation relative to the entrance pupil was observed in 85% of eyes with a mean distance of the center of ablation from the center of the entrance pupil of 0.51 mm.[24]

It has been recently demonstrated by Uozato and Sakurai in Japan that the center of the natural pupil can be used to optimally center refractive procedures in most cases.[25]

PHOTOTHERAPEUTIC USE OF THE EXCIMER LASER

Several phototherapeutic keratectomy trials have been reported from Australia and Asia. Rogers et al treated 11 patients with Reis–Bucklers' corneal dystrophy using a Summit laser in Sydney.[26,27] They found an improvement of visual acuity and a complete cessation of recurrent erosions in all their patients. They noted a hypermetropic shift of less than 2.0 D and little associated astigmatism with treatments using between 75 and 175 total pulses. Snibson et al from Melbourne, using a Visx laser, reported using PTK on 76 patients with a range of diagnoses: anterior corneal scarring (32%), recurrent corneal erosions (25%), calcific band keratopathy (13%), several corneal dystrophies (11%), and scarring after pterygium surgery (11%).[28] Ablations (5–10 µm) were sufficient to have a profound effect on the severity and frequency of recurrent erosions without loss of corneal transparency or the induction of significant hyperopia. Calcium deposition in band keratopathy was also effectively removed using this technique. The study noted that deeper ablations produced unwanted refractive changes and corneal haze.

Hahn et al in Seoul also reported the outcome of PTK in nine patients with superficial corneal diseases including corneal scarring, Reis–Bucklers' and granular dystrophies.[29] They demonstrated good results except for a mild hypermetropic shift, mild to moderate corneal haze and the recurrence of granular deposits in one case of granular dystrophy. Kim and Hahn, also in Seoul, have used the excimer laser therapeutically for the ablation of conjunctival epithelial melanosis without recurrence in two cases (Table 14.2).[30]

PHOTOREFRACTIVE SURGERY IN AUSTRALIA AND ASIA

Photorefractive surgery has been performed in both Australia and Asia during the past 5 years. The excimer laser has been used in the treatment of both myopia and myopic astigmatism.

Tan and Tan surveyed 106 patients in Singapore who had contact lens-related problems and asked about their interest in having a PRK after information about the procedure was given to them.[31] Altogether 44% indicated that they would consider PRK; 79% of these cited the convenience of not needing spectacles or contact lenses. Among the 56% who were not interested in PRK, 78% of these expressed fears about possible complications. The group of patients interested in PRK was comprised of more males and high myopic persons. Of particular interest is that in the next 3 months only two patients underwent PRK.

The degree of myopia in adults who underwent excimer laser treatment was studied by our group in Melbourne.[32] We found that those with higher degrees of myopia were more likely to undergo excimer laser treatment. In fact, based on the occurrence of myopia in the community, highly myopic and extremely myopic persons, respectively, were 10 times and 16 times more likely to have excimer laser treatment than lower myopic persons.

Table 14.2
Clinical results in the phototherapeutic use of the excimer

Author	Country	Technique	Number	Diagnosis of Eyes	Outcome	Complication
Lawless et al[27]	Sydney Australia	Summit 75 to 175 pulses	11	Reis–Bucklers'	Good: No erosions	Mild <2.00 D hyperopia
Snibson et al[28]	Melbourne Australia	Visx	76	Recurrent erosions scarring band keratopathy corneal dystrophy	Good	Recurrent erosion, mild hyperopia haze
Hahn et al[29]	Seoul Korea	Summit	9	Reis–Bucklers' granular dystrophy corneal scar band keratopathy	Good	Recurrence of granular deposits mild hyperopia moderate haze
Kim et al[30]	Seoul Korea	Summit 300 to 350 pulses	2	Conjunctival epithelial melanosis	Good	No recurrence

Performing bilateral PRK in one operative session was reported by MacRobert and Ho in Hong Kong.[6] This is usually avoided in most centers. They reported that the overall treatment time was shortened and there was only one experience of pain out of 28 eyes treated. The disadvantages noted included bilateral painful eyes, 2–3 weeks away from work, and the need for bilateral eye padding. One ophthalmologist described his personal experience with bilateral simultaneous PRK for contact lens intolerance.[6] His preoperative refraction was −2.75 D OD and −3.25 −0.50 × 60 OS. He was treated with a 5 mm ablation zone with an attempted correction of −2.30 D OD and −2.90 D OS. He experienced severe pain that required pethidine, a strong feeling of helplessness from the padding for three days, and intense photophobia on the fourth day. On the fifth day after his treatment he could see 6/6 with +2.50 OD and −1.00 OS. He had minimal haze at three weeks. He felt the difference in his life was remarkable and 3 months after his surgery his refraction was −0.25 OD and −0.75 OS.

An Australian ophthalmologist has also reported his own personal experience after PRK.[2] His preoperative refraction was −4.50 D and his attempted correction was −3.75 D. Postoperatively, glare was a problem especially with night driving for the first two weeks. His final refraction was reported to be within 0.50 D of attempted correction. He regretted he had not been fully corrected.

Subjective pain assessment was reported by our group in 64 patients who had PRK.[33] The peak self-reported pain was encountered 24 hours postoperatively. The degree of myopia and prior excimer experience were not related to the use of analgesia or self-reported pain. Patients who received topical non-steroidal anti-inflammatory drugs for 24 hours postoperatively reported less pain.

CLINICAL PHOTOREFRACTIVE RESULTS FOR LOW AND MODERATE MYOPIA

A number of prospective clinical studies from Australia and Asia have been reported. We will describe the results for the treatment of myopia and myopic astigmatism separately.

A comparison of the surgical outcome of comparable patients treated with three different excimer laser systems, Summit, Visx and LEI, was undertaken.[34] This is one of the very few studies to compare the results obtained with two or more lasers. Forty cases treated with each laser were matched for age and attempted corrections and compared. The group treated using

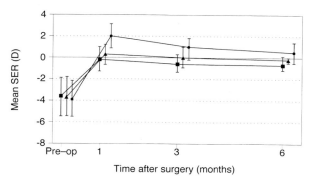

Comparison of three excimers

● Summit ▲ Visx ■ LEI(TELCO)

Figure 14.3 *Mean and standard deviation of spherical equivalent refraction (SER) before, and 1, 3 and 6 months after myopic excimer laser PRK using three different laser delivery systems. (Reproduced with permission from the* Australian and New Zealand Journal of Ophthalmology, *Kang et al. 1995;23:269[34]).*

the Summit system tended to be relatively overcorrected at 6 months and demonstrated significantly greater regression than the other groups. The Visx group were slightly undercorrected at 6 months after treatment, and the LEI group was even more significantly undercorrected. Overall, the results with the three different lasers were comparable in terms of refraction and visual acuities 6 months after myopic photorefractive keratectomy (Fig. 14.3).

The treatment of low and moderate myopia using a Summit laser with 12 month follow-up after PRK was reported by Lawless et al on their initial 50 treated eyes.[35] In this study, 90% were within 0.50 D and 94% were within 1.00 D of emmetropia. No patients had lost their best-corrected visual acuity, but one patient required retreatment at 12 months for haze and regression. A trace corneal haze was noted in 30% of eyes (Table 14.3).

Results of the treatment of low and moderate myopia with a Visx laser using a 6 mm zone have been reported by our group.[36] At 6 months in the initial group of 55 eyes, 88% receiving PRK were within 1.00 D of plano refraction. Similar results were seen with a larger group of patients.[37] At 1 year 96% of low myopic persons (less than −5.00 D) were within 1.00 D of the targeted refraction.[38]

Table 14.3
Clinical results in the treatment of myopia less than −7.00 D: one year follow-up

Author	Country	Laser	Refraction	Number of Eyes	Outcome	Complication
Lawless et al[35]	Sydney Australia	Summit 5 mm zone	−1.50 to −6.00 D (−3.90 D ± 1.51)	50	92%>6/6 98% >6/12	Trace haze
Kim et al[5]	Seoul Korea	Summit 5 mm zone	−2.00 to −7.00 D (−4.79 D ± 1.17)	135	−0.45 D ± 0.88	Blurred night vision
Shimizu et al[4]	Tokyo Japan	Summit 4.5 mm	−3.00 to −6.00 D (−3.90 D ± 1.51)	45	−0.89 D ± 1.23 decentration in 33%	Haze > 2 in 15.7% at 3 months
Snibson et al[38]	Melbourne Australia	Visx	Up to −5.00 D (−3.48 ± 1.00)	80	88% > 6/12 96% ± 1.00 D	Mild haze

In a similar study, Balakrishnan et al in Singapore reported on 6 months of follow-up of 31 eyes treated for myopia between −2.00 and −6.00 D from patients treated with a Summit laser.[39] Altogether 84% were within 1.00 D of emmetropia. Corneal haze did not pose a significant problem.

In a larger study of low and moderate myopia, Kim et al in Seoul reported their results with a Summit laser with a maximum attempted correction of −6.00 D using a 5 mm ablation zone in 202 myopic eyes.[5] Eyes with less than −7.00 D had a mean refraction of −0.45 ± 0.88 D at 1 year. Keratometry showed a mean reduction of 3.46 D at 1 year which underestimated the true refractive change (Fig. 14.4). They found that 91% were within 1.00 D of attempted correction, but 8% had a decrease in their best spectacle-corrected visual acuity and 21% had blurring or decreased vision in dim light or at night. With 2 year follow-up of 45 eyes, they reported uncorrected visual acuity of 6/7.5 in 89%.[40] Among these patients 17% were unsatisfied because of glare or halo at night and 78.3% reported decreased night vision.

This group also reported on problems associated with decreased visual acuity after PRK in 2920 treated eyes.[41] Corneal haze of grade two or more developed in 11 eyes of nine patients (seven male and two female), and decreased best-corrected visual acuity of two lines or more was seen in eight eyes with irregular astigmatism as one of the major causes. The total rate of all significant complications was 0.79% in their

study group at the end of 2 years. Recently, this group reported that corneal haziness is likely to be related to the cause of myopic regression following PRK and that an eye has a higher incidence of regression if the other previously treated eye experienced regression.[42]

A comprehensive study of 97 eyes with 1 year follow-up after Summit laser PRK was reported by

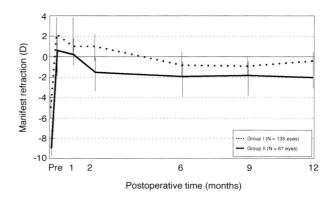

Figure 14.4 *Change in average manifest refraction one year after photorefractive keratectomy with a Summit laser. (Reproduced with permission of the American Society of Cataract and Refractive Surgery,* J Refract and Corn Surg, *Kim et al. 1993;9:S13[5]).*

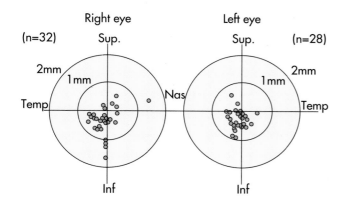

Figure 14.5 *Decentration reported after PRK with a Summit laser. The center of the ablation is plotted relative to the center of the pupil aperture. (Reproduced with permission of the American Society of Cataract and Refractive Surgery,* J Refract and Corn Surg, *Shimizu et al. 1994;10:S185[4]).*

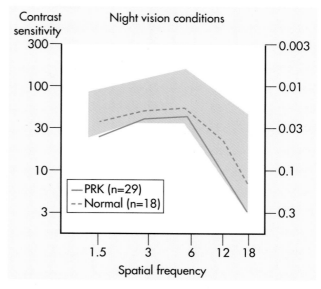

Figure 14.6 *Contrast sensitivity under night vision conditions after PRK with a Summit laser. (Reproduced with permission of the American Society of Cataract and Refractive Surgery,* J Refract and Corn Surg, *Shimizu et al. 1994;10:S186[4]).*

Shimizu et al in Tokyo.[4] They used a 4.5 mm diameter ablation. Pachymetry at 1 year showed thinning for all the groups, especially the moderate and high myopic persons. Specular microscopy showed no significant epithelium or endothelium changes. Corneal topography demonstrated decentration especially inferiorly, in 60% of eyes within 0.5 mm; in 33% within 0.5 to 1.0 mm; and in 5% within 1.0 to 1.5 mm. They believed that this was due to the laser operator's visual axis not being aligned coaxially to the laser beam. One eye that was somewhat decentered more than 1.5 mm had monocular diplopia (Fig. 14.5). Low illumination contrast sensitivity simulating night vision was only reduced, but 'day vision' contrast sensitivity was reduced in eyes with significant haze (Fig. 14.6). Significant haze (grade 2 or more) was noted in 16% of cases at 3 months, but this cleared by 1 year. Haze was thought more common in Asian eyes than reported in European eyes (Table 14.3).

PRK to correct residual myopia after radial keratotomy was reported by Hahn et al in Seoul.[43] Ten eyes were treated with the Summit laser using a 5 mm ablation zone single step treatment. The maximum attempted correction was –6.00 D. The mean residual pretreatment myopia was –5.06 D, which was reduced to –0.66 D at 9 months, showing that PRK can correct residual myopia after RK.

CLINICAL PHOTOREFRACTIVE RESULTS FOR HIGH AND EXTREME MYOPIA

The treatment of high myopia (> –10.00 D) has been reported by two separate groups in Australia. Rogers et al used a two zone ablation technique with the Summit laser (Table 14.4).[44] The 14 eyes followed for 12 months had a mean refraction of –1.91 D ± 3.87, but the range was very large (–11.00 to +2.50 D). The mean keratometric flattening did not correlate with the refractive change. Significantly, half of these eyes were reablated for significant scarring and regression. Corneal opacity and regression tended to occur in the second eye if it occurred in the first.[45] Opacity was more common in higher myopia and in males.[46]

The Melbourne group used a Visx laser with a different treatment allocation algorithm (Table 14.5).[47] At 6 months after surgery the mean postoperative refraction was within 1.00 D in 66.5% and within 2.00

Table 14.4

Clinical results in the treatment of myopia greater than −10.00 D: one year follow-up

Group	Country	Refraction	Number of Eyes	Technique	Results	Complications
Rogers et al[44]	Sydney Australia	−10.25 to −20.50 D (−13.23 D ± 2.55)	14	Summit 2 zone	−1.91 D ± 3.87	50% retreated Corneal haze regression
Taylor et al[47]	Melbourne Australia	−10.25 to −21 D	15	Visx 3 zone	−1.60 ± 2.59	27% retreated Central islands regression

D in 89.2% of the high myopic persons, and within 1.00 D in 37.7% and within 2.00 D in 49.0% of the extreme myopic persons. At 12 months, 89 high myopic eyes had a mean refraction of −0.80 D ± 1.06 and 15 extreme myopic eyes had a mean refraction of −1.60 D ± 2.59 (Fig. 14.7). Four eyes were reablated for undercorrection. Corneal haze (>= 2.0) occurred in 6% of the high myopic persons and 15% of extreme myopic persons but cleared over time (Fig. 14.8); one eye was reablated for grade 3 corneal haze. One patient noted monocular diplopia and another noted halos. Refractive results were better for the high myopic persons than the extreme myopic persons. Central islands and corneal haze were more common

Table 14.5

Treatment allocation for multizone treatment of myopia.

Author	Country	Laser	Degree of myopia	1st Zone Diameter	1st Zone Correction	2nd Zone Diameter	2nd Zone Correction	3rd Zone Diameter	3rd Zone Correction
Rogers et al[44]	Sydney Australia	Summit	> −10 D			5.0			
Taylor et al[47]	Melbourne Australia	Visx	< 5 D	6.0 mm	100%				
			5–10 D	5.0 mm	50%	6.0 mm	50%		
			> 10 D	4.5 mm	33%	5.0 mm	33%	6.0 mm	33%
Cho et al[48]	Seoul Korea	Summit	< 6 D	5.0 mm	100%				
			6–8 D	5.0 mm	6 D	4.5 mm	Up to 2 D		
			8–10 D	5.0 mm	6 D	4.5 mm	2 D	4.0 mm	Up to 2 D
J. Kim et al[49]	Seoul Korea	Summit	< 6 D	4.5 mm	100%				
			> 6 D	4.5 mm	6 D	5.0 mm	Remainder		
J. Yong et al[57]	Seoul Korea	Visx	< 5 D	6.0 mm	100%				
			5–8 D	6.0 mm	5 D	5.0 mm	Up to 3 D		
			> 8 D	6.0 mm		5.0 mm	3 D	4.5 mm	Remainder
P. Tong et al[50]	Hong Kong	Visx	< 5 D	6.0 mm	100%				
			5–8 D	5.0 mm	60%	6.0 mm	40%		
			> 8 D	4.5 mm	50%	5.0 mm	30%	6.0 mm	20%

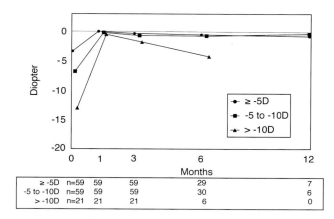

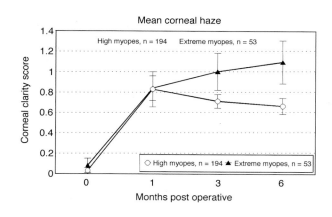

Figure 14.7 *Mean spherical equivalent for patients treated with PARK stratified by initial refractive error. The numbers at each examination are shown below the figure. (Reproduced with permission of the American Society of Cataract and Refractive Surgery, J Refract and Corn Surg. Taylor et al 1994:20;245[37]).*

Figure 14.8 *Mean corneal clarity score in high (n = 194) and extreme (n = 53) myopes treated with a Visx excimer laser surgery. (Reproduced with permission of the American Society of Cataract and Refractive Surgery, J Refract and Corn Surg. Taylor et al 1994:20;245[37]).*

in extreme myopic persons who often had a delay in the return of best-corrected visual acuity, although some had an increase in visual acuity (Table 14.4).

Recent studies from Asia have evaluated multizone PRK techniques for higher myopia.[48] Cho et al from Pusan, Korea reported their results with the Summit laser (Table 14.6). The mean attempted correction was −7.38 D and 6 months after surgery the mean refraction was −2.23 D, which represented an overcorrection. Little haze was noted (Figs 14.9 and 14.10). Kim et al from Seoul have also reported similar results (Tables 14.6 and 14.7).[49]

A recently published study from Hong Kong by Tong et al using the Visx laser with a similar multizone treatment method had comparable results. They noted a higher regression rate for more highly myopic eyes over time.[50]

In highly myopic eyes it appears that the use of corticosteroids has only a transient beneficial effect on the refractive outcome and corneal haze according to a recent study reported by Baek et al in Korea.[51] They noted that with the cessation of corticosteroids these differences were no longer significant.

Table 14.6
Clinical results in the treatment of myopia greater than −8 D: 6 month follow-up

Author	Country	Refraction	Number of Eyes	Technique	Results	Complications
Cho et al[48]	Seoul Korea	−8.87 to −16.99 (mean, −12.28 D)	19	Summit 3 zone	−2.23 D*	Trace haze
Kim et al[49]	Seoul Korea	−8.00 to −13.50 (mean, −9.77 D)	19	Summit 2 zone	−1.09 D	Trace haze
Tong et al[50]	Hong Kong	−8.25 to −23.00 (mean, −14.6)	32	Visx 3 zone	−3.27 D	Early regression

*(Note: attempted correction not always plano, maximum attempted correction −10.00 D)

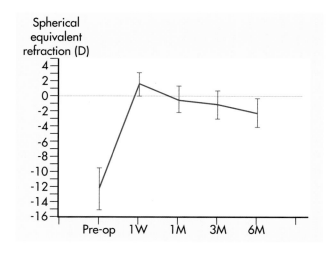

Figure 14.9 *Change in manifest refraction after multi-step photorefractive keratectomy (mean ±SD) using a Summit laser. (Reproduced with kind permission of the American Society of Cataract and Refractive Surgery, Cho et al. 1993;9:S39[48]).*

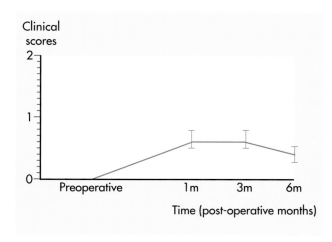

Figure 14.10 *Change in central corneal thickness over time after multi-step photorefractive keratectomy with a Summit laser. (Reproduced with permission of the American Society of Cataract and Refractive Surgery, Cho et al. 1993;9:S39[48]).*

CLINICAL PHOTOREFRACTIVE RESULTS FOR RETREATMENT

Retreatment for residual myopia and corneal opacity has also been studied by the two Australian groups. An overall retreatment rate of 4% (14 of 380 treated eyes) was reported in Summit treated eyes with at least 6 months follow-up (Table 14.7).[45] Transepithelial ablation was used as it was thought to give a smoother surface for ablation than that obtained by mechanical ablation. The Melbourne group had retreated 16% of eyes within 1 year (Table 14.7).[52,38] In their study retreatment appeared to be effective without increased risk of haze or other complications.

The Sydney group noted that 21% of retreated eyes developed corneal scarring of one eye.[53] Eyes retreated less than 6 months after initial treatment were more likely to develop corneal haze.

CLINICAL PHOTOREFRACTIVE RESULTS FOR MYOPIA COMBINED WITH ASTIGMATISM

Several studies from Asia and Australia have looked at the treatment of myopic astigmatism. One small study of four eyes by Balakrishnan et al in Singapore used the Summit UV200LA laser with an 'Emphasis Erodible Mask'.[54] The mask is a polymethylmethacrylate button attached to a quartz substrate mounted to an eyecup assembly. Decentered ablation zones were noted in all four patients that resulted in severe monocular diplopia in one. Problems noted included the use of a non-coaxial microscope, difficulty with alignment of the excimer laser beam due to the erodible mask and the central corneal zone, the inability to interrupt and restart the procedure due to ablation of the reference marks on the mask, and patient discomfort.

A group in New Zealand reported on a combined technique using transverse keratotomy and PRK with the Summit laser system.[55] Ring and co-workers reported 40 eyes with a preoperative range of myopia of −1.50 to −13.50 D and mean attempted spherical correction of −1.73 D (range −0.75 to −4.00 D). The timing of transverse keratotomy depended on the degree of astigmatism. For patients with less than 2.00 D of astigmatism the transverse keratotomy could be done at the same time as PRK. With astigmatism greater than 2.00 D it was found that the cornea required up to 3 weeks to stabilize before PRK to allow for the coupling effect of the transverse excisions and could not be done at the same time as PRK. The mean postoperative spherical equivalent was −0.01 D at 6 months, and the sight in 75% of their patients was 6/12 or better, uncorrected, at 6

Table 14.7
Retreatment by degree of myopia with 12-month follow-up

Group	Country	Refraction	Number of Eyes	Technique	Retreatment Rate	Complications
Lawless et al[45] n = 285	Sydney Australia	< −6.00 D −6.00 to −10.00 D > −10.00 D	4 8 9	Summit	1.8% 18.6% 37.5%	More scarring if treated within 6 months of initial treatment.
Snibson et al[52] n = 179	Melbourne Australia	< −5.00 −5.00 to −10.00 D > −10.00 D	8 11 10	Visx	9% 15% 56%	None significant

months. Vector analysis was not used in this study, so that any significant cylinder axis change would be difficult to assess (Fig. 14.11).

Choi et al in Seoul reviewed 136 eyes after PARK with the Visx laser.[56] Six months after the operation, the mean refractive cylinder decreased from 1.62 ± 0.88 D to 0.48 ± 0.48 D. The 'surgically induced refractive change' (SIRC) was determined by vector analysis. When the preoperative refractive cylinder was compared to the cylinder of the SIRC, the effect

of the cylindrical ablation was 93.9 ± 36.7%. The axial error of the cylinder was 5.9 ± 10.2% at 6 months (Table 14.8).

Similarly, Kim et al (Seoul) recorded comparable 6 month results with an elliptical program.[57] Spherical corrections up to 5.00 D were done with a 6 mm ablation zone, from 5.00 D to 8.00 D a 5.0 mm and 6.0 mm zone were used and for greater than 8.00 D 4.5 mm, 5.0 mm, and 6.0 mm zones were used. Vector analysis at 6 months showed 65.2% were within ± 0.50 and 91.0% were within ± 1.0 D of intended correction. Residual astigmatism after surgery was within 10° of the preoperative axis in 46.1% of eyes. However, 12.4% of eyes had an axis 80–90° away from the preoperative axis indicating overcorrection. Vector analysis revealed that 60.1% of the eyes had a postoperative axis less than 10° off the preoperative and intended axis (Tables 14.8 and 14.9).

One of the largest reports of PARK has come from Melbourne. We published our initial 6-month results for PARK with the Visx.[36] In this study 54 eyes underwent sequential PARK. The cylindrical correction was performed first and the spherical correction was reduced to compensate for the hyperopic shift. All treatment used a 6 mm zone. Altogether 85% were within 1 D of plano refraction. We subsequently published results from 139 consecutive eyes with PARK and a minimum of 3 months follow-up.[37] In this group 68% were within 1 D of plano refraction. We later presented the 12-month results of PARK (76 eyes) and PRK (74 eyes).[38] Overall 81% of all the eyes and 72% of the PARK-treated eyes were within 1 D of the intended correction. Vector analysis using the Alpins method showed a mean angle of error of −1.07

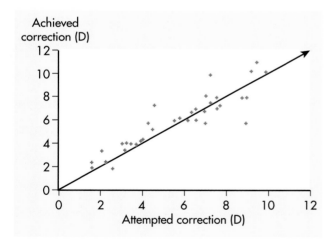

Figure 14.11 *Simple arithmetic analysis of attempted and achieved correction with transverse keratotomy and PRK. (Reproduced with permission of the American Society of Cataract and Refractive Surgery, Ring et al. 1994;10:S220[55]).*

Table 14.8

Clinical results in the treatment of myopia and astigmatism

Author	Country	Laser/ Technique	Number of Eyes	Refraction	Follow Up	Vector Analysis Results
Snibson et al[38]	Melbourne Australia	Visx Multizone Sequential 36% Elliptical 64%	76	up to −6.00 D cylinder and sphere was −1.25 to −14.50 D (−4.45 ± 2.06 D Seq)	1 year	72% within 1.00 D 82% within 2.00 D −1.07E ± 29.47 55% within 10° 72% within 20°
Yong et al[57]	Seoul Korea	Visx Multizone Elliptical	89	0.50 to 4.25 D cylinder (1.51 ± 0.81 D) and sphere was −2.50 to −17.25 D (−7.27 ± 2.66 D)	6 months	65.2% within 0.50 D 91.0% within 1.00 D Alignment not stated 60.1% within 10°
Choi et al[56]	Seoul Korea	Visx Elliptical	136	1.62 ± 0.88 D cylinder	6 months	Effect of cylindrical ablation was 93.9 ± 36.7% 5.9 degrees ± 10.2 Percent corrected not stated

degrees ± 29.47 with no significant difference evident between sequential and elliptical algorithms. The high degree of variation may have been due to either epithelial healing, decentration, or difficulty in accurate alignment of small residual cylindrical error.[58] Nine eyes (6%) had lost two or more lines of best-corrected visual acuity, but 14 eyes (9%) improved by two or more lines. Decentration of the ablation zone by more than 1 mm was noted in eight patients (15%). Central islands greater than 3 D were demonstrated in six patients (12%) 3 months after treatment. It was noted that central islands that were −3.00 D or less were seen more frequently than an absence of islands, suggesting these may be a normal postoperative topographic variation.[59] We concluded that PARK is safe and accurate for low and moderate degrees of myopia and astigmatism. The outcome was similar for PRK and PARK. Epithelial healing occurred faster in females and in eyes with more severe myopia.[60] Poorer postoperative best-corrected visual acuity occurred in older people with poorer initial acuity and in those with higher myopic prescriptions. The patient's data at a given time were the best predictors of subsequent outcome (Table 14.8).

CONCLUSION: A LOOK TO THE FUTURE

The Australia and Asia experience with the excimer laser has added a great deal to our understanding of the excimer with both pioneering excimer research and studies, and large prospective clinical studies looking at PRK, PARK, and PTK. This experience is currently one of the largest and most comprehensive in the world and it is estimated that in a few years over a million people will be treated with the excimer laser in Asia alone. Unfortunately, however, the outcome of treatment of many patients is either not followed or not reported. This is unfortunate as the results of treatment of large numbers of patients, especially those from different racial or ethnic backgrounds, would greatly enhance our knowledge of the effects of excimer laser surgery.

Current research from Australia and Asia demonstrates that the excimer may have additional therapeutic applications such as the treatment of glaucoma or conjunctival melanosis. Preliminary studies have also shown that corneal opacification may be reduced

Table 14.9

Net cylinder change (D) after excimer laser PARK

Group (cylinder)	Preoperative cylinder (mean)	Postoperative cylinder percentage		Improvement at 6 months
		3 months (n = 168)	6 months (n = 89)	
1 (0.50–0.75)	0.62 ± 0.13	0.49 ± 0.55	0.60 ± 0.54	4.8
2 (1.00–1.75)	1.28 ± 0.27	0.69 ± 0.53	0.60 ± 0.58	53.5
3 (2.00–2.75)	2.25 ± 0.23	0.77 ± 0.65	0.92 ± 0.69	59.1
4 (3.00–4.25)	3.33 ± 0.34	1.12 ± 0.59	1.04 ± 0.62	68.8

with topical interferon-alpha-2b and by avoiding a significant temperature rise in the cornea. We have also seen that the excimer laser can cause transient thermal damage to the stroma that might be of crucial importance in the induction of corneal haze.

High success rates in treating low and moderate myopia are reported in most studies from this region, some of which have included well over 1000 treated eyes. The more highly myopic eyes have had greater problems with regression and corneal haze and these problems may be reduced with changes in the treat-ment parameters including multiple zone treatments. There have also been reports that corneal haze may be more common in young males and in the Asian population, but more definitive studies are needed to assess this further. Several of the studies also indicate that decentration and decreased night vision are some of the other difficulties with PRK. Patients have had significant reduction in astigmatism after PARK, but a wide range in the mean angle of error is of some concern as well as the less satisfactory results in the more highly myopic eyes.

REFERENCES

1. van Saarloos PP, Constable IJ, Allan BD, Cooper RL, First Australian excimer laser keratectomy patients [letter], *Aust N Z J Ophthalmol* (1992) **20**:79–80.
2. Cohen P, Photorefractive keratectomy a personal insight, *Refract Corneal Surg* (1993) **9(Suppl)**:S121–2.
3. Guest CS, Taylor HR, The excimer laser in Australia [letter], *Med J Aust* (1992) **157**:436–7.
4. Shimizu K, Amano S, Tanaka S, Photorefractive keratectomy for myopia: one-year follow-up in 97 eyes, *J Refract Corneal Surg* (1994) **10(Suppl)**:S178–87.
5. Kim JH, Hahn TW, Lee YC, Joo CK, Sah WJ, Photorefractive keratectomy in 202 myopic eyes: one year results, Refract Corneal Surg (1993) 9(Suppl):S11--16.
6. MacRobert IJ, Ho SS, Bilateral simultaneous myopic PRK as experienced by an ophthalmologist, *Refract Corneal Surg* (1993) **9(Suppl)**:S121–2.
7. van Saarloos PP, Constable IJ, Bovine corneal stroma ablation rate with 193 nm excimer laser radiation: quantitative measurement, *Refract Corneal Surg* (1990) **6**:424–9.
8. van Saarloos PP, Reduced regression following excimer laser PRK [abstract], *Invest Ophthalmol and Vis Sci* (1995) **36**:S191.
9. Morlet N, Gillies MC, Crouch R, Maloof A, Effect of topical interferon alpha 2b on corneal haze after excimer laser photorefractive keratectomy in rabbits, *Refract Corneal Surg* (1993) **9**:443–51.
10. Gillies M, Garrett S, Shina S, Morlet N, Taylor H, Topical interferon alpha 2b of fibrosis after excimer laser photorefractive keratectomy. (Submitted for publication).
11. Allan BD, van Saarloos PP, Russo AV, Cooper RL, Constable IJ, Excimer laser sclerostomy: the in vitro development of a modified open mask delivery system, *Eye* (1993) **7**:47–52.
12. Allan BD, van Saarloos PP, Cooper RL, Keogh EJ, Constable IJ, 193 nm excimer laser sclerostomy using a modified open mask delivery system in rhesus monkeys with experimental glaucoma, *Graefes Arch Clin Exp Ophthalmol* (1993) **231**:662–6.
13. Allan BD, van Saarloos PP, Cooper RL, Constable IJ, 193 nm excimer laser sclerostomy in pseudophakic patients with advanced open angle glaucoma, *Br J Ophthalmol* (1994) **78**:199–205.
14. Brooks AMV, Martin S, Carroll N, Downie N, Taylor HR, Excimer laser filtration surgery photoablation of limbal tissue. (Submitted for publication).
15. Cherny M, Stasiuk R, Kelly P, Lee S, Golembo G, Taylor H, Computerised scheimpflug densitometry as a measure of corneal opacification following excimer laser surgery, *Ophthalmic Res* (1994) **26(Suppl)**:49–54.
16. Cano DB, Downie NA, Young IM, Carroll N, Pollock GA, Taylor HR, Excimer Laser Lamellar Keratoplasty, *Aust NZ J Ophthalmol* (1995) **23**:189–94.
17. Cano DB, Carroll N, Pollock GA et al, Endothelial Changes

with mid-stromal excimer laser ablations in human and porcine eyes, *Invest Ophthalmol and Vis Sci* (1995) **36**:S710.

18. Sano Y, Sakabe I, Ohki K, Tsuneoka H, Kitahara K, Effects of vibration on the corneal endothelium and Descemet's membrane in rabbits, *Invest Ophthalmol and Vis Sci* (1995) **36**:S712.

19. Niizuma T, Ito S, Hayashi M, Futemma M, Utsumi T, Ohashi K, Cooling the cornea to prevent side effects of photorefractive keratectomy, *J Refract Corneal Surg* (1994) **10(Suppl)**:S262–S266.

20. Tsubota K, Toda I, Itoh S, Reduction of subepithelial haze after photorefractive keratectomy by cooling the cornea [letter], *Am J Ophthalmol* (1993) **115**:820–1.

21. Toda I, Tsubota K, Itoh S, Endothelial change after excimer laser photorefractive keratectomy [letter], *J Refract Corneal Surg* (1994) **10**:379.

22. Amano S, Shimizu K, Tsubota K, Specular microscopic evaluation of the corneal epithelium after excimer laser photorefractive keratectomy, *Am J Ophthalmol* (1994) **117(3)**:381–4.

23. Amano S, Tanaka S, Shimizu K, Optical performance of the cornea following excimer laser myopic photorefractive keratectomy [abstract], *Invest Ophthalmol and Vis Sci* (1995) **36**:S711.

24. Amano S, Tanaka S, Shimizu K, Topographical evaluation of centration of excimer laser myopic photorefractive keratectomy, *J Cataract Refract Surg* (1994) **20**:616–8.

25. Uozato H, Sakurai I, Effect of pupil decentration on centering corneal surgical procedures [abstract], *Invest Ophthalmol and Vis Sci* (1995) **36**:S713.

26. Rogers C, Cohen P, Lawless M, Phototherapeutic keratectomy for Reis Bucklers' corneal dystrophy, *Aust N Z J Ophthalmol* (1993) **21**:247–50.

27. Lawless M, Cohen P, Rogers C, Phototherapeutic keratectomy for Reis Bucklers' dystrophy, *Refract Corneal Surg* (1993) **9(Suppl)**:S96–8.

28. Snibson GR, Murrell I, Taylor HR, Therapeutic applications of the excimer laser, (Unpublished).

29. Hahn TW, Sah WJ, Kim JH, Phototherapeutic keratectomy in nine eyes with superficial corneal diseases, *Refract Corneal Surg* (1993) **9(Suppl)**:S115–8.

30. Kim JH, Hahn TW, Excimer laser ablation of conjunctival epithelial melanosis, *J Cataract Refract Surg* (1993) **19**:309–11.

31. Tan DT, Tan JT, Will patients with contact lens problems accept excimer laser photorefractive keratectomy? *CLAO J* (1993) **19**:174–7.

32. Carson C, Taylor HR, Prevalence of myopia in adults: implications for refractive surgeons, *J Refract Surg* (1996) *In press*.

33. Carson CA, Garrett SKM, Aldred GF, Taylor HR, Subjective pain assessment following excimer laser photorefractive keratectomy for myopia and astigmatism, *J Refract Corneal Surg* (1996) **12**:365–9.

34. Kang HK, Beaumont PE, Taylor HR, van Saarloos PP, Constable IJ, Visual outcome of the excimer laser photorefractive keratectomy for myopia: a comparison of three laser delivery systems in Australia, *Aust NZ Ophthalmol* (1995) **23**: 265–72.

35. Lawless MA, Rogers C, Cohen P, Excimer laser photorefractive keratectomy: 12 months' follow-up, *Med J Aust* (1993) **159**:535–8.

36. Taylor HR, Guest CS, Kelly P, Alpins NA, Comparison of excimer laser treatment of astigmatism and myopia, *Arch Ophthalmol* (1993) **111**:1621–6.

37. Taylor HR, Kelly P, Alpins N, Excimer laser correction of myopic astigmatism, *J Cataract Refract Surg* (1994) **20(Suppl)**:243–51.

38. Snibson GR, Carson CA, Aldred GF, Taylor HR, One year evaluation of excimer laser photorefractive keratectomy for myopia and myopic astigmatism, *Arch Ophthalmol* (1995) **113**: 994–1000.

39. Balakrishnan V, Lim AS, Low CH, et al, Excimer laser photorefractive keratectomy in Singapore: a new treatment modality for myopia, *Singapore Med J* (1993) **34**:309–12.

40. Kim JH, Hahn TW, Lee YC, Sah WJ, Excimer laser photorefractive keratectomy for myopia: two year follow up, *J Cataract Refract Surg* (1994) **20(Suppl)**:229–33.

41. Kim JH, Sah WJ, Hahn TW Lee YC, Some problems after photorefractive keratectomy, *J Refract Corneal Surg* (1994) **10(Suppl)**:S226–S230.

42. Kim MS, Park CK, Sah WJ, Lee YC, Joo CK, Kim JH, Evaluation of factors influencing regression after photorefractive keratectomy, *Invest Ophthalmol and Vis Sci* (1995) **36**:S716 (abst).

43. Hahn TW, Kim JH, Lee YC, Excimer laser photorefractive keratectomy to correct residual myopia after radial keratotomy, *Refract Corneal Surg* (1993) **9(Suppl)**:S25–S29.

44. Rogers CM, Lawless MA, Cohen PR, Photorefractive keratectomy for myopia of more than 10 diopters, *J Refract Corneal Surg* (1994) **10(Suppl)**:S171–S173.

45. Lawless MA, Cohen PR, Rogers CM, Retreatment of undercorrected photorefractive keratectomy for myopia, *J Refract Corneal Surg* (1994) **10(Suppl**:S174–S177.

46. Lawless MA, Rogers C, Sutton G, Photorefractive keratectomy for high myopia: an analysis of risk factors, *International Society of Refractive Keratoplasty* 1994 Pre-American Academy of Ophthalmology Meeting Book, San Francisco, California, October 1994, 50 (abst).

47. Taylor HR, Carson CA, Excimer laser treatment for high and extreme myopia, *Trans Am Ophthalmologic Soc* (1994) **92**: 251–64.

48. Cho YS, Kim CG, Kim WB, Kim CW, Multistep photorefractive keratectomy for high myopia, *Refract Corneal Surg* (1993) **9(Suppl)**:S37–S41.

49. Kim JH, Hahn TW, Lee YC, Sah WJ, Clinical experience of two step photorefractive keratectomy in 19 eyes with high myopia, *Refract Corneal Surg* (1993) **9(Suppl)**:S44–S47.

50. Tong PP, Kam JT, Lam RH, et al, Excimer laser photorefractive keratectomy for myopia: Six-month follow-up, *J Cataract Refract Surg* (1995) **21**:150–5.

51. Baek SH, Kim WJ, Chang JH, Lee JH, The effect of topical corticosteroids on refractive outcome and corneal haze after excimer laser photorefractive keratectomy: comparison of the effects on low to moderate and high myopia groups, *Invest Ophthalmol and Vis Sci* (1995) **36**:S713 (abst).

52. Snibson GR, Taylor HR, Retreatment following laser photorefractive keratectomy, *Invest Ophthalmol Vis Sci* (1994) **35**:2019.

53. Lawless MA, Rogers C, Sutton G, Retreatment for scarring and regression following photorefractive keratectomy (PRK), *Br J Ophthalmol* (1995).

54. Balakrishnan V, Lim AS, Tseng PS, Hong LC, Decentered ablation zones resulting from photorefractive keratectomy with an erodible mask, *Int Ophthalmol* (1993) **17**:179–84.

55. Ring CP, Hadden OB, Morris AT, Transverse keratotomy combined with spherical photorefractive keratectomy for

compound myopic astigmatism, *J Refract Corneal Surg* (1994) **10(Suppl)**:S217–S221.

56. Choi YI, Min HK, Hyun PM, Excimer laser photorefractive keratectomy for astigmatism, *Korean J Ophthalmol* (1993) **7**:20–4.

57. Yong JK, Sohn J, Tchah H, Lee CO, Photoastigmatic refractive keratectomy in 168 eyes: six-month results, *J Cataract Refract Surg* (1994) **20**:387–91.

58. Alpins NA, A new method of analyzing vectors for changes in astigmatism, *J Cataract Refract Surg* (1993) **19**:524–33.

59. Levin S, Carson CA, Garrett SK, Taylor HR, Prevalence of central islands following excimer laser surgery, *J Cataract Refract Surg* (1995) **21**:21–26.

60. Carson CA, Snibson GR, Taylor HR, An analysis of clinical correlations one, three, six and 12 months after excimer laser photorefractive keratectomy, *Lasers and Light in Ophthalmol* (1994) **6**:249–57.

Chapter 15 Photoastigmatic refractive keratectomy (PARK)

Noel A Alpins, Geoffrey C Tabin and Hugh R Taylor

INTRODUCTION: DEFINING THE PROBLEM

Previous chapters have shown how the 193 nm excimer laser can treat myopia. However, a majority of patients seeking excimer laser photorefractive surgery for myopia have concomitant astigmatic refractive errors. In our experience, patients with moderate myopia (less than 5.0 D) averaged 1.04 D of associated cylinder at the corneal plane, while the high myopes (greater than 5.0 D but less than 10.0 D) averaged 1.20 D and the extreme myopes (greater than 10.0 D) 1.39 D. In order to achieve the goals of emmetropia, optimal uncorrected visual acuity, and maximum patient satisfaction, the refractive surgeon must address the problem of astigmatic errors. This chapter will review the role of the excimer laser in combating astigmatism.

Astigmatism can be one of the most difficult and frustrating problems in refractive surgery. First one must precisely quantify the astigmatism that is to be treated. Astigmatism can be measured objectively at the corneal plane via keratometry or corneal topography, or subjectively based on manifest refraction. The surgeon must weigh several options in deciding how to individualize treatment for each case. Moreover, ocular surgery in general, as well as refractive surgery, can create its own unintended induced astigmatic changes—Surgical Induced Astigmatism (SIA) vector.

ASTIGMATISM: SURGICAL AND OPTICAL CONCEPTS

Astigmatism is defined optically as 'the refractive anomaly in which no point focus is formed owing to the unequal refraction of the incident light by the dioptric system of the eye in different meridians'.[1] Curvature astigmatism of the anterior corneal surface occurs physiologically. The average normal cornea has a difference in refractive power between its principal meridians of 0.5–0.75 D, with a difference of 1.0 D being the upper limit of normal. 'Regular' astigmatism occurs when the principal meridians are at right angles to each other on the topographical map and equal in magnitude. Most younger people have the axis of least curvature in the horizontal plane and the axis of steepest curvature in the vertical plane. This has been termed 'with-the-rule' astigmatism. With age there is usually a gradual shift of axis, with a steepening of the horizontal and flattening of the vertical meridian, a configuration called 'against-the-rule' astigmatism.

However, the net 'refractive' astigmatic error is not entirely derived from an asymmetric anterior corneal surface. The posterior surface of a normal cornea usually shows an astigmatic error that varies from 0.25 to 0.5 D. The principal meridians of the posterior corneal astigmatism are usually opposite in orientation to the anterior surface, and partially neutralize the astigmatic error. There is also curvature astigmatism on both surfaces of the lens. These again usually have the greater curvature in the horizontal meridian and partially negate the anterior corneal astigmatism. In addition, the laminated zones of the lens are not always concentric and may vary considerably in their refractive indices. This variance in refractive power in different meridians induces a small net astigmatism. Astigmatism also arises from the decentering of the optical system. None of the optical surfaces of the eye is geometrically centered around the visual axis or has a true axis of symmetry. The fovea is not on the optical axis, but is usually situated 1.25 mm inferiorly to the temporal side; meanwhile, the central pupillary line and optical axis are generally eccentric to the nasal side of the cornea. Furthermore, there is usually some degree of inherent tilting of the retina. Following Gullstrand's model of 1911 which accepts an angle of 5° between the pupillary line and optical axis, there would be 0.1 D of astigmatism that exists as the result of the alignment of the optical axis with a 2 mm pupil. Finally, the visual cortical perception of the transmitted image can influence the readings that are measured by the subjective manifest refraction.

The astigmatism that is measured by the manifest refraction is the 'refractive astigmatism'. The astigmatism that is measured on the anterior corneal surface by topography is the 'topographical astigmatism'. The disparity between the refractive astigmatism as measured at the corneal plane and the topographical (or keratometric) astigmatism is the 'residual astigmatism'. The residual astigmatism is the sum of the effect of the astigmatic errors present on the posterior corneal surface, the lens surfaces and varying refractive indices of the media, and from decentration of the optical system. The residual astigmatism can be determined by vectorially subtracting the values of the topographical astigmatism from the refractive astigmatism at the corneal plane, or its magnitude can be measured directly by performing a subjective refraction with a spherical hard contact lens on the cornea. If the excimer laser were to create a spherical anterior corneal surface, the patient's residual astigmatism would remain as the refractive astigmatism. If the excimer laser is used to sculpt all the refractive astigmatism onto the cornea, then the topographical astigmatism remaining on the cornea would equal the residual astigmatism both in magnitude and axis, and would neutralize the astigmatism from the other refractive components of the eye.

Over a large series it was found that young adults averaged 1.04 D of corneal astigmatism and 0.61 D of residual astigmatism.[2] Some degree of detectable refractive astigmatism was found in 95% of eyes. The most common form of astigmatism was compound myopic (39%), with compound hypermetropic astigmatism (27%) being the next most frequent; simple hypermetropic (14%), mixed astigmatism (11%) and simple myopic astigmatism (10%) were slightly less common.

The amount of astigmatism varies greatly. Approximately 85% of people have less than 1.25 D of refractive astigmatism. An increase in spherical error is associated with a larger astigmatic error as mentioned above. Astigmatism results in both blurring and distortion of the visual image. Regular astigmatism, with the principal steep and flat meridians at right angles to each other, results in no single focused retinal image, but has two separate lines at right angles to each other, with an intervening ellipse of least confusion that has a diameter proportional to the degree of astigmatism (Figure 15.1). In hyperopic and mixed astigmatism, the patient will generally attempt to focus one of the lines

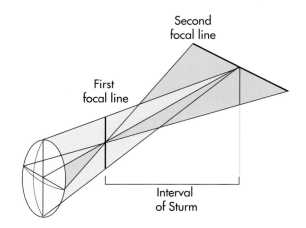

Figure 15.1 *Schematic of the Conoid of Sturm demonstrating that a spherocylindrical lens produces two focal lines separated by the interval of Sturm.*

via accommodation, preferring to have a distorted rather than blurred image. The myopic astigmatic patient will be unable to compensate with accommodation and will have a perpetually blurred image for distance vision. The adverse effect on uncorrected visual acuity, at least in terms of recognizing Snellen letters, is least for with-the-rule astigmatism, less for against-the-rule and perhaps greatest when the astigmatism is oblique. This will be discussed in more detail when we turn to surgical planning.

One diopter of astigmatic error will, on average, decrease uncorrected acuity to the level of 20/30 or 20/40 depending on the axis (versus 20/50 for 1.00 D of spherical myopia or absolute hyperopia.)[3] Other than simply blurred vision, astigmatism can cause glare, asthenopia, distortion, eye strain, headaches, monocular diplopia, a head tilt with neck pain from attempting to change an oblique axis closer to vertical, and continual squinting in an unconscious attempt to create a stenopeic slit to view only the paraxial rays of one meridian.

ADDRESSING THE PROBLEM: CONSIDERATIONS FOR PLANNING THE PROCEDURE

The refractive surgeon who wishes to provide optimal uncorrected vision has to address the complexities of

Residual astigmatism
magnitude (Diopters)

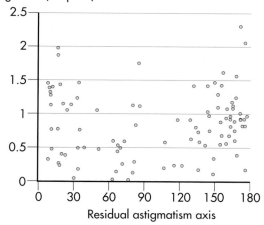

Figure 15.2 *Scatterplot of residual astigmatism: axis versus magnitude for 100 consecutive patients.*[38]

astigmatic errors. The corneal shape must be incorporated with the refraction into a specific surgical plan. This can best be done with vector analysis.[4] The first priority is to identify the goal of the treatment for each individual's eye according to the preoperative parameters of topography and refraction. Subjective refraction, modified if necessary by cycloplegic findings, and corneal topography are both obtained. Simply creating a spherical anterior corneal surface, guided by topography, will leave the residual error from the posterior surface of the cornea, the lens and decentration of the axis. This resultant astigmatism is often in an against-the-rule or oblique orientation, and it can be difficult for the patient to adapt to the new axis. However, using the refractive astigmatism, and sculpting a spherocylindrical lens into the cornea without regard for the sphericity of the cornea, may cause spherical aberration which increases in corneas with larger amounts of astigmatism.[5]

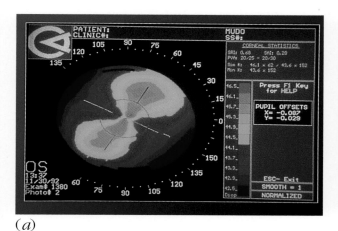

(a)

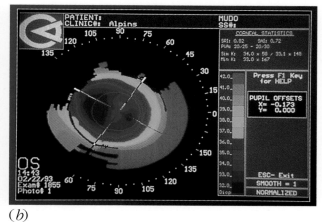

(b)

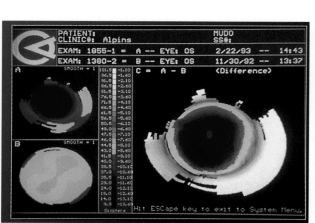

(c)

Figure 15.3 *Computerized corneal topographic maps. (a) Before PARK treatment showing bow tie regular astigmatism. (b) After PARK treatment showing uniform curvature of the central cornea. (c) Subtraction map showing the astigmatic change produced by the laser.*

The targeted final astigmatism is determined from the differences in the refractive and topographical astigmatism. As has been previously stated, 'with-the-rule' astigmatism is preferable to other orientations. Having the steepest meridian oriented vertically, in a case of simple astigmatism, places the clearest retinal image in the vertical meridian. Eggers has shown that this improves visual acuity as measured by Snellen type, as vertical strokes predominate in the English alphabet.[6] In addition, the nasotemporal overlap of ganglion cells that supply both optic tracts are bilaterally cortically represented. They lie on the vertical midline raphe of retinal receptors and neuronal fibers, centered on the fovea, with a width extending greater than 1° of arc.[7] This explains the much lower stereoscopic threshold for vertical objects than those oriented in any other meridian.

In eyes that have lost their accommodative powers, such as occurs in pseudophakia, it may also be advantageous to have a small amount of residual 'with-the-rule' astigmatism in association with a mild amount of myopia. Sawusch and Guyton calculated the cross-sectional area of Sturm's conoid for a schematic eye for given refractive errors and at fixed distances.[8] They found the optimal astigmatic error needed to obtain maximal depth of focus and least theoretical blur for any given spherical equivalent refractive error. The optimal depth of focus was obtained when the plus cylindrical component equalled the negative sphere minus 0.25 D, for example, +0.50D −0.75D × 180°. They then correlated these results with 10 pseudophakic patients who had better than 20/40 (6/12) Snellen uncorrected visual acuity for both near and distance vision.

In a personal series of 100 consecutive patients who underwent photorefractive astigmatic keratectomy, the calculated mean residual astigmatism of the group as determined by vector analysis was 0.81 D with a range of 0.01–2.32 D (Fig. 15.2). The residual astigmatism exceeded 1.00 D in 34 patients, and seven of these exceeded the preoperative magnitude of topographic astigmatism (simulated keratometry) as measured by videokeratography. In the surgical planning process, the surgeon should decide on the optimal manner in which to deal with the residual astigmatism. Using the dual guiding refractive principle that it is more favourable to have less corneal astigmatism with a bias to maintaining a with-the-rule orientation, the surgeon can choose to leave a calculated amount of residual astigmatism in the manifest refraction and reduce the amount of targeted corneal

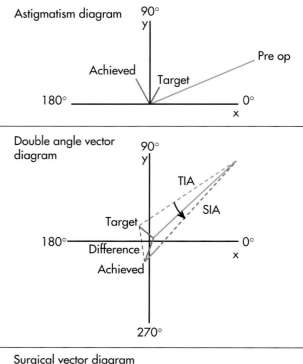

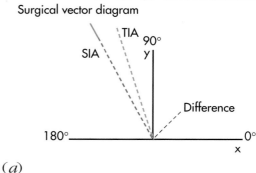

(a)

Figure 15.4(a) *Alpins' method of vector analysis utilizing doubled angles to calculate the surgical vector of change in astigmatism.*[4]

astigmatism. If the target spherical equivalent is achieved within range, the patient will no longer require spectacles but will benefit from less resultant corneal astigmatism.

Once the desired topographic and refractive targets have been chosen, a calculation is made to determine the desired targeted change in astigmatism in the corneal curvature. The force required to effect this change from the preoperative topographic and refractive condition is termed the 'Target Induced Astigmatism (TIA) vector'. The actual path taken is the SIA. This is the vector representing the actual change that occurs. By using the targeted corneal

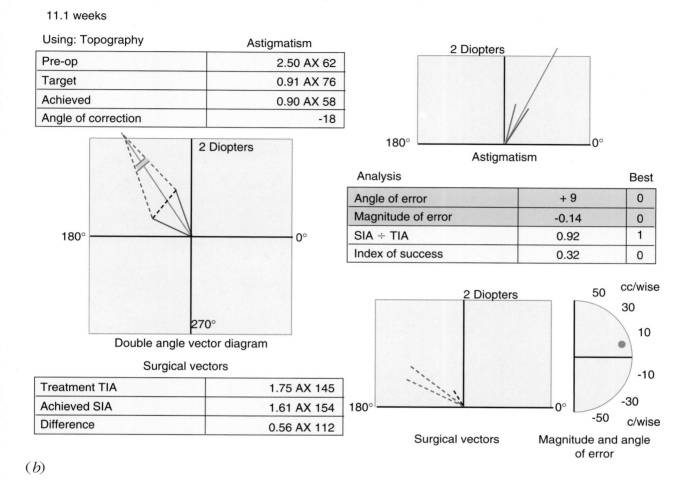

Alpins method

11.1 weeks

Using: Topography

	Astigmatism
Pre-op	2.50 AX 62
Target	0.91 AX 76
Achieved	0.90 AX 58
Angle of correction	-18

2 Diopters

180°   0°

Astigmatism

Double angle vector diagram

Surgical vectors

Treatment TIA	1.75 AX 145
Achieved SIA	1.61 AX 154
Difference	0.56 AX 112

Analysis		Best
Angle of error	+ 9	0
Magnitude of error	-0.14	0
SIA ÷ TIA	0.92	1
Index of success	0.32	0

Surgical vectors

Magnitude and angle of error

(*b*)

Figure 15.4 *(b) Vector analysis applied to the case shown topographically in Figure 14.3.*

astigmatism instead of one of the two preoperative astigmatism values, all astigmatism surgeons can operate under a single paradigm with parallel goals set on the optimal targeted result of surgery.[4,38]

Analyzing astigmatism results by topography as well as refraction is an essential step to enable the objective as well as the subjective evaluation of the results of the procedure. It is the various relationships between the SIA and the TIA that provide the necessary information as to whether too much or too little change was applied, how to adjust for it, and whether the treatment was on axis or off axis (Fig. 15.3). A topographic subtraction map is useful in demonstrat-

ing the point-by-point change in astigmatism, but it does not provide vector analysis of the changes.

Vector analysis enables the refractive surgeon to examine his or her results in no more complex a manner than a golfer analyzing his or her putting on a flat green. Was the ball hit too firmly or too softly? Was it on axis, or was it misdirected in a clockwise or counter-clockwise direction? If the hole was missed on the first putt, how long must the second putt be to land in the hole (the Difference Vector) and how does this length compare to the length of the first putt (Index of Success)?

Astigmatic Vector Terminology

TIA	— Target Induced Astigmatism, the planned astigmatic change expressed as a vector.
SIA	— Surgically Induced Astigmatism, the astigmatic change that results from surgery expressed as a vector.
Difference Vector	— Astigmatism change still required to achieve the initial goal of surgery.
Percentage of Astigmatism Corrected	— Correction Index (SIA/TIA) × 100.
Index of Success	— Difference Vector/TIA.

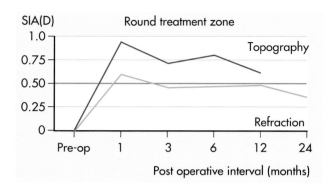

Figure 15.5 *Mean SIA magnitude after spherical PRK by topography and refraction in 60 patients followed for 2 years.[9]*

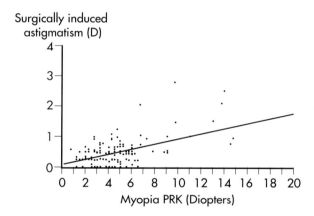

Figure 15.6 *SIA magnitude plotted against the amount of preoperative myopia for 155 PRK patients at 1-year follow-up: note the increasing inadvertently induced astigmatism with the treatment of larger amounts of myopia.[11]*

Because astigmatism is usually reported using polar coordinates in a 0–180° sense, certain changes can be difficult to quantify. For instance, a change in astigmatism from a preoperative value of 5° to a postoperative equal value of 175° appears numerically and graphically to be a counterclockwise change of 170°. It is, in fact, only a 10° clockwise change. Doubling the angles during the calculations ensures that results are examined in a 360° sense, so that rectangular coordinates may be used (Fig. 15.4). This method simplifies interpretation of changes between preoperative, desired, and achieved astigmatic values and is necessary to determine the magnitude and direction of surgical vectors.

It is important to assess how effective a treatment has been, that is how close the SIA is to the TIA. This will depend on the computer algorithm used for the laser, proper and steady centration and uniform epithelial healing. Remodelling of the anterior corneal surface may also result in changes in the astigmatic status. Spherical photorefractive keratectomy does not intend to induce astigmatism. However, the SIA from treating purely myopic refractive errors with spheric treatment zones is about 0.5 D by refraction and 0.6 D by topography at 12 months in our patients (Fig. 15.5). Alpins and Taylor reported a mean induced astigmatic change of 0.45 D in 42 eyes one year after spherical PRK treatments,[9] and Goggin and his associates report a mean cylinder power change of 0.75 D in 60 eyes.[10] Nine eyes had greater than 1.00 D of SIA. Tabin et al report a linear relationship, with increased inadvertently induced astigmatism with the treatment

of increasing amounts of spherical myopia (Fig. 15.6).[11] This inadvertent SIA must be considered when planning excimer laser surgery.

HOW IT WORKS: THE WAY VARIOUS EXCIMER LASERS CORRECT ASTIGMATISM

The first description of how the excimer laser can be used to create toric ablations for the correction of

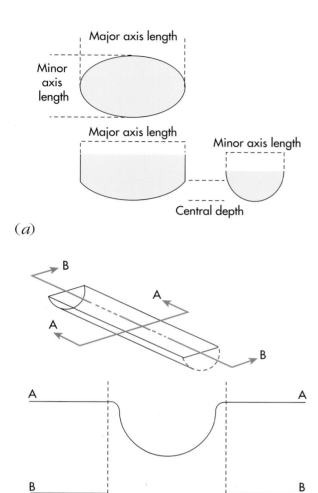

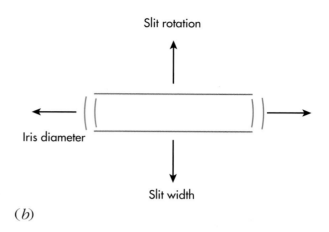

(a)

(b)

(c)

Figure 15.7 *Visx treatment of astigmatism. (a) Elliptical ablation geometry. (b) Astigmatism aperture mechanism. (c) Astigmatism ablation model.*

astigmatism was published in early 1991.[12] The techniques and computer programs for PRK to create a radially symmetric ablation with a greater depth centrally than peripherally in order to correct myopia were already well established. In general terms, utilizing incisional or laser techniques, one can correct corneal astigmatism by selective flattening of a steep meridian or steepening of a flat meridian. Munnerlyn and his associates modified the laser software to have a large diameter laser beam pass through an aperture created by a mobile set of parallel blades that the computer controls.[12] The width of the slit changes with the separation or narrowing of the blades in order to provide a controlled cylindrical ablation; the slower the blade movements for a constant pulse rate, the greater the astigmatic correction (Fig. 15.7). The cornea is relatively flattened in the meridian perpendicular to the long axis of the slit. This long axis is called the 'mechanical axis' and would ideally undergo no refractive change if only astigmatism were to be corrected. Initially the astigmatic correction was performed as a cylindrical ablation followed by a second, spherical, ablation to correct the residual myopia. This method has been termed the 'sequential' method of ablation, referring to performing the treatments for myopia and astigmatism in two phases.

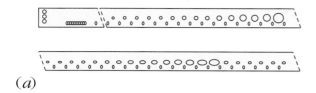

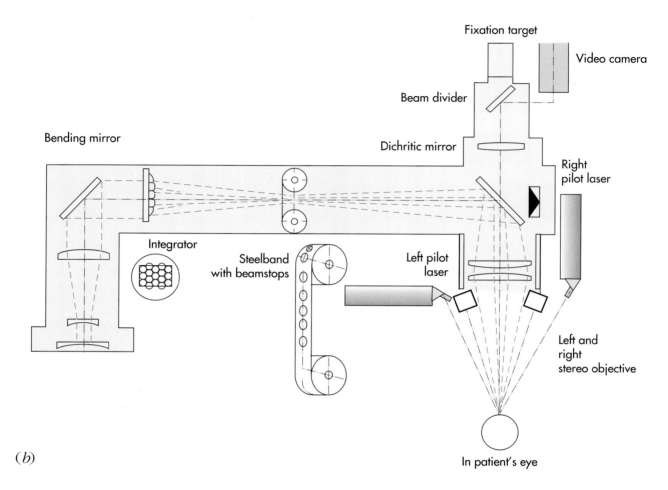

Figure 15.8 *Schwind treatment of astigmatism. (a) Maskenband. (b) Delivery system. The band passes through the delivery system like film through a projector controlling the contour of the laser ablation.*

The Visx software was further modified to combine expansion of the inner parallel blades with a controlled contraction of a round diaphragm.[12] This allowed the full myopic and astigmatic correction to be sculpted into the cornea in one, smooth ablation. This technique has been termed the 'elliptical' method. The elliptical program effectively avoids excessive narrowing of the minor axis of the ellipse, as the surgeon is precluded from treating astigmatism in excess of the amount of spherical myopia.

The Schwind excimer laser controls its beam profile by means of a series of apertures on a revolving band that pass between the laser and the eye, much like film running through a movie projector (Fig. 15.8). Round apertures are employed to guide their purely myopic ablations, and an oval or slit aperture aligned at the appropriate axis to treat astigmatic errors.[13]

Another approach that allows the excimer laser to correct astigmatism is to use an erodible mask to control the shape transfer.[14] A polymethylmethacrylate button, of a specific shape determined by the refractive error of the patient, is placed between the beam and the cornea. The ablation rate of the button

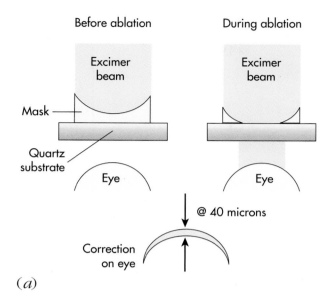

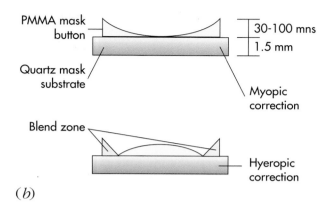

Figure 15.9 *(a) An ablatable mask is inserted between the laser and the eye. (b) The mask transfers the preset astigmatic contours onto the cornea. This is the technique being used by the Summit laser.*

is similar to that of the cornea. The treatment is performed using the maximal aperture of the laser diaphragm so that the button is simultaneously ablated over its entire surface. When the thinnest part of the button has been ablated, the laser begins to sculpt the cornea. This process effectively reproduces the mask's shape onto the cornea producing the desired astigmatic correction. This is the technique that is currently being developed for the Summit laser (Fig. 15.9).

A different mask technique is being employed by the Aesculap–Meditech MEL 60 excimer laser. Dausch and his associates developed a rotating mask with an hourglass-shaped opening over a slit delivery system that uses a scanning process rather than a broad beam exposure (Fig. 15.10).[15] If the mask is rotated in equidistant angular steps over 360°, a symmetric ablation is achieved. However, if the mask is held in one position longer than another, the ablation depth will be increased in a desired meridian. Thus, by selectively allowing more time in a specific meridian during the rotation, astigmatism can be corrected. By altering the mask aperture Dausch and co-workers are able to treat hyperopic astigmatism.[15] For mixed astigmatism they used the same technique in a two-stage process, correcting first the myopic cylinder followed by a spherical hyperopic correction, or by correcting first the hyperopic cylinder and then the residual myopia (Fig. 15.11).

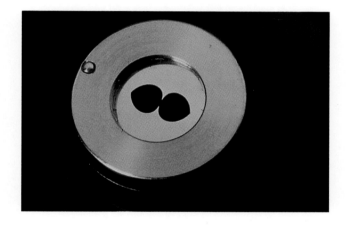

Figure 15.10 *Meditech treatment of astigmatism utilizes a rotating mask. By controlling the time the mask spends in different alignments during the rotation, an ablation can be performed to treat both myopic and hyperopic astigmatism.*

The Technolas (Fig. 15.12), Nidek (Fig. 15.13) and Lasersight lasers all employ a scanning mechanism to correct astigmatic errors. The Technolas model has the laser beam move along the axes of astigmatism with an increasing diameter. The Lasersight and

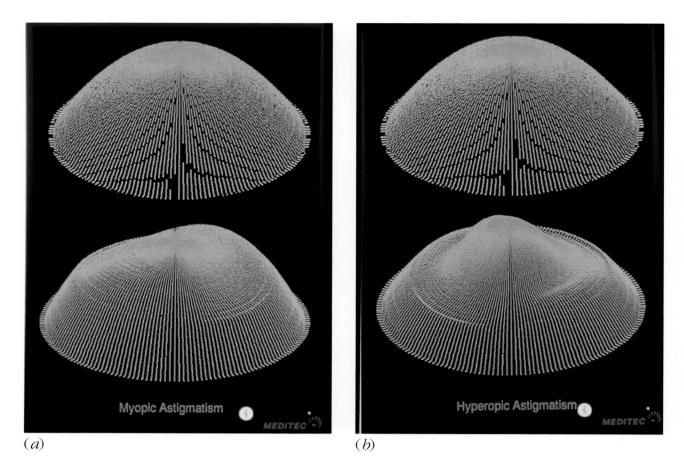

(a) (b)

Figure 15.11 (a) Schematic contour map of a cornea after a Meditech laser ablation for myopic astigmatism. (b) Schematic contour map of a cornea after a Meditech laser ablation for hyperopic astigmatism.

The laserbeam moves along the axis of the astigmatism (negative convention) with increasing diameter

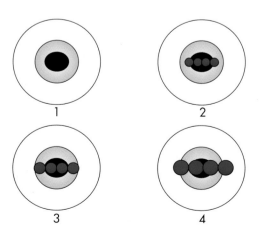

Figure 15.12 The Chiron Technolas scanning mechanism alters the diameter of the laser beam as it moves along the axes of astigmatism to carve an astigmatic ablation.

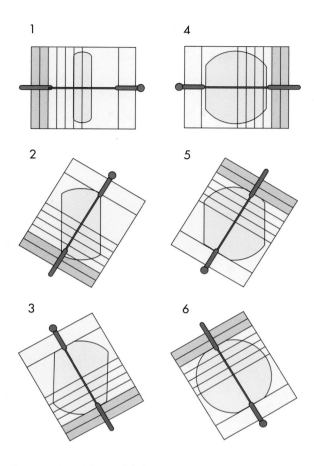

Figure 15.13 *The Nidek laser uses a scan and rotate model to create astigmatic changes in the corneal topography.*

Nidek lasers utilize a similar concept in their rotating scanning beam. Recent innovations by Technolas and Lasersight have introduced the technique of a flying spot facilitating treatment of hyperopic astigmatism by selective ablation for steepening at the flat axis.

Astigmatic keratotomy, which uses a knife to create a partial thickness cut in the cornea on the steepest axis, has been used to combat astigmatism since 1885 when Schiotz described a penetrating limbal incision in a post-cataract patient with high astigmatism.[16] Fyodorov[17] popularized modern anterior corneal keratotomy techniques that have been refined over the past 25 years. Agapitos and Lindstrom recently reported on the state of arcuate keratotomy and found the results to be only 'reasonable' and often 'unpredictable'.[18] There is no published vector analysis of results of astigmatic keratotomy and thus quantitative comparison with PARK is not possible. Despite the

unpredictability of the results, Lipschitz et al[19] and Ring et al[20] have both advocated a two-step procedure combining both incisional and laser surgery. To treat compound myopic astigmatism these authors first use an incisional astigmatic keratotomy that is followed by a spherical photorefractive keratectomy.

All of the above methods are used to treat regular astigmatism. The initial surgical plans to correct astigmatism with the excimer laser were based on the refractive astigmatic error converted to the corneal plane as the sole determinant of treatment. By the early 1990s, advances in corneal topographic mapping gave new parameters to guide the corneal refractive surgeon, but the quantitative information provided has not been fully utilized. We advocate the consideration of corneal topography when developing the surgical plan to treat regular astigmatism to reduce the amount of resultant corneal astigmatism and to optimize its meridian.[4,38]

Astigmatism that is not regular cannot be treated by the application of any simple geometric pattern of tissue removal. However, with computerized topography, the surgeon can identify high, steep areas of the cornea. These areas then can be selectively ablated with small, circular focal treatments, as would be done for a phototherapeutic keratectomy (PTK).[21] This can be followed by a PRK centered over the entrance pupil. The overall effect minimizes the differences between steeper and flatter areas on the topographical map, reduces the irregular astigmatism and improves the optical quality of the cornea.

RESULTS: THE EFFECTIVENESS OF THE EXCIMER LASER IN CORRECTING ASTIGMATISM

MYOPIC ASTIGMATISM

The first clinical report of the excimer laser creating toric ablations to treat cylindrical errors was published by McDonnell and colleagues in 1991.[22] Four patients with compound myopic astigmatism were successfully treated. An average of 83% ±17% of the refractive astigmatism was corrected. These initial good results led many surgeons around the world to start treating myopic astigmatism with the excimer laser.

In Melbourne there are now data on 343 patients who have had more than a 1 year follow-up after excimer laser correction of myopic astigmatism.[23] Myopic astigmatism was treated by using either the sequential or elliptical method. In the sequential method, the amount of minus sphere to be treated is calculated by first determining the expected hyperopic shift. This is calculated by subtracting 1.00 D from the amount of cylinder and then halving the remaining amount of cylinder to provide a spherical equivalent.[24] This amount of expected hyperopic shift is then subtracted from the spherical component to give the residual spectacle myopia to be treated. With the elliptical method, no correction for hyperopic shift is required.

The PARK procedures were divided into single or multiple treatment zone sizes according to the amount of correction. For corrections of −5.00 D or less spherical equivalent (SE) (low myopia), we used a single 6.0 mm zone; for corrections > −5.00 D SE and ≤ to −10.00 D SE (high myopia), we used two zones (5.0 mm and 6.0 mm); for corrections > −10.00 D (extreme myopia), we used three zones (4.5 mm, 5.0 mm and 6.0 mm).[23] The myopic correction was divided equally into each zone. When an elliptical astigmatic correction was performed, the cylindrical correction, which did not exceed 80% of the spherical dioptric correction for the zone, was entered into the largest (6.0 mm) zone size. When the cylinder exceeded 80% of the sphere to be treated in the 6.0 mm zone, the astigmatic correction was shared equally between the 5.0 mm and 6.0 mm zones in order to prevent overlapping boundaries and create concentric ellipses and evenly contoured ablation zones. No astigmatism was corrected in the 4.5 mm zone when this zone was employed for the correction of > −10.0 D spherical equivalent.

Our results indicate that both the myopic (Table 15.1) and the astigmatic components of myopic astigmatism can be effectively treated with the excimer laser (Table 15.2). Postoperatively, 68% of the patients had a spherical equivalent within 1.00 D of plano and 77% within 2.00 D of plano at 6 months.[23] If one looks only at patients whose preoperative refraction was −10.00 D or less the results improve to 73% within 1.00 D and 87% within 2.00 D. Seventy-two per cent of these patients had an uncorrected visual acuity equal to or better than 20/40.

Vector analysis was used to assess the change in both topographic and refractive astigmatism. When comparing the targeted change in astigmatism with both the elliptical and sequential methods for the treatments prior to April 1993, the SIA, both by refraction and topography, showed an undercorrection. Therefore, a calculated adjustment of 1.2 was factored into all our subsequent astigmatic treatments. This adjustment has now been incorporated

into the Visx software and has led to less undercorrection with the SIA closer to the TIA (Fig. 15.14) and a correction index closer to 1.0.

When measuring the success of the procedure at 12 months, the index improved from 0.55 to 0.43, which means that nearly 60% correction of the astigmatism is being achieved. When this is stratified into three groups of spherical myopia, 0–5 D, 5–10 D and 10–15 D, the index of success by refraction shows that there were fairly equivalent results between the groups. However, the visual outcome was worse for the extreme myopes.[25]

Although the magnitude of correction remained excellent, results in Melbourne for extreme myopes showed a less successful visual result than for low or high myopes. We have 1 year follow up on 58 extreme myopes who have had PARK. We had a post-treatment mean spherical equivalent of −1.91 D

Table 15.1

Accuracy of refraction

| | 12 Months | | | |
| | PRK | | PARK | |
	±1D	±2D	±1D	±2D
Low	90.6%	99.1%	84.9%	98.8%
High	75%	95.5%	62%	88.3%
Extreme	77.8%	77.8%	28.2%	50%

Table 15.2

Mean correction index × 100 (per cent)
Alpins' method
95% confidence limits

| Coefficient 1.0 | | | |
Elliptical		Sequential	
Low (n = 52)	77 (66, 91)	Low (n = 22)	71 (58, 86)
High (n = 63)	78 (64, 97)	High (n = 9)	74 (59, 93)
Extreme (n = 13)	104 (60, 189)	Extreme	–

| Coefficient 1.2 | | | |
Elliptical		Sequential	
Low (n = 70)	101 (88, 115)	Low (n = 16)	82 (59, 96)
High (n = 66)	86 (79, 99)	High (n = 1)	69
Extreme (n = 18)	74 (35, 153)	Extreme	–

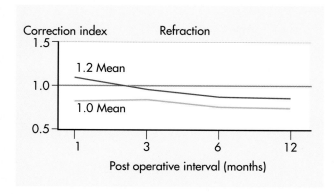

Figure 15.14 *Correction index, showing SIA/TIA for PARK before and after the 1.2 adjustment with the Visx laser as measured by refraction at the corneal plane. We are now closer to our goal.*[40]

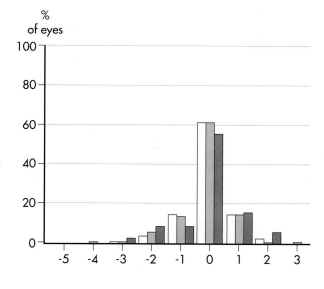

Figure 15.15 *Graph showing the loss and gain in best corrected visual acuity for 333 PARK patients.*[40]

and a mean astigmatism of −1.06 D ±0.97. Refraction within 1.00 D of emmetropia was achieved in 39% of the patients and 56% were within 2.00 D. The mean angle of error was −6.16° ±17.3°. Retreatment was required in 30% of the patients. The mean haze score remained 1.0 at one year, and 15% of the eyes lost one line of best corrected acuity, with 8% losing two or more lines (Fig. 15.15).

There was also a difference in the undercorrection between the patients treated with an elliptical ablation, and sequential treatments of a plano-cylindrical treatment followed by a spherical treatment. The SIA is closer to the TIA for the elliptical treatments (Fig. 15.16). However, the sequential method was used for more difficult patients, where the amount of cylinder was larger relative to the spherical error.

Our magnitude of correction has become satisfactory. However, our overall index of success was only 0.43. This can be explained by the angle of error. Although the mean angle of error measured by both refraction and topography is near zero, the standard deviation is 30° wide. This can be confirmed on scatter plots (Fig. 15.17) which show a wide distribution from −90° to +90° with the greatest variation being with low levels of attempted astigmatic correction. The subjective test of refraction shows a predictable peak at the zero axis. There is a potential for future improvement in astigmatism surgery by

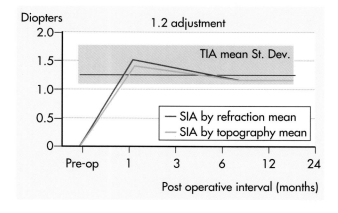

Figure 15.16 *SIA compared to TIA by both refraction and topography after the Visx 1.2 systematic adjustment.*[40]

improving the accuracy in the axis of applied treatment. This is achievable by better identification of the steepest corneal axis at the time of surgery, more accurate laser beam alignment, and ensuring completeness of epithelial removal.

Other important factors in unwanted astigmatic change are the irregularity of epithelial healing and

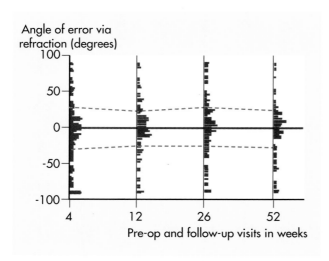

Figure 15.17 *Angle of error of treatment. The mean axis misalignment is close to zero and constant over time. However, the scatter is wide with a wide standard deviation band.*

thickening and the excessive synthesis of collagen and glycosaminoglycans by keratocytes in the treatment zone. These may lead to a thickening over the ablation zone and irregular topography causing optical aberrations and decreased postoperative vision.[26] Developments in antimitotic[27] and non-steroidal anti-inflammatory therapy[28] may help smooth the healing process and improve the outcome for high myopes and the accuracy of PARK.

Our visual results are similar to those of other groups using the Visx Twenty/Twenty laser to treat myopic astigmatism. Pender reported 1 year follow up on six patients who were treated for low or moderate myopia and astigmatism.[29] All had uncorrected visual acuities of 20/50 or better, and 62.5% had better than 20/40 vision. Two patients lost one line of best corrected vision and in six of the eight eyes they noted a change in axis postoperatively of greater than 5° from the preoperative cylinder.

Kim et al in Korea reported on 168 eyes that had treatment for myopic astigmatism with the Visx system.[30] Their mean preoperative astigmatism was 1.51 D. Their results showed, by simple analysis, a decrease in astigmatism of 56%. By comparing the preoperative and postoperative refractive astigmatism axis, they found that the axis of astigmatism changed > 10° in 54% of the eyes. However, there is limited value in simply comparing pre- and postoperative

axis of astigmatism without undertaking vector analysis. Their visual results were excellent, with 91% of the patients having an uncorrected visual acuity of 20/40 or better at 6 months and 60% seeing 20/25 or better. However, the majority of their patients had low to moderate myopia.

The Summit ablatable mask technique effectively treated myopic astigmatism in rabbits.[31] Hersh and Patel recently reported the initial results of the FDA phase 2b clinical trial on 10 patients who had toric corrections for myopic astigmatism.[32] Their patients all had less than 6.0 D of sphere and less than 2.75 D of astigmatism. The mean astigmatism decreased from 1.48 D preoperatively to 0.86 D postoperatively, with 63% achieving an uncorrected visual acuity of 20/40 or better. Their follow up was only for 2–4 months and vector analysis was not performed. Cherry et al also reported 3 month data on 34 eyes who were treated with the Summit ablatable mask for myopic astigmatism.[33] They found a reduction of approximately 50% in refractive astigmatism. Significantly, the objective changes of keratometry were reported to show less change than the subjective values of refraction. Again, the lack of vector analysis means it is not possible to assess the efficacy of the Summit lasers in treating astigmatism.

Dausch et al report 3-month results with the Meditech MEL 60 laser. They treated 29 patients with myopic astigmatism.[15] The mean preoperative cylindrical refraction was −2.10 D with a range from −1.0 D to −5.0 D. Postoperatively the mean astigmatism was reduced to −0.10 D with a range from 0 to −2.25 D. They also report a mean shift in axis of 2.0°, with a maximum change of 19°. The uncorrected visual acuity improved from a mean of 20/180 to 20/25 after laser surgery. However, 15% of these patients lost one line of best corrected acuity and 3% lost two Snellen lines, while 12% gained one line of best corrected vision. Again, vector analysis was not provided, making comparison with other systems difficult.

An initial report of 27 eyes that underwent PARK with the Coherent–Schwind Keratom gives promising visual results.[34] Eighty-two per cent of the eyes had an uncorrected visual acuity of 20/40 or better with 46% seeing 20/25. However, 40% of their patients were overcorrected by 1.0 D or more and 9% of their patients lost two or more lines of Snellen best corrected acuity. No mention of the vector changes in astigmatism or amount of refractive astigmatism was made.

As of June 1996, we are not aware of published data for the Technolas, Lasersight, and Nidek scanning laser treatment of astigmatism.

HYPEROPIC ASTIGMATISM

Dausch and Klein treated 23 patients with stable hyperopia of less than +8.00 D with stable astigmatism of less than −6.50 D.[15] Thirteen patients had hyperopic astigmatism and 10 had mixed astigmatism. They used the Meditech laser, and aimed for emmetropia in all cases.

For their group with compound hyperopic astigmatism, the mean preoperative spherical equivalent was +4.00 D ±1.28 D. After three months this value averaged −0.88 D ±1.73 D. The mean cylinder changed from −2.70 D ±1.23 D preoperatively to −0.40D ±0.13 D at 3 months. They reported that the postoperative refractive axis of astigmatism was within 10° of the preoperative axis in all eyes. Best corrected vision remained the same with three eyes gaining one Snellen line of best spectacle correction and three eyes losing one line of best acuity. The mean uncorrected acuity improved from 20/150 preoperatively to 20/50 at 3 months, with 61.5% obtaining an uncorrected acuity of 20/40 or better. However, two partially sighted eyes did not have the potential of 20/40 vision.

Their patients with mixed astigmatism were treated first with a myopic cylindrical ablation followed by a hyperopic spherical correction. They treated 10 eyes with an average preoperative spherical equivalent of + 0.47 D ±1.08 D and a mean preoperative cylinder of −5.02 D ±0.77 D. Three months after treatment the mean spherical equivalent was −0.22 D ±0.96 D and the mean cylindrical refraction was −0.25 D ±0.60 D. Seven of the 10 patients had an uncorrected visual acuity of 20/40 or better and two eyes did not have 20/40 potential.

The technique used for hyperopic astigmatism leaves the central cornea, including Bowman's layer, intact. Thus haze across the visual axis is less likely. Despite the small number of patients treated and the short follow up period, these results are encouraging.

POSTSURGICAL ASTIGMATISM

We used the Visx laser to treat patients with astigmatism remaining as the result of surgical procedures.[35] There is now 6-month data on 51 eyes in this group. Sixteen of these patients were post-penetrating keratoplasty, 14 had astigmatism induced from cataract surgery, nine were treated for post-radial keratotomy, three had corneal scars, and three were treated for astigmatism induced by glaucoma or retinal procedures. The treatment technique was divided, with 58% done with the sequential program and 42% with the elliptical method.

The post-keratoplasty patients had a wide range of spherical equivalents from −19.25 D to +2.50 D and astigmatism that varied from −1.5 D to −8.0 D with a mean of −5.02 D. Six months postoperatively the mean spherical equivalent was +0.10 D ±2.71 with a mean astigmatism of −3.04 D. Overall, the correction index was 0.73 showing that 73% of the planned astigmatic correction was achieved with a mean angle of error of +12.5° (counterclockwise).

Despite the promising numerical results, the visual outcomes were disappointing. Many of these patients had irregular astigmatism that decreased visual acuity beyond what would be expected from the spherical equivalent and amount of astigmatism. Only two patients gained an unaided visual acuity of 6/12 or better. Seven had an acuity worse than 6/18 and four remained worse than 6/60. The mean grading of corneal haze was 1.08, with 15% having grade 2+. Three patients went on to have a failed graft from irreversible rejection, four were retreated with the excimer laser and two had astigmatic keratotomy performed. Four became hyperopic by more than 1.00 D. The problem of irregular astigmatism was ineffectively treated and may be partially responsible for the poor visual results.

The post-cataract patients fared slightly better. However, they also had less myopia and less astigmatism. The mean spherical equivalent was −2.75 D ±2.27, with a mean astigmatism of −3.86 D ±1.22. Postoperatively, 43% had an unaided visual acuity of better than 6/12, and 92% were within 2.00 D of the planned refraction with a mean astigmatism of −1.56 D ±1.08. Haze was minimal, with a mean score of 0.46. Half of the patients were greater than 1.00 D hyperopic. The mean postoperative spherical equivalent was +1.36 D ±1.96.

The patients who were treated for astigmatism resulting from radial keratotomy had results which approached that of primary PARK. They also had less myopia and astigmatism to correct. The group had a mean spherical equivalent of −3.75 D ±2.18, with a mean astigmatism of −1.72 D ±1.66. Postoperatively all had an unaided acuity of better than 6/18, with one-third seeing 6/6 or better. One patient required retreatment and none developed severe haze.

IRREGULAR ASTIGMATISM

Gibralter and Trokel reported two patients with postoperative irregular myopic astigmatism.[21] They identified steep areas by corneal topography, and performed phototherapeutic ablations in overlapping confluent 4.0 mm zones at depths of 10 or 20 microns, centered over the localized steep areas. This was followed by a spherical correction with a 6.0 mm zone. They obtained a change of 4.00 D of localized refractive change with a 20 micron ablation of 4 mm in diameter.

These initial results suggest that the excimer laser can be used to treat irregular astigmatism, although currently this is a rather crude technique. Improvements in topographical analysis of the corneal surface will allow more accurate predictions of the size and depth of the areas to be ablated. In the future we can expect that the excimer laser will be able to convert an irregular central corneal surface into a predetermined regular and symmetric curved surface employing asymmetrical ablation patterns.[36] This holds promise for patients with irregular central corneal astigmatism of an idiopathic type, but also after trauma, scarring, pterygia excision, penetrating keratoplasty, or other surgical procedures.

CONCLUSION AND FUTURE DIRECTIONS

There has been significant success in correcting astigmatism with the excimer laser. The benefits provided by vector analysis of outcomes enable the results of astigmatic treatment to be separated from those of the concurrent spherical changes induced by surgery.[37] Planning astigmatism surgery, with the assistance of vector planning,[38] helps the surgeon approach a complex subject, and may provide the direction necessary to improve the capabilities of excimer laser machines and enhance the visual results of surgery.

The introduction of corneal topography data into the surgical plan raises new complexities concerning the optimal treatment of astigmatism. These issues include optimizing corneal shape and astigmatic orientation,[38,39] and the potential application of topographical mapping to guide asymmetrical ablations.[36] Alignment of treatment and corneal axis is likely to be improved by the ability to view a real-time topographical image through the surgical microscope at the time of surgery. The quantitative data provided by computer-assisted videokeratography are likely to play an increasing role in the objective assessment of astigmatism surgery.[40]

Irregularities of corneal epithelial healing are currently difficult to control or predict and can create their own axes of irregular astigmatism. As our topographical analysis improves, our ability to modulate corneal healing expands, and new laser technologies are developed, we will be better able to create the exact astigmatic results we desire.

EXCIMER LASER TREATMENT OF ASTIGMATISM – KEY POINTS

- Vector analysis is essential in evaluating astigmatic changes.
- The excimer laser is effective in carving astigmatic ablations on the cornea.
- Visual results after PARK are similar to those of PRK.
- Irregular epithelial healing after any excimer ablation induces a random, inadvertent astigmatic change that affects the outcome of PARK, particularly when treating small amounts of astigmatism.

REFERENCES

1. Duke-Elder S, *System of Ophthalmology*, Vol.5 274 (Henry Kimpton: London, 1970.)
2. Jackson S, Epidemiology of refractive errors, *J Am Med Ass* (1935) **105**:1412.
3. Duke-Elder S, *System of Ophthalmology* Vol.5 282 (Henry Kimpton: London, 1970).
4. Alpins N, A new method of analysing vectors for changes in astigmatism, *J Cataract Refract Surg* (1993) **19**:524–33.
5. Seiler T, Reckman W, Maloney R, Effective spherical aberration of the cornea as a quantitative descriptor in corneal topography, *J Cataract Refract Surg* (1993) **15**:155–65.
6. Eggers H, Measuring visual acuity, *Arch Ophthalmol* (1945) **33**:23.
7. Fukada Y, Sawaii H, Watanabe M, et al, Nasotemporal overlap of crossed and uncrossed retinal ganglion cell projections in the Japanese monkey, *J Neuroscience* (1989) **9**:2353–73.

8. Sawusch MR, Guyton D, Optimal astigmatism to enhance depth of focus after cataract surgery, *Ophthalmology* (1991) **98**:1025–29.

9. Alpins N, Taylor HR, Surgically induced astigmatism with the excimer laser, *Current Research: Refractive and Corneal Surgery Symposium* (1993) **88** (abst).

10. Goggin M, Algawi K, O'Keefe M, Astigmatism following photorefractive keratectomy for myopia, *J Refract Corneal Surg* (1994) **10**:540–4.

11. Tabin G, Alpins N, Aldred G et al, Astigmatic change one year after treatment of myopia and myopic astigmatism with the excimer laser, *J Cat Refract Surg* (1996) **22**:924–31.

12. McDonnell PJ, Moreira H, Garbus J et al, Photorefractive keratectomy to create toric ablations for correction of astigmatism, *Arch Ophthalmol* (1991) **109**:710–3.

13. Shimmick J, Bechtel L, Elliptical ablations for the correction of compound myopic astigmatism by photoablation with apertures, *SPIE Ophthalmic Technologies* (1992) **1644**:32–9.

14. Brancato R, Carones F, Traabucchi G et al, The erodible mask in photorefractive keratectomy and astigmatism, *J Refract Corneal Surg* (1993) **9(supp)**:125–30.

15. Dausch D, Klein R, Landesz M, Schröder E, Photorefractive keratectomy to correct astigmatism with myopia or hyperopia, *J Cataract Refract Surg* (1994) **20(supp)**:252–7.

16. Schiotz H, Ein Fall von hochgradigen Hornhautastigmatismus nach Starextraction. Besserung auf operativum Wege, *Arch f Augenhilk* (1885) **15**:178–81.

17. Thornton S, Astigmatic keratotomy: A review of basic concepts with case reports, *J Cataract Refract Surg* (1990) **16**:430–5.

18. Agapitos PJ, Lindstrom RL, Astigmatic keratotomy, *Ophthalm Clin North Am* (1992) **5**:709–15.

19. Lipschitz I, Lowenstein A, Lazar M, Astigmatic keratotomy followed by photorefractive keratectomy in the treatment of compound myopic astigmatism, *J Refract Corneal Surg* (1994) **10(supp)**:282–4.

20. Ring C, Hadden O, Morris A, Transverse keratotomy combined with spherical photorefractive keratectomy for compound myopic astigmatism, *J Refract Corneal Surg* (1994) **10(supp)**:217–21.

21. Gibralter R, Trokel S, Correction of irregular astigmatism with the excimer laser, *Ophthalmology* (1994) **101**:1310–15.

22. McDonnell P, Moreira H, Clapham T, et al, Photorefractive keratectomy for astigmatism: Initial clinical results, *Arch Ophthalmology* (1991) **109**:1370–3.

23. Taylor HR, Kelly P, Alpins N, Excimer laser correction of myopic astigmatism, *J Cataract Refract Surg* (1994) **20(supp)**:243–51.

24. Taylor HR, Guest CS, Kelly P, Alpins NA, Comparison of excimer laser treatment of astigmatism and myopia, *Arch Ophthalmol* (1993) **111**:1621–6.

25. Taylor HR, Carson CA, Aldred GF, Predictability of excimer laser treatment of myopia, *Arch Ophthalmol* (1996) *In press.*

26. McDonnell P, Excimer laser corneal surgery: New strategies and old enemies, *Invest Ophthalmol Vis Sci* (1995) **36**:4–8.

27. Talamo JH, Gollamudi S, Green WR, et al, Modulation of corneal wound healing after excimer laser keratomileusis using topical mitomycin C and steroids, *Arch Ophthalmol* (1991) **109**:1141–6.

28. Phillips AF, Szerenyi K, Campos M, et al, Arachidonic acid metabolites after excimer laser corneal surgery, *Arch Ophthalmol* (1993) **111**:1273–8.

29. Pender P, Photorefractive keratectomy for myopic astigmatism: Phase 2A of the Federal Drug Administration study (12 to 18 months follow up), *J Cataract Refract Surg* (1994) **20(supp)**:262–4.

30. Kim Y, Sohn J, Tchah H, Lee C, Photoastigmatic refractive keratectomy in 168 eyes: Six month results, *J Cataract Refract Surg* (1994) **20**:387–91.

31. Maloney R, Friedman M, Harmon T, et al, A prototype erodible mask delivery system for the excimer laser, *Ophthalmology* (1993) **100**:542–9.

32. Hersh P, Patel R, Correction of myopia and astigmatism using an ablatable mask, *J Refract Corneal Surg* (1994) **10(supp)**:250–4.

33. Cherry P, Tutton M, Bell A, et al, Treatment of myopic astigmatism with photorefractive keratectomy using an erodible mask, *J Refract Corneal Surg* (1994) **10(supp)**:239–45.

34. Cantu-Charles C, Talamo JH, Excimer PRK for myopia and astigmatism with the Coherent-Schwind Keratom, *ARVO* (1995) S190 (abst).

35. Snibson G, Taylor HR, SARK-excimer laser treatment of post surgical astigmatism (1996) *In press.*

36. Alpins NA, The treatment of irregular astigmatism, (1997) *In press.*

37. Alpins NA, Simple and vector analysis of astigmatism for cataract and refractive surgery, (1997) *In press.*

38. Alpins NA, A new method of targeting vectors for the optimal treatment of astigmatism, *J Cat Refract Surg* (1997) **23**.

39. Alpins NA, Vector analysis of astigmatism changes by flattening, steepening and torque, (1997) *In press.*

40. Alpins NA, Tabin GC, Adams L, Aldred GF, Taylor HR, Success achieved in excimer laser treatment of astigmatism, (1996) *In press.*

Chapter 16 High and extreme myopia

Cathy A McCarty, Ronald M Stasiuk and Hugh R Taylor

INTRODUCTION

Following several scientific studies reporting good results obtained with excimer surgery for low myopia, the use of excimer surgery for high myopia has increased dramatically in the last few years.[1–30] In Melbourne we have found that high and extreme myopes are in fact 10- and 16-times more likely, respectively, to undergo excimer laser correction of their myopia than low myopes (Taylor HR and McCarty CA, unpublished data), perhaps because the perceived benefits of excimer surgery are greater for people with a higher degree of myopia (Fig. 16.1).

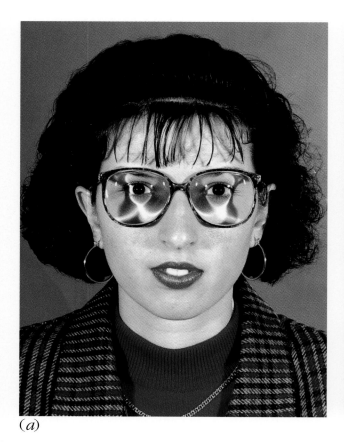
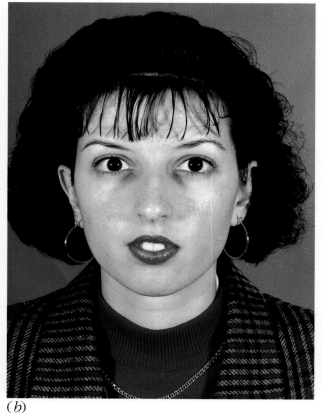

(*a*)   (*b*)

Figure 16.1 *People with high myopia (in this instance 15 D) may be encouraged to undergo excimer laser correction for cosmetic reasons or because of contact intolerance.*

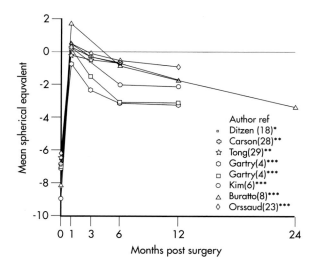

Figure 16.2 *Published results of excimer laser surgery for high myopia (–5.00 D to –10.00 D) with cohorts of at least 20 patients.*

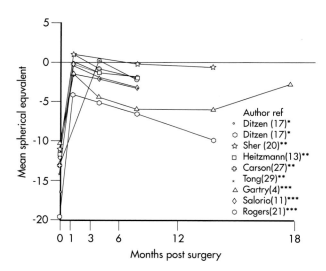

Figure 16.3 *Published results of excimer laser surgery for extreme myopia (> –10.00 D) with cohorts of at least 20 patients.*

DEFINITION

There is no uniform agreed definition of high myopia. Spherical equivalent at the spectacle plane is usually used to distinguish high myopia from low myopia and to establish the treatment algorithm for multizone procedures, but the magnitude of myopia is quite variable.

The following spherical equivalent lower cutoff points have been used to define 'high myopia': (1) –5.00 D,[12,18,27] (2) –6.00 D,[2,7,8,11,16,17,22–25] (3) –7.00 D,[6] (4) –8.00 D,[3,9,10,13,19,20,29] and (5) –10.00 D.[14,21,28] The degree of high myopia is often further subdivided at –10.00 D and –15.00 D. The definition employed by laser companies to secure FDA approval has been –6.00 D.

Uniformity in the classification and reporting of degree of myopia would facilitate both research and communication. However, this may alter treatment regimens because multizone treatments are determined by the degree of myopia. As a result of the current discrepancies in defining high myopia, this chapter will summarize the results of excimer surgery for high myopia using the most conservative definition currently employed, a spherical equivalent of –5.00 D.

RESULTS

Results of excimer laser surgery for high myopia have been more variable than for low myopia and it has been suggested that treatment of high myopia should be considered a multistage procedure. This is supported by the fact that high myopia is associated with more regression after the initial treatment and is one of the most common indications for excimer laser retreatment.[31–35]

The more variable outcomes observed in higher degrees of myopia could be due to several factors. Obviously, the depth of the ablation is greater in higher corrections and with larger ablation zone diameters. However, the latest studies of the treatment of higher myopia have frequently employed several zones (multizone) with a large number of steps in an attempt to both decrease the depth of treatment and smooth the ablation edges. Some surgeons also suggest the correction of high myopia in stages. The different ablation profiles employed for high myopia may theoretically lead to irregular epithelial healing and regression.

A summary of the refractive data from published studies with at least 20 patients is presented for high myopia, –5.00 D to –10.00 D, and extreme

Table 16.1

Results of excimer laser surgery for high myopia employing the Summit laser

Author, year (ref)	Laser model	Size of ablation zone(s)	Definition of high myopia (D)	Number of eyes	Length of follow-up	Percentage within 1 D /2 D target
Gartry, 1992 (4)	Excimed UV200	4.0 mm	a) −5.00 b) −6.00 c) −7.00	a) 20 b) 20 c) 20	12 months	a) 50%/NA b) 40%/NA c) 20%/NA
Kim, 1993 (6)	Excimed UV200	5.0 mm	−7.25 to −13.50	67	12 months	52%/NA
Machat, 1993 (7)	Excimed UV200	5.0 mm	−6.00 to −8.75	28	3–16 months	61%/93%
Buratto, 1993 (8)	UV200	single 4.3 mm or 4.5 mm	−6.00 to −10.00	40	24 months	35%/NA
Salorio, 1993 (11)	NA	5.0 mm	<−6.00	88	3–18 months	NA/NA
Shimizu, 1994 (22)	Excimed UV200LA	4.5 mm	<−6.00 to −14.00	41	12 months	44%/71%
Orssaud, 1994 (23)	Excimed UV200LA	5.0 mm	−6.00 to −8.50	33	1–12 months	43%/NA
Murta, 1994 (25)	Omnimed	single 4.5–4.9 mm	a) −6.12 to −9.00 b) <−9.00	a) 29 b) 10	3 months	a) 80%/93% b) 60%/90%
Cho, 1993 (9)	Excimed UV200	2–3 zones 5.0 mm, 4.5 mm, 4.0 mm	−8.87 to −16.99	19	6 months	32%/53%
Kim, 1993 (10)	Excimed UV200LA	4.5 mm and 5.0 mm	−8.00 to −13.50	19	6 months	74%/NA
Rogers, 1994 (21)	Excimed UV200LA	3.6–4.5 mm or 5.0 mm	−10.25 to −20.50	27	3–16 months	75% at 12 months/NA

Table 16.2

Results of excimer laser surgery for high myopia employing the Visx laser

Author, year (ref)	Laser model	Size of ablation zone(s)	Definition of high myopia (D)	Number of eyes	Length of follow-up	Percentage within 1 D /2 D target
Sher, 1991 (2)	2015	single 5.2–6.0 mm	−6.00 to −12.00	19	6 months	16%/42%
Sher, 1992 (3)	2015	single 5.5, 5.6 or 6.0 mm	−8.62 to −14.50	16	6 months	NA/69%
Sher, 1994 (20)	2015/2000	single 5.5–6.2 mm	−8.00 to −15.25	48	12 months	40%/64%
Heitzmann, 1993 (13)	2020	4.0, 5.0 and 6.0 mm	−8.00 to −19.50	23	1–12 months	39%/65%
Carson, 1995 (27)	2020	2–3 zones 4.5, 5.0, 6.0 mm	a) −5.00 to −10.00 b) −10.25 to −21.00	a) 194 b) 53	6 months	a) 67%/89% b) 38%/49%
Krueger, 1995 (28)	2020	6, 5, 4 mm or 6, 5.5, 5 mm	−10.37 to −24.50	14	6 months	NA/21%
Tong, 1995 (29)	2020	2–3 zones 4.5, 5.0, 6.0 mm	a) −5.25 to −8.00 b) −8.25 to −23.00	a) 23 b) 36	6 months	a) 70%/100% b) 19%/47%

myopia, greater than −10.00 D (Figs 16.1–16.3). These data reveal no obvious difference in outcome by the type of laser employed, but demonstrate that preoperative refraction appears to be associated with outcome at the furthest time point after surgery. This chapter will summarize, by type of laser, published results of the initial treatment for high myopia only (Tables 16.1–16.3). For a review of outcomes after retreatment, see Chapter 24.

Table 16.3

Results of excimer laser surgery for high myopia employing the Meditec laser

Author, year (ref)	Laser model	Size of ablation zone(s)	Definition of high myopia (D)	Number of eyes	Length of follow-up	Percentage within 1 D/ 2 D target
les Jardins, 1994 (16)	MEL 60	5.0 mm	−6.00 to −9.00	12	6 months	41%/74%
Ditzen 1994 (17)	MEL 60	5.0 mm	a) −6.25 to −10.00	a) 97	12 months	NA
			b) −10.25 to −15.00	b) 87		
			c) <−15.25	c) 48		
Dausch, 1993 (14)	MEL 60	tapered transition zone	−12.00 to −24.00	6	12 months	NA

SUMMIT LASER

SINGLE ZONE

There are many reports of the outcome of excimer laser correction of high myopia employing a single ablation zone with a Summit laser.[4,6–8,11,22–25] Ablation zone size varies from 4.0 to 5.0 mm. In a study by Gartry et al in which a 4.0 mm zone was employed for 60 patients with myopia >−5.00 D (maximum treatment of −7.00 D), initial overcorrection postoperatively was noted to be higher than in low myopes and regression over time was greater.[4] Topical corticosteroids were tapered over 3 months. Significant symptoms of halo persisted in 10% of the cohort at 12 months. In another study, 67 patients with myopia between −7.25 D and −13.50 D were followed for 12 months after treatment with a 5.0 mm zone to correct 6.00 D of myopia.[6] A pressure patch and topical corticosteroids were used until the epithelium healed. Corneal haze was noted to be greater with higher degrees of myopia and haloes were reported by 78% of patients; they were troublesome or problematic in 10% of patients. The authors suggested that higher myopia (>−7.00 D) may require a two-step (repeated) procedure to achieve target refraction because of the myopic regression in this group.

Machat and Tayfour reported results of a 5.0 mm zone to treat 28 patients with myopia ranging from −6.00 D to −8.75 D.[7] The epithelium was removed mechanically, and dexamethasone was tapered over 3 months. Follow-up time ranged from 3 to 16 months. Interestingly, preoperative astigmatism was noted as the primary cause of reduced uncorrected visual acuity in the high myopia group, rather than

myopic regression. In contrast, Buratto and Ferrari employed a zone of 4.3 mm or 4.5 mm to treat 40 patients whose myopia ranged from −6.00 D to −10.00 D preoperatively.[5] The epithelium was removed mechanically and dexamethasone was tapered over 3 months. Twenty-four months after surgery, regression was still occurring in 65% of the patients such that the authors supported the use of alternate techniques in myopia of this degree.

In a larger study of 88 patients with preoperative myopia >−6.00 D treated with a 5.0 mm zone and 3 months of postoperative fluoromethalone (FML), more overcorrection and less predictable results were noted compared to low myopia.[11] FML drops were tapered over 3 months and follow-up ranged from 3 to 18 months.

Shimizu et al followed a cohort of 41 Japanese patients with preoperative myopia <−6.00 D for 12 months.[22] A 4.5 mm zone was employed to correct between 2.00 D and 7.50 D of myopia, the epithelium was mechanically removed and FML drops were tapered over 2 months. Predictability of refraction decreased with higher myopia with the authors hypothesizing that post-PRK subepithelial haze is actually more common in Asian eyes. Orssaud et al, in a variant of this procedure, used a 5.0 mm zone and two-step procedure performed in the same day to treat 33 patients with preoperative myopia ranging from −6.00 D to −8.50 D.[23] Initial overcorrection was higher and more regression was observed in the group with higher preoperative myopia.

A 4.5 mm zone was used by Murta et al to treat myopia up to −9.00 D while a single zone of 4.6–4.9 mm was used to treat myopia ranging from −6.12 D to −9.00 D.[25] The epithelium was manually removed, a pressure patch was applied and FML drops were dosed based on the regression of myopia. Although corticosteroids appeared to modulate the regression in most patients, follow-up was limited to 6 months and many patients were still on topical steroids at that time.

In summary, the results of excimer laser surgery for high myopia employing a single ablation zone with a Summit laser reveal greater variability than for low myopia, significant postoperative corneal haze, and significant myopic regression. These results led researchers to use multiple zones for high myopia in an attempt to smooth the deeper ablation zone (Fig. 16.1).

MULTIPLE ZONES

The amount of tissue ablated through excimer surgery is a function of the diameter of the ablation zone(s) and the targeted refraction. Because of a demonstrated association between depth of ablation, and haloes, corneal scarring and regression, many groups have experimented with multiple zones for higher degrees of myopia to minimize adverse healing responses.[9,10,13,14,18,21,27–29] The majority of the papers have appeared in journal supplements and have not been subjected to the peer-review process. Although algorithms for the amount of myopia treated in each zone vary, the basic procedure reported for Visx and Summit machines is similar, with smaller central ablation zones being used for higher degrees of myopia (Fig. 16.4). The decreasing diameter for the multizone procedures allows for a tapered transition zone and a smoother edge to the ablation.

Four studies of excimer laser PRK results after using multiple ablation zones for high myopia with a Summit laser have appeared in the literature.[9–11,21] In a study by Cho and colleagues,[9] nineteen myopes between –8.87 D and –16.99 D were treated and followed for 6 months. The maximum attempted correction was 10.00 D and two or three ablation zones were used: (1) 5.0 mm to correct 6.00 D, (2) 4.5 mm to correct myopia within 2.00 D, and (3) 4.0 mm to correct myopia up to a further 2.00 D. A bandage contact lens was in situ for an average of 4 weeks and FML drops were tapered over 6 months. Mean manifest refraction continued to regress at the 6-month examination, with only 32% of the cohort within 1.00 D of plano.

Emmetropia was the goal for 19 eyes with preoperative refraction of –8.00 D to –13.50 D in a study by Kim et al.[10] Up to 7.00 D of myopia was treated in a 4.5 mm ablation zone and the remainder was treated

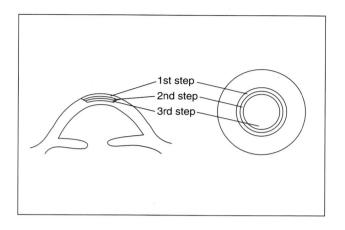

Figure 16.4 *Diagram of photorefractive keratectomy involving multiple zones.*

in a 5.0 mm zone. The eyes were patched for 3 days after surgery and prednisolone drops were used for 1 month or adjusted according to regression and corneal haze. The change in mean regression was not significant between 3 and 6 months postoperatively, with 14 of 19 patients within ±1.00 D of emmetropia at 5 months.

Two ablation zones were used by Rogers et al to treat patients with myopia >–10.00 D.[21] The first ablation zone size ranged from 3.6 to 4.5 mm in diameter, with the aim to correct two thirds of the myopia. The remaining myopia was corrected with a 5.0 mm zone assuming that this ablation would lead to 1.00 D more correction than intended because Bowman's layer would not be present. The epithelium was manually removed, the eye was patched after surgery, and dexamethasone drops were tapered over a period of 4–5 months. Ten of fourteen eyes (71%) with 12-month follow-up were within ±1.00 D of emmetropia. Seven eyes were retreated because of regression and scarring and have returned to at least their preoperative best corrected acuity.

VISX LASER

SINGLE ZONE

One group (Sher et al) has reported the results after 12 months of using a single ablation zone with a Visx

2015/2000 laser to treat high myopia.[2,3,20] An ablation zone of 5.5–6.2 mm was used after mechanical removal of the epithelium, postoperatively, a bandage contact lens was placed over the operated eye for 3 days, and FML drops were tapered over 4 or 5 months. Regression had slowed, but was still continuing, between 12 and 18 months (–0.83 during that time) in the 14 eyes with that amount of follow-up. Irregular astigmatism and/or corneal haze contributed to a loss of two lines best corrected visual acuity in 15% of the patients at 12 months.

MULTIPLE ZONES

Four groups have reported the results of using multiple ablation zones for treatment of high myopia with a Visx laser.[13,18,27–29] In the first group, three zones (4.0, 5.0 and 6.0 mm) were used to treat 23 patients with a Visx 2020 excimer laser.[13] Myopia ranged from –8.00 D to –19.50 D. Fifty per cent of the refractive error was treated in the smallest zone, 30% in the middle zone, and 20% in the largest zone. The epithelium was removed mechanically, a pressure patch was used until the epithelium healed and FML drops were tapered over 6 months. At 6 months, 55% of eyes were within 1.00 D of attempted correction. Major changes in refractive stability were not noted after six months and only two of 23 eyes lost two lines of best corrected acuity. The authors suggested that retreatment should be considered for correction of high myopia.

Six-month results after excimer surgery with a Visx 2020 have been reported for 194 high myopes and 53 extreme myopes.[27] Intended spherical correction was divided equally between two ablation zones (5.0 mm, 6.0 mm) for high myopia and three ablation zones (4.5, 5.0, 6.0 mm) for extreme myopia, which did not exceed 15.00 D. The epithelium was mechanically removed, a bandage contact lens was used in 28 patients and FML drops were tapered over 4 months. Refraction was still regressing between 3 and 6 months, although it had slowed for the high myopes. Eighty-nine per cent of the high myopes and 49% of the extreme myopes were within ±2.00 D of emmetropia at 6 months, while 71% and 31% had uncorrected acuity of 6/12 or better, respectively. Loss of two or more lines best corrected visual acuity (13% in both groups) was associated with corneal haze in most cases.

Three ablation zones (6.0, 5.0, 4.0 mm or 6.0, 5.5, 5.0 mm) and a Visx 2020 were used to treat 14 eyes ranging from –10.37 D to –24.50 D preoperatively.[28] A pressure patch or bandage contact lens was used and FML drops were within 2 D of attempted corrections. Four (29%) of the eyes were eventually retreated because of myopic regression. Three (21%) eyes experienced a loss of two or more lines best corrected acuity that was associated with moderate to severe corneal haze. Myopic regression was noted to be more common with nitrogen gas blowing to remove debris during the procedure.

Slightly better results were obtained in Hong Kong using two ablation zones (5.0, 6.0 mm) for 23 moderate (–5 to –8 D) myopes and three ablation zones (4.5, 5.0, 6.0 mm) for 36 high (>–8 D) myopes.[29] A bandage contact lens or pressure patch was used and FML drops were tapered over 2–4 months. Six months after surgery, 70% of the moderate myopes and 19% of the high myopes were within 1 D of intended correction, while 35% of the moderate myopes and none of the high myopes could see 6/12 or better unaided. None of the moderate myopes and 10% of the extreme myopes lost two or more lines best corrected visual acuity. The amount of corneal haze observed did not vary significantly between groups. At 6 months, seven patients reported occasional haloes.

MELBOURNE EXCIMER LASER GROUP EXPERIENCE

In the first 38 months of operation, the Melbourne Excimer Laser Group treated 513 high (–5.01 D to –10.00 D) myopes and 116 extreme myopes (>–10.00 D) with a Visx 2020 excimer laser following the protocol mentioned previously.[27] The maximum amount of myopia treated was –15.00 D.

Forty-one extreme myopes and 189 high myopes were followed for 12 months. Refractive data noted more overcorrection initially and more myopic regression in the extreme myopes (Fig. 16.5). The percentage of high myopes within 1 and 2 D of emmetropia at 12 months was 57% and 90%, respectively, while the corresponding percentages for extreme myopes were 39% and 56%. Preoperatively, 214 (90%) of the high myopes were legally blind uncorrected, 18 (8%) had 6/60 vision, and the remaining six (2%) had vision of 6/36 or 6/48. At 12 months, 48 (25%) of the high myopes had uncorrected vision of 6/6 or better, 135 (71%) 6/12, and 165 (87%) 6/18. Preoperatively, all of the extreme myopes were legally blind without correction. At 12 months, one (2%) had uncorrected vision of 6/6, 11 (27%) 6/12, and 22 (54%) 6/18. At all time points,

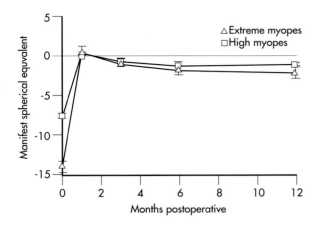

Figure 16.5 *Mean spherical equivalent (±95% confidence limits) before and after surgery for high (n=189) and extreme (n=41) myopia with a Visx laser (Melbourne Excimer Laser Group.)*

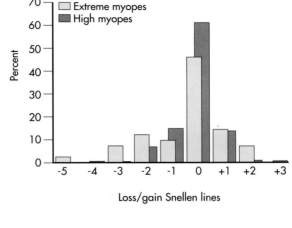

Figure 16.6 *Lines of best-corrected vision gained/lost 1 year after surgery for high (n=189) and extreme (n=41) myopia with a Visx laser (Melbourne Excimer Laser Group.)*

uncorrected visual acuity was significantly better for the high myopes. Preoperatively, 231 (97%) of the high myopes and 45 (78%) of the extreme myopes had best corrected vision of 6/12 or better. At 12 months, 181 (96%) of high myopes and 28 (68%) of extreme myopes had best corrected vision of 6/6 or better. Fifteen (8%) of the high myopes and nine (22%) of the extreme myopes had lost two or more lines of best corrected visual acuity at 12 months (Fig. 16.6). Extreme myopes were significantly more likely to lose best corrected visual acuity ($\psi^2 = 0.08$, p = 0.008). Preoperatively, seven (12%) of the high myopes and 24 (10%) of the extreme myopes had faint corneal haze. Mean corneal haze peaked 1 month postoperatively in the high myopes and 3 months postoperatively in the extreme myopes (Fig. 16.7) Twelve months postoperatively, seven (4%) high myopes and one (2%) extreme myope had corneal haze scores ≥ grade 2 in the anterior stroma.

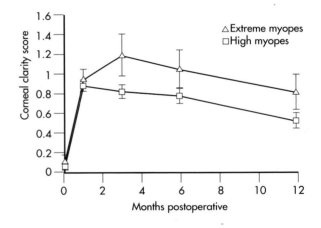

Figure 16.7 *Mean corneal clarity score (±95% confidence limits) before and after surgery for high (n=189) and extreme (n=41) myopia with a Visx laser (Melbourne Excimer Laser Group.)*

CASE STUDY

Collective results are obviously important but mask individual responses to laser treatment. The following is the case report of a high myope who obtained very good results following one excimer laser treatment. In contrast, a case example of a high myope who required retreatment because of myopic regression is illustrated elsewhere (see Chapter 24).

Ms. M is a 24-year-old accountant who has worn glasses since the age of 5 years, requiring correction of −5.00 in the right eye and −2.00 in the left eye initially. Her myopia progressed until the age of 21. She was intolerant of both hard and soft contact lenses and desired excimer correction of her high myopia to 'get out of her thick (myopic) glasses'.

Table 16.4

The clinical results of the right eye of a patient after undergoing excimer surgery with a Visx 2020 excimer laser reveal the excellent visual and refractive results achieved with a single procedure

Time point	Uncorrected acuity	Best-corrected acuity	Sphere (D)	Cylinder (D)	Axis	Spherical equivalent (D)
Preoperative	HM	6/9.6	−12.50	−4.50	180	−14.75
1 month	6/18.9	6/15	0	−1.75	60	−0.88
3 months	6/12	6/9.6	−0.50	−0.50	80	−0.75
6 months	6/12	6/9.6	−1.00	−0.50	80	−1.25
12 months	6/10	6/7.5	−1.25	−0.50	5	−1.50

Table 16.5

The clinical results of the left eye of a patient after undergoing excimer surgery with a Visx 2020 excimer laser reveal the excellent visual and refractive results achieved with a single procedure

Time point	Uncorrected acuity	Best-corrected acuity	Sphere (D)	Cylinder (D)	Axis	Spherical equivalent (D)
Preoperative	HM	6/12	−14.00	−2.50	180	−15.25
1 month	6/12	6/12	0.50	−0.50	140	0.25
3 months	6/15	6/9.6	−1.50	0	0	−1.50
6 months	6/15	6/12	−0.25	−0.50	10	−1.75
12 months	6/12	6/12	−1	−0.25	135	−1.13

Upon examination, uncorrected acuity in both eyes was hand movements and best corrected acuity was 6/9.6 in the right eye and 6/12 in the left eye. Spherical equivalent was −12.50/−4.50 at 180° in the right eye and −14.00/−2.25 at 180° in the left eye. She initially underwent PARK with a Visx 2020 excimer laser in the non-dominant eye, her left, and subsequently had the right eye corrected 8 months later. For both eyes, the target refraction following excimer surgery was −0.50 D and the spherical correction was equally divided into three ablation zones of 4.5, 5, and 6 mm diameter. For the left eye, the cylindrical treatment was divided equally between the two largest zones and for the right eye, all of the cylindrical error was treated in the largest zone. The epithelium was removed manually and the eye was patched after surgery. She had no complications or adverse reactions and the epithelium in both eyes healed by day three. FML drops were tapered over 4 months. At 12 months, she had slight corneal haze in the right eye, had a spherical equivalent of −1.50 D, had 6/45 uncorrected and 6/7.5 best corrected vision

(Table 16.4). She saw 6/12 both corrected and uncorrected in her left eye at 12 months, with a spherical equivalent of −1.13 D and mild residual corneal haze (Table 16.5). The subtraction and corneal topography maps prior to and 12 months after excimer surgery for the right and left eyes are demonstrated in Figs 16.8 and 16.9, respectively. They reveal the decreased central dioptric power of the cornea after treatment and good centration of the procedures. She occasionally wears a pair of glasses with a minor correction for night driving. Ms. M was obviously delighted with the results of her excimer surgery.

MEDITEC LASER

SINGLE ZONES

Two papers reporting the results of the Meditec laser to treat high myopia with a single ablation zone have

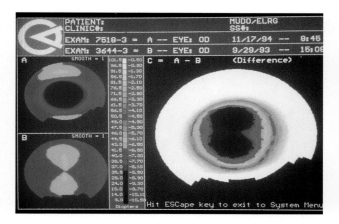

Figure 16.8 *Corneal topography maps of the right eye of a patient prior to and 12 months after excimer laser correction of high myopia with a Visx 2020 excimer laser.*

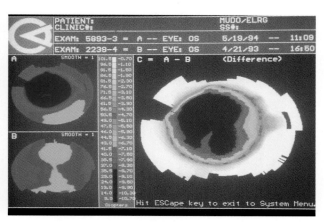

Figure 16.9 *Corneal topography maps of the left eye of a patient prior to and 12 months after excimer laser correction of high myopia with a Visx 2020 excimer laser.*

appeared in the literature.[16,17] In the first study,[16] 12 eyes with preoperative refraction of −6.00 D to −9.00 D were followed for 6 months. The epithelium was removed with alcohol, a single 5.0 mm ablation zone was used, and FML drops were tapered over a maximum of 3 months. In eyes with significant undercorrection, haze or regression, drops of dexamethasone or FML with flurbifropen were prescribed for up to 6 months. At 6 months, 41% and 74% of the high myopes were within 1 D and 2 D of targeted refraction, respectively. The mean haze was considerably higher for the high myopes at 6 months (2.80 as compared with 1.85 for the low myopes). For those patients with 12 months follow-up, the mean regression between 6 and 12 months was minimal, from −1.50 D to −1.60 D.

In a larger study involving the Meditec laser to treat high myopia,[17] 232 people with preoperative myopia <−6.25 D were followed for 12 months. Maximum attempted correction was −13.00 D and eyes with more than 2.50 D cylinder were excluded. The epithelium was mechanically removed, a single 5.0 mm ablation zone was employed, a pressure patch was used until the epithelium healed and FML drops were tapered over 3 months. The regression rate was twice as high in the groups with higher degrees of myopia. Ablation depth and time to epithelial healing were associated with haze; no corneas were clear in eyes that took 8–9 days for the epithelium to heal.

TAPERED MULTIZONE

A tapered transition zone with a Meditec laser was also used to treat six patients with high myopia.[14] The treatment algorithm for the tapered transition zone is based on a parabolic equation, with a theoretical angle of the resulting ablated edge curvature of 0°. The diameter of the refraction corrected area was 4.0 mm and the diameter of the final transition zone did not exceed 7.0 mm. Targeted correction ranged from 10.00 to 13.00 D so that the patients could wear weaker glasses. Bandage contact lenses were fitted for 10 days and FML drops were tapered over 5 months. Twelve months after surgery, none of the six patients reported haloes or glare sensitivity at night. Detectable haze was still present in three of the eyes. With the exception of 1 patient, refraction was fairly stable after one month in this group, although it is not clear what percentage of intended myopic correction was achieved (Fig. 16.5).

MULTIPASS MULTIZONE PRK (MP–PRK)

Although several centers have been employing multipass multizone PRK and PARK (MP–PRK) to treat varying levels of myopia, only one substantial study has been published upon this interesting variant of the standard PRK technique. Mihai Pop, using a Visx laser, commenced a prospective MP–PRK study of 315 eyes, with a wide range of preoperative myopia, in November 1993.[36] This technique involves fractionating the intended myopic correction into a series of 'passes' (up to seven in total) in multiple zones from 3.5 to 6.9 mm diameter. Between each pass, which is limited to a single ablation zone (with a maximum of 4 D correction within each zone), there is a 25–60 second delay. The major clinical advantages to this technique are: the facility to correct fixation at each interval, thus improving centration, equilibration of surface temperature and hydration may (theoretically) occur between passes, by employing multiple zones, which are not exactly superimposed, subsequent ablation steps will tend to smooth preceding ones leading to a smoother ablation bed, and possible intrinsic advantages offered by this modified multizone algorithm.

The six-month results, including data upon 170 eyes with low myopia (<–6.00 D), 105 highly myopic eyes (–6.00 D to –10.00 D) and 40 extremely myopic eyes (–10.00 D to –27.00 D), were published in November 1995.[36] The refractive and visual outcomes were broadly similar to best results already outlined, with 92.0% and 60.0% of the high and extremely myopic eyes obtaining 20/40 or better unaided vision, respectively. However, mean corneal haze at 1 month was similar for all treatment subgroups and at 6 months haze values were 0.14, 0.35, and 0.59 for the low, high and extremely myopic groups respectively. In contrast the mean haze values were significantly higher in a control group treated by a single pass multizone technique. At 6 months 6.2%, 15.2% and 29.0% of the respective subgroups exhibited undercorrection by greater than –1.00 D and might therefore be potential candidates for retreatment. However, only 2% of eyes with high myopia and 6% of eyes with extreme myopia lost two lines or more of best corrected Snellen acuity. The authors contend that this is a superior technique which produces less haze, less regression, and fewer eyes with significant loss of best corrected visual acuity. These preliminary results are certainly encouraging but longer term follow-up data is obviously essential.

SUMMARY OF EXCIMER LASER RESULTS FOR HIGH MYOPIA

Preoperative, surgical, and postoperative care of patients with high and extreme myopia varies a great deal. Regardless of the type of excimer laser, the postoperative corticosteroid regimen or the number of zones employed, more regression is observed after excimer laser surgery for high myopia. The role of corticosteroids in the management of regression after excimer surgery for high myopia remains controversial and the subject of ongoing investigations. The majority of high myopes have improved unaided vision and require a weaker myopic spectacle correction after a single laser procedure. Loss of best corrected vision in a significant minority of high myopes (range 0–38%) is distressing and warrants further investigation. Ongoing controlled studies of the treatment of high myopia are essential, both to improve refractive results and to attempt to identify which highly myopic patients are less likely to have favorable outcomes.

Key points of published research
- Excimer laser results more variable for high myopia
- No marked differences in results by type of laser
- Percentage within 1 D of emmetropia ranged from 16 to 80%
- Percentage with 6/12 unaided vision ranged from 25 to 79%
- Percentage losing two or more lines best corrected acuity ranged from 0 to 38%
- Use of corticosteroids to control corneal haze is controversial
- Use of multiple zones and/or multipass, to limit depth of ablation and create smooth ablation surface the current focus of research
- Irregular epithelial thickening (epithelial hyperplasia) may cause both loss of best corrected vision and regression

---

FUTURE DIRECTIONS

The perfect surgical solution for the treatment of high myopia has yet to be developed. However, the future for successful excimer laser surgical correction of high myopia is promising with the key developments likely in the following areas:

ABLATION SHAPE

More sophisticated aspheric shapes with gentle tapering peripheral (transition) zones are required to avoid sharp changes in curvature that may encourage epithelial thickening to fill in the ablated areas. Further refinements in multizone construction, automatic multipass software, and improved software algorithms continue apace.

PRK PHARMACOLOGICAL REFINEMENTS

Various pharmacological agents may theoretically be useful to modulate epithelial healing, reduce haze and regression (see Chapter 25). Several new pharmacological agents show promise in reducing corneal haze following excimer laser PRK. Morlet and colleagues found a significant reduction in corneal haze following excimer laser PRK in rabbits with postoperative use of topical interferon-alpha-2b eyedrops.[37] Plasmin and plasminogen-activator inhibitors may help prevent postoperative regression and haze in a concept proposed by Lohmann and Marshall, although results to date have been disappointing.[38]

COMBINED TECHNIQUES

This may be necessary for extreme myopia such as a combination of laser in-situ keratomileusis (up to −16 D) with a secondary PRK of the lenticle (up to −8 D).[30]

LASER IN-SITU KERATOMILEUSIS

A safer more accurate surgical cut of the lenticle by improved automatic microkeratomes, or laser-assisted lamellar dissection, combined with LASIK specific algorithms may see the increasing emergence of LASIK in the treatment of extreme myopia (see Chapter 18).

CONCLUSION

Excimer laser PRK for low myopia is now highly safe and reliable. Further research, clinical trials, and evaluation are needed to find the most effective way of correcting high myopia. Irregular epithelial healing and epithelial thickening are likely causes of problematic corneal haze and myopic regression, thus research needs to be directed toward controlling the exaggerated healing response after excimer laser PRK for high myopia. Changes in the aspheric contours of the ablated area may reduce irregular epithelial thickening and improve the predictability of the results.

The ultimate refractive technique selected to correct high myopia needs to be safe, simple, reproducible, inexpensive, with good results and preferably extraocular. Perhaps several techniques should be combined for full correction of the high myopia. Safe and effective surgical correction of high myopia is the greatest challenge currently facing refractive surgeons.

REFERENCES

1. Zabel RW, Sher NA, Ostrov CS, et al, Myopic excimer laser keratectomy: a preliminary report, *Refract Corneal Surg* (1990) **6**: 329–34.
2. Sher NA, Chen V, Bowers RA, et al, The use of the 193-nm excimer laser for myopic photorefractive keratectomy in sighted eyes. A multicenter study, *Arch Ophthalmol* (1991) **109**: 1525–30.
3. Sher NA, Barak M, Daya S, et al, Excimer laser photorefractive keratectomy in high myopia. A multicenter study, *Arch Ophthalmol* (1992) **110**: 935–43.
4. Gartry DS, Muir MGK, Marshall J, Excimer laser photorefractive keratectomy. 18-month follow-up, *Ophthalmology* (1992) **99**: 1209–19.
5. Buratto K, Ferrari M, Genisi C, Myopic keratomileusis with the excimer laser: one year follow-up, *Refract Corneal Surg* (1993) **9**: 12–19.
6. Kim JH, Hahn TW, Lee YC, et al, Photorefractive keratectomy in 202 myopic eyes: one year results, *Refract Corneal Surg* (1993) **9**: S11–S16.
7. Machat JJ, Tayfour F, Photorefractive keratectomy for myopia: preliminary results in 147 eyes, *Refract Corneal Surg* (1993) **9**: S16–S19.
8. Buratto L, Ferrari M, Photorefractive keratectomy for myopia from 6.00 D to 10.00 D, *Refract Corneal Surg* (1993) **9**: S34–S36.
9. Cho YS, Kim CG, Kim WB, et al, Multistep photorefractive keratectomy for high myopia, *Refract Corneal Surg* (1993) **9**: S37–S41.
10. Kim JH, Hahn TW, Lee YC, et al, Clinical experience of two-step photorefractive keratectomy in 19 eyes with high myopia, *Refract Corneal Surg* (1993) **9**: S44–S47.
11. Salorio DP, Costa J, Larena C, et al, Photorefractive keratectomy for myopia: 18-month results in 178 eyes, *Refract Corneal Surg* (1993) **9**: S108–S110.
12. Taylor HR, Guest CA, Kelly P, et al, Comparison of excimer laser treatment of astigmatism and myopia, *Arch Ophthalmol* (1993) **111**: 1621–26.
13. Heitzmann J, Binder PS, Lassar BS, et al, The correction of high myopia using the excimer laser, *Arch Ophthalmol* (1993) **111**: 1627–34.

14. Dausch D, Klein R, Schröder E, et al, Excimer laser photorefractive keratectomy with tapered transition zone for high myopia. A preliminary report of six cases, *J Cataract Refract Surg* (1993) **19**: 590–94.

15. Piebenga LW, Matta CS, Deitz MR, et al, Excimer photorefractive keratectomy for myopia, *Ophthalmology* (1993) **100**: 1335–45.

16. les Jardins Sl, Auclin F, Roman S, et al, Results of photorefractive keratectomy on 63 myopic eyes with six months minimum follow-up, *J Cataract Refract Surg* (1994) **20**: 223–28.

17. Ditzen K, Anshütz, Schröder E, Photorefractive keratectomy to treat low, medium and high myopia: a multicenter study, *J Cataract Refract Surg* (1994) **20**: 234–38.

18. Taylor HR, Philip P, Alpins N, Excimer laser correction of myopic astigmatism, *J Cataract Refract Surg* (1994) **20**: 243–51.

19. Maguen E, Salz JJ, Nesburn AB, et al, Results of excimer laser photorefractive keratectomy for the correction of myopia, *Ophthalmology* (1994) **101**: 1548–57.

20. Sher NA, Hardten DR, Fundingsland B, et al, 193-nm excimer photorefractive keratectomy in high myopia, *Ophthalmology* (1994) **101**: 1575–82.

21. Rogers CM, Lawless MA, Cohen PR, Photorefractive keratectomy for myopia of more than −10 diopters, *J Refract Corneal Surg* (1994) **10**: S171–S173.

22. Shimizu K, Amano S, Tanaka S, Photorefractive keratectomy for myopia: one-year follow-up in 97 eyes, *J Cataract Refract Surg* (1994) **10**: S178–S187.

23. Orssaud C, Ganem S, Binaghi M, et al, Photorefractive keratectomy in 176 eyes: one year follow-up, *J Refract Corneal Surg* (1994) **10**: S199–S205.

24. Sabetti L, Spadea L, Fuecese L, et al, Measurement of corneal thickness by ultrasound after photorefractive keratectomy in high myopia, *J Refract Corneal Surg* (1994) **10**: S211–S216.

25. Murta JN, Proenca R, Velze RAV, et al, Photorefractive keratectomy for myopia in 98 eyes, *J Refract Corneal Surg* (1994) **10**: S231–S235.

26. Gomes M, Keratamileusis-in-situ using manual disection of corneal flap for high myopia, *J Refract Corneal Surg* (1994) **10**: S255–S257.

27. Carson CA, Taylor HR, Excimer laser treatment of high and extreme myopia, *Arch Ophthalmol* (1995) **113**: 431–36.

28. Krueger RR, Talamo JH, McDonald MB, et al, Clinical analysis of excimer laser photorefractive keratectomy using a multiple zone technique for severe myopia, *Am J Ophthalmol* (1995) **119**: 263–74.

29. Tong PPC, Kam JTK, Lam RHS, et al, Excimer laser photorefractive keratectomy for myopia: six-month follow-up, *J Cataract Refract Surg* (1995) **21**: 150–55.

30. Pallikaris IG, Siganos DS, Excimer laser in situ keratomileusis and photorefractive keratectomy for correction of high myopia *J Refract Corneal Surg* (1994) **10**: 498–510.

31. Seiler T, Derse M, Pham T, Repeated excimer laser treatment after photorefractive keratectomy, *Arch Ophthalmol* (1992) **110**: 1230–33.

32. Lawless MA, Cohen PR, Rogers CM, Retreatment of undercorrected photorefractive keratectomy for myopia, *J Refract Corneal Surg* (1994) **14**: S174–S177.

33. Epstein D, Tengroth B, Fegerholm P, et al. Excimer retreatment of regression after photorefractive keratectomy, *Am J Ophthalmol* (1994) **117**: 456–61.

34. Snibson GR, Taylor HR, Retreatment following excimer laser photorefractive keratectomy, *Invest Ophthalmol Vis Sci* (1994) **35**:S2019.

35. Gartry DS, Larkin DFP, Flaxel CJ, Ficker LA, Steel ADMcG, Retreatment for significant regression following excimer laser photorefractive keratectomy (PRK)—a prospective, randomized, double-masked trial, *Invest Ophthalmol Vis Sci* (1995) **36**: S190.

36. Pop M, Aras M, Multizone/multipass photorefractive keratectomy: Six month results, *J Cataract Refract Surg* (1995) **21**: 633–43.

37. Morlet N, Gillies MC, Crouch R, et al, Effect of topical Interferon-Alpha 2b on corneal haze after excimer laser photorefractive keratectomy in rabbits, *Refract Corneal Surg* (1993) **4**: 443–51.

38. Lohmann CP, Marshall J, Plasmin – and plasminogen – activator inhibitors after excimer laser photorefractive kerarectomy: a new concept in prevention of post-operative myopic regression and haze, *Refract Corneal Surg* (1993) **9**: 300–2.

Chapter 17 The surgical and laser correction of hypermetropia

Charles N J McGhee, Con N Anastas, Lyn Jenkins, Christopher M Rogers and Jean-Pierre Danjoux

INTRODUCTION

The treatment of myopia and myopic astigmatism, initially by radial keratotomy (RK) techniques and more recently by 193 nm excimer laser photorefractive keratectomy (PRK) or photo-astigmatic refractive keratectomy (PARK), is well established. However, the treatment of hypermetropia currently represents a far greater challenge for the refractive surgeon. Indeed, the successful and permanent treatment of low-to-moderate hypermetropia is regarded by many as one of the last great frontiers of refractive surgery.

Although this relatively greater frequency of hypermetropia in many Western populations has been long established (Fig. 17.1),[3] the surgical treatment of hypermetropia has never enjoyed the widespread popularity and acceptance, amongst patients or practitioners, that RK and PRK for myopia has achieved. Indeed, the surgical treatment of hypermetropia is fraught with technical difficulties as, in general terms, it appears to be relatively easier to surgically flatten rather than steepen the axial cornea.[4]

PREVALENCE OF HYPERMETROPIA

In childhood and early adulthood many hypermetropic individuals, unlike their myopic cousins, can manage very successfully without a refractive correction but the incidence of hypermetropia in the general community is actually greater than that of myopia, although this obviously varies with the age and race of the population studied.

In Britain the most informative statistics are those of Harman,[1] who studied 30 000 subjects aged 16 years or over, who presented for ocular examination (emmetropic individuals and small errors were therefore absent). The distribution of refractive errors was noted to be: myopia 27%, hypermetropia 56% and mixed astigmatism 2.25%.

In the United States the distribution of refractive error is somewhat comparable, although myopia has previously appeared to be less frequent. However, the most recent large study (1994),[2] involving a study population of 4533, revealed an approximately 2:1 ratio of hypermetropic, compared to myopic, refractive errors (49.0% versus 26.2%).

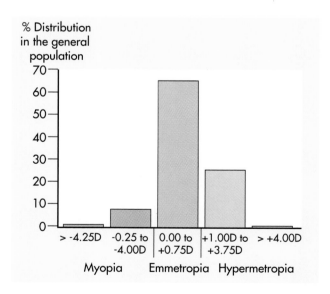

Figure 17.1 *The distribution of refractive errors in a normal population demonstrates a preponderance of hypermetropic refractive errors. Notably more than 96% of the population exhibits refractive errors between −4.00 D and +4.00 D. (After Stromberg.[3])*

SURGICAL OPTIONS IN THE CORRECTION OF HYPERMETROPIA

Many authorities cite the animal experiments of Lans in 1898 as the first faltering step on the route to surgical correction of hypermetropia. Lans[5] produced increased corneal power by utilizing superficial radial burns in rabbit corneas and, thus, the first thermokeratoplasties were documented. However, although Lans and his contemporary, William Bates, created the principles of incisional and thermorefractive surgery, after completing his experimental thesis with Snellen, Lans failed to pursue the surgical correction of refractive errors further.

HEXAGONAL KERATOTOMY

Following the widespread success of RK in the treatment of myopia, it is unsurprising that a variety of incisional methods have been suggested to correct hypermetropia. Yamashita,[6] developed an eight-sided incisional technique, subsequently termed hexagonal keratotomy (hex), as a potential method of correcting RK overcorrections. By decreasing the diameter of the hex, greater steepening of the central cornea was obtained. Others developed this technique to tackle naturally occurring hypermetropia, since, theoretically, by reducing the diameter of the hex from 7.5 mm to 4.5 mm up to 4.0 D of hypermetropia could be corrected. One of the major problems with this initial approach of six overlapping incisions, since the incisions essentially decouple the central cornea biomechanically from the periphery, was of excessive wound gape and associated irregular astigmatism. Thus, despite promise in cadaver models,[7,8] early clinical trials reported limited success due to problems of unpredictable induced astigmatism, loss of best spectacle corrected visual acuity (BSCVA) and the problems common to incisional surgery.[9,10]

Vociferous opposition to the technique emerged in the USA in the early 1990s[11,12] but modifications of the technique (Fig. 17.2) continue to be practised by a number of skilled surgeons, with apparently acceptable results. In 1995 Grandon et al, reporting upon a spiral-hex technique, recorded a mean 1.6 D reduction in hyperopia, from a preoperative mean of +2.7 D to +1.1 D, in 184 eyes. In this series 51% of eyes were within ±1.0 D of emmetropia and 55% achieved

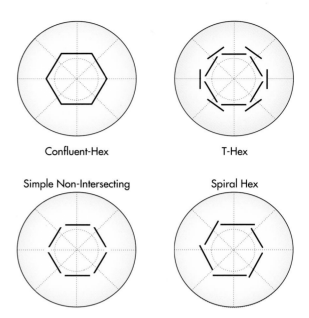

Figure 17.2 *Modifications upon the incisional technique of hexagonal keratotomy using 4.5–6.00 mm diameter optical zones. Inner circle (dotted line) represents an optical zone of 4.5 mm diameter.*

6/12 (20/40) or better uncorrected visual acuity; however, 32% of eyes lost one line of corrected Snellen acuity, 4% lost two or more lines and 23% demonstrated an increase in refractive cylinder of more than 1.0 D.[13]

RADIAL THERMOKERATOPLASTY AND LAMELLAR TECHNIQUES

Radial thermokeratoplasty (TKP) was revived for treatment of hypermetropia in the early 1980s by Fyodorov.[14] The technique employed the application of a series of superficial peripheral corneal burns in a pattern similar to RK. However, in direct contrast to the biomechanical effects of RK, these superficial burns flattened the corneal periphery and steepened the central cornea (Fig. 17.3). This technique of superficial heat application was rapidly supplanted

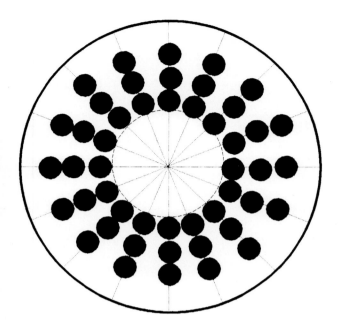

Figure 17.3 *Pattern of intrastromal burns used in the radial TKP technique developed by Fyodorov. Three to four applications, using a nichrome wire probe at 600°C inserted to 80% corneal thickness, were placed in the peripheral cornea along 16 radial marks.*

by the insertion of a nichrome wire probe to 80% depth of the cornea in a similar treatment pattern. The probe reached temperatures of 600°C with subsequent necrosis of corneal tissue adjacent to the probe and shrinkage of collagen on the periphery of the coagulation zone. Fyodorov's group presented data on 117 eyes that had undergone this technique, with a mean reduction in hyperopia of –3.84 D and an improvement in 6/12 unaided vision from 10% preoperatively to 53% 1 year post-treatment.[15] However, because of instability of refraction – associated with marked regression – and the overall unpredictability of results, radial TKP has not been widely used to treat hypermetropia.[16–18]

Hyperopic correction with lamellar techniques, such as keratophakia and keratomileusis, or with donor lenticules, as in epikeratophakia, have enjoyed limited success because of procedural difficulty, predictability and complications.[4,19] More invasive techniques, such as clear lens extraction with intraocular lens implantation in normally sighted hyperopic

eyes,[20] have yet to gain widespread acceptance and are largely reserved for extenuating circumstances.

HOLMIUM:YAG THERMAL KERATOPLASTY (LTK)

In an attempt to refine the basic concept – reawakened by Fyodorov in the form of radial TKP – of steepening the central cornea by heat-induced collagen shrinkage, several groups and manufacturers began to look at laser sources in the late 1980s. The holmium:YAG laser, generating infrared energy, is a flashlight-pumped solid-state laser with a pulse length of 200–300 μs and variable pulse repetition rate, producing an emitted wavelength of 2.1 μm, which produces a fluence in the range of 19 mJ per pulse. This modality has been used to induce paracentral corneal stromal coagulation, in a similar but more controlled manner than TKP, in order to cause central corneal steepening. By applying a train of 5–25 pulses to each location, theoretically, the underlying cornea is heated in a controlled manner to 60°C, thereby causing focal corneal shrinkage without the tissue necrosis associated with radial TKP.[21]

In 1990, Seiler and co-workers[22] published results of their pioneering work in this field. Treatment consisted of eight focal applications to the cornea, on the circumference of two concentric circles that were centred on the optical axis. It was noted that the induced refractive change was inversely related to distance of treatment application from the centre of the cornea and directly related to laser pulse energy. A small blind eye study by the same workers[23] demonstrated that the parameters evaluated in cadaver eyes could be transferred to living eyes and clinical trials on partially sighted and sighted eyes were commenced in 1991.[24]

Significant regression of induced refractive change was noted to occur during the first postoperative months and regression of effect has continued to plague more recent trials.[21,25] Long-term regression, even after 2 years, has been reported.[4]

Tutton et al,[26] reported on the 2-year follow-up of 22 eyes treated with a Summit Technology Omnimed holmium laser, utilizing two rings of eight laser spots at 6.5 mm and 9.0 mm diameter zones, applied by a hand-held quartz fibreoptic hand piece, focused by a disposable sapphire tip (Fig. 17.4). Preoperative hypermetropia ranged from +1.75 to +4.75 D and in

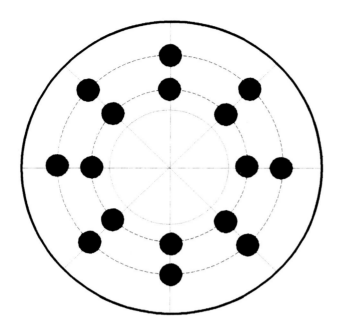

Figure 17.4 *Holmium:YAG laser thermokeratoplasty pattern using Summit treatment protocol. Two rings, each of eight laser coagulation spots, at 6.5 and 9.0 mm radius centred on the visual axis. The inner circle (dotted line) represents a 4.5 mm optical zone.*

all subjects a +4.00 D correction was attempted. A mean reduction in hypermetropia of –2.17 D was obtained at 2 years, but only 25% of eyes were within ±1.00 D of intended correction and 23% of eyes required retreatment for induced astigmatism. The authors noted that the average refraction did not actually stabilize until 21 months after treatment (Fig. 17.5).

It has been shown that a precision in application – to within 0.1 mm of the intended diameter – is necessary for successful and predictable hypermetropic LTK treatment. Therefore, following preliminary cadaver studies,[27,28] non-contact methods, rather than direct application, were suggested as a technical modification likely to achieve greater likelihood of success.

Sunrise Technologies Corneal Shaping system (CSS) utilizes a non-contact, slit-lamp delivery system to produce holmium LTK (Fig. 17.6). This system has obvious theoretical benefits over hand-held techniques, particularly in terms of accurate positioning of the laser spots by simultaneous delivery of eight uniform beams in a well-defined geometric pattern. The procedure is extremely fast, typically taking 2–4 seconds per application. However, 1-year results with this technique have also demonstrated

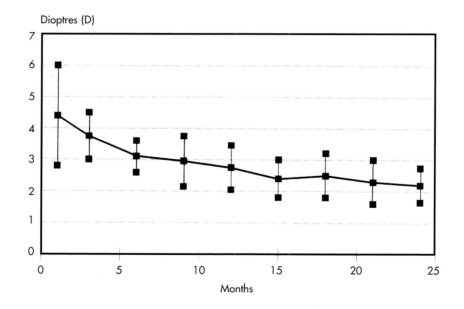

Figure 17.5 *Total induced refractive change (±1 SD) followed a +4.00 D holmium:YAG LTK using a Summit Omnimed system (n=17) is plotted against time. A continual decay in induced refractive effect, to approximately 50% of the 1 month mean refractive outcome, is noted during the first 2 years post-LTK. (After Tutton and Cherry[26].)*

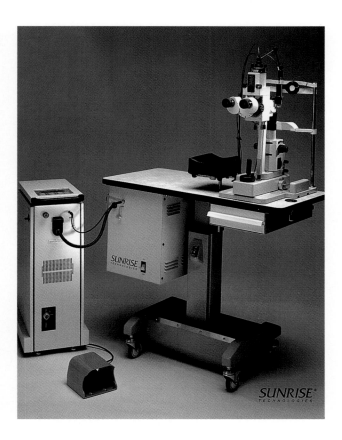

Figure 17.6 *Sunrise Technologies Corneal Shaping System (CSS) non-contact, slit lamp delivery, holmium:YAG thermal keratoplasty unit. (Courtesy Sunrise Technologies.)*

significant regression. In the USA Food and Drug phase IIa trial, all nine hypermetropic eyes treated with the Sunrise Technologies system, using a single-ring or two-ring treatment (Fig. 17.7), demonstrated a significant regression of induced steepening over the first 90 days post-treatment.[29] In the group treated with a single ring, mean change (reduction) in spherical equivalent (SE) of subjective manifest refraction decreased from −2.05 D at day 1 to −0.59 D at 1 year, whereas the group treated with a two-ring technique evidenced less marked decay of induced refractive effect, with respective values of −2.56 D and −1.41 D at 1 day and 1 year respectively.

It would appear, depending on further long-term clinical data, that the niche role for holmium:YAG non-contact LTK in refractive surgery will largely be restricted to low hypermetropes (+0.75 to +2.50 D) in the presbyopic age group or the small group of overcorrected myopic PRK subjects.

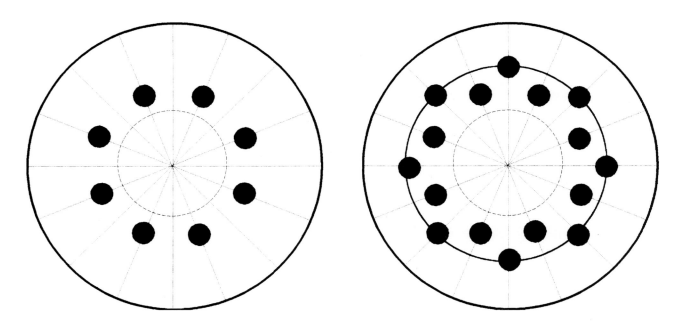

Figure 17.7 *One-ring and two-ring patterns for hypermetropic treatment using the Sunrise Technologies non-contact holmium:YAG LTK procedure. The inner circle (broken line) represents a 4.5 mm optical zone.*

DEVELOPMENT OF AN EXCIMER LASER FOR HYPERMETROPIA

PRECLINICAL STUDIES

Following the initial clinical promise of excimer laser PRK for myopia and myopic astigmatism, and taking into consideration the limitations of the foregoing treatment modalities for hypermetropia, developing excimer laser algorithms for hypermetropia was a logical progression. The principle of hypermetropic

PRK correction is to steepen the anterior corneal curvature and the theoretical recontouring of the cornea for hypermetropic PRK was first described by L'Esperance in 1983.[30] The cornea is sculpted into a steeper convex lens by creating a furrow-like ring zone in the corneal periphery. For the creation of such an annulus of tissue removal a larger ablation zone than in myopic PRK is necessary (Figs 17.8, 17.9).

Laser delivery can generally be divided into scanning- or broad-beam delivery and a variety of methods have been utilized (Fig. 17.10) to create the hypermetropic profile from these existing laser

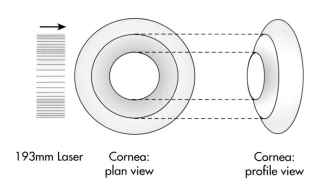

193mm Laser   Cornea: plan view   Cornea: profile view

Figure 17.8 *Hypermetropic PRK achieves a central steepening of the cornea by creating a midperipheral corneal trough, which blends into the central optical zone and outwards to the corneal periphery.*

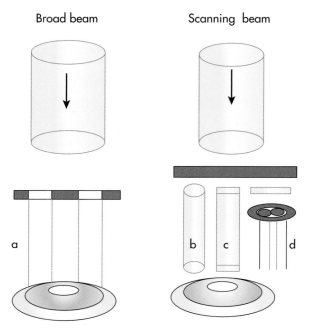

Figure 17.10 *The various methods by which broad beam and scanning beam lasers can create hypermetropic ablations are highlighted in diagrammatic form. Broad-beam lasers such as Summit and Schwind create the correct beam profile by utilizing an ablatable or non-ablatable mask (a). Other broad-beam systems achieve a similar result by creating a smaller circle beam, or spot, using an iris diaphragm (Technolas, LEI), or small slit beam, utilizing iris and parallel plate diaphragms (Visx) (b,c) and then scan this smaller beam in a circular fashion. The scanning slit-beam system of Meditec incorporates a rotating non-ablatable mask to create the correct profile (d). Small spot scanning lasers such as the Autonomous Technology system or the new Technolas 217 system already utilize small 'flying spot' beam technology, which can be scanned in a circular fashion.*

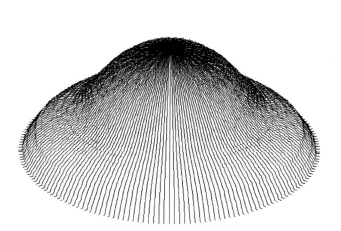

Figure 17.9 *A wire diagram highlights the central steepening of the cornea following hypermetropic PRK. (Courtesy of Aesculap–Meditec.)*

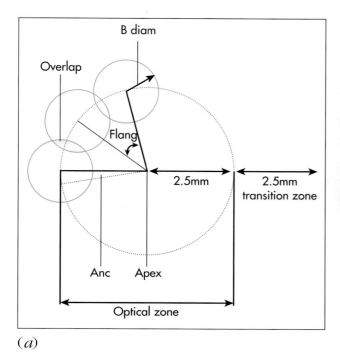

(*a*)

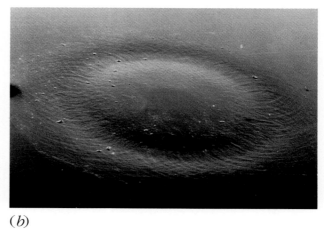

(*b*)

Figure 17.11 (*a*) *The Lions Eye Institute laser system (LEI) from Perth, Western Australia is a broad-beam system that uses an iris diaphragm and mirrors to scan a smaller beam of varying diameter to create a hypermetropic ablation. (b) A PMMA plate demonstrating a hypermetropic correction created by scanning a small circular beam. (Courtesy of Paul van Saarloos PhD, Lions Eye Institute, Perth, W A.)*

systems, including non-erodible masks (Meditec), erodible masks (Summit), rotating scanning spot (Technolas, Autonomous, LEI systems) (Figs 17.11a,b), rotation of an expanding slit (VisX) and variable aperture bands and fractal masks (Schwind) (Figs 17.12a–c).

Reports of *in vivo* excimer PRK for hypermetropia began with Del Pero[31] who performed +6.00 D treatments on five cynomolgus monkeys and found a mean refractive change of −5.20 D at 1 year. The earliest clinical studies of human hypermetropic PRK were presented by Dausch and colleagues,[32] and Anschütz and Ditzen.[4]

EARLY CLINICAL STUDIES

Dausch and colleagues,[32] utilizing a scanning-mode MEL 60 (Aesculap–Meditec) 193 nm excimer laser and a rotating spiral mask, treated 23 hypermetropic patients in a prospective study with 1 year follow-up. In group 1, consisting of 15 hypermetropic eyes with preoperative refractions of +2.00 D to +7.50 D, (+4.7 ± 1.6 D, mean ± standard deviation [SD]), 80% were within ±1.00 D of the intended correction and 80% had 6/12 unaided visual acuity or better at 1 year, whilst one eye lost two lines BSCVA. In a second group, consisting of eight aphakic eyes, with a mean refractive error of +13.1 D (SD ± 2.0 D), only 37% were within ±1.00 D of the intended correction, whilst 25% achieved 6/12 unaided visual acuity or better at 1 year. Two (25%) in this latter group lost two or more lines of BSCVA. Loss of BSCVA in every case was attributed to decentration of the ablation zone. All eyes exhibited a transient ring of corneal haze and suffered reduced visual acuity under glare conditions, both conditions being more common in the greater attempted corrections of the aphakic group. Significant regression was seen at all time points in both groups but again much more so in the latter group.

Anschütz and Ditzen,[4] also utilizing a scanning-mode MEL 60 (Aesculap–Meditec) 193 nm excimer laser, treated 81 hypermetropic patients with 1 year follow-up. In group 1, consisting of 49 eyes with preoperative refractions between +2.00 D and +5.75 D, 66% of eyes were within ±1.00 D of the intended correction, with a mean regression of +1.00 D posthypermetropic PRK. In

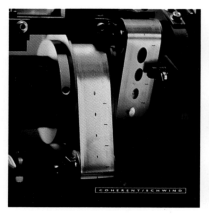

(a)

Circular apertures for correction of myopia and PTK

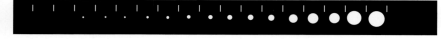

Elliptical apertures for correction of astigmatism

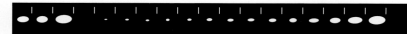

Opposite sector apertures for correction of hyperopia

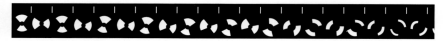

(b)

Fractal mask patterns for hyperopia correction

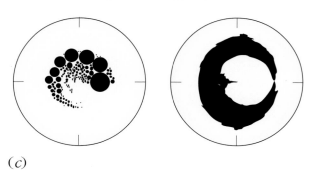

(c)

Figure 17.12 *(a) The Coherent:Schwind excimer laser shapes a broad beam to the desired profile for myopic, astigmatic or hypermetropic correction by interposing a perforated steel band in the path of the laser beam. (b) These bands act in a similar fashion to an iris diaphragm to control the width and shape of the beam reaching the cornea and a zoom lens is used to smooth the transition between each aperture. (c) Complex fractal mask designs are presently being investigated as an alternative method of producing a transition free corneal ablation for hypermetropia. (Courtesy Coherent:Schwind.)*

group 2, consisting of 32 more highly hypermetropic eyes (preoperative refractions +6.00 D to +10.0 D), only 38% were within ±1.00 D of the intended correction post-treatment. Notably, 15% of patients in this latter group demonstrated a loss of three Snellen lines of BSCVA. In this study, loss of BSCVA was once more attributed to decentration of the ablation zone in each case. A further 2-year study by Anschütz[4] begun in 1991 followed 51 eyes in two groups, defined as in the first study, in addition to an aphakic group (preoperative refractions +10.00 D to +15.00 D). The results of this study, despite some changes in treatment protocol, were essentially similar to the preceding Meditec studies but continued regression of induced refractive effect was noted in the second year, with 62% of group 1 within ±1.00 D but only 28% of group 2 within ±1.00 D of intended correction. The aphakic group in this study exhibited a final refractive result that was poorer than in the initial study by Dausch.[32]

From these earliest preclinical and clinical studies it became apparent that wider ablation zones with smoother transition profiles gave more stable and predictable results, and that centration of the treatment zone was more critical than in myopic PRK if loss of BSCVA was to be avoided.

PROSPECTIVE STUDIES OF HYPER-METROPIC CORRECTION IN THE UK

A prospective study at the Chiltern Hospital, England, has been co-ordinated by one of the authors (LJ), utilizing an Aesculap–Meditec scanning-beam excimer laser with a non-erodible mask to correct hypermetropia (Figs 17.13a,b). This study emphasizes some of the practical difficulties in establishing reproducible criteria for the assessment of outcome following hyperopic PRK.

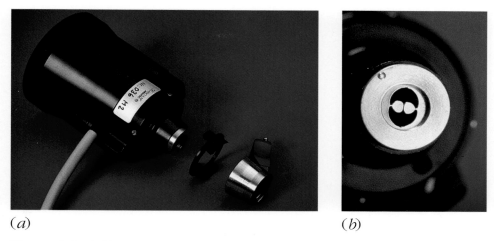

(a)　　　　　　　　　　　　　　　(b)

Figure 17.13 *(a,b) A second generation Aesculap–Meditec hand-held rotating mask for the treatment of hypermetropia. (Courtesy Aesculap–Meditec.)*

Thirty hypermetropic PRK treatments were performed and observed prospectively over an 18-month period, with data available for 25 cases at 1 year post-treatment. A non-erodible rotating mask for hypermetropia was used in all cases. The Meditec hypermetropic mask has gone through three stages of development and the second and third versions of the mask, exhibiting a 7.0 mm and 8.0 mm aperture, respectively, were used in this study (Fig. 17.14). However, scanning excursion of the Meditec laser beam is limited to 7.0 mm vertically and 10.0 mm horizontally; therefore, a maximum 7.0 mm by 8.0 mm ablation zone is feasible.

(a)　　　　　(b)　　　　　(c)

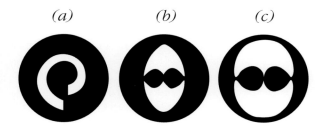

Figure 17.14 *Three generations of non-erodible rotating masks created by Aesculap–Meditec for the treatment of hypermetropia by excimer laser PRK. (a) Initial spiral-shaped mask, (b) second-generation mask with 7.00 mm ablation zone, (c) third-generation mask providing an 8.00 mm hypermetropic ablation zone.*

Centration of treatment proved to be a problem in the initial group of patients. The Meditec laser at that time relied on positioning of the eye suction ring to achieve centration, and a handpiece containing a mechanized mask was then fitted onto the suction ring before treatment was commenced. As the mask obscured the centre of the cornea (in order to prevent ablation of the central cornea) it was not possible to confirm that the centration of the suction ring had been maintained until the moment of treatment. In addition, the initial centration of the suction ring depended upon the operating ophthalmologist estimating the centre of an 8 mm aperture. Later modifications to this system – incorporating a centration device – allow more accurate positioning of the suction ring, whilst the use of a wider mask enables the pupil margin to be visualized prior to treatment to confirm accurate centration has been maintained (Figs 17.15a,b).

In analyzing the results of PRK treatment for hypermetropia for the first time the ophthalmologist may find the refraction confusing. Firstly, retinoscopy is very unreliable as a single linear reflex from a streak retinoscope is not visible through the pupil. Secondly, the patient will accept a large range of lenses without any apparent change in visual acuity and the normal blur point – used to check for myopic overcorrection – is not obvious in these patients. Patients will often accept plus lenses, almost up to their preoperative refraction, before there is a significant decline in visual acuity. It is, therefore, in many ways, more important to measure unaided vision for

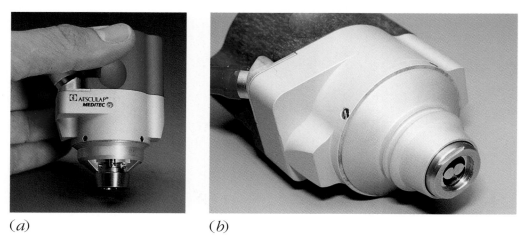

(*a*)   (*b*)

Figure 17.15 *The Aesculap–Meditec hand-held rotating mask for hypermetropia demonstrating (a) relative size and (b) current mask shape. (Courtesy Aesculap–Meditec.)*

far and near, both before and after treatment, than it is to measure subjective refraction.

An example of the discrepancy between the change in unaided vision and refractive change is highlighted by the following case history. A 57-year-old patient preoperatively achieved less than 6/60 unaided vision with uncorrected near vision of N36, but obtained a best corrected distance vision of 6/5 with +4.75 Dioptic Sphere (DS) and N5 with a reading add of +1.50. Two months after a +4.75 PRK for hypermetropia his unaided vision had improved to 6/12 and best corrected vision with +2.00 DS was 6/6. Unaided near vision was a remarkable N5 and was not improved with corrections between +2.00 DS to +4.00 DS. Five months postoperatively, whilst still exhibiting a manifest refractive error of +2.00 D, the patient enjoyed unaided vision of 6/7.5 and N8, respectively. The explanation for this omnifocal phenomenon must be the increased asphericity of the central cornea following excimer laser PRK for hypermetropia. This may account for the range of positive lenses tolerated without reduction in BSCVA (for the pseudoaccommodation effect, whereby good near vision coexists with reasonable distance acuity), the lack of a clearly defined end point to refraction using the +1.00 D blur test (see Chapter 8) and the poor retinoscopic image.

The postoperative progress is, therefore, much more difficult to monitor by refraction, when compared to myopic PRK, and computerized video-keratography (CVK) becomes more important in

assessing the amount of regression. As the peripheral trough produced by the hypermetropic excimer laser ablation 'fills in' during regression, the induced refractive effect is reduced, the amount of asphericity decreases and sensitivity to correcting lenses increases (Fig. 17.16). Significant regression of the effect can be identified by CVK maps over the first 3 months, although this appears to stabilize between 6 and 12 months post-treatment (Figs 17.17, 17.18). Probably the most reproducible way to monitor the regression process following correction of hypermetropia is to correlate corneal power on the CVK plots at various time points post-treatment.[29] Perhaps the easier method of accomplishing this is to record keratometric power at the apex – and at set distances from the corneal apex – by averaging values from the major and minor axes at these set distances (Figs 17.19–17.21).

Nonetheless, purely in terms of unaided vision, whilst only 35% of treated eyes obtained 6/6 or better unaided vision, the vast majority in this study (87%) achieved 6/12 or better unaided vision at a mean follow-up of 1 year post-treatment (range 5–18 months) (Fig. 17.22). However, this improved unaided acuity was at the expense of loss of Snellen lines of BSCVA in a large number of cases (Fig. 17.23).

The haze resulting from the treatment is greater than that found with PRK treatments for myopia of similar magnitude, but since it does not affect the central cornea it has less effect on visual acuity. Glare

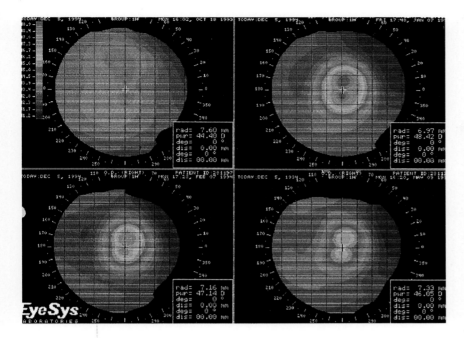

Figure 17.16 *CVK maps of a 56-year-old patient with a preoperative hypermetropia of +5.50 D (top left). One month posthypermetropic PRK using a Meditec laser, the CVK map (top right) demonstrates markedly increased central power and the patient obtained 6/12 unaided vision. However, 2 months postlaser (bottom left) moderate regression of central steepening is noticeable. Five months post-PRK the CVK map (bottom right) demonstrates loss of more than 2.5 D of central power, compared to the 1 month map, and there is considerable filling in of the midperipheral trough with associated regression of induced refractive effect. Unaided vision was 6/36 at this time with BSCVA of 6/6 with a +4.00 D sphere. The subject subsequently underwent retreatment.*

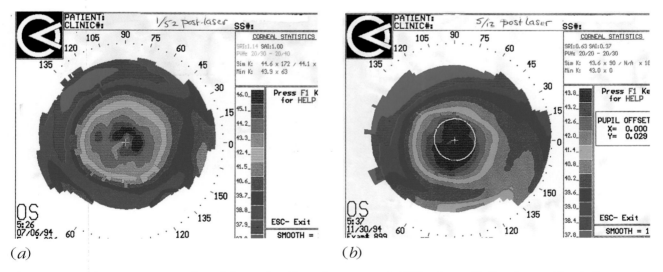

(a)   (b)

Figure 17.17 *CVK maps at 1 week and 5 months after a hypermetropic PRK using a Meditec laser with rotating mask. In the left CVK map (a) the ablation has created a central zone of increased power and a midperipheral zone of decreased corneal power, with a mean power over the central 3.0 mm of approximately 44.4 D at this 1-week stage (surface regularity index (SRI) 1.14, surface asymmetry index (SAI) 1.00. The map becomes more regular, but maintains the central increase in power at 5 months post-treatment, with a mean central power of 43.8 D (SRI) 0.63, (SAI) 0.37 (right CVK map (b)).*

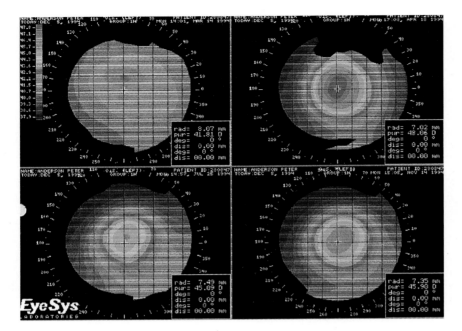

Figure 17.18 *CVK maps of a 46-year-old subject following hypermetropic PRK with a Meditec excimer laser. Unaided vision was 6/24 with BSCVA of 6/4 with a +5.50 D spherical correction (top left). At 1 month post-PRK, a pronounced increase in central corneal power is evident (top right) but topographic regression of effect is evident at 4 months post-treatment (bottom left), although topographic stability appears to have been reached between 4 and 7 months (bottom right). Interestingly, despite an approximate regression of 2.00 D in central CVK corneal power during this period, the patient maintained 6/9 unaided vision and the manifest refraction at 1 month (+1.50 D), with which the subject obtained BSCVA of 6/6, was not significantly different at 7 months (+1.00 D)*

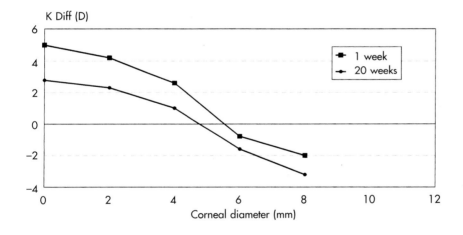

Figure 17.19 *Example of the use of difference in keratometry (K) values before and at time intervals post hypermetropic PRK to monitor refractive effect. Difference in K values (K Diff D) were calculated from CVK maps, using measurements at the apex and fixed diameters from the vertex of the cornea. This case illustrates a +6.0 D attempted correction, demonstrating an increase in central corneal power of +5.0 D, and midperipheral decrease in power of −3.2 D at 1 week post-PRK. At all corneal diameters a decay in induced refractive effect is noted with time (20 weeks) and this effect is maximal centrally.*

at night, however, still proves to be problematic. It was also notable in these early studies that the visual acuity for distance was better in bright light, sometimes by as much as three lines, than in low-light conditions. Since using an 8.0 mm ablation mask with a 7.0 × 8.0 mm ablation zone, the width of the optical component of the treatment zone centred over the pupil has significantly increased and this has resulted in less difference between light versus dark acuities and a decrease in the pseudoaccommodative effect compared to earlier studies; however, there was no corresponding improvement in loss of BSCVA

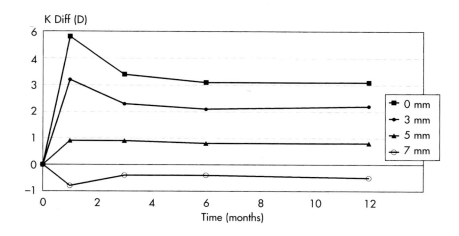

Figure 17.20 *Using calculated difference in keratometry from CVK analysis (K Diff D), these data can be plotted for various corneal diameters against time (months) following 7.00 mm hypermetropic PRK ablations with the Aesculap–Meditec excimer laser (n=20 eyes). Marked decay in induced refractive change is noted in the first 3 months for apex power and at 3 mm corneal diameter. Little change in mean K Diff D values is noted at greater diameters. Refractive change appears stable between 6 and 12 months post-treatment.*

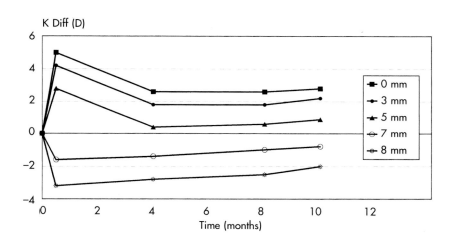

Figure 17.21 *Utilizing a wider hypermetropic zone ablation (8.0 mm) with the Aesculap–Meditec laser appears to produce earlier stabilization of induced refractive effect, as demonstrated by this case. Plot of change in keratometry (K Diff D, calculated from pre- and post-treatment CVK maps) against time post-treatment (months) at various corneal diameters (mm). Attempted correction of +6.00 D using third-generation rotating mask and 8.00 mm ablation zone.*

Figure 17.22 *Unaided vision at 1 year post-treatment, following correction of low-to-moderate hypermetropia utilizing an Aesculap–Meditec excimer laser at two ablation diameters.*

Attempted Correction Hypermetropic PRK	No Eyes	Unaided vision post PRK		
		6/6	6/12	N8
7.00mm ablation zone				
+2.00D to +4.00D	4	75%	100%	100%
+4.25D to +6.50D	9	11%	88%	33%
8.00mm ablation zone				
+2.00D to +4.00D	4	75%	100%	100%
+4.50D to +7.50D	6	17%	66%	50%
+2.00D to +7.50D	23	35%	87%	61%

Diameter of Ablation		Loss of Snellen lines of BSCVA			
Hypermetropic PRK	Eyes	0 Lines	1 Line	2 Lines	3 Lines
7.0mm zone	13	55%	23%	15%	7%
8.0mm zone	10	40%	10%	40%	10%

Figure 17.23 *Loss of lines of Snellen BSCVA, at 1 year, following attempted correction of +2.00 D to +7.50 D of hypermetropia using an Aesculap–Meditec laser with rotating mask at two ablation diameters.*

at this larger diameter. This centre near effect is presumably caused by the isolation of the maximally curved cornea over the centre of the entrance pupil, when the pupil constricts during near synkinesis. The relative size of the pupil in relation to the optical component of the ablation zone might similarly explain the improvement in distance acuity in brighter light.

In general this pilot study demonstrated that excimer laser treatment for hypermetropia will significantly improve unaided vision, for both near and far sight, with 87% of eyes achieving 6/12 unaided vision and almost two-thirds (61%) enjoying N8 unaided reading vision. However, it is notable, despite the fact that the majority of subjects were very happy with this outcome, that 35% of eyes lost two or more lines of Snellen BSCVA. The amount of sacrifice is not decreased by increasing the ablation zone width. However, there is a noticeable pseudoaccommodative effect, which benefits presbyopic individuals and improves the quality of reading vision when uncorrected. Unlike distance visual acuity, the quality of corrected near vision, possibly due to pupillary constriction, does not seem to be adversely affected when compared to preoperative BSCVA for near vision.

On the basis of these preliminary results in low hypermetropia the study was extended to treat 10 eyes with iatrogenic hypermetropia secondary to myopic PRK overcorrection. Attempted corrections varied from +2.00 D to +7.50 D (Fig. 17.24). All 10 eyes were corrected to within 1 D of intended correction at latest follow-up. No patients lost BSCVA and there were no cases of significant corneal haze at any stage. Interestingly, these secondary hypermetropic PRK procedures, upon previous myopic PRK ablation zones, did not result in an obvious increase in central power on CVK map analysis, but rather produced an apparent enlargement of the ablation zone (Fig.

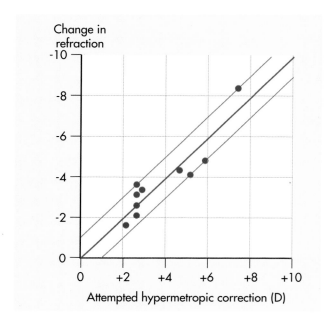

Figure 17.24 *Hypermetropic photorefractive keratectomy (H-PRK) appears to be successful in treating hypermetropia that has resulted from myopic PRK overcorrection, as demonstrated by this graph which highlights 10 H-PRK procedures in subjects with +2.10 to +7.50 D overcorrections following myopic PRK. Following H-PRK all eyes were within ±1.00 D of emmetropia at 6 months post-treatment.*

17.25). A possible explanation for the superior success of these treatments, compared to hypermetropic PRK procedures on virgin corneas, is that these eyes are self selected for lack of regression after PRK by virtue of the fact that they remained overcorrected after the primary myopic PRK procedure.

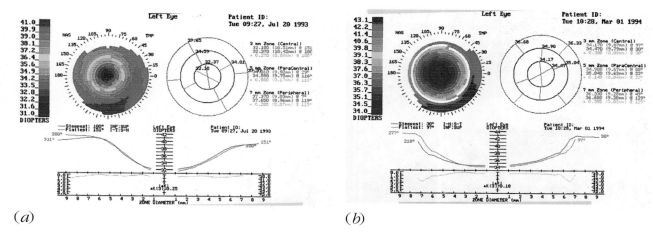

(*a*)   (*b*)

Figure 17.25 (*a*) *CVK map of an eye with a refraction of +3.00/0.75 at 20° following a myopic PRK. The central 3.0 mm power is fairly uniform at 32.1 D to 32.37 D. The patient underwent a deliberate hypermetropic-PRK overcorrection (to allow for regression of effect) of +5.50/1.00 at 20° using an Aesculap–Meditec laser with a rotating mask providing a 7.0 mm diameter ablation zone. (*b*) Nine months later the central CVK map power has increased from +34.17 to +34.47 at 3.00 mm diameter, with an apparent widening of the ablation zone and a more gentle rate of change in power from periphery to apex. Refraction stabilized at −1.25/−0.50 at 40°, providing 6/6 BSCVA.*

PRK CORRECTION OF HYPERMETROPIA WITH THE SUMMIT SVS APEX PLUS SYSTEM

Early attempts to treat astigmatism and hypermetropia using an ablatable mask[33] proved to be unpredictable, largely due to difficulties in centration of the hand held mask system. To obviate this difficulty the Summit SVS Apex Plus system (previously named the Summit SVS Apogee Laser) has now incorporated the ablatable mask into a cartridge, which is inserted, in rail, into the path of the laser beam (Figs 17.26a–c). Two of the authors (CMR and JPD) have been involved in the preliminary assessment of this new approach to hypermetropic correction.

To facilitate the treatment of hypermetropia by a 10 mm diameter treatment zone, Summit Technologies has also developed the Axicon lens. The treatment of hyperopia is carried out in two stages. Initially, a 6.5 mm diameter hypermetropic correction is created using the appropriate ablatable mask in rail; this produces maximum ablation at 6.5 mm diameter and minimum ablation over the centre of the pupil, thus creating increased anterior corneal curvature (Figs 17.27a–d). The used ablatable mask is

then replaced, in rail, by the Axicon lens. This lens diverges the 6.5 mm diameter excimer beam into an annular beam of 6.5 mm internal diameter and 9.4 mm external diameter (Fig. 17.28).

Because of the design of the Axicon lens, virtually no energy is delivered to the central 6.5 mm of cornea where the hypermetropic optical zone has been ablated; indeed, maximal energy is distributed at the 6.5 mm junction, with a tapering off of this energy delivery towards the 9.4 mm outer diameter. The maximal ablation achieved at 6.5–7.0 mm creates a corneal trough which extends, via a gentle blend, or transition zone, to 9.4 mm diameter (Figs 17.29a–b) The number of pulses delivered via the Axicon lens is related to the attempted hypermetropic correction. Theoretically, this wider treatment and transition zone should lead to greater stability of refractive effect, with less marked regression and fewer visual side-effects related to decentration.

In the prospective study conducted by the authors, 11 patients with varying degrees of hypermetropia were recruited, after fully informed consent, to undergo PRK hypermetropic correction with the Summit Apex Plus system. Ten of the subjects were phakic and one aphakic, with a mean age of 42.1

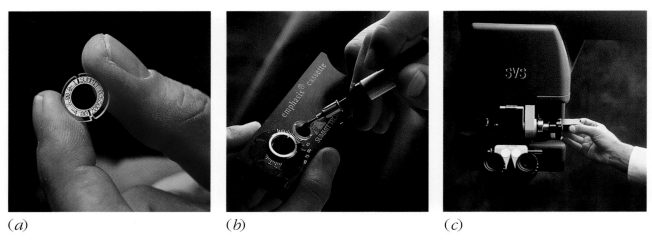

(*a*)   (*b*)   (*c*)

Figure 17.26 (*a*) *The single use Summit emphasis erodible mask, or laser disc, consists of an erodible polymethylmethacrylate (PMMA) component, and a supporting quartz disc, which allows transmission of the 193 nm excimer wavelength. The PMMA component can be precisely shaped to correct astigmatism and hypermetropia. (b) The Summit emphasis erodible mask is carefully placed into a cassette or cartridge prior to insertion into the laser. (c) Once the erodible mask has been inserted into a cassette, the cassette is positioned 'in-rail' in the Summit SVS Apex Plus laser, such that the mask is accurately positioned in the path of the excimer beam. (Courtesy Summit Technology.)*

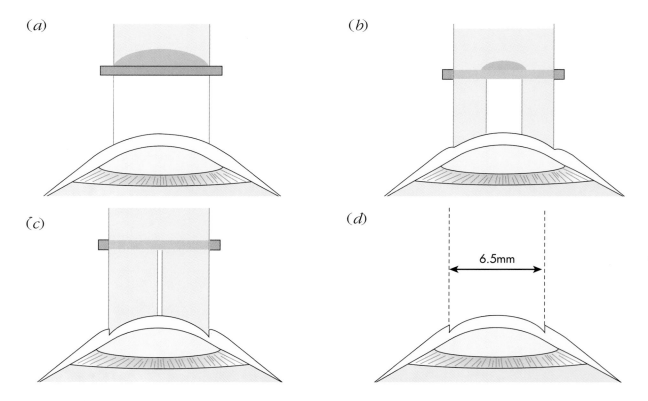

Figure 17.27 (*a–d*) *The Summit Emphasis erodible mask is positioned in the laser path prior to commencing hypermetropic PRK. The PMMA portion absorbs energy from the 193 nm beam and is slowly ablated or eroded, whereas the quartz substrate transmits the laser beam without absorption. As the PMMA template is ablated its contour is replicated upon the underlying corneal stroma, creating a 6.5 mm diameter area of central corneal steepening. (Courtesy Summit Technology.)*

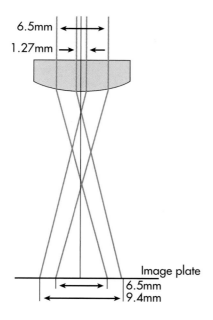

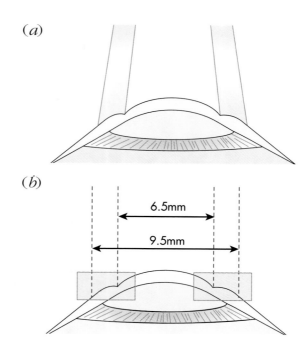

Figure 17.28 *The reusable Axicon lens uses prismatic design to diverge the standard 6.5 mm diameter laser beam to create an annular beam of 6.5 mm inner and 9.4 mm outer diameter.*

Figure 17.29 *(a) After a central hypermetropic zone of 6.5 mm is created using an emphasis erodible mask the Axicon lens is utilized to create the peripheral corneal component of the hypermetropic correction. (b) The effect of the Axicon lens is to create a midperipheral corneal trough with a large blend transition zone extending to 9.4 mm diameter. (Courtesy Summit Technology.)*

years (range 25–67 years). One eye per patient was treated and preoperative assessment included cycloplegic refraction, BSCVA, manual keratometry, CVK and a full ocular examination.

Preoperative preparation involved instillation of topical pilocarpine 2% and amethocaine (tetracaine) drops. With the subject positioned on the laser couch, the corneal epithelium was manually debrided with a hockey blade, leaving a small peripheral cuff adjacent to the limbus. As the cornea in the hypermetropic eye tends to have a smaller diameter than the myopic eye, and the intended treatment zone extends to 9.4 mm diameter, it is essential to leave only a small peripheral cuff of intact epithelium.

With the patient self-fixating a flashing green target light, a +2.0 D, +3.0 D or +4.0 D correction was performed using a hypermetropic mask in rail. The hyperopic mask was than replaced with the Axicon lens and after a 20 second delay the peripheral component of the ablation was completed. The number of pulses performed via the Axicon lens varied from 177 pulses with a +2.00 D correction to 372 pulses with a +4.00 D correction. Cyclopentolate 1% and chloramphenicol 0.5% drops were instilled in the eye and the eye patched for 36 hours. Once the epithelium had healed, by day 4 postoperatively in all cases, fluorometholone 0.1% drops were applied three times daily for 1 week then once daily for 1 month.

Postoperative data was collected at 4, 8, 12, 26 and 39 weeks. This included refraction, BSCVA, manual keratometry, CVK analysis (Fig. 17.30) and grading of corneal haze.

Preoperative refraction ranged from +2.50 D to +8.38 D (SE) with a mean of +5.36 ± 1.81 D (mean ± SD) at the spectacle plane, which equates to +5.80 ± 2.10 D at the corneal plane. The mean attempted hypermetropic correction was +3.09 D at the corneal plane. Refractive results for the group as a whole demonstrated an initial overcorrection at 4 weeks, with subsequent regression

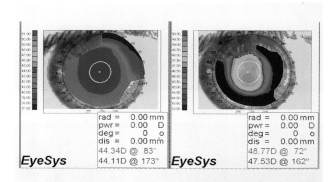

Figure 17.30 *Corneal CVK maps before (left) and after (right) a +4.00 D hypermetropic PRK correction using an emphasis erodible mask and Axicon lens. Marked increase in central power surrounded by a mid-peripheral reduction in dioptric power are clearly seen (right).*

until about 12 weeks post-treatment; thereafter, no statistically significant fluctuation in mean refraction occurred (Figs 17.31 and 17.32). The degree of initial overcorrection and subsequent regression was greater in the higher attempted corrections.

Induced astigmatism was calculated by computer using vector analysis. Magnitude and axis of induced astigmatism were assessed, taking into account pre-existing astigmatism. Calculations utilized both keratometric and refractive data. Approximately +0.75 D of with-the-rule cylinder was induced, as estimated by refraction and +1.00 D, again with-the-rule, based on keratometry data. BSCVA was 6/6 in all 10 phakic eyes and 6/0 in the aphakic eye prior to treatment. No eye lost two Snellen lines or more of BSCVA at any time point post-PRK. At the 9 month (latest) review, 10 eyes obtained BSCVA equal to preoperative values and one eye gained one line of BSCVA. Corneal haze was visually insignificant, being limited to the midperipheral cornea (Fig. 17.33).

The results of this pilot study suggest that the degree of correction obtained when measured by refraction is greater than attempted. However, changes in both manual and CVK keratometry mirrored the attempted correction much more closely than the refraction. The algorithms will certainly need adjustment and fine tuning, probably in the number of pulses delivered via the Axicon, but these results suggest that PRK for hypermetropia up to +4.00 D appears to be a relatively safe procedure, with acceptable visual and refractive outcome using ablatable mask technology.

Change in mean refraction after hyperopic PRK

	preop	4 weeks	8 weeks	12 weeks	26 weeks	39 weeks
All patients (mean correction +3.09 dioptres) SECP (dioptres)	+5.80 (SD 2.10)	-0.47 (SD 0.84)	+0.19 (SD 0.74)	+0.83 (SD 0.96)	+0.93 (SD 1.10)	+0.93 (SD 0.94)
+2 dioptre treatment group SECP (dioptres)	+3.44 (SD 0.75)	-0.24 (SD 0.90)	-0.20 (SD 0.89)	+0.06 (SD 1.32)	-0.08 (SD 0.76)	-0.43 (SD 0.71)
+3 dioptre treatment group SECP (dioptres)	+5.35 (SD 0.62)	-0.42 (SD 1.04)	+0.45 (SD 0.38)	+0.67 (SD 0.49)	+1.35 (SD 0.47)	+1.45 (SD 0.38)
+4 dioptre treatment group SECP (dioptres)	+8.03 (SD 1.20)	-0.69 (SD 0.77)	+0.21 (SD 0.95)	+1.57 (SD 0.58)	+1.49 (SD 1.10)	+0.91 (SD 1.31)

SECP = spherical equivalent corneal plane
SD = standard deviation

Figure 17.31 *Change in mean refraction after hypermetropic PRK (n=11) using emphasis erodible masks, Axicon lens and a Summit SVS Apex Plus laser. As a group the mean preoperative refraction of +5.80 D was reduced by 4.87 D to a mean of +0.93 D following an average attempted correction of +3.09 D at the corneal plane.*

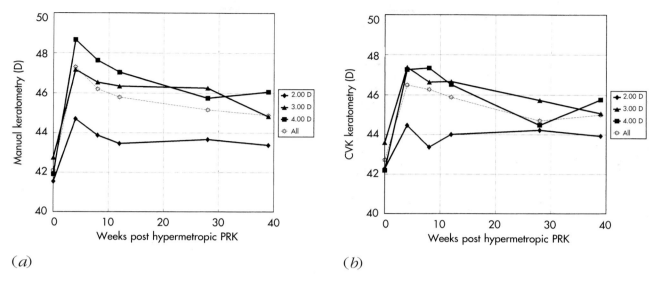

(*a*)   (*b*)

Figure 17.32 *Manual (a) and CVK-derived (b) keratometry demonstrate early overcorrection in all eyes (n=11) following hypermetropic PRK. However, keratometry values stabilize by 12 weeks in the eyes that underwent an attempted correction of +2.00 D, whereas +3.00 D and +4.00 D corrections show a continued reduction of induced refractive effect until 6 months post-treatment. The group as a whole appear to have reached refractive stability between 6 and 9 months, as measured by manual and CVK-derived keratometry.*

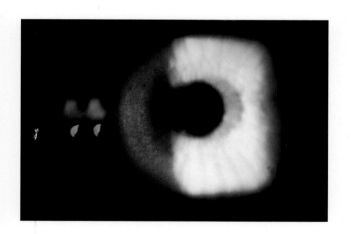

Figure 17.33 *An annulus of mild corneal haze is seen in the midperiphery of a cornea 3 months after a +4.00 D hypermetropic correction with an emphasis erodible mask and Axicon lens.*

HYPERMETROPIC-ASTIGMATISM CORRECTION (H-PARK)

Little has been published on hypermetropic-astigmatic PARK. However, to obtain the intended correction it is necessary to perform an oval furrow-like ring zone in the steep meridian. Such ablative profiles are created by appropriate mask design, in combination with varying rotation speeds to increase ablation depth in any desired meridian.[3,26] Results for astigma-

tism in combination with low-to-moderate hypermetropia (up to +6.50 D) show promise[4,34] (Fig. 17.34).

COMPLICATIONS

All complications pertaining to excimer laser PRK for myopia in terms of debridement, lasering, healing

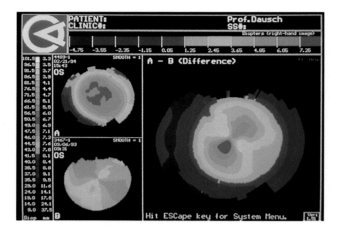

Figure 17.34 *CVK map of a left eye after a hypermetropic astigmatic (H-PARK) correction of +7.25/–3.75 at 56°. Preoperative astigmatism is highlighted in the lower left map and the 3 month post-PARK appearance is shown in the upper left map, which shows a regular round or oval topographic appearance. A difference map (right) highlights the induced topographic change. Refraction at 3 months post-H-PARK was –0.75/–0.50 at 55°. (Courtesy Prof D Dausch MD and Aesculap–Meditec.)*

and pharmacology apply to excimer laser PRK for hypermetropia and are discussed in full in Chapter 23. As can easily be gleaned from the above studies, two main complications in regard to hypermetropic PRK warrant special attention:

- Treatment zone centration is critical, far more so than with PRK for myopia and this is highlighted in the above studies where loss of BSCVA is attributed almost solely to this.[4,32] Suggested improvements in this area include meticulous attention to intraoperative detail, enlargement of the ablation zone, and other technological advances, such as passive and active laser tracking of ocular movements.[35]

- Regression of effect is also highlighted by the above studies[3,25] and it appears that this occurs to a much greater extent than for a myopic PRK of similar magnitude. Suggested improvements in this area focus around an enlarged ablation

diameter (necessitating deeper peripheral sculpting), together with a more gradual transition zone to the periphery in order to facilitate an attenuated healing response. Such refinements are obviously quite technologically demanding but are currently under investigation.[36,37]

It is worth reiterating that the haze induced by PRK for hypermetropia, which is maximal at the junction of the central refractive zone and the peripheral transition zone (corresponding to the area of deepest sculpting), may be worse than that for a myopic PRK of similar magnitude, but appears to follow the same sort of time course towards resolution. However, as it is in the form of a peripheral ring that does not affect the axial cornea, it is likely to have much less effect on vision than haze associated with myopic PRK.

CONCLUSIONS

Hexagonal keratotomy is now in its twilight and holmium:YAG LTK increasingly appears to be limited to the correction of low level hypermetropia. It therefore appears likely that the treatment of moderate hypermetropia, between +2.00 D and +6.00 D, may be the last challenge to surface-based excimer PRK techniques.

However, unlike PRK and PARK for myopia, hypermetropic PRK is still in its infancy on the steep upward slope of development. Further research is currently underway, with particular emphasis on ablation zones of 9.0–10.0 mm diameter. The creation of a wider central optical zone should further improve the quality of unaided and best corrected vision, although the pseudoaccommodative effect previously noted in presbyopes may be diminished and it may be that, ultimately, different ablation diameter treatments could be offered to subjects of differing age and visual requirement. Theoretically, these wider zones with smooth transition elements should be more stable and less likely to develop regression of effect.

Development of active eye tracking systems to improve centration is certainly going to be of greater importance in hypermetropic correction than corresponding myopic corrections of similar magnitude. This is particularly so for those lasers that utilize a scanning system, for several reasons. Firstly, the increased time to perform the ablation compared to comparable myopic ablations increases the likelihood of decentration; secondly, unlike an expanding broad-beam ablation, a scanning system that essentially creates a corneal trough provides fewer visual clues to the surgeon in respect of accurate centration; and, finally, the smaller optical zones in hypermetropic corrections are more prone to produce symptomatic problems, when decentred, than larger myopic ablation zones.

Late 1995 and early 1996 saw the arrival of the long-awaited FDA approval for Summit and Visx lasers for the treatment of low-to-moderate myopia. Animal studies using Visx lasers to treat hypertropia were reported by Keates et al in January 1992 and in the summer of 1993 the Visx hypermetropic-

PRK study of mild-to-moderate hypermetropia began at three US centres.[38] Summit Technologies have pursued diverging technologies in the treatment of hypermetropia – holmium:YAG LTK using the contact method as previously discussed and hypermetropic PRK using the emphasis erodible mask and Axicon lens. The latter studies commenced in 1995 and have produced encouraging preliminary results from three non-US centres – Sydney, Calgary and Milan – at the time of writing.[39–41] However, in light of the experience with myopic PRK, it appears that several more years will elapse before excimer laser technology for the correction of hypermetropia reaches FDA approval for use in the USA.

REFERENCES

1. Duke-Elder S, Abrams D, Anomalies of the optical system. In: Duke-Elder S, ed, *System of Ophthalmology, Vol. 5* (Henry Kimpton: London, 1970) 234–9.
2. Wang Q, Klein BE, Klein R, Moss RE, Refractive status in the Beaver Dam Study, *Invest Ophthalmol Vis Sci* (1994) **35**:4344–7.
3. Stromberg S, Refraction and axial length of human eyes, *Acta Ophthalmol* (1936) **14**:281–5.
4. Anschütz T, Laser correction of hyperopia and presbyopia, *Int Ophthalmol Clin* (1994) **42**:139–43.
5. Lans LJ, Experimentelle Untersuchungen über die Entstehung von Astimatismus durch nicht-perforirende Corneawunden, *Albrecht Von Graefes Arch Klin Exp Ophthalmol* (1898) **45**:117–21.
6. Yamashita T, Schneider M, Fuerst D, Pearce W, Hexagonal keratotomy reduces hyperopia after radial keratotomy in rabbits, *J Refract Surg* (1986) **2**:261–4.
7. Gilbert ML, Friedlander M, Aiello JP, Granet N, Hexagonal keratotomy in human cadaver eyes, *J Refract Surg* (1988) **4**:12–14.
8. Vrabec MP, Durrie DS, Hunkeler JD, Arcuate keratotomy for the correction of spherical hyperopia in human cadaver eyes, *Refract Corneal Surg* (1992) **9**:388–91.
9. Neumann AC, McCarty GR, Hexagonal keratotomy for correction of low hyperopia: preliminary results from a prospective study, *J Cataract Refract Surg* (1988) **14**:265–9.
10. Jensen R, Hexagonal keratotomy: clinical experience with 483 eyes, *Int Ophthalmol Clin* (1991) **31**:69–73.
11. Nordan LT, Maxwell WA, Avoid radial keratotomy with small optical zones and hexagonal keratotomy (Letter), *Refract Corneal Surg* (1992) **8**:331.
12. Harr D, Sparring over hexagonal keratotomy, *Refract Corneal Surg* (1992) **8**:266–7.
13. Grandon SC, Sanders DR, Anello RD, Jacobs D, Biscaro M, Clinical evaluation of hexagonal keratotomy for the treatment of primary hyperopia, *J Cataract Refract Surg* (1995) **21**:140–9.
14. Fyodorov S, Corneal curvature change using energy of laser radiation, Russian Patent 1980; no. 822407.

15. Neumann AC, Fyodorov S, Sanders DR, Radial thermokeratoplasty for the correction of hyperopia, *Refract Corneal Surg* (1990) **6**:404–11.
16. Neumann AC, Sanders D, Raanan M, DeLuca M, Hyperopic thermokeratoplasty: clinical evaluation, *J Cataract Refract Surg* (1991) **17**:830–8.
17. Charpentier DY, Nguyen-Khoa JL, Duplessix M, Colin J, Denis P, Intrastromal thermokeratoplasty for correction of spherical hyperopia: a 1-year prospective study, *Journal Francais d' Ophtalmologie* (1995) **18**:200–6.
18. Feldman ET, Ellis W, Frucht-Perry J, *et al*, Regression of effect following radial thermokeratoplasty in humans, *Refract Corneal Surg* (1989) **5**:288–91.
19. Seiler T, Wollensak J, Refractive surgery of the cornea: corneal surgery – an alternative to optical aids? *Fortschritte der Medizin* (1991) **109**:579–81.
20. Siganos D, Siganos CS, Pallikaris IG, Clear lens extraction and intraocular lens implantation in normally sighted hyperopic eyes, *Refract Corneal Surg* (1994) **10**:117–21.
21. Thompson VM, Seiler T, Durrie DS, Cavanaugh TB, Holmium:YAG laser thermokeratoplasty for hyperopia and astigmatism: an overview, *Refract Corneal Surg (Suppl)* (1993) **9**:S134–S137.
22. Seiler T, Matallana M, Bende T, Laser thermokeratoplasty by means of a pulsed holmium:YAG laser for hyperopic correction, *Refract Corneal Surg* (1990) **6**:99–102.
23. Seiler T, Matallana M, Bende T, Laser coagulation of the cornea with a holmium:YAG laser for correction of hyperopia, *Fortschritte der Ophthalmologie* (1991) **88**:121–4.
24. Seiler T, Ho:YAG laser thermokeratoplasty for hyperopia, *Ophthalmol Clin North Am* (1993) **5**:773–80.
25. Durrie DS, Schumer DJ, Cavanaugh TB, Holmium:YAG laser thermokeratoplasty for hyperopia, *Refract Corneal Surg* (1994) **10(Suppl)**:S277–S280.
26. Tutton MK, Cherry PMH, Holmium:YAG laser thermokeratoplasty to correct hyperopia: two years follow-up, *Ophthalmic Surgery and Lasers* (1996) **27(Suppl)**:S521–S524.

27. Parel JM, Ren Q, Simon G, Noncontact laser photothermal keratoplasty I: biophysical principles and laser beam delivery system, *Refract Corneal Surg* (1994) **10**:511–18.

28. Simon G, Ren Q, Parel JM, Noncontact laser photothermal keratoplasty II: refraction effects and treatment parameters in cadaver eyes, *Refract Corneal Surg* (1994) **10**:519–28.

29. Kohnen T, Husain SE, Koch DD, Corneal topographic changes after holmium:YAG laser thermal keratoplasty to correct hyperopia, *J Cataract Refract Surg* (1996) **22**:427–35.

30. L'Esperance FA Jr, Warner JW, Telfair WB, Yoder PR Jr, Martin CA, Excimer laser instrumentation and technique for human corneal surgery, *Arch Ophthalmol* (1989) **107**:131–9.

31. Del Pero RA, Gigstad JE, Roberts AD, et al., A refractive and histopathological study of excimer laser keratectomy in primates, *Am J Opthalmol* (1990) **109**:419–29.

32. Dausch D, Klein R, Schröder E, Excimer laser photorefractive keratectomy for hyperopia, *Refract Corneal Surg* (1993) **9**:20–8.

33. Maloney RK, Friedman M, Harman T, et al., A prototype erodible mask delivery system for the excimer laser, *Ophthalmology* (1993) **100**:542–9.

34. Dausch D, Klein R, Landesz M, Schröder E, Photorefractive keratectomy to correct astigmatism with myopia or hyperopia, *J Cataract Refract Surg* (1994) **20(Suppl):**252–7.

35. Preussner PR, Leukefeld J, Automatic tracking system for laser surgery of the human cornea, *Biomedizinische Technik* (1992) **37**:218–21.

36. Seiler T, McDonnell PJ, Excimer laser photorefractive keratectomy, *Surv Ophthalmol* (1995) **40**:80–118.

37. Ramirez-Florez S, Koons SJ, Shimmick JK, Telfair WB, Correction of hyperopia with excimer laser PRK, *Invest Ophthalmol Vis Sci* (1994) **35(Suppl):**2023.

38. Macy JI, Nesburn AB, Salz JJ, Laser correction of hyperopia: VisX blind eye study United States results. In: Salz JJ, ed, *Corneal Laser Surgery* (Mosby: St Louis, 1995) 256–60.

39. Gimbel HV, Correction of hyperopia using the Summit Apogee laser, *Ophthalmic Surgery and Lasers* (1996) **27(5):**S530(1) (abst).

40. Rogers CM, Hyperopic correction with the Axicon lens, *Ophthalmic Surgery and Lasers* (1996) **27(5):**S530(2) (abst).

41. Carones F, Venturi E, Gobbi PG, Brabcato R, Hyperopia correction using an erodible mask in-the-rail excimer laser delivery system, *Ophthalmic Surgery and Lasers* (1996) **27(5):**S531 (abst).

Chapter 18 Excimer laser in situ keratomileusis (LASIK)

George O Waring III

INTRODUCTION

Excimer laser in situ keratomileusis under a hinged flap is known most commonly by the acronym LASIK (Table 18.1), a term initially suggested by Pallikaris and colleagues.[1] This versatile surgical technique for correcting myopia and astigmatism—and potentially hyperopia—can correct from approximately −2.00 to −20.00 D of myopia. LASIK combines two advanced refractive surgical technologies, a microkeratome that creates a plano anterior corneal flap and an excimer laser that does photoablation. This combination gives a surgeon the advantage of automated technology,

provides the patient rapid, virtually painless, recovery of vision, produces good refractive stability, and allows for repeated surgery for residual myopia.

DEVELOPMENT OF LASIK

The history and development of keratomileusis span some 40 years of innovation and advancement (Tables 18.2[1–7] and 18.3[8–13]). After José Barraquer introduced the term refractive keratoplasty in 1949, he developed the microkeratome for excising a plano

Table 18.1
Terminology of keratomileusis

Term	Definition
Keratomileusis	Carving the cornea. Procedures that use a microkeratome or other instrument to create a corneal flap or disc as part of refractive keratoplasty.
Myopic keratomileusis	Keratomileusis to treat myopia
Hyperopic keratomileusis	Keratomileusis to treat hyperopia.
Cryolathe keratomileusis	Keratomileusis for myopia or hyperopia using a cryolathe to change the curvature of the back of the corneal disc.
Planar, non-freeze keratomileusis	Keratomileusis for myopia or hyperopia using a microkeratome and a set of dies to change the curvature of the back of the disc.
Excimer laser keratomileusis	Keratomileusis using the excimer laser to make the refractive cut on the back of the disc.
In situ keratomileusis	Keratomileusis for myopia with refractive cut made in the corneal stromal bed.
Automated lamellar keratoplasty	Neologism for keratomileusis in situ in which a mechanically propelled microkeratome makes the flap or disc and the refractive cut.
Laser in situ keratomileusis (LASIK)	Useful abbreviation for keratomileusis in situ performed with the excimer laser. May be done with a corneal disc or corneal flap.

Table 18.2

Techniques and development of keratomileusis

	Early clinical publications	Location and shape of stromal refractive cut	Approximate thickness of disc (µm)	Disc tissue injury	Sutures	Complexity of equipment (1+ to 4+)	Complexity of surgical procedures (1+ to 4+)
Cryolathe on disc	Barraquer (1964)[2]	Disc, lenticular	300	Freeze	Yes	4+	4+
Planar, non-freeze on disc	Krumeich and Swinger (1987)[3]	Disc, lenticular	300	Mechanical desiccation	Yes	3+	3+
In-situ*; manual and automated microkeratome	Ruiz and Rowsey (1988)[4]	Bed, plane	160	Desiccation	Yes or No	2+	2+
In-situ, flap technique	Barraquer (1980)[5]	Bed, plane	160	Minimal	No	2+	2+
Excimer laser on disc	Buratto et al (1992)[6]	Disc, lenticular	300	Desiccation	Yes	4+	3+
In-situ, excimer laser	Pallikaris et al (1990)[1]	Bed, lenticular	160	Minimal	No	4+	3+

1+ = minimal; 2+ = mild; 3+ = moderate; 4+ = severe (author's personal estimates)
*Automated lamellar keratoplasty, also designated ALK

disc of cornea (a disc with parallel surfaces) with which he performed two types of refractive keratoplasty in the early 1960s: keratophakia (Gk. keras, horn, cornea + fakos, lens) and keratomileusis (Gk. keras, horn, cornea + smileusis, to sculpt or carve), the latter term being attributed to Professor John Charamais of Athens, Greece.[14] Today, the term keratomileusis designates any refractive keratoplasty technique that combines a lamellar resection of the cornea performed with a microkeratome or other instrument and an additional technique to change the corneal radius of curvature: cryolathe, microkeratome excision, or excimer laser ablation. The LASIK procedure uses an excimer laser to create a spherocylindrical ablation in the stromal bed (in situ), which effects a refractive change.

Surgical procedures that seem new often have an historical antecedent; LASIK is no exception. The concept of creating a corneal flap and removing tissue from the underlying stromal bed was first described by Pureskin[8] in 1967; he demonstrated that a smaller diameter of the resected stromal tissue creates a larger refractive change; he referred to this operation as

stromectomy. Pureskin used a trephine to manually remove stroma from the bed and demonstrated in a series of 93 eyes that an 8.0 mm diameter disc resection could induce 2.50 D of corneal flattening, whereas a 4.0 mm diameter disc resection could induce approximately 12 D of corneal flattening.

José Barraquer[14] tried this idea, using a microkeratome to remove a layer of stromal tissue from the bed, but abandoned the technique in favor of cryolathe keratomileusis on the back of the disc itself. In the late 1980s, Ruiz[4] revived the idea of keratomileusis in situ, using the plano resection principles of Krumeich, resecting two plano discs—one at the anterior surface and the other from the stromal bed. Ruiz varied the depth and diameter of the in situ excision to flatten the central cornea. Ruiz never published a series of cases and the technique underwent a number of changes, including changing nomograms. It was plagued with poor predictability and produced mild irregular astigmatism. To increase the accuracy of the procedure, Ruiz designed a mechanically advanced microkeratome. The Chiron Vision Corporation manufactured the Corneal Shaper

Table 18.3
Phases in development of in situ keratomileusis for myopia

Phase	Designation	Originator	Instrument for Creation of Anterior Plano Disc	Instruments for Refractive Cut	Type of Refractive Cut	Methods of Attaching Disc
Phase I	Partial stromectomy	Pureskin[8]	Manual	Manual trephine	Circular button	Hinged flap, sutures
Phase II	In situ keratomileusis	Ruiz[4,9]	Manually advanced microkeratome	Manually advanced microkeratome	Plano lenticule	Sutured disc
Phase III	Lamellar automated refractive keratoplasty (LARK)	Ruiz	Automated microkeratome— early models	Automated microkeratome— early models	Plano lenticule	Sutured disc
Phase IV	Automated lamellar keratoplasty (ALK)	Ruiz, Guimerez[10]	Automated microkeratome— refined models	Automated microkeratome— refined models	Plano lenticule	No-suture disc
Phase V	Excimer laser in situ keratomileusis (LASIK)	Pallikaris[1,11]	Custom-designed microkeratome	Excimer laser, ArF spherical myopia	Spherical ablation	Hinged-sutured flap
Phase VI	Excimer laser in situ keratomileusis (LASIK)	Slade, Ruiz[12]	Automated microkeratome— refined models	Excimer laser, ArF compound myopic astigmatism	Sphero-cylindrical ablation	Hinged flap, no suture

and launched an international educational and sales campaign that combined the talents of surgeons and marketeers, renaming keratomileusis in situ 'automated lamellar keratoplasty (ALK)'. In spite of the heavy promotion, the procedure remained intrinsically restricted by the fact that the refractive cut was not truly lenticular, but depended on the resection of a plano disc of tissue. The procedure gradually fell into disuse as LASIK techniques emerged.

In 1985, Peyman applied for a patented method of laser stromal surgery and in 1989, in rabbit eyes, used an erbium–YAG laser to remove corneal tissue from the stromal bed.[15] The patent has been licensed to the Chiron Vision Corporation. Pallikaris, working in Heraklion, Crete, developed LASIK clinically. In 1988, Pallikaris and colleagues[1] carried out their initial study in rabbit eyes and performed LASIK in blind human eyes in 1989[16]; in 1994 they demonstrated that LASIK was superior to photorefractive keratectomy (PRK) for the correction of high myopia.[11] The procedure was further refined and developed by Ruiz et al,[12] by Salah et al,[17] and by Guell.[18] In 1995, Waring,

Thompson and Stulting commenced a large clinical series in the United States at the Vision Correction Group, Emory Vision Correction Center in Atlanta (Waring GO. Excimer laser in-situ keratomileusis (LASIK) for myopia. Investigational Device Exemption Application, FDA, 1995). At the same time, LASIK was becoming popular among refractive surgeons around the world.

ADVANTAGES OF LASIK

THIRTY YEARS OF CLINICAL EXPERIENCE

The first cryolathe keratomileusis procedure was performed on humans in the early 1960s, giving approximately 30 years of experience with the evolving techniques of keratomileusis. Although there is minimal long-term data published about the stability of keratomileusis,[19] the basic technique of keratomileusis has remained extant for three decades and continues to progress and improve. Thus, there is little chance of unexpected long-term complications, such as marked regression or progression of the refractive change, late scarring in the stromal bed, progressive development of irregular astigmatism, or long-term structural changes in the cornea from the procedure.

CORRECTION OF MOST AMETROPIAS

The refractive change is created by the spherical or spherocylindrical ablation of the excimer laser, initially designed for PRK on the corneal surface and therefore improvements in the PRK technology can be transferred to the LASIK procedure with the ablation in the bed. LASIK has been documented to correct myopia from −2.00 to −20.00 D,[17] and as the algorithms and technology of excimer laser photoablation improve, the reliability of such corrections will probably improve. It is likely that compound myopic astigmatism can be corrected by LASIK, since it can be corrected with PRK. The correction of hyperopia has not yet been well documented, but it is also probable that once large diameter flaps and ablations with appropriate corneal contours are developed, hyperopia can be corrected as well. If these projections are true, the LASIK procedure can become a 'one technique fits all' approach to refractive surgery, making it easier for the surgeon who needs only to master one technique and for patients who need to understand only one approach, in contrast to the current situation in which multiple refractive surgical procedures are available.

OUTPATIENT SURGERY

One of the most attractive features of LASIK is also common to PRK and refractive keratotomy—outpatient surgery under topical anesthesia. This makes it user friendly for both the patient and the surgeon, since it can be performed in a clean office setting, often in a facility separate from that of standard ophthalmic practice that allows a more custom-tailored approach for refractive surgery patients, who have higher demands for service than the average eye patient. When done efficiently, the process can be completed in less than an hour of the patient's time, and the surgery procedure takes less than 15 minutes from start to finish, including a 5 minute waiting time for the flap to dry on the cornea. The design of contemporary excimer lasers allows enough working room between the objective lens of the microscope and the eye for the entire procedure to be carried out under the excimer laser, obviating patient movement from one location to another. The patient leaves without a patch and—since the epithelium is preserved—with improved although blurred vision.

EXTRAOCULAR SURGERY

LASIK shares the feature of extraocular (intracorneal) surgery with other corneal refractive procedures. However, safety should not be taken for granted, since it is possible to create severe corneal distortion—particularly if the flap is damaged or lost—that can produce marked visual disability for the patient. The remote risk of bacterial keratitis should not be forgotten. Current studies report no damage to the corneal endothelium.

AUTOMATED INSTRUMENTS

Although the term automated is a misnomer (the surgeon must still perform the surgery correctly), microkeratomes that advance mechanically and programmable excimer lasers make the procedure easier and above all ensure a greater uniformity. These advantages become more obvious when compared to earlier techniques of keratomileusis, with manually advanced microkeratomes and cryolathes or dies used to shape the corneal disc. The automated features of microkeratomes will improve with better mechanical advances, integrated suction ring-microkeratome systems, improved visibility of the cornea during surgery, and better ergonomics. Similarly, the automated features of excimer lasers will improve, with improved centering or tracking devices, and improved methods of calibrating the laser beam prior to surgery.

HINGED CORNEAL FLAP

The hinged corneal flap provides numerous advantages. First, the flap remains attached to the cornea, which decreases the chance of damage or loss. Second, the hinge allows the flap to be placed back in its original anatomic position decreasing irregular astigmatism. Third, the hinge helps obviate the need for sutures that distort the cornea and produce astigmatism. Fourth, if the flap comes loose postoperatively, it can remain attached at the hinge so it is not lost. Fifth, the flap can be repositioned within a few seconds after the last laser pulse, reducing the chance of deposit of particles with epithelium in the stromal bed. Sixth, the dimensions of the flap do not have to be exact, since it does not contribute to the refractive outcome; if it is slightly decentered, slightly thicker or thinner, or slightly smaller or larger than the prescribed dimensions, the refractive outcome will not be affected. Seventh, the flap can be lifted months to years after surgery, which allows repeated in situ ablation.

RAPID POSTOPERATIVE RECOVERY

The features that will drive LASIK into popularity among patients are the minimal postoperative pain and rapid recovery of visual function. Since the epithelium is disturbed minimally during the procedure and because the central Bowman's layer remains intact, damage to the naked nerve endings is minimal and patients often require no analgesia after surgery. The central ocular surface remains intact, so that improved vision can be appreciated shortly after surgery, as occurs with refractive keratotomy, and within 24 hours, most patients see well if the refractive correction has been successful. There is still some fluctuation of vision in the first few weeks after surgery as the flap settles. These events are in stark contrast to what occurs after PRK, in which topical or systemic analgesics and a soft contact lens are often used to blunt the pain resulting from the 6.5–7 mm epithelial defect and in which 3–5 days must pass before clear vision begins to return.

SPHEROCYLINDRICAL REFRACTIVE CUT

The refractive ablation performed by the laser is lenticular—that is, a spherocylindrical shape can be etched into the stromal bed, theoretically with submicron accuracy, although in reality the saccadic eye movements and fluid shifts in the tissue blunt this accuracy. Such a lenticular cut is an advance when compared to the plano refractive resection of keratomileusis in situ done with a microkeratome (automated lamellar keratoplasty, ALK) and with the indirect flattening of the central cornea produced by refractive keratotomy.

WOUND HEALING

In PRK, the damaged epithelium and ablated stromal bed are in contact with each other; the epithelium relays molecular cytokine messages to the stromal keratocytes, which become fibroblasts and secrete new extracellular matrix that may manifest clinically as subepithelial haze (see Chapters 4 and 23). There is essentially no haze in the lamellar bed after LASIK and no subepithelial haze. Therefore, topical corticosteroids are not necessary after surgery, eliminating the chance of drug-induced elevations of intraocular pressure (IOP) and cataract, as well as the variability induced by modulation of corneal wound healing by the steroids. The central epithelium is not disrupted by the LASIK procedure, and if the corneal contours created by the ablation are gradual, epithelial hyperplasia should not play a role in the outcome. Theoretically, the reduced role of corneal wound healing should increase predictability of refractive outcome with LASIK as compared to refractive keratotomy or PRK, but this postulate requires clinical verification.

PRESERVATION OF BOWMAN'S LAYER

The central Bowman's layer is not disturbed during LASIK. This increases the chance of having a smooth corneal surface and reduces the chance of irregular astigmatism, assuming a smooth cut is made by the microkeratome. It also eliminates direct epithelial–stromal interaction, which decreases stromal wound healing. For example, in a study by El-Maghraby and colleagues,[20] patients received LASIK in one eye and PRK in the other eye during the same surgical session using the same techniques. Although the refractive outcome was identical for the two eyes at one year after surgery, statistically more patients saw 20/20 with the LASIK eye than with the PRK eye and the subjective judgement about the quality of vision was better in the LASIK eye than the PRK eye. The authors attributed some of these differences to an intact Bowman's layer.

SHORT-TERM AND LONG-TERM STABILITY

Although there is some initial loss of effect within the first few weeks after LASIK, the refractive correction probably stabilizes within the second month after surgery, and seems to remain stable thereafter, although refractive stability has not been studied and reported for more than one year. It is likely that the refractive result remains stable indefinitely, although it is possible that over a period of many years, some steepening of the cornea could occur because the 160 μm deep lamellar keratotomy could weaken the overall biomechanical structure of the cornea. Documenting this will require a decade or two of meticulous follow-up. Certainly, the cornea is more stable than after radial keratotomy (RK), where approximately half of the eyes show a hyperopic shift of 1 D or more within 10 years after surgery with full length incisions (see Chapter 19).

MINIMAL CHANGE IN THE MECHANICAL STRUCTURE OF THE CORNEA

The cornea is not substantially physically weakened by LASIK or PRK, thus eliminating the chance of rupture of the cornea from severe direct trauma when compared to incisional refractive techniques.

REPEATED LASIK FOR RESIDUAL MYOPIA

In cases of undercorrection, a repeated LASIK is possible and relatively easy. The edge of the flap can be broken with an intraocular lens hook and the flap folded back. A repeated ablation is done in the bed and the flap repositioned. It is possible in the future that algorithms for correcting residual astigmatism, induced hyperopia, and maybe even presbyopia may become available. If so, LASIK would be an easily adjustable procedure. This is in contrast to PRK in which a new large epithelial defect with stromal wound healing occurs after every retreatment (see Chapter 24).

DISADVANTAGES OF LASIK

CREATING THE CORNEAL FLAP

The most dangerous part of the LASIK procedure is creating the corneal flap with the microkeratome or other instrument. This requires considerable surgical skill, and makes the procedure more complex than PRK and refractive keratotomy. This is particularly important because the microkeratome operates in front of the entrance pupil, so that complications such as an irregular flap can severely reduce visual acuity.

TECHNICAL COMPLEXITY

Both the microkeratome and the excimer laser are technically complex. A talented, well-trained operat-

ing staff is necessary to maintain a microkeratome in good working condition and to ensure its proper assembly without damage to the blade prior to each case. Of course, the surgeon must double check the instrument before every case. New designs may make maintenance, assembly and use easier. A service technician or engineer must be available to provide ongoing maintenance for the excimer laser, such as changing optical elements and mirrors when they wear out, changing the laser gas tanks, and maintaining alignment of the laser and delivery system. They must also be available to solve problems that arise during clinical use, such as failure of the laser to put out enough energy. These responsibilities are beyond the ability of medically trained personnel.

The surgeon is dependent on the manufacturer. The quality of the microkeratome blade and its cutting action is central to creating a smooth bed and a proper corneal flap. The excimer laser ablation rate, beam homogeneity, pulse energy, uniformity of ablation, and stability of the laser beam are the responsibility of the manufacturer; they can be minimally verified and controlled by the surgeon.

Creating the anterior corneal flap—whether with a microkeratome as done currently or with a laser or waterjet as may be done in the future—requires high technical competence of the surgeon and increases the risk for the patient. An irregular flap, partial cut, lost cap, missing plate with an incision into the anterior chamber, and other complications can permanently reduce visual function.

LACK OF INTRAOPERATIVE CONTROL

The surgeon cannot monitor or modulate the details of the procedure intraoperatively and has control only at the grossest level. Once the chiron corneal shaper microkeratome begins advancing across the cornea, the surgeon can stop it if there is difficulty, but the bed and the flap cannot be observed in detail as they are being cut. During the excimer laser ablation, the laser beam is invisible and the configuration of the ablation on the stroma cannot be detected by visual inspection. Thus, the surgeon is at the mercy of technology—an uncomfortable position.

CHANGING SURGICAL ALGORITHMS

The ablation algorithms are undergoing constant evolution and improvement: increasing diameter, more complex ablation curvatures, and the correction of astigmatism and hyperopia. For example, the simple term 'multizone' is almost meaningless, given the wide variety of multiple diameter and blended types of ablations that are available. The surgeon must remain alert to these changing algorithms and their effect on the refractive outcome in different models of one brand of laser and among different laser manufacturers.

CHANGING INSTRUMENTS

Microkeratomes continue to change in their design and function, placing considerable responsibility on the surgeon. The surgeon must not only learn to use a given model, but also spend money and time learning to use new models. Not only are increasingly complex excimer lasers appearing—with scanning beams and eye trackers—but solid state lasers are also undergoing clinical trials. The situation is analogous to that in the late 1970s when intraocular lens designs were changing rapidly.

EXPENSIVE EQUIPMENT

With an excimer laser costing approximately $500 000, its maintenance costing between $50 000 and $100 000 annually, and a microkeratome costing approximately $40 000, this is not a technology easily acquired by an individual private practising ophthalmologist. Thus, business interests have taken a leadership role in delivering excimer laser refractive surgical care, increasing the complexity of financial dealings for the surgeon.

LESS THAN DESIRABLE ACCURACY OF CORRECTION

Only approximately 50–60% of eyes with −2.00 to −20.00 D of myopia have a refractive outcome within 0.50 D of the desired result. The LASIK procedure is less predictable than spectacles or contact lenses, which it portends to replace. In spite of high patient acceptance, LASIK must achieve improved accuracy and adjustability before it can be considered the equal of optical correction.

SURGICAL TECHNIQUE FOR LASIK

Detailed below are the practical steps in the LASIK surgical procedure, with specific reference to the Chiron Automated Corneal Shaper and the Summit Apex (Omnimed) excimer laser. The steps are summarized in Table 18.4 and illustrated in Figures 18.1–18.6.

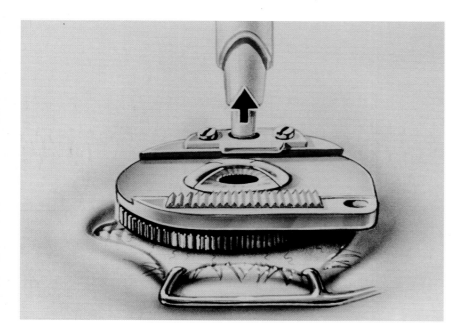

Figure 18.1 *The eyelashes are sequestered beneath an adhesive drape. A four radial marker (or alternatively a Ruiz marker) creates alignment lines on the cornea. The suction ring is applied to the globe (arrow). The drawing shows an adjustable suction ring that creates a corneal flap 7.2–7.5 mm in diameter; a non-adjustable ring that makes an 8.5 mm diameter flap is preferable. (Courtesy Salah T, Am J Ophthalmol.)*

Table 18.4

Summary checklist for a LASIK procedure

(Instruments: Chiron Automated Corneal Shaper and Summit Apex [Omnimed] Laser)

1. Confirm preoperative refraction, desired refractive change, refraction to be entered into the laser, diameter of ablation, and other laser parameters, and post them on the laser in an easily visible form.
2. Verify the laser calibration by ablating the Wratten filter and the PMMA disc and checking the high voltage and laser pressure on the printout.
3. Position the patient under the microscope, prepare with povidone iodine, drape, insert lid speculum, and grossly align the laser.
4. Check the function of the suction ring and microkeratome. Suction should read 23 inches of mercury with good adhesion on thumb; verify thickness plate number as 160 μm (or 130 μm for corrections greater than 15 D). Verify the presence of the blade, listen to sound of motor and observe microkeratome travel in both directions, verifying the function of the stopper. Inspect the edge of the blade under the microscope to detect any irregularities.
5. Program the laser and bring out of test to ensure laser will function properly.
6. Mark the cornea with three or four radial ink marks.
7. Apply the suction ring oriented with the toe of the plate temporal and with slight nasal decentration.
8. Dry the cornea and confirm that intraocular pressure is greater than 65 mmHg with meniscus well within the circle of the applanation tonometer.
9. Moisten surface of cornea and suction ring with two or three drops of BSS.
10. Insert microkeratome into suction ring and seat gears in track.
11. Verify no impediment to microkeratome movement (speculum, drape, lid, etc.).
12. Depress forward foot pedal and advance microkeratome to stopper, but don't jam.
13. Depress reverse foot pedal and remove microkeratome.
14. Release suction and lift ring from globe.
15. Focus laser on cornea and center on pupil with two red HeNe beams at 3 and 9 o'clock at edge of pupil.
16. Fold flap back on the surface of globe and hold with surface tension.
17. Focus and center laser with good patient fixation on fixation light.
18. Depress laser pedal and complete ablation. Stop immediately if centration is lost, have patient refixate, and then complete ablation.
19. Place flap back onto dry bed immediately after last laser pulse.
20. Float the flap completely up on a layer of balanced salt solution and align radial marks, or leave in position dry.
21. Wait 2–5 minutes for flap to dry in place with eye open, depending on technique.
22. Verify flap adhesion by depression of peripheral cornea.
23. Remove speculum and drapes, and verify flap adhesion again by blinking.
24. Inspect cornea with slit-lamp microscope and look for microslip, flap wrinkles or dislocation of flaps.
25. Apply postoperative antibiotics and nonsteroidal anti-inflammatory drug.

PREOPERATIVE MEDICATION

Apply one or two drops of topical anesthetic (e.g. proparacaine 0.5%) to anesthetize the conjunctiva and cornea. Excessive dosing will damage, soften, and loosen the corneal epithelium. Instill pilocarpine 1% to constrict the pupil, making the patient less sensitive to the microscope lights and assisting in centering the ablation (also see Chapters 9 and 13). Instill one drop of diclofenac or ketorolac to decrease postoperative pain and inflammation. Instill one or two drops of topical antibiotic, such as tobramycin or ciprofloxacin, to help in prophylaxis against infection.

ADJUST THE MICROSCOPE AND FOOT PEDALS

Adjust the pupillary distance, the position and tilt of the microscope and its height with respect to the surgeon's stool, to ensure comfort for the surgeon. Arm rests on the stool help stabilize the surgeon's arms.

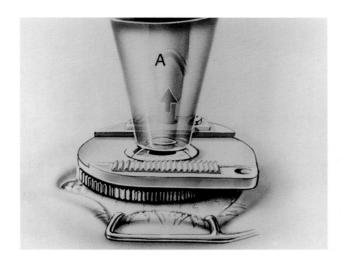

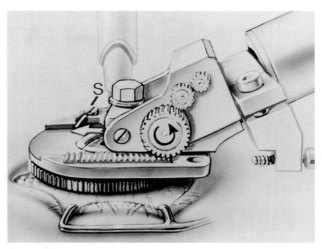

Figure 18.2 *The intraocular pressure is verified as greater than 65 mmHg with an applanation tonometer (A) by having the meniscus of the dried corneal surface within the circle etched on the tonometer. (Courtesy Salah T, Am J Ophthalmol.)*

Figure 18.3 *The surgeon inserts the microkeratome (with a baseplate that creates a 160 µm thick flap) into the dovetail of the suction ring. Activating the foot pedal advances it forward (large arrow) with the gear mechanism (circular arrow) until the edge of the blade is aligned with the screw head (S) at which point the stopper screw halts the forward advance of the microkeratome. (Courtesy Salah T, Am J Ophthalmol.)*

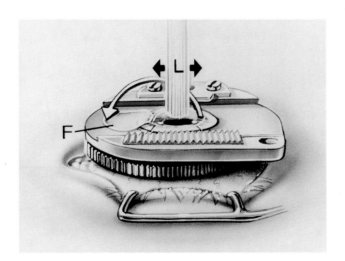

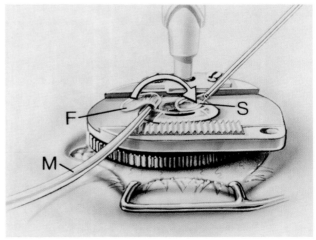

Figure 18.4 *The surgeon turns off the suction, steadies the eye with the suction ring, turns back the corneal flap (F), focuses and centers the excimer laser (L) that ablates the bed with an expanding diaphragm (solid arrows) to correct myopia. Alternatively the suction ring is removed from the eye and patient fixation is used for centration. (Courtesy Salah T, Am J Ophthalmol.)*

Figure 18.5 *The flap (F) is flipped back into place with a blunt instrument (M). Balanced salt solution (S) is injected beneath the flap until it floats on the bed with the fiduciary marks properly aligned or the flap is rolled back into position dry. (Courtesy Salah T, Am J Ophthalmol.)*

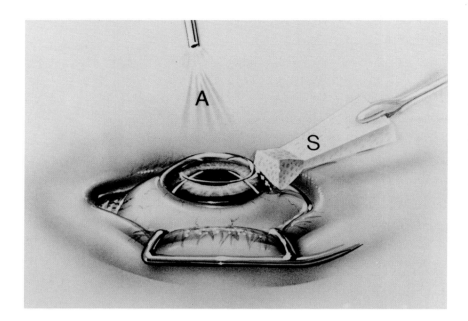

Figure 18.6 *At this point, the author prefers not to touch the flap at all, letting it adhere to the surface with 5 minutes of exposure to room air. Other surgeons use a microsponge (S) to remove fluid from the edge of the flap or blow filtered humidified oxygen (A) onto the cornea for approximately 30 seconds from a distance of approximately 6 inches. (Courtesy of Salah T, Am J Ophthalmol.)*

Arrange the foot pedals. There are numerous pedals and switches involved in the procedure. Each should be accessible without the surgeon looking at them.

- The pedals that control the position of the patient's chair or table in the X, Y, and Z directions are needed to center the patient under the microscope.
- The off/on switch that controls the suction ring works like a light switch, so that when it is depressed the suction turns on and stays on without continued pressure on the foot pedal. The foot pedal must then be depressed a second time, like turning off a light switch, in order to stop the suction.
- The toggle foot switch for the microkeratome activates the microkeratome when depressed and stops it when released. It has two directions: the switch at the end advances the microkeratome and the switch near the entry of the power cord reverses the microkeratome.
- A toggle foot switch for the excimer laser is in a safety housing to prevent inadvertent depression. It activates the laser upon depression and stops the laser when released, allowing the surgeon to stop the ablation instantly, in the middle of the procedure, reposition the patient and continue the ablation by again depressing the pedal.

All these pedals must be arranged in a way that is practical and ergonomic for the surgeon. In some operating rooms, the surgeon operates all four pedals; in others, a nurse or technician will operate the pedal for the suction ring to make it easier for the surgeon. The surgeon must personally operate the pedals for the microkeratome and the excimer laser.

VERIFY THE CALIBRATION OF THE LASER

Each laser manufacturer has a specific technique of calibrating the instrument. For example, with the Summit Apex (Omnimed) laser, a 100 μm thick Wratten filter is ablated, using the phototherapeutic program with a diameter of 6.0 mm. About 550–650 pulses are required to break through the filter and another 250 pulses to remove 90% of the filter, if the laser is properly calibrated. This calibration helps estimate the pulse energy of the laser. In addition, the high voltage reading on the Summit Apex laser should be between 20 000 and 25 000 volts. If it is higher than that, the laser is having trouble getting enough energy to the last energy monitor, and there may be some problems in the laser or the delivery system. Ablation of a polymethylmethacrylate disc, which can be sent to Summit for profilometry, can verify the uniformity of the ablation, but of course this must occur a few days before the actual treatment; ablating an unexposed Polaroid film allows the surgeon to see the uniformity and centration of the energy distribution; when compared to the centration of the initial breakthrough of the Wratten filter, the surgeon can estimate the homogeneity of the energy in the large area ablation. These steps are done before each series of cases. (Newer techniques of dosimetry will improve the surgeon's ability to monitor the laser's function before each case.)

VERIFY THE INFORMATION TO BE ENTERED INTO THE LASER'S COMPUTER

The surgeon and the laser operator should verify together the refractive correction, ablation diameter, multizone components of the ablation, and other variables to be entered into the laser's computer, taking the information from the patient's record or the preoperative planning form and ensuring that it is properly entered into the laser. At this point, test firing of the laser is done and the surgeon must verify that the laser passes calibration and test firing before the microkeratome is applied to the eye.

ATTIRE THE SURGEON

Powderless gloves are preferred. Wearing cap, mask, scrubs, and a gown are optional.

VERIFY THE FUNCTIONS OF THE MICROKERATOME AND SUCTION RING

Each type of microkeratome has a different preoperative check-out procedure. The one described here is for the Chiron Automated Corneal Shaper.

- Test the suction ring on your thumb and be sure that a suction of 23–27 inches of mercury is read on the console, and that the ring adheres to the thumb.
- Test the motion—the advance and retreat—of the microkeratome in the dovetails of the suction ring. Listen to the microkeratome and check the voltmeter in the console to be sure the blade is translating smoothly.
- Be sure the blade is in place, is new, is undamaged, and translates smoothly.

- Verify the thickness, plate number, and location to ensure proper thickness of the flap. A plate that creates a flap 130–160 µm thick is preferred.
- If an automatic stopping mechanism is used, verify the setting on the stopper to ensure an appropriate size for the flap hinge.

CALM THE PATIENT WITH PRACTICAL HYPNOTIC SUGGESTION

The patient should have been instructed preoperatively in the basic steps of the operation, particularly the sensations at the time of applying the suction ring, so there are no surprises intraoperatively. The surgeon speaks in a slow, calm voice. 'Take in a slow deep breath, let it out as slowly as you can, let each part of your body go loose... etc'. The important phrase 'You will feel me working, but nothing I do will bother you' has a great calming effect on the patient.

ANESTHETIZE THE CONJUNCTIVA

Anesthetizing the cornea is easy, one or two drops of topical anesthetic does the job for the duration of the case. Anesthetizing the conjunctiva is difficult and often requires direct application of anesthetic on a saturated microsponge or ring for 5–10 seconds. Application into the fornix decreases the sensation of the lid speculum and increases the patient's comfort. Application around the limbal and bulbar conjunctiva decreases the sensation of the suction ring. The surface of the conjunctiva is then dried to give better adhesion of the suction ring.

POSITION THE SURGEON COMFORTABLY

From this point on it is unnecessary for the surgeon to look up from the operating microscope, because the assistant can hand everything to the surgeon, who saves time by maintaining gaze through the microscope.

POSITION OF THE PATIENT

The patient's head should be positioned with the neck hyperextended slightly so that the globe centers between the lids, making application of the suction ring easier. Adjust the chair or table so that the eye is positioned properly beneath the operating microscope and the patient can view the fixation lights. After the preparation and drape, the patient should be repositioned.

PREPARE AND DRAPE THE PATIENT

Preparation of the skin, lids, and lashes with povidone iodine solution will help prevent infection. An adhesive drape is applied. The goal here is to be sure that the lashes and eyelids do not interfere with the surgical procedure. Some surgeons simply apply a circular drape around the lid skin. Some use the drape or steristrips to hold back the lashes, and others wrap the drape around the lid margin as is commonly done with cataract surgery. The lid speculum is inserted, one strong enough to open the lids widely and to give plenty of room for the suction ring. Some patients may develop postoperative ptosis, possibly from crushing of the levator aponeurosis. The lashes and the drape must be completely removed from the area of the suction ring so as not to interfere with the movement of the microkeratome.

CONFIRM LASER STATUS

Before touching the cornea, the surgeon must confirm that the laser has been programmed properly, that it has passed test firing, and that it is ready to do the refractive ablation.

PLACE ALIGNMENT MARKS ON THE CORNEA

Use a four-bladed RK marker or some other marker that creates a series of methylene blue-marked lines that straddle the edge of the flap. Three marks are helpful to orient the flap as close to its natural preoperative position as possible, and to help orient the disc in case it is cut off completely. Ink is applied directly to three of the four radial ridges. Multiple marks make it easier to accurately position the flap throughout its circumference and are preferred to a single tangential mark (Fig. 18.1).

PASS THE INSTRUMENTS

When the technician passes the suction ring and microkeratome to the surgeon, they should be passed in the orientation in which they will be used. For the left eye of a patient, the suction ring is passed to the surgeon's right, with the handle oriented toward the head of the patient. When the microkeratome is passed, it is placed in the surgeon's hand in the position he/she desires. These manoeuvers allow the surgeon to avoid looking up from the microscope and speed the procedure.

APPLY THE SUCTION RING

This is probably the most difficult part of the procedure for the patient, and some reassuring words from the surgeon will help the patient remain calm. After the ring is inserted between the lids and the lid speculum and is pressed firmly onto the surface of the globe, suction is applied. At this point only a gentle depression of the handle of the suction ring is necessary and the globe does not have to be retropulsed. The ring must be free of the speculum, drapes, and eyelashes. It is more difficult to fit a suction ring into a small palpebral fissure or on to an eye that is recessed into the orbit. A gentle touch and calm, relaxed persistence allows the ring to be applied to almost every globe. For the right eye, the surgeon holds the suction ring in the left hand and spreads the eyelid speculum, if necessary, with the right hand. For the left eye, he holds the suction ring in the right hand and spreads the speculum with the left. The surgeon can verify adequate adhesion of the suction ring by moving the ring slightly to be sure that the globe is adherent. Pulling up briskly on the suction ring may break the suction. Because only one diameter flap is used in LASIK—approximately 8.2 mm—there is no need for an adjustable suction ring.

Since refractive surgical procedures should be centered around the entrance pupil, one might think that the suction ring should be centered around the entrance pupil as well, but this is not always true, because the position of the plano flap minimally affects the refractive result. A flap centered on the pupil may place the hinge too close to the ablation zone, especially if the pupil is displaced slightly nasally, if a 6.5 mm or larger diameter ablation zone is used, and if the flap is smaller than 8.5 mm. Therefore it is useful to displace the suction ring approximately 1 mm nasally so that the hinge is more likely to remain out of the ablation zone.

Position the globe properly in the ring before applying suction, because suction creates an indentation and groove in the bulbar conjunctiva to which the suction ring returns every time it is reapplied.

When the suction is turned on, the globe commonly shifts 0.5–1.0 mm, because the suction ring seats itself in a more 'comfortable' position on the conjunctival limbus. Therefore, the surgeon may apply a finger to the surface of the cornea and move the eye under the ring to position it into the desired location, holding it there while suction is applied. If the ring positions itself too eccentrically, release suction immediately, rub the conjunctiva with a microsponge to flatten the groove, wait a few minutes, and then reapply the suction ring in the desired position.

The suction ring may cause conjunctival hemorrhages, and the patient should be informed of these at the conclusion of the procedure.

DRY THE SURFACE OF THE CORNEA

If no moisture has been applied to the corneal surface from the time the alignment marks are made until now, the corneal surface will be dry and no wiping or manipulation is necessary. If the surface is moist, it must be dried, so that the Barraquer surgical applanation tonometer applied to the surface will read accurately, and the reading will not be confounded by a meniscus of fluid. The surgeon applies the tonometer to the cornea and ensures that the meniscus circle is well inside the circle etched on the tip of the tonometer, indicating a pressure greater than 65 mmHg (Fig. 18.2). The tonometer is suspended in a circular ring, which allows it to be balanced on the cornea, its weight providing the applanation pressure. This essential step cannot be omitted, because inadequate suction will give a lower pressure and an incorrectly sized flap, a partial flap, an eccentric flap, or no flap at all.

If the meniscus is outside the tonometer circle, the pressure in the globe is too low because of poor adhesion of the suction ring. In some cases, it is possible for the conjunctiva to be pulled up in the suction ring so that the ring is adherent to the surface of the globe, but the episcleral tissues are not pulled up, so the pressure in the globe is not elevated enough to allow an appropriate flap.

There are other clues to confirm appropriately high pressure in the globe: a change of the sound of the suction console when good adhesion is achieved, digital palpation of the cornea, a firm feel as the applanation tonometer is lowered onto the cornea and the patient's loss of vision. Some microkeratome systems supply an applanation lens to

verify the diameter of the flap, but this step is not essential for the LASIK procedure.

MOISTEN THE SURFACE

The surface of the suction ring and globe must be wet to ensure that the microkeratome will slide easily. Two or three drops of balanced salt solution are spread over the cornea with the surgeon's finger to lubricate the surface. Too much fluid creates spattering when the microkeratome passes.

INSERT THE MICROKERATOME INTO THE SUCTION RING GROOVES

This is harder than it looks. Each surgeon must develop a foolproof manual technique. The one the author prefers for the Chiron Automated Corneal Shaper is to grasp the handle of the microkeratome palm down, place the first finger on the top of the microkeratome head, and lift the elbow to align the forearm with the long axis of the microkeratome handle; this helps align the microkeratome base parallel to the surface of the suction ring. Insert one edge of the microkeratome into the long dovetail of the suction ring by tilting the microkeratome and sliding it sideways into position (Fig. 18.3). Lower the microkeratome on to the surface of the suction ring and engage the second edge against the other side of the groove. Advance the microkeratome forward manually, engaging both edges beneath the lips of the dovetails. Slide the microkeratome forward until the gear has firmly engaged the track. Tilt the microkeratome back and forth gently by rotating it between the fingers to ensure that both edges are secure within the dovetails. Release the microkeratome handle and support the distal end of the motor at the junction of the power cord gently with one finger; excessive lifting or depressing of the handle may cause the microkeratome to bind in the ring. In this position, the microkeratome and the blade have been advanced to the edge of the opening in the ring.

INSPECT THE SURGICAL FIELD

Ensure that nothing will impede the advance of the microkeratome, including the lid speculum, the drape, eyelashes, eyelid skin, the movable flange on the suction ring handle, and the like. Ensure that the microkeratome is fully advanced forward to engage the gears in the track.

ACTIVATE THE MICROKERATOME

The surgeon steps on the forward end of the foot pedal lever and gears propel the microkeratome forward across the cornea. If the microkeratome does not advance, explore the following problems:

- The gears are not properly meshed in the track: slide the microkeratome slightly backward and then advance it to engage the gears in the track.
- The surgeon is holding the microkeratome with too much upward or downward pressure and should simply relax the support for the microkeratome by gently placing one finger beneath the power cord.
- The microkeratome is jammed in the suction ring track, which is dirty or has particulate matter in it—a problem that should not occur because of testing the microkeratome advance in the suction ring immediately before the surgery.
- The microkeratome is improperly positioned in the dove tails, a circumstance that should not occur because of visual inspection and manual checking of the security of the microkeratome and the suction ring.

ADVANCE THE MICROKERATOME AND CREATE THE CORNEAL FLAP

Ordinarily the microkeratome advances smoothly until the stopper abuts on the suction ring and stops it, at which moment the surgeon quickly releases the foot pedal. On the Chiron Automated Corneal Shaper, the surgeon can verify the proper stopping position of the microkeratome, because the leading edge of the blade is aligned with the center of a second surface screw on the suction ring. At this time, the flap slides up onto the inner surface of the microkeratome and is somewhat wrinkled. This may contribute to some of the small wrinkles and folds that are seen postoperatively; ideally the flap should remain completely flat. There is no need to manipulate the flap within the microkeratome, since the microkeratome will be reversed and the flap will flatten out on the corneal surface.

PROBLEM SOLVING DURING THE ADVANCE OF THE MICROKERATOME

If the microkeratome jams part way across the advance, the surgeon should release the pedal immediately. If the advance was stopped by an external impediment, such as the lid speculum, the microkeratome can be freed gently, and the advance of the microkeratome continued to complete the flap. This may leave a small line where the microkeratome stopped, but generally this does not seriously affect the outcome. Alternatively, if the microkeratome is jammed or malfunctioning so that the advance cannot be continued, turn off the microkeratome switch and the suction and remove both the suction ring and the microkeratome together from the cornea, moving in a temporal direction to let the cut part of the flap slide out of the microkeratome and reposition itself on the surface of the cornea. The surgeon floats the partial flap up with balanced salt solution to ensure a proper position, and the procedure is terminated, to be repeated in approximately 3 months.

If the microkeratome completes its excursions, but the surgeon observes an irregular bed and the flap is cut irregularly, is button-holed, or is cut off completely as an irregular disc of any thickness or configuration, the disc or flap should be repositioned and left to heal for approximately 3 months. If a complete disc has been cut, the tissue can be identified between the cutting end of the blade and the plate, whence it can be teased gently onto the surface of the plate. Avoid pulling the tissue up from the inside of the microkeratome, because it is hard to visualize and the edge of the blade might cut the tissue further. Smooth the tissue on the plate, moisten it, slide it onto a wide spatula (such as a Paton corneal transplant spatula), place it on the bed, and orient it to align the epithelial marks. If it is a normal thickness complete disc with acceptably regular margins, the operation can proceed as planned. This method avoids confusing the stromal and epithelial surfaces because the disc is never picked up from the microkeratome. In any case, the surgeon can identify the epithelial side by the presence of the inked alignment marks and the shiny reflectivity that is not present on the stroma. If this manoeuver is done quickly, it is unnecessary to irrigate the bed and the tissue before reapplying the disc (as described below). If the tissue approximates the bed smoothly and uniformly, it can be left to dry in place for 5 minutes and no sutures are necessary. Edge-to-edge sutures should be avoided if possible because they further distort the tissue and create more astigmatism; however, if the tissue does not approximate well, or is highly irregular, it can be sutured in place with either an x-shaped overlay suture or interrupted 10-0 nylon sutures that are tied gently to avoid tissue compression and astigmatism. Generally, irregular flaps or discs will heal in place with minimal scarring and good surface contours, so that the LASIK procedure can be completed at a later time, usually after 3 months of healing.

If a complete disc with acceptable thickness, diameter and shape is cut, it can be left in the microkeratome or on the plate with one drop of balanced salt solution (BSS) to moisten it; it is unnecessary to manipulate it by putting it into a dish or chamber. The technician holds the microkeratome during the excimer laser ablation, which takes less than 1 minute; no significant damage occurs to the disc during that time. Avoiding manipulation of the disc will help to decrease the chance of epithelial implantation in the bed, of getting the two surfaces of the disc confused, and of attracting foreign bodies to the surface of the disc. The disc can be lifted off the microkeratome with a broad spatula or a pair of fine forceps or tying forceps and transferred back to the bed, where it is positioned and adheres without sutures after 5 minutes.

REVERSE THE MICROKERATOME

The surgeon steps on the reversing end of the foot switch and the microkeratome gears propel it back across the cornea, laying the flap down smoothly on the surface. Some microkeratomes reverse automatically. The microkeratome can be slid out of the track and then the suction ring released, or the suction can just be turned off and then the ring and microkeratome removed from the eye as one unit and handed to the technician.

If a mechanical stopper is used to halt the advance of the microkeratome, the microkeratome sometimes jams in the advanced position. A slight 'jiggle' of the microkeratome and a couple of taps on the reverse end of the foot pedal will usually loosen it to move in the reverse direction.

To stabilize the eye during the ablation, some surgeons leave the suction ring on the eye after the microkeratome is removed, without the suction being active. Others remove the ring and use patient fixation to center the eye (Fig. 18.4).

CENTER THE LASER

During the microkeratome cut, the eye loses its centration, so the surgeon must realign the chair, place the cornea in focus, and center the laser over the pupil (not over the light reflection off the surface of the cornea). This should be done before the flap is turned back, to decrease changes in hydration in the stromal bed and to decrease the time of exposure of the bed to foreign particles. With the Summit laser, the surgeon focuses the two helium neon beams that converge from the right and left on a single point on the surface of the cornea and aligns them at 3 and 9 o'clock at the edge of the pupil, which has been constricted with pilocarpine. The patient is then asked to look at the fixation light and to train his gaze there for the remainder of the procedure even though the light may become blurred.

TURN BACK THE FLAP

This is done easily with a pair of toothless forceps that grasp the flap at the temporal margin and fold it back to lie on the surface of the conjunctiva or the surface of the suction ring nasally. The surgeon takes care to avoid folding the edge of the flap onto its stromal surface. Alternatively, a blunt-angled spatula or sweep can be slipped beneath the flap (avoiding folding the edge under) and the flap swept nasally. A cyclodialysis spatula, which is slightly flat and has a somewhat more pointed flattened edge to it, is ideal for this manoeuver. The flap will adhere to the conjunctiva by surface tension. During this manoeuver, avoid scraping the spatula on the stromal bed, where it could create irregularities—a problem avoided by lifting the flap with forceps. If an edge of the flap is folded, it should be opened immediately with the forceps or sweep. If the flap springs back onto the cornea, one drop of BSS on the conjunctival or suction ring surface will increase the surface tension and allow the flap to remain folded back.

PERFORM THE REFRACTIVE ABLATION

During the ablation, it is often helpful to dim the room lights and the operating microscope lights, making alignment lights and fixation light easier to see and decreasing glare for the patient.

The surgeon confirms the focus and centration of the laser, gently holds the patient's head to steady and guide it during the procedure, and adds verbal reassurance to the patient that everything is fine and the surgeon is in complete control as long as the patient looks at the light. The surgeon steps on the foot pedal and fires the laser. During the entire ablation, the surgeon using a Summit laser looks directly at the helium neon beams on the surface of the iris, keeping them positioned at 3 and 9 o'clock by gentle slight movements of the patient's head or of the suction or fixation ring. If the beams leave their position, stop the ablation immediately, reassure the patient that 'everything is okay', reposition the eye by having the patient observe the fixation light and by moving the head so that the helium neon beams are back at 3 and 9 o'clock, and complete the ablation. Stopping the ablation requires a quick response from the surgeon, who should resist the desire to continue firing the laser with the false feeling that the procedure may almost be over. The surgeon should not watch the enlarging ablation on the stromal surface, the ejection plume, or the edge of the hinge—just watch the alignment beams on the iris. If the laser has no alignment beams, the surgeon should attempt to keep the ablation centered over the pupil. It is not helpful to ask the patient to 'find the fixation light' during the ablation because the patient may look around in an attempt to see it more clearly; therefore, once the ablation is commenced, it is best to tell the patient he is 'doing fine' and to move his head to maintain centration (see Chapter 13).

Some surgeons will observe the stromal bed, and if a central fluid pool forms, will stop the ablation and gently wipe the bed with a Merocel sponge to remove the fluid and to decrease the chance of creating a central steep island.

If the edge of the ablation extends slightly onto the hinge, it is probably best to allow the ablation to continue. This may create a small step nasally, but generally it is at the 5.5–6.0 mm zone and probably will not substantially affect the refractive or functional outcome (see Chapter 8).

REPOSITION THE FLAP

As soon as the last laser pulse is fired, the technician hands the surgeon an angled instrument or forceps, and the flap is replaced immediately on the dry bed. Some surgeons irrigate and wipe the flap and the stromal bed at this point, but that should be avoided, because copious irrigation and wiping often leave more particles and debris in the bed than a simple dry reapplication of the flap. If a fiber or foreign material is observed on the bed, this can be picked off before the flap is repositioned. The surgeon can slip an angled spatula or irrigating canula under the epithelial side of the flap at the base of the hinge and briskly sweep the flap back onto the surface of the bed. The flap usually does not position itself with good alignment of the radial lines at this point. Alternatively, the surgeon can nudge the stromal surface of the flap forward gradually, pulling the flap back into place without irrigation.

A 27-gauge, long, angled, blunt canula on a syringe or bottle of BSS is then inserted beneath the flap and the entire bed is irrigated, so the flap floats up on to a layer of fluid. When the last attachment of the flap to the dry bed is released, the flap automatically repositions itself with good alignment of the lines (Fig. 18.5). The irrigation is not designed to wash material out of the bed, but simply to lift the flap up so it will float into its most biomechanically neutral position. If the flap is not in the proper position, it should be floated up again on a layer of BSS and allowed to snap in place. If a complete disc has been removed, it can be lifted off the plate of the microkeratome with a spatula and repositioned onto the eye. It is then floated onto a layer of BSS and mechanically positioned so that the lines match between the disc and the peripheral cornea. Putting methylene blue ink on only three of the four lines of the RK marker makes it easier to line up a disc, avoiding the problem of possibly misaligning the four lines, which sometimes may be symmetrical, although they are usually asymmetrical enough that there is only one orientation of the disc that will align all four lines.

The lid speculum is left in place so the eye remains open for 2–5 minutes, allowing good adhesion of the flap (Fig. 18.6). The surgeon should avoid the following:

- Poking the edge of the flap with microsponges.
- Wiping the surface of the flap with a moist microsponge.
- Massaging the flap with an instrument.
- Mechanical repositioning of the edge of the flap (unless it remains out of alignment or is folded).
- Air drying the flap (although this will reduce the 5 minute waiting time to approximately 1 or 2 minutes, the air will cause the edge of the flap to retract slightly and create a wider area of epithelial stromal contact with a wider peripheral scar that remains more visible). Reducing mechanical manipulation of the flap will reduce the number of cracks in Bowman's layer, the severity of fine striae that can appear postoperatively, and the amount of irregular astigmatism.

ENSURE ADHESION OF THE FLAP

There are at least four factors that allow the flap or disc to adhere to the surface of the bed without sutures.

- Surface tension
- The stickiness of the molecules (e.g. the glycosaminoglycans) in the stroma
- The 'sucking' pressure created by the corneal endothelial pump
- The mechanical approximation of the tissues.

Verify the adhesion of the flap by indenting the peripheral cornea with a blunt instrument and demonstrating that the wrinkles are transmitted into the flap.

If the surgeon is concerned that the flap or disc is not adhering properly, an overlay X-shaped suture can be placed by using 10-0 nylon and taking a bite parallel to the tangent of the limbus at 12 o'clock and 6 o'clock (or at 3 o'clock and 9 o'clock) approximately 50% deep in the peripheral stroma, and then tying the suture gently over the surface of the cornea.

REMOVE THE SPECULUM

After removing the speculum and drapes, the surgeon manually moves the eyelid over the flap and has the patient blink to be sure the flap is adherent. It is better to detect dislocation of the flap at this point, where it can be replaced easily, rather than later at the slit-lamp microscope.

APPLY TOPICAL MEDICATION

Topical antibiotics, such as ciprofloxacin or tobramycin and topical non-steroidal anti-inflammatory drugs such as diclofenac or ketordac are applied immediately at the end of surgery. In general, topical corticosteroids are unnecessary, but can be used in the form of dexamethasone or prednisolone acetate at the surgeon's discretion. No patch is necessary. The patient is warned not to rub the eye.

INSPECT THE CORNEA

With a slit-lamp microscope, the surgeon inspects the cornea 5–15 minutes after surgery to be sure the flap has not come loose. If the flap is not properly aligned, if one edge of the wound is wider than another, or if large foreign bodies are in the bed (e.g. a fiber), the patient is returned to the operating microscope of the laser or is positioned securely at the slit-lamp microscope and the flap is floated up and adjusted perfectly. Reassurance and final instructions are given to the patient at this time.

CLEAN THE MICROKERATOME AND SUCTION RING

At the end of each procedure, the technical staff clean the microkeratome and suction ring meticulously, according to the manufacturer's instructions, to prevent the build up of debris and possible future malfunction.

REPEATED LASIK SURGICAL TECHNIQUE

IDENTIFY THE EDGE OF THE FLAP

If the scar at the edge of the previous flap or disc is faint, it is difficult to see under the operating microscope of the laser. Therefore, inspect the cornea with a slit-lamp microscope immediately before surgery and mark the location of the edge of the flap with a surgical marking pen. Alternatively, the edge of the flap may be gently dissected at the slit-lamp microscope and lifted with a bent 25-gauge hypodermic needle or a Sinskey-style IOL hook. Or the surgeon can scrape a Sinskey hook centrally from the limbus until it picks up the edge of the flap.

FOLLOW THE PRIMARY LASIK PROCEDURE

Follow the same procedures as for the primary LASIK procedure in terms of calibrating, programming and testing the laser, aligning the patient's eye, and centering around the pupil.

LIFT THE FLAP

Once a 1.0 mm long break in the edge of the flap is created and the flap is slightly undermined, it can be lifted with a pair of fine-tooth forceps, taking great care to avoid tearing the edge of the flap. It is probably safer, however, to insert a blunt spatula, such as an iris sweep or a cyclodialysis spatula into the lamellar bed and sweep it back and forth to loosen the flap. The epithelium around the edge of the flap is then broken from the inside out, to avoid wiping any epithelium into the bed. The flap is then either lifted and folded back with forceps or flipped back with the spatula, and held on the surface of the conjunctiva with surface tension.

CENTER THE LASER AND COMPLETE THE ABLATION

The procedure is now identical to the laser ablation in the primary LASIK procedure.

REPOSITION THE FLAP

Reposition the flap in the same manner used for the primary LASIK procedure, and instill postoperative topical medications.

RESULTS OF LASIK

At the time of writing, early results of LASIK are beginning to be published, but none with a follow-up of more than 1 year.

One of the earliest publications was that of Pallikaris and Siganos[11] in which they compared the results of PRK with those of LASIK in two groups of 10 eyes each. They used the Meditech laser in both groups and the Draeger Lamellar Rotor Keratome in the LASIK group. The mean attempted correction in the LASIK group was 11.40 D (8.00–16.00 D) and in the PRK group 11.72 D (–8.80 to –17.60 D), using a 9 mm diameter flap and 4.9 mm diameter ablation zone for the LASIK and a 6.0 mm ablation zone for PRK. The major difference in the outcome was a fairly stable refraction in the LASIK eyes, with a mean achieved correction of –10.32 D at 1 month and 10.96 D at 12 months. In contrast, the PRK eyes had a mean correction of –15.78 D at 1 month which underwent regression to –7.17 D at 12 months. At 12 months, the mean haze score in the cornea was 0.25 for LASIK and 1.20 for PRK. They concluded that LASIK was more predictable than PRK in this higher range of myopia.

Table 18.5

Postoperative refractive astigmatism in 87 myopic eyes at a mean of 5 months after LASIK. (Salah and colleagues)[17]

| | *Eyes* | |
Astigmatism* (D)	Number	(%)
0.00	25	28.4
0.25	6	6.8
0.50	17	19.3
0.75	12	13.6
1.00	10	11.4
1.25	5	5.7
1.50	5	5.7
1.75	3	3.4
2.00	2	2.3
2.25	1	1.1
2.50	0	0.0
2.75	0	0.0
3.00	1	1.1
4.00	1	1.1

*Mean ± S.D. 0.70 ± 0.72 diopter.

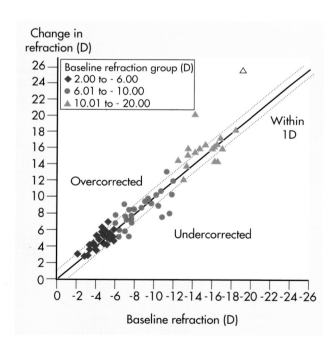

Figure 18.7 *Scattergram from Salah and colleagues[17] displays the spherical equivalent of the manifest refraction in three baseline refraction groups (D) at a mean of 5 months after LASIK in 88 eyes. Dotted lines indicate ± 1.00 D.*

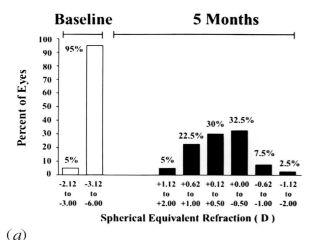

(a)

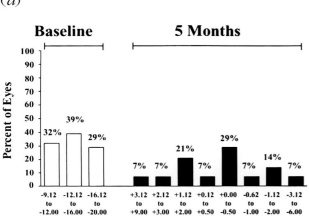

(c)

Figure 18.8 *Bar graphs from Salah and colleagues[17] display the spherical equivalent of the manifest refraction in 88 eyes at a mean of 5 months after LASIK in three baseline refractive groups: lower group of 40 eyes (top left), middle group of 29 eyes (top right) and higher group of 19 eyes (bottom left). The heights of the bars represent the percentage of eyes in each range of refraction.*

Salah and colleagues[17] studied retrospectively 88 eyes with spherical myopia between –2.00 and –20.00 D (mean, –8.24 D) treated with the Chiron Automated Corneal Shaper and the Summit Omnimed Laser using two algorithms, one with a 6.0 mm diameter ablation zone and the other with approximately a 4.5 mm diameter ablation zone. With a goal of emmetropia in all eyes, the mean spherical equivalent refraction after surgery was +0.22 ± 1.42 D (range +6.50 to –4.50 D). Of the 40 eyes with a baseline refraction from –2.00 to –6.00 D, 25 eyes (63%) had a refractive outcome within ±0.50 D of emmetropia and 37 eyes (93%) within ± 1.00 D. In 29 eyes with a baseline refraction of –6.12 to –12.00 D, postoperative refraction was within ± 1.00 D in 19 (65%) eyes. Of the 19 eyes with a baseline refraction of –12.10 to –20.00 D, postoper-

ative refraction was within ± 1 D in 8 (43%) of 19 eyes (Table 18.5; Figs 18.7 and 18.8). There was minimal induced refractive astigmatism, only two eyes showing an increase of more than 1.00 D, although 20 eyes (22%) showed a surgically induced refractive astigmatism by vector analysis of more than 1.00 D. In this study, both eyes were operated at the same time in 32 patients, with good symmetry of outcome; refractive asymmetry between the two eyes of the same patient of 2.01–5.87 D was present in 51 patients (15.6%) at baseline but in only three patients (9.4%) after LASIK. The authors emphasized the advantage of treating a wide range of myopia with essentially the same refractive surgical procedure, and also emphasized the need for modification and improvement of surgical algorithms.

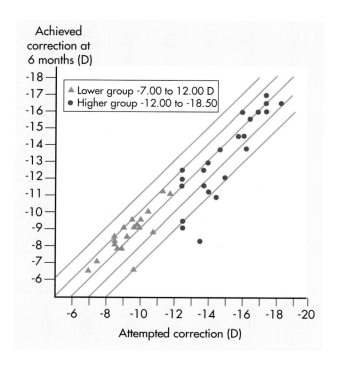

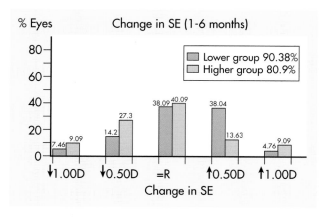

Figure 18.10 *Change in spherical equivalent (SE) between the first and the sixth month after surgery.*[18]

Figure 18.9 *Attempted correction (D) versus achieved correction (D) at 6 months after LASIK in 43 eyes. There were no overcorrections.*[18]

Guell and Muller[18] reported 43 consecutive eyes that received LASIK using the Chiron Automated Corneal Shaper and the Chiron Keracor 116 Excimer Laser, using a multizone modified algorithm and an ablation zone of 6.8 mm. They reported 6 month results (Figs 18.9 and 18.10) of 21 eyes with a preoperative refraction of −7.00 to −12.00 D, 11 eyes (52.3%) had a refraction of plano to −0.50 D and 18 eyes (85.7%) had a refraction of plano to −1.00 D. Of 22 eyes with a baseline refraction of −12.25 to −18.00 D, three eyes (13.6%) had a refraction of plano to −0.50 D, nine eyes (40.9%) a refraction of plano to −1.00 D, and 14 eyes (63.6%) a refraction of plano to −2.00 D. There were no overcorrections. They demonstrated good stability, 80 to 90% of the eyes changing by less than 0.50 D from the first to the sixth month. The endothelial cell count was stable between preoperative and 6 months postoperative measurements (see Chapter 13).

LASIK VS PRK IN THE SAME INDIVIDUAL

El Maghraby[20] conducted a prospective bilateral randomized comparison of LASIK and PRK in 33 patients, one eye being treated with LASIK and the other with PRK, both eyes being treated in the same surgical session by the same surgeon using the Summit Omnimed Laser with a 6.0 mm diameter ablation and the Chiron Automated Corneal Shaper. He randomized eyes to receive each type of surgery and the sequence of the procedures. Preoperative myopia ranged from −2.50 to −8.00 D. Results were reported at 1 year with 92% follow-up. There was a marked difference between the two procedures in the early postoperative period, 81% of patients reporting no pain in the LASIK eye and all patients reporting pain in the PRK eye. Baseline spectacle corrected visual acuity recovered in 1 week in eyes that received LASIK and in 1 month in eyes with PRK.

Overall, there was no statistically significant or clinical difference in the refractive outcomes, with 22 (73%) of the LASIK eyes and 20 (67%) of the PRK eyes achieving a refraction within ± 0.50 D of the intended outcome. Visual acuity outcome was also similar, at 1 year, with 20 (67%) eyes after LASIK and 16 (53%) eyes after PRK seeing 20/20 or better and 29 (97%) eyes in each group seeing 20/40 or better uncorrected. However, patients reported a higher

Table 18.6
Comparison of refractive outcome of corneal surgical procedures for myopia of approximately −2.00 to −20.00 D.

Surgical technique	First author	Range (mean) of preoperative refraction (D)*	Follow-up time (yr)	Number of eyes	Number of eyes (%) within ±1.00
Barraquer cryolathe keratomileusis	Nordan[21]	−4.25 to −14.00 (−8.51)	1.0	74	38 (51)
BKS 1000 non-freeze keratomileusis	Laroche[22]	−6.25 to −28.00 (−14.24)	1.0	82	21 (26)
Corneal shaper automated in situ keratomileusis (ALK)	Ibrahim[13]	−3.75 to −28.00 (−11.97)	1.0	63	22 (35)
Refractive keratotomy (deepening incisions) (RK)	Bauerberg[23]	−6.00 to −12.00 (−7.83)	1.0	167	97 (58)
Visx 20/15 excimer laser photorefractive keratectomy (PRK)	Sher[24]	−8.00 to 15.00 (−11.18)	0.5	48	20 (40)
Summit excimer laser keratomileusis on the disc	Buratto[25]	−11.20 to −24.50 (−17.90)	1.0	30	13 (33)
Aesculap-Meditec excimer laser in situ keratomileusis (LASIK)	Pallikaris[11]	−10.62 to 25.87 (−16.61)	1.0	10	6 (67)
Summit excimer laser in-situ keratomileusis (LASIK)	Salah[17]	−2.00 to −20.00 (−8.24)	0.5	88	64 (73)

*Spherical equivalent refraction

subjective satisfaction with the LASIK treated eyes than with the PRK treated eyes at 1 year. In addition, glare, halos or flare were reported in only six (19%) of the LASIK-treated eyes as compared to 11 (33%) of the PRK-treated eyes at 1 year. In addition, there was a statistically significant difference in the corneal topography, which was studied in 13 of the patients, central corneal distortion being present more commonly after PRK than after LASIK. The author found that early recovery of vision is faster after LASIK and that the long-term quality of vision may be better after LASIK, possibly because of the preservation of Bowman's layer. Both procedures gave similar refractive outcomes. Other authors (Table 18.6) have also reported results with LASIK.[26–29]

COMPLICATIONS OF LASIK RELATED TO THE FLAP

Most authors' reported complications of LASIK are usually from the microkeratome while making the corneal flap. For example, Guell and Muller[18] reported one complete severing of a disc, which was repositioned without complications, one epithelial ingrowth that required removal, and a few eyes with epithelial ingrowth at the edge of the flap that did not require removal. Salah and colleagues[17] reported three eyes with complete severing of the flap into a disc; two were sutured in place and one was repositioned without sutures; none had an abnormal postoperative course. In three eyes the microkeratome stopper jammed after the flap was fully created, requiring that the suction ring and the microkeratome be removed together. One eye lost two lines of spectacle corrected visual acuity from 20/20 to 20/30 because of irregular compound hyperopic astigmatism. Two eyes of the same patient had preoperative myopic macular degeneration (Fuchs' spot) that progressed during the 5 months postoperatively, so that the visual acuity fell from 20/40 preoperatively to 20/200 postoperatively. The cause of the progression was unknown. El Maghraby[20] reported no serious complications in the eyes treated with PRK, but one eye treated with LASIK had a dislocated corneal flap immediately after surgery, with epithelial implantation in the bed that required removal and resulted in symptomatic permanent irregular astigmatism. Three other eyes lost two or three lines of spectacle corrected visual acuity, to levels of 20/25, 20/30 and 20/50.

Other complications using the microkeratome can include excision of an irregular thin disc because of poor suction or the wrong plate, excision of a disc or flap with a buttonhole in the center because of a damaged blade or a cornea with markedly abnormal curvature (for example, after a penetrating keratoplasty for keratoconus), incision into the anterior chamber because of the absence of a thickness plate, partial excision of a flap because the microkeratome jams during its excursion across the cornea, and extreme damage to or loss of a corneal disc, requiring either a 'capless' procedure or the use of a disc from a donor cornea.

Clearly, surgeons who perform LASIK must be proficient in the use of the microkeratome, and this proficiency requires the usual steps in training: reading about the procedure, understanding the principles of operation of the microkeratome, taking a lecture and laboratory course with hands on practice, observing videotapes and live surgery of cases, and having an expert surgeon assist in early cases.

OTHER COMPLICATIONS OF LASIK

Complications may also occur from the excimer laser, but they are not as serious as those with the microkeratome. Decentration of the ablation in the bed can produce multifocal optics over the pupil. If the hinge of the flap is not displaced nasally somewhat, and if the pupil is displaced nasally somewhat, the laser ablation may overlap the hinge, creating a step. Among the most serious complications from the excimer laser is an asymmetrical ablation because of an inhomogeneous or unstable beam. Manufacturers should provide a mechanism by which beam calibration—including homogeneity of the beam used in large area ablations—can be tested prior to each case in a practical and efficient manner. Of course, if abnormalities are found, the remainder of cases that day must be cancelled, unless a laser engineer or repair technician is on site.

One of the most disturbing complications to patients is simply a broken laser—one that will not calibrate properly, will not come out of the testing procedure properly, or becomes unusable during a series of cases. This requires cancellation and rescheduling of patients, which is seen as a complication by the patient, although it is not a complication for the eye.

LASIK AND PRK

It is not my intention in this chapter to analyse both LASIK and PRK, but a few comparative remarks are appropriate. An analogy can be drawn: LASIK is to PRK for the correction of myopia as phaecomulsification with an internal corneal valve incision and topical anesthesia is to extracapsular cataract extraction with a sutured incision and intraorbital anesthesia for cataract extraction. PRK and extracapsular cataract extraction are the simpler, more time proven, safer techniques in the hands of the average surgeon. LASIK and phaecomulsification are the more expensive, more technically demanding, and riskier techniques; but these offer the advantages of more rapid visual rehabilitation, improved quality of vision, and greater patient acceptance. It is likely that all four techniques will remain as part of the surgical resources of the well-trained anterior segment surgeon for the foreseeable future.

UNFINISHED BUSINESS

LASIK has considerable potential for the treatment of ametropia, and numerous improvements are being introduced. Improved designs of microkeratomes to make them safer and easier to use are appearing gradually. Modifications of the ablation algorithms specifically for the LASIK procedure are being tested, utilizing the improvements of larger diameter ablation zones and more gradual blending of the surface to create more physiologically acceptable corneal contours as designed for PRK, and introducing LASIK-specific algorithms that adjust the ablation for its location in the stromal bed rather than on the surface of Bowman's layer and the anterior stroma. Early trials of the correction of compound myopic astigmatism and hyperopia are also being carried out.

Where LASIK will end up among refractive surgical procedures remains to be seen. In the future, there will certainly be many different surgical techniques to manage ametropia—including LASIK.

REFERENCES

1. Pallikaris J, Papatsanaki M, Stathi E, Frenschock O, Georgiadis A, Laser in situ keratomileusis, *Lasers Surg Med* (1990) **10**:463–8.
2. Barraquer, J, Queratomileusis para la correccion de la miopia, *Arch Soc Am Oftalmol Optom* (1964) **5**:27–48.
3. Krumeich J, Swinger C, Non-freeze epikeratophakia for the correction of myopia, *Am J Ophthalmol* (1987) **103**:397–403.
4. Ruiz L, Rowsey J, In situ keratomileusis, *Invest Ophthalmol Vis Sci* (1988) **29(suppl)**:592.
5. Barraquer J, *Queratomileusis y Queratofaquia* (Instituto Barraquer de America: Bogota, 1980) 79.
6. Buratto L, Ferrari M, Rama P, Excimer laser intrastromal keratomileusis, *Am J Ophthalmol* (1992) **113**:291–5.
7. Salah T, Waring GO, El-Maghraby A, Excimer laser keratomileusis, Pt I. In: Salz JJ, McDonnell PJ, McDonald MB, eds, *Corneal Laser Surgery* (Mosby: St. Louis, 1995) 187–95.
8. Pureskin N, Weakening ocular refraction by means of partial stromectomy of cornea under experimental conditions, *Vestnik Oftalmologii* (1967) **80**:1–7.
9. Arenas-Archila E, Sanchez-Thorin JC, Naranjo-Uribe JP, Hernandez-Lorano, Myopic keratomileusis in situ: a preliminary report, *J Cataract Refract Surg* (1987) **17**:424–35.
10. Rozakis GW, *Refractive Lamellar Keratoplasty*. (Slack Inc: Thorofare, 1994) 70–74.
11. Pallikaris IG, Siganos DS, Excimer laser in situ keratomileusis and photorefractive keratectomy for correction of high myopia, *J Refract Corneal Surg* (1994) **10**:498–510.
12. Ruiz L, Slade S, Updegraff S, Excimer laser keratomileusis: Bogota experience, Pt II. In: Salz JJ, McDonnell PJ, McDonald MB, eds, *Corneal Laser Surgery*. (Mosby: St Louis, 1995) 195.
13. Ibrahim O, Waring GO, Salah T, El Maghraby A, Automated in situ keratomileusis for myopia, *J Refract Surg* (1995) **11**:431–41.
14. Barraquer JI, *Chirugia Refractiva de la Cornea, Vol 1* (Instituto Barraquer de America: Bogota, 1989) 40–41.
15. Peyman GA, Corneal ablation in rabbits using an infrared (2.9 µm) erbium:YAG laser, *Ophthalmology* (1989) **96**:1160–70.
16. Pallikaris IG, Papatzanaki ME, Siganos DS, Tsilimbaris MK, A corneal flap technique for laser in situ keratomileusis, *Arch Ophthalmol* (1991) **145**:1699–1702.
17. Salah T, Waring GO, El Maghraby A, Moadel K, Grimm S, Excimer laser in situ keratomileusis under a corneal flap for myopia of 2 to 20 diopters, *Am J Ophthalmol* (1996) 121:143–55.
18. Guell J, Muller A, Laser in situ keratomileusis (LASIK) for myopia from −7 to −18 diopters, *J Refract Surg* (1996) **12**:222–28.
19. Barraquer JI. Long-term results of myopic keratomileusis— 1982. *Arch Soc Am Oftal Optom* (1983) **17**:137–42.
20. El Maghraby A, Prospective randomized bilateral comparison of laser-assisted in-situ keratomileusis and photorefractive keratectomy for myopia, *Ophthalmology* (1995) **102(suppl)**:99.
21. Nordan LT, Fallor MK, Myopic keratomileusis: 74 consecutive non-amblyopic cases with one year of follow-up. *J Refract Corneal Surg* (1986) **2**:124–8.
22. Laroche L, Gauthier L, Thenot JC, Lagoutte F, Nordmann JP, Denis P et al, Nonfreeze myopic keratomileusis for myopia in 158 eyes. *J Refract Corneal Surg* (1994) **10**:400–12.
23. Bauerberg J, Stvzovsky M, Brodsky M, Radial keratotomy in myopia of 6 to 12 diopters using full-length deepening incisions, *J Refract Corneal Surg* (1989) **5**:150–4.
24. Sher NA, Hardten DR, Fundingsland B, DeMarchi J, Carpel E, Doughman DJ, 193-nm excimer photorefractive keratectomy in high myopia. *Ophthalmology* (1994) **101**:1575–82.
25. Buratto L, Ferrari M, Genesi C, Myopic keratomileusis with the excimer laser: one-year follow up. *J Refract Corneal Surg* (1993) **9**:12–9.
26. Bas A, Onnis R, Excimer laser in situ keratomileusis for myopia, *J Refract Surg* (1995) **11(suppl)**:S229–S233.
27. Fiander DC, Tayfour F, Excimer laser in situ keratomileusis in 124 myopic eyes, *J Refract Surg* (1995) **11(suppl)**:S234–S238.
28. Gomes M, Laser in situ keratomileusis for myopia using manual dissection, *J Refract Surg* (1995) **11(suppl)**S239–S243.
29. Kremer F, Dufek M, Excimer laser in situ keratomileusis, *J Refract Surg* (1995) **11(suppl)**:S244–S247.

Chapter 19 · Radial keratotomy and transverse astigmatic keratotomy

Geoffrey J Crawford

INTRODUCTION

Procedures that have been designed to correct myopia in patients without lenticular or corneal pathology by means other than the use of the excimer laser, have taken many different approaches and methods to achieve the same endpoint — flattening of the anterior corneal curvature. These different surgical procedures can be categorized into five major groups:

- Incisional   radial keratotomy, astigmatic keratotomy
- Lamellar   keratomileusis, automated lamellar keratectomy (ALK)
- Inlays   intracorneal ring, intracorneal lens
- Onlays   epikeratoplasty
- IOLs   phakic intraocular lens

Descriptions of techniques relating to shortening of the eye have not been included in this chapter as they are regarded as extremely experimental and potentially very dangerous.

Despite the increasingly widespread availability of excimer laser facilities, many of these procedures still have their place in refractive surgery, and ophthalmologists advising patients and practising refractive surgery should have a sound knowledge and understanding of available alternative techniques besides excimer laser. Despite our aspirations and hopes for excimer laser, no single procedure is, or will be, the panacea for all refractive problems.

RADIAL KERATOTOMY

The aim in surgery for the correction of myopia is to achieve flattening of the central corneal curvature, which radial keratotomy achieves by the placement of deep peripheral radial incisions. These radial

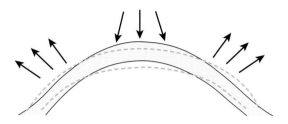

Figure 19.1 *Following radial incisions, there is 'bulging' of the peripheral cornea resulting in flattening of the central cornea.*

incisions weaken the paracentral and peripheral cornea, allowing the normal intraocular pressure to 'bulge' the peripheral cornea outward (Fig. 19.1). Since the cornea remains relatively fixed at the limbus, this peripheral bulge results in central corneal flattening. The amount of central flattening depends on the interaction between the surgery performed and the response of the individual eye to these incisions (Fig. 19.2).

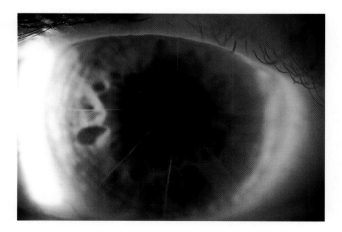

Figure 19.2 *Eight-incision radial keratotomy.*

It is now a matter of history that Lans in the late 1800s performed experiments in rabbits which formed the basis for modern radial keratotomy.[1] He elucidated the following principles:

- radial incisions in the anterior surface of the cornea flatten the cornea in the meridian in which they are made
- deeper incisions produce a greater flattening of the cornea
- the cornea steepens during healing, reversing some of the effect of the incisions.

It was largely the work of the Russians, Yenaliev[2] in the late 1960s and Fyodorov[3] in the 1970s that improved the predictability of the procedure; while various American workers in the late 1970s and 80s have brought greater safety to the techniques, as well as improved predictability.[4,5]

The surgical variables that influence the outcome of radial keratotomy are well recognized, although the outcome is still not completely controllable, largely related to factors involved in corneal wound healing. These surgical variables are:

- Incision number — four, six or eight incisions are suggested.
- Incision depth — deep incisions appear to be a major contributor to outcome.
- Shallow incisions give little effect.
- Diameter of Central Clear (Uncut) Zone — this is the means of adjusting the effect of radial keratotomy.

Besides the variables in surgical technique, variations posed by individual patient characteristics must also be considered in the outcome of the procedure. The factors that most seem to have an influence on outcome are age, sex, baseline refraction, and intraocular pressure.

PROSPECTIVE EVALUATION OF RADIAL KERATOTOMY

Radial keratotomy has been very closely scrutinized as a surgical procedure with evaluation in many well-organized series. In 1980, the National Eye Institute funded the Prospective Evaluation of Radial Keratotomy (PERK) study group in the United States.[6] The objective of the PERK study was to evaluate the safety and efficacy of the surgical procedure including outcome predictability and long-term stability.

The technique used was rigidly standardized using radial incisions directed centrifugally, from the optical zone to the limbus, known as the American method of incision. The protocol did not allow corrections for astigmatism nor take into account the patient's age, and postoperative enhancements generally were not carried out. Nevertheless this study has provided a large amount of well-organized scientific data especially with regard to safety and long-term stability.

In October 1994, the 10-year results of the PERK study were released.[7] Of the 427 patients (793 eyes that underwent RK) originally enrolled into the study, 374 patients (693 eyes), or 88%, returned for the 10 year examination. Thirty-eight per cent of eyes had a final refractive error within ±0.50 D and 60% within ±1.00 D. Uncorrected visual acuity was 6/6 or better in 53% of eyes and 6/12 or better in 85% of eyes. Among 310 patients with bilateral RK, 70% reported not wearing spectacles or contact lenses for distance vision at 10 years. Loss of best-corrected visual acuity of two lines or more on a Snellen chart occurred in 3% of all eyes that underwent surgery. Eighteen per cent lost one or more Snellen chart lines. Between 6 months and 10 years, the refractive error of 43% of eyes changed in the hyperopic direction by 1.00 D or more. The average rate of change was +0.21 D per year between 6 months and 2 years and +0.06 D per year between 2 and 10 years.

The major concern with radial keratotomy has become the long-term stability, and in particular the continued refractive effect in the direction of hypermetropia with time. The above results confirm this concern, but it is important to remember that these are all eight-incision RKs and not the four-incision technique used more frequently at the present time. In addition there is no breakdown of the amount of hyperopic shift experienced in each of the different preoperative refractive subgroups, whereas in all series the degree of hyperopic shift is much less or absent in the lower levels of myopia.

RECENT EVOLUTION OF RADIAL KERATOTOMY

Over the past two decades, and especially since the time of adoption of the standard technique by the PERK study, there has been continued evolution of the procedure of radial keratotomy. This has included improvement in instrumentation, surgical technique, predictive factors and nomograms, as well as our understanding of corneal wound healing.

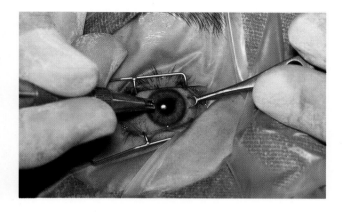

Figure 19.3 *The radial incisions may be directed away from the optical zone (American method) or toward it (Russian method).*

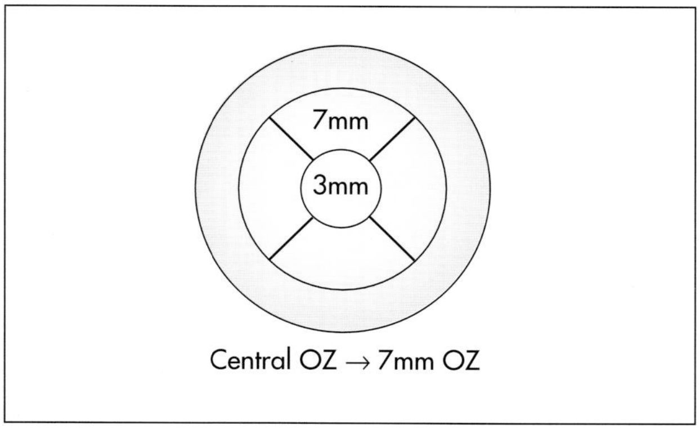

Figure 19.4 *In mini-RK, the incisions extend from the selected optical zone to the 7.0 or 8.0 mm optical zone.*

Incision direction

It is now recognized that centripetally directed (uphill or Russian method) incisions provide greater effect with consistently deeper incisions than the American method (Fig. 19.3).[8] However, the reduced safety of the Russian method still exists, especially for novice refractive surgeons. The incisional method, known as the *combined technique* (Genesis method), is now preferred by many RK surgeons.[9] The technique combines the safety of the centrifugal method with the efficacy of the centripetal method of making radial keratotomy incisions. The knife initially enters the cornea at the central clear optical zone margin and then the usual centrifugal or limbal directed incision is made to within 1 mm of the limbus. Then, without removing the diamond knife from the incision groove, the surgeon reverses direction, returning back 'uphill' or centripetally to the central clear zone, obtaining a good depth effect at the edge of the optical zone before removing the blade.

Number of incisions

There is a trend to the lowest number of incisions that can be used and also to a concept of 'staged' procedures. Having started with the 32 incisions made by Yenaliev, the number has decreased to 16, to eight (as used in PERK study), to the four incisions now used. The smaller number of incisions reflects the observation that most of the corneal flattening occurs with the first four incisions and that the

proportional contribution of further incisions declines as their numbers increase. On the basis of these findings, most surgeons advocate performing radial keratotomy initially with only four incisions for patients with less than 4 D of myopia.[10] If an undercorrection should occur then a secondary procedure can be performed. This induces less trauma to the cornea and reduces the incidence and amount of overcorrection. New nomograms have been developed to take into account the reduced number of incisions and the 'staging' concept.

Mini-RK

Another variation on incision size is the so called mini-RK or minimally invasive radial keratotomy technique introduced by Lindstrom.[11] This technique essentially uses four or eight incisions from the preferred central optical zone to the 7.0–8.0 mm optical zone, rather than fully extending the radial incisions to the standard RK length (Fig. 19.4). This is used for low to moderate myopia and is based on the observation that incisions made with an optical zone of 6.00–7.00 mm or larger do not correct any myopia. This technique is said to reduce the invasiveness of radial keratotomy and hopefully reduce the long-term instability resulting in diurnal fluctuation and progression of hypermetropia. In 1995 Lindstrom published results on 100 patients with myopia of −1.00 to −6.00 D. Ninety-two per cent of eyes were within ±1.00 D of emmetropia and 94% had 6/12 or better uncorrected visual acuity. None was overcorrected more than 1.00 D. Long-term results to confirm the claim of improved stability were not available. Again new nomograms were presented. Chen and Lindstrom also suggest that the four incisions be placed obliquely to reduce glare post-operatively and allow equivalent length incisions.[12]

RK knife design

Several variations of diamond knife are available — but the overall tendency is for a thinner width diamond blade of less than 150 microns and a broader footplate. Both front and back blades are sharp. Dedicated calibration microscopes are available but have not been shown to improve on surgical outcome. Many of the newer aspects of instrument design, technique and nomograms have been incorporated and marketed as total incisional surgery packages such as the Casebeer System.[13]

STABILITY OF POSTOPERATIVE REFRACTION

The problem of long-term stability following radial keratotomy has perhaps represented the greatest concern to RK surgeons. An early observation after radial keratotomy was the partial decrease or loss of corrective effect as the surgical wounds healed — a phenomenon referred to as regression. The amount of this regression is greater for the higher levels of myopia. Although early observations suggested that refraction stabilized by 3 months after surgery, further experience has documented continued changes in refraction for up to 10 years after surgery.[7]

In the PERK study, between 6 months and 1 year after surgery,[14] approximately 75% of the eyes remained stable within ±0.50 D. The other 25% continued to change, most showing a continued decrease in the amount of myopia; that is, a progressive effect of the operation. Dietz and Sanders[15,16] first described this phenomenon in 1985 and called it 'progressive hyperopia' or more accurately 'a change in the hyperopic direction'. They reported that 31% of 225 eyes operated with a metal blade showed a decrease in minus power (a continued surgical effect) of 1.00 D or more between 1 and 4 years after surgery. All subsequent studies of stability have confirmed this finding, with various studies of the same time frame showing a rate of 'hyperopic shift' of between 17 and 31% for all levels of myopia treated.

In the PERK study, between 6 months and 4 years,

23% of the eyes showed 1.00 D or more decrease in minus power, whereas 74% changed less than 1.00 D.[17] Between 6 months and 10 years, 43% of eyes changed refractive power in the hyperopic direction by 1.00 D or more.[7] The mean change was approximately 1.00 D of hyperopic shift. The mean rate of change was approximately 0.10 D per year (0.21 D per year during the first 2 years; and 0.06 D per year between 2 and 10 years). The higher levels of attempted myopic correction display a higher level of hyperopic shift. At this stage there is no published evidence that the hyperopic shift will stop at an identifiable time after surgery.

Most refractive keratotomy surgeons now aim for a final refractive error of −0.50 D rather than emmetropia. This low residual myopia allows patients to retain good uncorrected visual acuity, delays the onset of symptomatic presbyopia, and hedges against a continued increase in the effect of the surgery, although it may reduce night vision in some patients.

PERSISTENT DIURNAL VARIATION

Another effect of corneal instability, although not as commonly observed, is fluctuation in refraction from morning to evening within a 24-hour period. There are no studies that attempt to evaluate the incidence of diurnal fluctuation in a total study population; however, within the PERK study, 52 eyes were examined both morning and evening 3.5 years after surgery.[18,19] These were all patients who were selected because of their specific complaints of diurnal fluctuations. Thirty-one per cent had an increase in the minus power of the manifest refraction of 0.50 to 1.50 D, 19% had a decrease in uncorrected visual acuity by two to five Snellen lines, and 29% showed central corneal steepening with a keratometry reading of 0.50 D to 1.00 D. This level of fluctuation was, however, less at 3.5 years compared to 1 year in the same group.

MacRae and colleagues[20] showed in their small study group of eight patients with diurnal fluctuation that the major correlation was with corneal thickness, as measured by central ultrasonic pachometry. Operated corneas were significantly thicker (5.7%) in the morning than in the afternoon, when compared with controls (1.7% thicker). There was no correlation with change in intraocular pressure. Again the patients suffering from this problem came from the higher levels of attempted myopic correction.

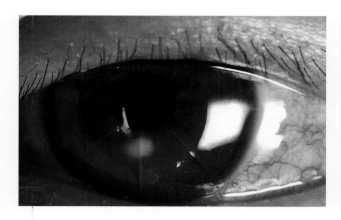

Figure 19.5 *Bacterial keratitis in a corneal wound 5 days following radial keratotomy.*

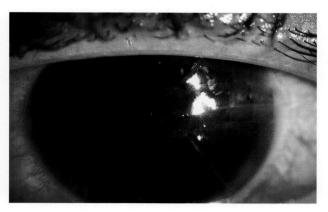

Figure 19.6 *Right cornea repaired following traumatic wound rupture 4 weeks after radial keratotomy.*

VISION-THREATENING COMPLICATIONS

A number of complications have occurred following radial keratotomy that have caused, or have the potential to cause, a reduction in vision permanently. The incidence of severe complications is not accurately known because complications occur sporadically and are not usually reported in the literature. In the author's own experience the incidence is less than 0.5%. The complications capable of causing permanent visual loss that have been reported are cataract formation, endophthalmitis, bacterial keratitis (early and delayed), irregular astigmatism, disabling glare and traumatic rupture of the globe (Figs 19.5 and 19.6).

PERTH RADIAL KERATOTOMY SERIES

In 1985, the author commenced a controlled prospective series of radial keratotomy which now numbers 3265 procedures with follow-up of up to 10 years, with all procedures being performed by a single surgeon. All post-operative visual acuities and refractions were done by an independent observer and not by the surgeon. The surgical technique has remained fairly consistent throughout this period although there have been some variations which were seen as improvements, such as the use of the 'combined incision technique' (described previously) and the shift to four-incision procedures. Except for 14 cases of 16 incisions, all other cases have been either four or eight incisions, using a micrometered KOI or Meyco

diamond knife and a self-formulated nomogram based initially on a hybrid of early formulas.

There are 1930 eyes with 5 years or more follow-up. Ninety-two per cent, or 1776 eyes, were reviewed at 5 years and all these cases are included. The population in Western Australia is a fairly stable one and so follow-up is fairly good. The male-to-female ratio was approximately equal, 52% were male and 48% were female, with an average age of 38.1 years at the 5-year examination.

Using the PERK preoperative baseline refractive groupings, the Perth Series results were as follows (Figs 19.7 and 19.8):

Refraction (± 1.00 D of emmetropia)	
−1.00 to −3.12D	93%
−3.25 to −4.37D	74%
−4.50 to −8.00D	68%
Overall	75%
Uncorrected visual acuity (6/12 or better)	
−1.00 to −3.12D	100%
−3.25 to −4.37D	93%
−4.50 to −8.00D	80%
Overall	88%

In this series of 1776 cases, the following vision-threatening complications occurred:

- three cases of bacterial keratitis (all early)
- one case of traumatically induced wound rupture (4 weeks post-RK)

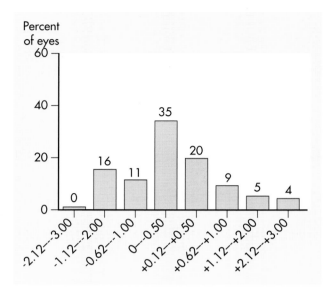

Figure 19.7 *The Perth Radial Keratotomy Series — refraction (D) at 5 years.*

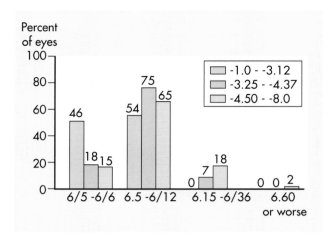

Figure 19.8 *The Perth Radial Keratotomy Series — unaided visual acuity at 5 years.*

- one case of disabling glare reducing vision
- two cases of retinal detachment (unrelated to RK surgery).

Since this 5-year review, there has been a further case of bacterial keratitis (delayed) and a further case of wound rupture following trauma 6 years after RK.

Reviewing the refractive stability of the group, the following progressive hyperopia was noted:

Decrease in minus power of >1.00 D

−1.00 to −3.12D	0%
−3.25 to −4.37D	5%
−4.50 to −8.00D	22%

From these results, there is definite hyperopic shift but this is more common in the higher levels of myopia corrected and is not present in the mild degrees of myopia. (Crawford GJ, unpublished work.)

The author has found from experience that the patients who are most unhappy following radial keratotomy are those who obtain an overcorrection of greater than +2.00 D postoperatively. While this is fortunately uncommon, especially with present techniques, these patients dislike their hypermetropia more than they disliked their previous myopia,

especially if they are in the presbyopic range. If overcorrection occurs in their first eye, they are often disillusioned and therefore do not correct their second eye, with resultant problems of anisometropia. There are a number of procedures to correct their overcorrection, including suturing of the central end of the incisions or a double purse-string intrastromal nylon suture, but none of these are highly predictable. Excimer laser hyperopic correction may eventually play a role in these cases.

THE ROLE OF RADIAL KERATOTOMY AT PRESENT

In those countries where excimer laser photorefractive keratectomy is freely available, the number of radial keratotomy procedures performed is declining, as excimer laser surgery increases, but is there any role for incisional surgery in the correction of myopia? This is a difficult and rather controversial question to answer. Eventually many would expect that excimer laser photorefractive keratectomy will take over, but there is still a cogent argument for the use of RK in the treatment of myopia below −3.00 D.

First, the predictability of radial keratotomy is excellent in this low level — 100% 6/12 or better in the author's personal series. Secondly there is no hyperopic shift or persistent diurnal fluctuation in this range, with a low risk of other vision-threatening complications. Then there are some other factors which can have an influence on the patient's choice. The recovery time, or time to visual rehabilitation, can be as rapid as 24–48 hours and certainly within 1 week. This becomes important with busy patients with limited time for recovery and reduced vision. Higher levels of astigmatism can be corrected better in this lower level of myopia with RK than PRK. The time between procedures is usually less with RK, the length of follow-up is usually less with RK, and the amount of postoperative pain is certainly less with RK. The use of topical steroids is not required for as long post-RK compared to many PRK protocols.

The possibility of combining the use of both radial keratotomy and excimer laser PRK has been suggested by several authors to correct larger amounts of myopia. This would theoretically increase the level of myopia that could be corrected but reduce the complications of each individual procedure modality. This, however, may be the domain of LASIK in the future. So far, there are only a small number of papers on a combined approach, and these all relate to using the excimer laser to correct residual myopia after previous radial keratotomy.[21] The author's experience of utilizing PRK to treat residual myopia after RK has also been encouraging.

Conversely, the author has also performed three cases of radial keratotomy after inadequately corrected myopia following PRK. In all three cases, the PRK was slow to settle and so the patient requested subsequent RK to correct the residual myopia rather than having to wait for a further PRK to settle. All three RKs successfully corrected the residual myopia effectively.

Radial keratotomy will have a reduced role in the world of excimer laser, but the author believes it will still maintain a place in refractive surgery.

ASTIGMATIC KERATOTOMY

Even though the surgical correction of astigmatism motivated the development of refractive keratotomy in the 19th century, the development of incisional surgery for astigmatism is still behind that for the correction of spherical myopia. In addition, there is still considerable difference in opinion about surgical techniques and patterns of astigmatic keratotomy.

Astigmatic keratotomy can be used for:

- Primary astigmatism
- Astigmatism post cataract surgery
- Astigmatism post keratoplasty.

PRINCIPLES OF ASTIGMATIC KERATOTOMY

The basic principles of astigmatic keratotomy apply to all types of astigmatism.[22]

- Keratotomy for astigmatism is placed in the steep corneal meridian, which is the meridian that is parallel to the plus cylinder refraction axis, that has the greatest power on central keratometry, and that crosses the short direction of the ellipse seen on keratography.
- Planning for astigmatic keratotomy is done on the basis of the minus cylinder refraction.
- Transverse incisions across the steep meridian will flatten that meridian and steepen the unincised meridian 90° away, until an arc length of 100–120° is reached.
- Semi radial incisions flatten both the parallel operated meridian and the meridian 90° away.
- In general, transverse incisions closer to the centre of the cornea (i.e. a smaller clear optical zone) produce greater change in astigmatism.
- More than two pairs of transverse incisions across the same meridian do not significantly increase the amount of change in astigmatism.
- The depth of a transverse incision should not exceed approximately 80% of the corneal thickness to prevent excessive uplift of the central edge of the incision.

Patterns of AK

For the correction of astigmatism alone, a number of different patterns have been suggested, but the main component is the 'transverse incision', sometimes called a 'tangential incision', or a 'T-cut'. For the correction of primary astigmatism, these transverse incisions may be straight or arcuate, single or multiple, but always perpendicular to the axis of steepness. Most commonly used now are two symmetrical arcuate transverse incisions (Fig. 19.9).

Astigmatic correction can be combined with radial keratotomy. Large amounts of astigmatism can be corrected independently of the degree of spherical myopia. Three basic combined patterns have evolved:

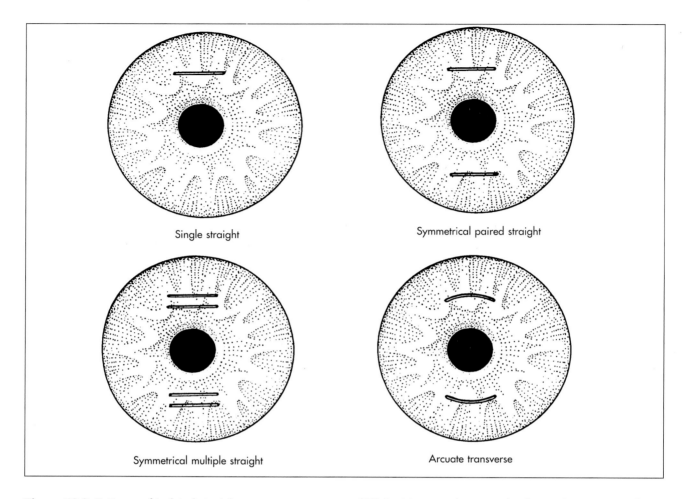

Single straight

Symmetrical paired straight

Symmetrical multiple straight

Arcuate transverse

Figure 19.9 *Patterns of isolated straight or arcuate transverse ('T') incisions made perpendicular to the steep meridian (90°) to treat astigmatism alone.*

- Transverse incisions between radial incisions
- Transverse incisions between semi radial incisions (trapezoidal, Ruiz)
- Interrupted transverse incisions (jump-T, flags) or interrupted radial incisions (jump radial).

Each of these three patterns has a complex set of interactions, particularly when considering the 'coupling phenomenon'. At the present time the most commonly used pattern is the straight or arcuate transverse incision between radial incisions — usually two, but maybe three or four — without any intersection (Fig. 19.10). The trapezoidal pattern has largely been abandoned.

Intersecting incisions

Originally transverse incisions intersected with the radial incisions in a variety of patterns until it was realized that these incisions created excessive wound gape, delayed wound healing, accentuated scarring, and a variable surgical result. It is now recommended that there be no intersection of incisions to avoid these problems in the long term.

The coupling effect

Simply, the 'coupling phenomenon' following transverse incisions means there is flattening of the incised

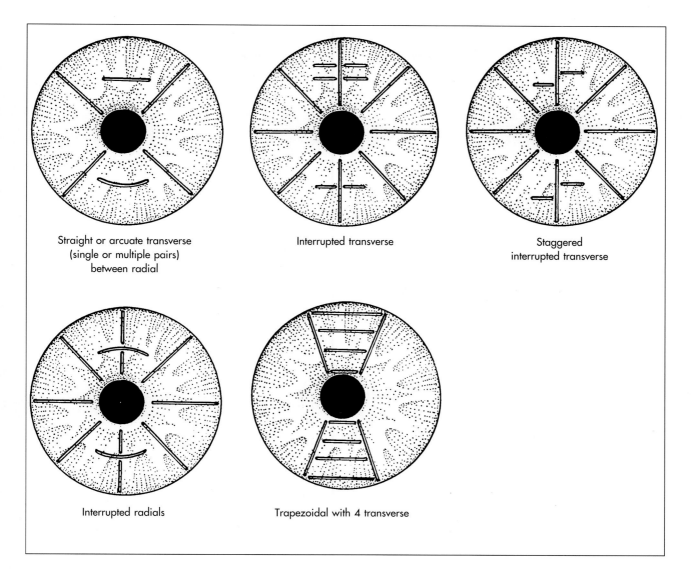

Straight or arcuate transverse
(single or multiple pairs)
between radial

Interrupted transverse

Staggered
interrupted transverse

Interrupted radials

Trapezoidal with 4 transverse

Figure 19.10 *Combined radial incisions and transverse ('T') incisions in the steep meridian (90°) to reduce astigmatism. Non-intersecting incisions are now used exclusively. Trapezoidal patterns are rarely used*

meridian and at the same time steepening of the unincised meridian 90° away. This effect is offset or reduced by adding radial incisions or by making the straight transverse incision long enough to become semi-radial.

STRAIGHT VERSUS ARCUATE INCISIONS

Thornton has been instrumental in the introduction and acceptance of arcuate incisions rather than straight incisions.[23] He points out that all straight lines on a three-dimensional spherical surface are curved, and that straight transverse incisions are actually inverse arcs on the corneal surface. Concentric arcuate incisions, on the other hand, are parallel to the limbus and transverse to the meridian and therefore have greater effect on the meridian transversed.

Thornton states that arcuate incisions, precisely following the curve of the circular optical zone, have the potential for greater effect because the chord length is the same as straight transverse incisions, but

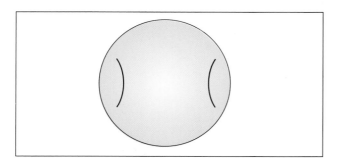

Figure 19.11 *Inverse arc incisions have both transverse and radial components and have the potential to reduce astigmatism and myopia.*

Holmium:YAG laser treatment of hyperopic astigmatism

Another modality that has been used to correct hyperopia and hyperopic astigmatism is thermokeratoplasty and in particular Holmium:YAG laser thermokeratoplasty (LTK).[27] This solid-state laser emits infrared radiation at 2.06 μm which is capable of heating and thus shrinking corneal collagen. The laser energy is focused with a sapphire tip and, if placed in the appropriate axis of astigmatism, it can steepen the flat axis of astigmatism and thereby correct the existing astigmatism. US FDA trials began in July 1992 for this modality, but as yet no approval has been granted.

the actual length is 10–15% longer on the curve, and the entire length of the incision is at the calculated optical zone.

Inverse arc incisions

Again, Thornton[24] has suggested that an exaggerated inverse arc could be used in cases of myopic astigmatism alone, without having to place additional radial incisions (Fig. 19.11). He has calculated that one can reduce the induced myopic spherical equivalent by one-half the amount of the cylinder corrected by using inverse arc incisions.

Depth of transverse incision

The depth of transverse incision required is believed to be less than required for radial incisions. Ruiz[25] has stated that incision depths greater than 90% commonly lead to overcorrections and that incision depths shallower than 70% commonly lead to undercorrection, suggesting a preferred incision depth of 80%. However, Deg and Binder[26] have demonstrated that the incision depth of astigmatic cuts tends to be shallower than the radial cuts using the same depth or length of blade.

The concern with deeper and longer incisions is the resultant 'central lift' as seen on corneal topography. This can reduce wound healing, create irregular astigmatism and glare, and often contribute to an overcorrection. This 'uplift' can be likened to anterior wound slippage after a penetrating keratoplasty.

CORNEAL RELAXING INCISIONS POST KERATOPLASTY

High levels of astigmatism following penetrating keratoplasty can be corrected by incisional surgery. Levels up to 15 D can be corrected with appropriately executed corneal incisions combined with compression sutures in the axis 90° to the axis of incisions, if required. This is not performed until all sutures are removed from the graft and only if the patient does not wish to attempt contact lens use, or is unable to obtain a comfortable contact lens fit.

While there is generally improvement in the degree of astigmatism, the outcome is relatively unpredictable for individual eyes — although the results can be enhanced by adhering to a standard technique. Surgical technique varies considerably in the literature. The author used a standardized graded incremental technique under an operating microscope in an operating theatre. The procedure is planned preoperatively after obtaining refraction, keratometry and corneal topographical mapping. The incisions are performed within the graft–host interface for 2–3 hours, depending on the level of astigmatism, in the axis of the steepest meridian. These incisions are usually paired and opposing each other, although if the astigmatism is asymmetrical, as indicated by corneal topography, then the incisions are positioned according to this asymmetry. The depth of incisions is titrated against the effect of astigmatic correction as judged by qualitative keratoscopy. The end point is apparent sphericity on intraoperative keratoscopy. Four compression sutures are then inserted at 90° to the incisions to cause 2–3

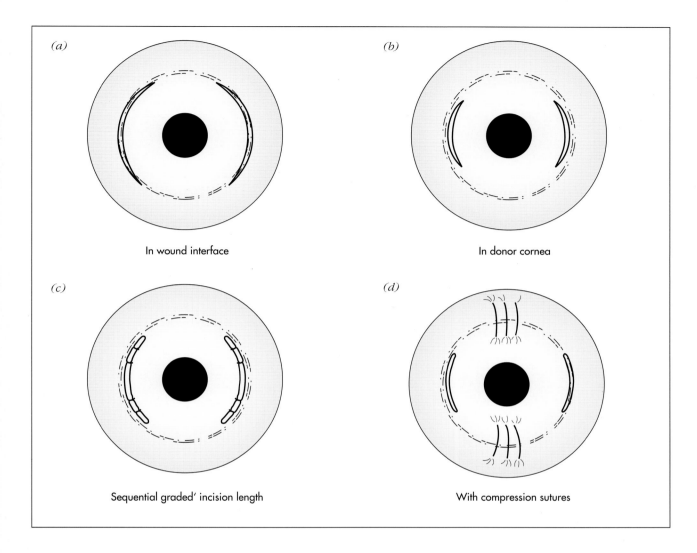

In wound interface

In donor cornea

Sequential graded' incision length

With compression sutures

Figure 19.12 *Arcuate transverse keratotomy or corneal relaxing incisions to reduce astigmatism after penetrating keratoplasty. (a) Incisions placed in the wound interface ('classic' technique). (b) Incisions placed in the donor can produce greater effect, but often increase photophobia. (c) A titrated approach in which incisions are lengthened or deepened to obtain the required effect as judged by intraoperative keratoscopy. (d) Compression sutures added in the original flat axis can enhance the effect of the incisions made in the steep axis.*

D of overcorrection. These sutures are removed at between 2 and 8 weeks depending on the degree of overcorrection postoperatively (Fig. 19.12).

The results of a personal series of 45 such cases demonstrate a mean reduction in post keratoplasty astigmatism from 10.23 D ±3.20 D to 3.69 D ±2.05 D, an empirical reduction in astigmatism of 64% and a vector corrected reduction of 95%. Eyes with preoperative astigmatism greater than 12.00 D (mean 16.83 D ±3.31 D) exhibited the greatest reduction in corneal cylinder with a mean empirical reduction of 76% and a vector-corrected surgically induced astigmatism of 108% (McGhee CNJ, Crawford GJ, unpublished data).

REFERENCES

1. Lans LJ, Experimentelle Untersuchungen uber Entstehung von Astigmatismus durch nicht-per-forirende Corneawunden, *Albrecht von Graefes Arch Ophthalmol* (1898) **45**:117–52.

2. Yenaliev FS, Experience in surgical treatment of myopia, *Vestn Oftalmol* (1974) **30**:841–5

3. Fyodorov SN, Durnev VA, Surgical correction of complicated myopic astigmatism by means of dissection of circular ligament of cornea, *Ann Ophthalmol* (1981) **13**:115–18.

4. Waring GO, The changing status of radial keratotomy for myopia, Part I, *J Refract Surg* (1985) **1**:81–6.

5. Waring GO, The changing status of radial keratotomy for myopia, Part II, *J Refract Surg* (1985) **1**:119–37.

6. Waring GO, Moffitt SD, Gelender H, et al, Rationale for and design of the National Eye Institute Prospective Evaluation of Radial Keratotomy (PERK) study, *Ophthalmology* (1983) **90**:40–58.

7. Waring GO, Lynn MJ, McDonnell PJ, et al, Results of the Prospective Evaluation of Radial Keratotomy (PERK) study 10 Years After Surgery, *Arch Ophthalmol* (1994) **112**:1298–308.

8. Melles GRJ, Binders PS, Effect of radial keratotomy incision direction on wound depth, *J Refract Corneal Surg* (1990) **6**:394–403.

9. Assil KK, Schanzlin DJ, Radial keratotomy surgical technique and protocol, In: Assil KK, Schanzlin DJ, eds, *Radial and astigmatic keratotomy: a complete handbook for the successful practice of incisional keratotomy using the combined technique*, (Slack: Thorofare, 1994), 87–110.

10. Salz JJ, Villasenor RA, Elander R, et al, Four-incision radial keratotomy for low to moderate myopia, *Ophthalmology* (1986) **93**:727–33.

11. Lindstrom RL, Minimally invasive Radial Keratotomy: Mini-RK, *J Cataract Refract Surg* (1995) **21**:27–34.

12. Chen V, Lindstrom RL, Oblique orientation of incisions in four-incision radial keratotomy, *Ophthalmic Surg* (1992) **23**:359.

13. Casebeer JC, *Casebeer Incisional Keratotomy* (Slack: Thorofare, 1993).

14. Waring GO, Lynn MJ, Gelender H, et al, Results of the Prospective Evaluation of Radial Keratotomy (PERK) study one year after surgery, *Ophthalmology* (1985) **92**:177–96.

15. Deitz MR, Sanders DR, Progressive hyperopia with long-term follow-up of radial keratotomy, *Arch Ophthalmol* (1985) **103**:782–4.

16. Deitz MR, Sanders DR, Raanan MG, Progressive hyperopia in radial keratotomy: long-term follow-up of diamond-knife and metal-blade series, *Ophthalmology* (1986) **93**:1284–9.

17. Waring GO, Lynn MJ, Fielding B, et al, Results of the Prospective Evaluation of Radial Keratotomy (PERK) Study 4 years after surgery for myopia, *JAMA* (1990) **263**:1083–91.

18. Santos VR, Waring GO, Lynn MJ, et al, Morning to evening change in refraction, corneal curvature, and visual acuity 2 to 4 years after radial keratotomy in the PERK study, *Ophthalmology* (1988) **95**:1487–93.

19. Schanzlin DJ, Santos VR, Waring GO, et al, Diurnal change in refraction, corneal curvature, visual acuity, and intraocular pressure after radial keratotomy in the PERK study, *Ophthalmology* (1986) **93**:167–75.

20. MacRae S, Rich L, Phillips D, et al, Diurnal variation in vision after radial keratotomy, *Am J Ophthalmol* (1989) **107**:262–7.

21. Ribeiro JC, McDonald MB, Lemos MM, et al, Excimer laser photorefractive keratectomy after radial keratotomy, *J Refract Surg* (1995) **11**:165–9.

22. Binder PS, Waring GO, Keratotomy for Astigmatism, In: Waring GO, *Refractive Keratotomy for myopia and astigmatism*, (Mosby-Year Book: St Louis, 1992), 1087–8.

23. Thornton S, Astigmatic keratotomy: a review of basic concepts with case reports, *J Cataract Refract Surg* (1990) **16**:430–5.

24. Thornton S, Inverse Arcuate Incisions, a new approach to the correction of astigmatism, *J Refract Corneal Surg* (1994) **10**:27–30.

25. Ruiz LA, The astigmatic keratotomies (Ruiz procedures), In: Boyd B, ed, *Highlights of ophthalmology, Vol 2, refractive surgery with the masters*, (Coral Gables: Florida, 1987), 162–93.

26. Deg JK, Binder PS, Wound healing after astigmatic keratotomy procedures in human eyes, *Ophthalmology* (1987) **94**:1290–8.

27. Thompson VM, Seiler T, Durrie DS, et al, Holmium: YAG laser thermokeratoplasty for hyperopia and astigmatism: an overview, *J Refract Corneal Surg* (1993) **9(supp)**: 5134–7.

Chapter 20 Alternative surgical techniques in the correction of high myopia

Ronald M Stasiuk, Cathy A McCarty, Hugh R Taylor and Charles N J McGhee

ALTERNATIVE METHODS FOR CORRECTING MYOPIA

Essentially these can be grouped into either intraocular or extraocular procedures. No totally satisfactory technique has yet been achieved and the correction of myopia continues to present a challenge to the refractive surgeon.[1] Some of these techniques are covered in more detail elsewhere (see Chapter 17 for excimer techniques in LASIK).

INTRAOCULAR PROCEDURES

The three main intraocular procedures for correcting myopia are:

- Clear lensectomy with or without an intraocular lens.
- Anterior chamber phakic intraocular lens.
- Intraocular contact lens.

CLEAR LENSECTOMY

With recent improvements in cataract surgery techniques, including small incisions, viscoelastics, capsulorhexis, and phacoemulsification of a clear soft nucleus, clear lensectomy offers a reasonable alternative treatment in the correction of high myopia. However, several major complications, particularly retinal detachment, endophthalmitis, and loss of accommodation, inhibit widespread application of clear lensectomy for high myopia. Two recent reports with a short follow-up time provided favorable results. Using the clear lensectomy technique in 31 eyes, Lyle and Jin found excellent visual acuity results and the absence of retinal detachments; 77% of eyes achieved 6/12 or better uncorrected vision during a 20 month mean follow-up.[2] A higher posterior capsular opacification rate than anticipated, of 58%, occurred in this follow-up period, with posterior chamber lens implantation for high myopia.

Koch and co-authors found the incidence of retinal detachment in eyes with an axial length of 25.0 mm or more was 10% following YAG laser capsulotomy.[3] Therefore, caution with clear lensectomy needs to be taken in the long term. A second report by Colin and Robinet presented similar results to Lyle, with special attention to retinal management and argon laser prophylaxis for retinal pathology. No cases of retinal detachment were reported in the 1 year follow-up period.[4] A controlled prospective study with a long-term longitudinal follow-up is needed to permit definitive conclusions about the safety and benefit-to-risk ratio.[1]

ANTERIOR CHAMBER PHAKIC INTRAOCULAR LENS

There are two *common* types used:

- the BAIKOFF angle supported intraocular lens
- the WORST iris-claw, iris supported intraocular lens.

Even though recent modifications have improved refractive predictability with fewer complications, progressive endothelial cell loss has been reported by several authors, which in the long term may result in corneal decompensation.[5-7] Recently, Menezo and colleagues reported a 5.5% endothelial cell loss rate at 1 year and 7.6% at 2 years in a study involving 90 eyes using the iris-claw phakic lens, with no significant detectable morphological changes.[5] Other authors, Mimouni et al and Saragoussi et al, found significant endothelial damage from use of anterior chamber phakic intraocular lenses.[6,7]

Interestingly, the theoretically 'normal' 0.5% (14 cells/mm²) per year endothelial cell drop out rate would need to be increased by only 1.0–1.5% (28–42 cells/mm²) per year in order for 70 years of anterior chamber, phakic intraocular lens exposure to result in complete corneal decompensation. Consequently, the future success of phakic intraocular lenses would appear to depend upon minimizing cumulative endothelial cell loss, and until this happens their future remains controversial in the correction of high myopia. The more recent third generation Baikoff anterior chamber multiflex myopic lens implants appear to have a lower endothelial cell loss. Allermann et al described a method using ultrasound biomicroscopy to assess suitable patients for the Baikoff lens, by measuring the iris to endothelium distance, where a minimum of 2.3 mm was recommended at 3.7 mm from the scleral spur to minimize endothelial cell loss.[26]

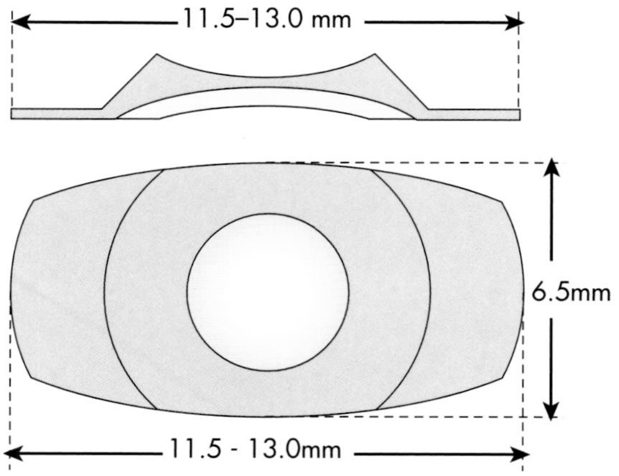

Figure 20.1 *Dimensions of an intraocular contact lens (courtesy of Chiron Adatomed).*

INTRAOCULAR CONTACT LENS

Fyodorov introduced this novel concept in 1986, in the form of a silicone intraocular contact lens. This is placed through a 3 mm clear corneal incision in the space between the iris and anterior lens surface. The lens rests on a layer of prelenticular aqueous.

Two companies are involved in intraocular contact lens research and development. Starr AG is developing a foldable, hydrophilic, collagen-silicone copolymer (COLLAMER), while Chiron-Adatomed GmbH is concentrating on a silicone model (Fig. 20.1).

The major potential complications, although unlikely, are endophthalmitis and retinal detachment. In a series of 1300 eyes, implanted with phakic posterior chamber lenses over 7 years, no such complications have been reported.[9] Possible posterior iris surface rub could potentially lead to iris pigment dispersion, iritis and secondary pigmentary glaucoma, as previously observed with early sulcus fixated posterior chamber lens implants. Marinho et al reported good results in 40 myopic eyes (range: –8.00 D to –26.00 D) using the silicone intraocular contact lens in the posterior chamber (Chiron-Adatomed) in a 2 year period to May 1995. Eighty-eight per cent of eyes were within ± ID with no loss of any line of best corrected vision. However, two eyes developed severe uveitis and two lenses were explanted because of intense glare.[27]

Zaldivar analyzed 76 cases with similar lenses (–12.0 to –19.0 DS); 65% achieved 20/40 or better uncorrected at one month. After three months 73% gained two lines or more of best corrected vision, while 2.7% lost one line.[28]

The simplicity of surgical implantation and the reversibility makes the intraocular contact lens appealing, especially with further improvements and if complications are minimal in the long term.

EXTRAOCULAR PROCEDURES FOR CORRECTION OF HIGH MYOPIA

Following the original work by Sato and Fyodorov with radial keratotomy, and Barraquer's keratomileusis, a number of extraocular techniques have evolved, with no ideal method for correction of high myopia.

These techniques may be classified on a historical and technical basis (Table 20.1).

RADIAL KERATOTOMY

Radial keratotomy (RK) has been effective in correcting up to –5.0 D myopia, but a significant number of patients have demonstrated progressive hyperopia. However, excimer photorefractive keratotomy (PRK) can be combined as a second procedure to either treat undercorrected RK, or to correct high myopia in two stages.[8,10–12]

Table 20.1

Classification of extraocular procedures for correction of high myopia

I *Incisional*
   Radial keratotomy
   Keratomileusis
   Automated lamellar keratoplasty
II *Corneal lenses*
   Epikeratophakia
   Intracorneal lenses
   Intracorneal rings
III *Laser ablation*
   Surface excimer photorefractive keratectomy and photoastigmatic refractive keratectomy
   Excimer keratomileusis
   Intrastromal

Table 20.2

Excimer laser PRK results after undercorrected radial keratotomy.

	Group 1	Group 2
Original myopia	Less than −6.0 D	More than −6.0 D
% within ± 1 D at 6 months	100%	54%
% within ± 0.5 D at 12 months	80%	23%

Azar and colleagues reported PRK as an effective second procedure in eyes undercorrected by RK, especially in patients with less than −6.0 D of myopia pre-RK.[11] Thirty-nine patients were treated, with a follow-up of 6–24 months. Group 1 had myopia of −6.0 D or less, while Group 2 had more than −6.0 D of original myopia. The mean original refractive error was −8.02 ± 2.99 D (range −2.0 to −17.0 D), and the mean pre-excimer refractive error was −3.98 ± 2.31 D (range −2.0 to −8.6 D). Results are shown in Table 20.2.

KERATOMILEUSIS

The evolution of keratomileusis has been refined since Barraquer introduced the lathing of a frozen corneal lenticle over 30 years ago for correction of high myopia.[13] Krumeich improved on this method by introducing the non-freeze lenticle to reduce corneal haze, but both methods produced only moderate predictability and required considerable surgical dexterity.[13]

Ruiz and Barraquer created an in-situ keratomileusis technique that involved two keratectomies. The primary keratectomy produced a plano corneal lenticle, followed by a second refractive keratectomy of the stromal bed. The superficial plano lenticle was then repositioned by a non-suture method. This has now been refined by the use of an automated geared microkeratome and the procedure is now described as automated lamellar keratoplasty (ALK).[14]

AUTOMATED LAMELLAR KERATOPLASTY

A recent prospective multicentre clinical trial to evaluate ALK for correction of myopia by Slade and co-workers showed encouraging results.[15] One hundred eyes with myopia ranging between −4.0 and −16.25 D were enrolled in a 2-year study. Postoperatively (10–14 months), uncorrected vision was 6/12 or better for 67% of patients with 59% within ± 1 D and 79% within ± 2 D of emmetropia.

However, there are several reports of significant complications with this technique, which appear to be due to instrument variability. Some of these complications include significant under- and over-corrections, induced regular and irregular astigmatism, lost and decentered lenticles, interface foreign bodies, infection, corneal ectasia requiring penetrating keratoplasty, hole in the flap, haze, and even anterior chamber perforation with secondary anterior segment trauma.

Mechanical failure, loss of suction during keratome activation, and variable sharpness of blades or warpage are some of the problems related to the instrument variability. Some of these complications appear to become less frequent with experience and with the use of a geared automatic microkeratome.[16]

EPIKERATOPHAKIA

This technique has lost appeal due to the need for donor material, extended recovery periods with irregular astigmatism, and especially poor predictability. There is limited use in some cases of pediatric aphakia and selected keratoconus. Panda recently reported onlay lamellar keratoplasty utilizing plano lenticles, prepared from fresh McCarey-Kaufman (M-

K) medium preserved corneas. Twenty eyes studied showed early visual improvement within 8 weeks and a mean astigmatism of 3.0 D in all eyes in a long-term study.[17] Undercorrection with epikeratophakia can be treated with a secondary excimer laser PRK. For further discussion see Chapter 12.

INTRACORNEAL LENSES

Intracorneal lenses (ICLs)—manufactured from Polysulfone or Hydrogel—have yet to live up to initial expectations, with sub-optimal material compatibility and variable results. McDonald and co-workers assessed the long-term corneal response to Hydrogel intrastromal lenses implanted in monkey eyes for up to 5 years.[18] They found minimal tissue reaction. Histopathological changes to the cornea included epithelial thinning anterior to the thickest portion of the ICL, fibroblastic activity along the ICL–stromal interface, and the deposition of an amorphous extra-cellular material adjacent to the intracorneal lens. Werblin found that initial human experience with Hydrogel ICLs gave significant undercorrection in five human patients.[19] Polysulfone corneal lenses have produced several complications, including both visually and non-visually significant interface opacities, lens extrusion, anterior corneal necrosis, refractile particles, and epithelial thinning, in a study by Lane and colleagues involving animal eyes.[20]

INTRASTROMAL CORNEAL RING

The intrastromal corneal ring (ICR®) is an optically transparent split ring composed of polymethyl-methacrylate (PMMA). When inserted into the mid-peripheral corneal stroma at approximately two-thirds depth, the ring flattens the anterior corneal curvature, without direct surgical intervention to the optical zone. Cadaver eye studies show that a direct relationship exists between increasing ICR thickness and greater degrees of corneal flattening; for each 0.027 mm increase in ICR thickness, approximately an additional 1.0 D of flattening can be achieved.

The initial US Phase I non-functional eye study indicated that a 0.30 mm thick ICR resulted in about 2.7 D of flattening.[21] A further Phase II FDA clinical trial involving 90 patients with varying ICR thickness (0.25–4.5 mm) is showing similar results with no significant postoperative complications.[22]

The most commonly observed complications were peripheral corneal haze, lamellar channel

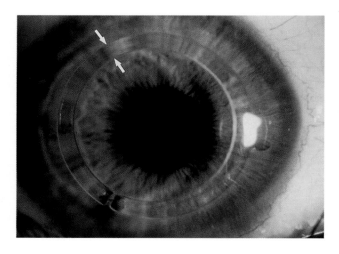

Figure 20.2 *Intrastromal corneal ring. (Courtesy of Kera Vision Inc).*

deposits, collagen/proteoglycan deposits in the ICR suture holes, and fluorescein staining at the incision site.[23]

To date, it appears the ICR will only correct low myopia and possibly some astigmatism using modified ICR segments. The ICR can be easily removed to reverse the refractive effect. The insertion technique is lengthy and may take up to 1 hour to perform. Its future appears to be limited to low myopia (Fig. 20.2).

Patel et al presented a mathematical model for deriving the optical performance of an intracorneal ring, and concluded that the maximum correction was −4.0 DS of myopia, otherwise significant ocular aberration and visual impairment would result if greater correction were attempted.[29]

EXCIMER LASER KERATOMILEUSIS

In 1989, Buratto combined ALK with excimer laser to sculpt the back of the lenticle (cap) or the stromal bed in situ; this is excimer laser keratomileusis (ELK).

Pallikaris, in 1990, further refined this by creating a primary hinged corneal flap and then sculpting the stromal bed with excimer laser. This has been variously termed excimer laser myopic keratomileusis, laser in situ keratomileusis (LASIK), or the 'Flap and Zap' technique (see Figs 20.3 and 20.4).[30]

The preliminary results of the latter two techniques appear encouraging, with a rapid visual stabilization

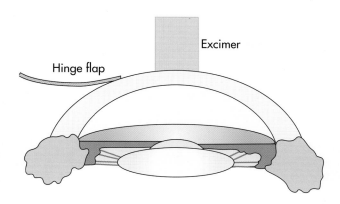

Figure 20.3 *Diagram showing laser in situ keratomileusis with a hinged superficial corneal flap and excimer laser ablation of the stromal bed*

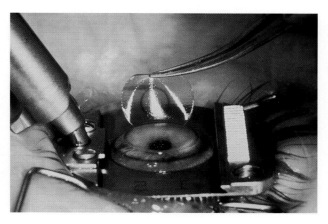

Figure 20.4 *Surgical photograph shows automated microkeratome ring in position with a hinged superficial corneal flap (courtesy of Chiron).*

by 1–2 months, few symptoms postoperatively, and insignificant regression or haze compared to conventional PRK in the treatment of high myopia.[13,14]

Several reports, although with small numbers and a short follow-up period, are encouraging. For further information refer to Chapter 11. Brint and colleagues reported 6 month results of the multicentre phase I study of laser keratomileusis in 57 eyes of 57 patients.[14] The mean preoperative spherical equivalent was –10.7 D with a postoperative result at 6 months of –0.63 D; 66% of patients achieved uncorrected vision of 6/12 or better. Fifteen per cent of eyes lost two lines of best corrected visual acuity but only 6.4% lost three or more lines. An optic zone of 4.5–5.0 mm was used, with a mean ablation depth of 90.7 μm (range 61–167 μm). Apart from two perforated lenticles, complications were minimal. Seven cases had a trace of deposits at the interface.

Williams recently reported a comparative study of excimer laser intrastromal keratoablation (Buratto technique) to one eye and PRK treatment to the second eye of six patients. Six highly myopic patients underwent correction with the Buratto technique, with a mean preoperative correction of –15.75 D (range –12.0 to –19.5 D). The second eye was treated using a three-step multizone PRK treatment with the Visx 2020 excimer laser; the mean preoperative myopia was –15.50 D (range –11.5 to –19.5 D). Results were similar in both groups, with a patient preference for PRK.

Buratto studied 40 eyes in 37 patients, correcting myopia from –6 to –10 D over a 24 month period.[13]

He used a Summit Excimed UV 200 laser with single ablation zones between 3.9 and 4.5 mm diameter, an older technique that results in significant regression. The PRK results demonstrated that 35% of eyes achieved a final refractive outcome within ±1 D compared to 63% of the LASIK patients (20 cases each). Seventy-two per cent of PRK procedures showed significant regression after 6 months, while LASIK demonstrated stability of vision by 1–3 months. Eighty-four per cent of eyes in the PRK group had a corneal haze of greater than +1 D, compared to all LASIK cases being clear by 3 months.

Pallikaris' report of 10 patients receiving PRK and 10 patients treated by LASIK in 1994 showed results that were similar to Brint and Buratto.[13,14] A Meditec MEL60 excimer laser was used with an unreported optic zone size. Ten per cent of PRK eyes achieved a final refractive outcome within ±1 D of emmetropia compared to 66% of eyes treated by LASIK, whilst 33% of PRK eyes were within ±2 D, and 88.8% in the LASIK group. The mean regression for PRK was >5 D for 6 months, while the LASIK group demonstrated only 1.5 D for 12 months. Interestingly, specular microscopy showed a small loss of endothelial cells in both groups; a mean of 10.6% with PRK and 8.6% in the LASIK group.

In all three reported LASIK series, the theoretical advantages advocated over PRK were:

- minimal immediate post-operative pain
- rapid visual recovery and stability within 1–3 months

- minimal corneal haze
- no hyperopic shift
- better visual acuity results
- fewer cases with loss of best corrected visual acuity.

Of concern are the possible serious complications that may occur with the microkeratome. They include:

- perforation of the corneal lenticle (2 out of 57 eyes in the Brint series)[14]
- perforation of the globe (1 out of 10 in Pallikaris' report)
- possible future central corneal ectasia and secondary keratoconus with deep ablations resulting in thin central corneas
- more endothelial cell loss if excimer laser ablation is performed closer to endothelium (8.6% in the Pallikaris series).

Larger series with longer follow-up periods are needed to interpret which techniques will ultimately provide superior results. Furthermore, PRK techniques continue to improve, and advances in techniques that were not utilized in the above series include:

- multizone ablation
- larger optic zones
- tapered transition zones
- multipass techniques
- improved software algorithms.

FUTURE DIRECTIONS IN THE TREATMENT OF HIGH MYOPIA

The future for successful surgical correction of high myopia is very promising with the key developments in the following areas:

PRK REFINEMENTS

Various pharmacological agents may be useful in reducing haze and regression, as well as the refined techniques of multizones, tapered transition zones and improved software algorithms. Several new pharmacological agents show promise in reducing corneal haze following excimer laser PRK. Morlet and co-workers found a significant reduction in corneal haze following excimer laser PRK in rabbits with postoperative use of topical Interferon-Alpha 2b eyedrops.[24]

Plasmin and plasminogen-activator inhibitors may help prevent postoperative regression and haze in a concept proposed by Lohmann and Marshall.[25]

COMBINED TECHNIQUES

This may be necessary for extreme myopia such as a combination of LASIK (up to −16D) with a secondary refining PRK of the lenticle. Undercorrection by RK or epikeratophakia can also be enhanced with PRK.[10]

LASER IN SITU KERATOMILEUSIS (LASIK)

A safer and more accurate surgical cut of the lenticle by a laser-assisted lamellar dissection, or improved automatic microkeratomes, would enhance the LASIK procedure. Lenticle problems such as irregular astigmatism and epithelial ingrowths need to be minimized.

INTRASTROMAL LASER ABLATION

Newer lasers that accurately ablate within the stroma with accurate automatic eye tracking may supersede LASIK techniques (e.g. ISL laser).

INTRAOCULAR CONTACT LENS

This perhaps shows the greatest promise of all the intraocular procedures, with recent reports showing improved results.[27,28] This method does not affect the cornea, but it has yet to reach its potential.

ANTERIOR CHAMBER PHAKIC INTRAOCULAR LENSES

Newer designs have reduced endothelial cell loss, but this complication is still a concern.

CONCLUSION

Further research, clinical trials and evaluation are needed to find the most effective way of correcting high myopia, as no single technique stands out. Pharmacological control of corneal haze and regression may hold the key for successful laser ablation.

The technique selected needs to be safe, simple, reproducible, inexpensive, with good results and preferably remain extraocular.

Perhaps, techniques should be combined for full correction of the high ametropia, but presbyopia must always be considered in this exciting, newly emerging field of refractive surgery.

KEY POINTS OF ALTERNATIVE METHODS FOR HIGH MYOPIA

- Excellent visual results with clear lensectomy, but several major complications
- Anterior chamber phakic intraocular lenses can result in endothelial cell loss
- Intraocular contact lenses have yet to live up to their promise
- Keratomileusis has been refined to Automated Lamellar Keratoplasty (ALK)
- ALK complications due primarily to instruments and inexperience
- Epikeratophakia requires donor material
- Intracorneal lenses have produced undercorrection and complications
- Intrastromal corneal ring probably limited to low myopia
- Excimer laser keratomileusis is promising, but with significant complications associated with the microkeratome and epithelial downgrowths
- Different or combined methods may be indicated
- No single technique stands out

REFERENCES

1. Obstbaum SA, Clear lens extraction for high myopia and high hyperopia, *J Cataract Refract Surg* (1994) **20**:271 (edit).

2. Lyle WA, Jin JC, Clear lens extraction for the correction of high refractive error, *J Cataract Refract Surg* (1994) **20**:273–6.

3. Koch DD, Liu JF, Fill EP, Parke DW, Axial myopia increases the risk of retinal complications after neodymium–YAG laser posterior capsulotomy, *Arch Ophthalmol* (1989) **107**:986–90.

4. Colin J, Robinet A, Clear lensectomy and implantation of low power posterior chamber intra-ocular lens for the correction of high myopia, *Ophthalmology* (1994) **101**:107–12.

5. Menezo JL, Cisneros AL, Cervera M, Harto M, Iris Claw Phakic Lens—Intermediate and longterm corneal endothelial changes, *Eur J Implant Ref Surg* (1994) **6**:195–9.

6. Mimouni F, Colin J, Koffi V, Bonnet P, Damage to corneal endothelium from anterior chamber intra-ocular lenses in phakic myopia, *Refract Corneal Surg* (1991) **7**:277–81.

7. Saragoussi JJ, Cotinas J, Renard G, Savoldelli MI, Abenhain A, Pouliquen Y, Damage to the corneal endothelium by minus power anterior chamber lenses, *Refract Corneal Surg* (1991) **7**:282–90.

8. Werblin TP, Discussion Section—Management of patients with high ametropia who seek refractive surgical correction, *Eur J Implant Ref Surg* (1994) **6**:299–301.

9. Grabow HB, Discussion Section—Management of patients with high ametropia who seek refractive surgical correction, *Eur J Implant Ref Surg* (1994) **6**:302–4.

10. Meza J, Perez-Santonja JJ, Moreno E, Zato MA, Photorefractive keratectomy after radial keratotomy, *J Cataract Refract Surg* (1994) **20**:485–9.

11. Azar DT, Hardten D, Aquavella J, et al, Excimer laser photorefractive keratectomy after undercorrected radial keratotomy, *ISRK* (1994) Oct:51 (abst).

12. Nordan LT, Amalgram Refractive surgeons signature, *ISRK* (1994) Oct:113 (abst).

13. Buratto L, Ferrari M, Photorefractive keratectomy or keratomileusis with excimer laser in surgical correction of severe myopia: which technique is better? *Eur J Implant Ref Sur* (1993) **5**:183–6.

14. Brint SF, Ostrick DM, Fisher C, et al, Six month results of the multicenter phase I study of excimer laser myopic keratomileusis, *J Cataract Refract Surg* (1994) **20**:610–15.

15. Slade SD, Gordon JF, Dru RM, A prospective multicentre clinical trial to evaluate automated lamellar keratoplasty (ALK) for the correction of myopia, *ISRK* (1994) Oct:79 (abst).

16. Neumann AC, Automated lamellar keratoplasty ALK complications: avoidance and management, *ISRK* (1994) Oct:80 (abst).

17. Panda A, Epikeratoplasty utilising manually prepared plano lenticule from fresh M-K preserved corneas (a longterm study), *ISRK* (1994) Oct:**75** (abst).

18. McDonald MB, McCarey BE, Storie B, et al, Assessment of the longterm corneal response to Hydrogel intrastromal lenses implanted in monkey eyes for up to five years, *J Cataract Refract Surg* (1993) **19**:213–22.

19. Werblin TP, Patel AS, Barraquer JI, Initial human experience with Permalens myopic Hydrogel intracorneal lens implants, *Refract Corneal Surg* (1992) **8**:23–26.

20. Lane SL, Lindstrom RL, Cameron JD, et al, Polysulfone corneal lenses, *J Cataract Refract Surg* (1986) **12**:50–60.

21. Durrie DS, Schanzlin DJ, Asbell PA, et al, The ICR® (Intra stromal corneal ring): theory and surgical technique, *ISRK* (1994) Oct:38 (abst).

22. Durrie DS, Schanzlin DJ, Asbell PA, et al, The ICR® (Intra stromal corneal ring): Phase II Update, *ISRK* (1994) Oct:39 (abst).

23. Williams KD, A comparative study of excimer laser intrastromal keratoablation (Buratto technique) to one eye and PRK treatment alone to the second eye of six patients, *ISRK* (1994) Oct:118 (abst).

24. Morlet N, Gillies MC, Crouch R, et al, Effect of topical

Interferon-Alpha 2b on corneal haze after excimer laser photorefractive keratectomy in rabbits, *Refract Corneal Surg* (1993) **9**:443–51.

25. Lohmann CP, Marshall J, Plasmin and plasminogen activator inhibitors after excimer laser photorefractive keratectomy: a new concept in prevention of post-operative myopic regression and haze, *Refract Corneal Surg* (1993) **9**:300–2.

26. Allemann N, Chamon W, Campos M, Safety prediction in Baikoff lenses for high myopia correction using ultrasound biomicroscopy, *ISRS* (1995) Oct:59–60 (abst).

27. Marinho AA, Neves M, Pinto M, et al, Posterior chamber IOLS (silicone) in myopic phakic eyes: 2 year experience, *ISRS* (1995) Oct: 58 (abst).

28. Zaldivar R, Hypernegative intraocular lenses in the posterior chamber of phakic eyes for the correction of high myopia, *ISRS* (1995) Oct:58 (abst).

29. Patel S, Marshall J, Fitzke III FW, Model for deriving the optical performance of the myopic eye corrected with an intracorneal ring, *J Refract Surg* (1995) **11**:248–52.

Chapter 21   Early phototherapeutic keratectomy studies in the United Kingdom

David S Gartry

INTRODUCTION

Following early laboratory and animal studies, which demonstrated the exquisite precision with which the 193 nm excimer laser could remove corneal tissue, the potential for such a 'laser scalpel' in the management of superficial corneal scars and opacities was readily apparent to the pioneers of photoablative laser surgery. Although photorefractive keratectomy (PRK) has become the more widely utilized excimer laser modality, in parallel with the advances in refractive technique and the demand for such surgery, a number of ophthalmic surgeons have continually probed the boundaries of phototherapeutic keratectomy (PTK) application. Phototherapeutic keratectomy now successfully replaces lamellar keratoplasty for certain conditions and has been applied successfully to recurrent corneal erosion syndrome and band-shaped keratopathy. These advances have been made in both the laboratory and the clinical setting. This chapter highlights some of the early laboratory and clinical studies while the next chapter provides an overview of contemporary applications of PTK.

LABORATORY STUDIES OF PTK AT ST THOMAS' HOSPITAL, LONDON

BACKGROUND

Prior to the treatment of overt corneal pathology with the excimer laser, it was necessary to elucidate the possible techniques of PTK in the laboratory setting in order to determine whether the laser could be used for wide area ablations to remove opacities and to produce smooth corneal surfaces. Since photoab-lation occurs across the entire area exposed, it was anticipated that, with repeated pulses, the original surface contour would be reproduced in the base of the ablated disc. In order to avoid reproducing irregular surfaces, it was, therefore, necessary to devise a means of smoothing an uneven surface during ablation. The simplest method of achieving this is to apply a liquid with approximately the same ablation properties as the cornea. The surface tension of such a liquid should ensure that if any elevated irregularities in the corneal surface have a different ablation rate to that of the surrounding tissue (for example, the dense calcium deposits in rough band keratopathy), the underlying, intervening tissue would be shielded by the liquid whilst the crystalline peaks underwent ablation. Three main laboratory models of corneal irregularity were commenced in 1986 at St. Thomas' Hospital, London, to assess the efficacy of the laser in smoothing non-uniform surfaces.

EXCIMER LASER ABLATION IN CADAVER EYES

Smoothing the relief patterns produced by the laser

The aim of these experiments was to create a geometric irregular surface in cadaver corneas and then to determine whether the excimer laser could be used to smooth these irregularities. An area of stroma was masked by placing a piece of bent wire (template) on the corneal surface in the path of the beam. This resulted in excavation of the stromal surface in areas not shielded by the wire; however, in areas directly beneath the wire, ridges of original tissue remained. The next objective was to attempt removal of the induced pattern with the excimer laser to restore a smooth surface across the entire ablation zone. The template wire was removed and the previously excavated areas 'masked' with a 1 or 2% solution of hydroxypropylmethycellulose (HPMC) to prevent their further ablation. These tear substitutes have a high water content and were, therefore, assumed to have similar ablation rates to corneal stroma.

Removal of a cylindrical 'facet'

In this experiment, the excimer laser was used to create a cylindrical excavation 1 mm in diameter and 100 µm deep (approximately one-fifth the normal axial corneal thickness). The beam diameter was then increased to 3 mm, the ablated cylinder filled with HPMC 1%, and the surrounding stromal surface carefully dried. Ablation of the cadaveric corneal surface then commenced and was continued until the surrounding stroma had been ablated to the same depth as the original cylinder. In practice, the progress was monitored by changes in tissue and fluid fluorescence.

Excimer laser smoothing of surgical lamellar keratectomy beds

This experiment was designed to assess the potential of excimer laser radiation, in combination with masking agents, to smooth irregular corneal surfaces similar to those encountered in clinical practice. Surgical lamellar keratectomies were carried out on human donor eyes. The initial incision was made with a disposable 6 mm trephine and the lamellar dissection was performed using a steel blade and Paufique's knives, beginning at the base of the trephine cut. Hydroxypropylmethylcellulose was then applied to the keratectomy bed and its amount and distribution adjusted while multiple overlapping ablation zones were produced until the bed was apparently smooth.

RESULTS OF PRELIMINARY LABORATORY STUDIES IN CADAVER EYES

Smoothing of relief patterns produced by the laser

The bas-relief pattern produced on the cornea by shielding the underlying stroma with bent wire was

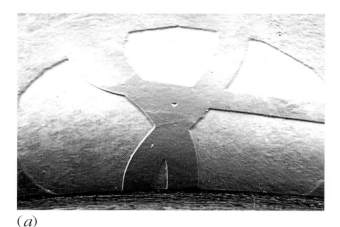

(*a*)

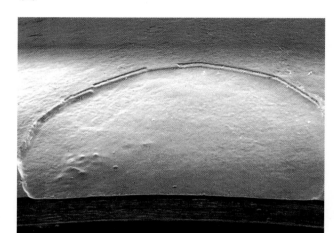

(*b*)

Figure 21.1 *Scanning electron micrographs of the surface of human donor corneas after excimer laser irradiation. (a) The pattern created by shielding stroma with a piece of bent wire during irradiation is shown. The ablated surface adjacent to the non-ablated ridges is smooth and the ridges themselves are sharply demarcated. The sides of these ridges are perpendicular as is the edge of the ablated zone. (b) A pattern similar to that in (a) has now been ablated leaving an almost totally smooth surface. A small peripheral annulus indicates that there has been a slight shift in the position of the eye prior to the final smoothing ablation. (Courtesy of* The British Journal of Ophthalmology *(1991)* **75***:258–69 and DS Gartry, MG Kerr Muir and J Marshall.)*

best demonstrated by scanning electron microscopy (Fig. 21.1a). The smoothness of the ablated surface was comparable to Bowman's layer on the non-ablated ridges and the stromal architecture was obscured by a continuous membrane-like structure.

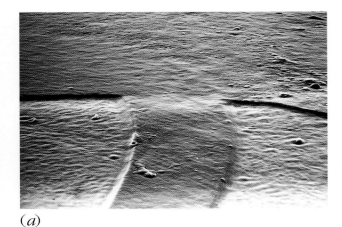

(*a*)

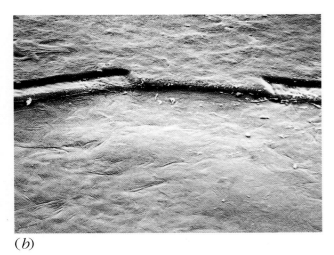

(*b*)

Figure 21.2 *High power scanning electron micrographs of the ridges created and removed by excimer laser irradiation. (a) Shows the magnitude and edge quality of the ridge seen in Fig. 21.1a. (b) Shows the residual portion of a ridge after a smoothing procedure. The ablation depth involved in generating the initial pattern and that involving its removal can be clearly distinguished as a result of displacement of the globe between the two procedures. (Courtesy of* The British Journal of Ophthalmology *(1991)* **75***:258–69 and DS Gartry, MG Kerr Muir and J Marshall.)*

By utilizing tear substitute masking agents, the ridges, which exhibited smooth perpendicular walls, were successfully ablated to produce a homogeneous, optically smooth surface (Fig. 21.1b). In some specimens, the ablation zone that produced the initial pattern and the subsequent smoothing ablation were not exactly coincident because of a slight shift in eye fixation. This resulted in a small peripheral annulus in which the ridges could still be seen (Figs 21.2a and b).

The most suitable masking liquid was HPMC 1% since it was easy to apply and remove and filled the troughs between surface projections. Hydroxypropyl-methycellulose fluoresced a bright blue when irradiated and the corneal stroma fluoresced a dark blue/black. There was, thus, a clear indication of the three-dimensional geometry of stroma undergoing ablation. When HPMC 1% flooded the surface, an even, bright blue fluorescence was noted across the entire target area with each pulse. As the masking agent was ablated, corneal stromal irregularities projected through the surface of the HPMC and were ablated, as dark blue, almost black, 'islands' within the bright blue HPMC 'sea' of fluorescence. As ablation proceeded, so the pattern and surrounding masking agent were removed until a common depth was reached, at which point HPMC once again spread throughout the 3 mm zone, indicated by uniform-homogeneous bright blue fluorescence. Further ablation beyond the original depth of 10–12 µm removed the little remaining HPMC and the entire area appeared dark blue/black with each pulse, confirming that the pattern had been completely removed. If further pulses were applied then the 3 mm zone of ablation was uniformly increased in depth.

With relief patterns in excess of 30 µm it was more difficult to achieve uniform smoothness because of a meniscus effect where the masking agent met the vertical sides of the ridges of non-ablated tissue. It was found that blotting the edges with cellulose (Weck-cell) sponges reduced this effect.

Removal of a cylindrical 'facet'

In this series, the 1 mm diameter facet experimentally created in the corneal stroma was initially filled with HPMC. On ablating the area around the cylinder, there was differential fluorescence – the central spot (HPMC) fluoresced bright blue while the surrounding stroma, in contrast, appeared dark blue/black. The end-point was reached when the blue disappeared and the entire area of ablation became uniformly black, that is, the surrounding stroma had been ablated to exactly the same depth as that of the original cylinder.

Excimer laser smoothing of surgical lamellar keratectomy beds

Scanning electron microscopy of the base and walls of a surgical lamellar keratectomy showed surfaces with a marked degree of destruction and dissociation of cellular and extracellular components (Fig. 21.3a). The walls of such sites demonstrated stratification with alternating layers of compression and shearing. There was an annulus in which epithelial cells were

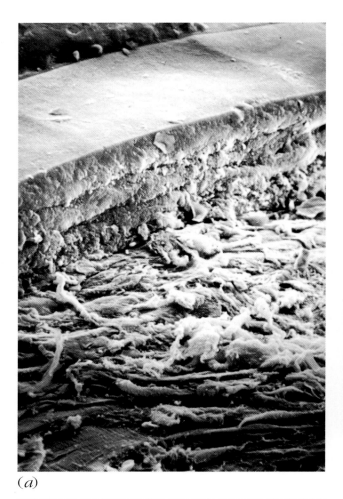

(a)

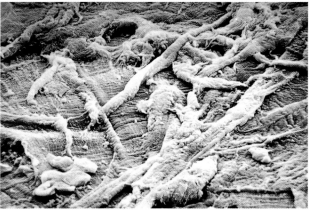

(b)

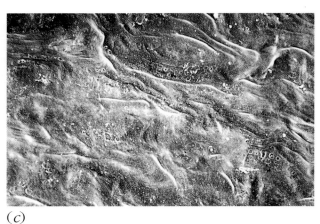

(c)

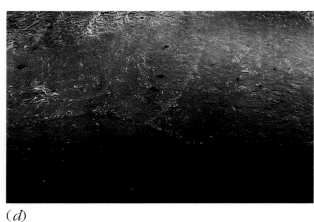

(d)

Figure 21.3 *Scanning electron micrographs of the corneal surface subsequent to (a) surgical lamellar keratectomy; (b) and (c) excimer laser irradiation. (a) The bed of a lamellar keratectomy showing rough, disorganized and torn tissue. The circular margin with vertical-sided walls represents the edge produced by the trephine. (b) High power of the keratectomy bed. (c) A surgical lamellar keratectomy bed smoothed by excimer laser irradiation. The surface has a confluent membrane-like quality seen as wrinkles and folds produced during preparation for scanning electron microscopy. (d) A lamellar keratectomy bed smoothed by application of multiple overlapping zones of excimer laser radiation. The slight discontinuities between different zones are seen as variations in ablation depth and defined by arcuate boundaries. (Courtesy of The British Journal of Ophthalmology (1991) **75**:258–69 and DS Gartry, MG Kerr Muir and J Marshall.)*

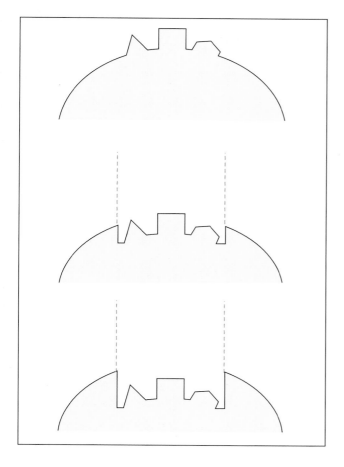

Figure 21.4 *The effect of excimer laser radiation on an unmasked irregular surface. (a) The unexposed surface. (b) After minimal exposure the surface irregularity is repeated deeper into the material, since a uniform layer of equal thickness is ablated across the entire exposed surface with each pulse. (c) The end result is a faithful representation of the original surface topography produced deep in the material. (Courtesy of* The British Journal of Ophthalmology *(1991)* **75***:258–69 and DS Gartry, MG Kerr Muir and J Marshall.)*

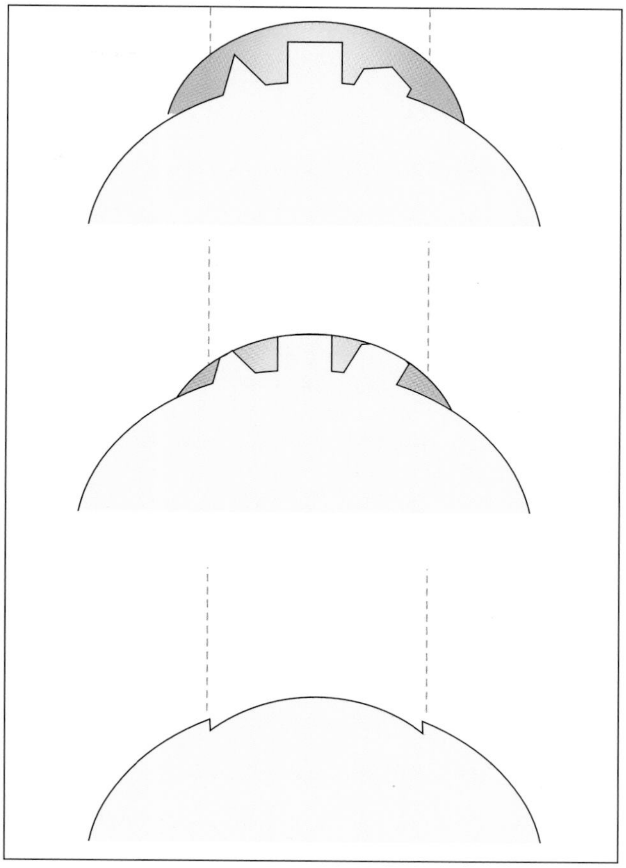

Figure 21.5 *Production of a smooth surface by excimer laser radiation utilizing 'masking' with HPMC. (a) The irregular surface, analogous to a rough corneal surface, is covered with a masking liquid. (b) After initial exposure to excimer laser radiation both the masking liquid and surface projections have been partially ablated—the normal stroma between projections having been shielded from unnecessary ablation. (c) The resultant smooth surface at the end of the procedure (determination of the end-point is assisted by observation of a uniform fluorescence. (Courtesy of* The British Journal of Ophthalmology *(1991)* **75***:258–69 and DS Gartry, MG Kerr Muir and J Marshall.)*

wiped away from Bowman's layer because the surface tissue was displaced and compressed against and within the barrel of the trephine and debrided as the trephine rotated. The floor never displayed a smooth cleavage plane and always consisted of ripped, torn lamellae and displaced ruptured keratocytes (Figs 21.3a and b).

The most appropriate method of smoothing lamellar keratectomy beds was by frequent application of small amounts of masking agent, with constant readjustment of the 'local distribution' of the liquid with cellulose (Weck-cell) sponges. This enabled removal of multiple small corneal surface projections without the unnecessary removal of deeper stroma. The resultant surface was smooth with some wrinkles and folds, suggesting a surface membrane (Fig. 21.3c). Multiple overlapping ablation zones were used to smooth the entire lamellar keratectomy base (Fig. 21.3d). Zones already smoothed were masked with HPMC to avoid unnecessary ablation. This technique was important in establishing criteria for treating large areas of stroma in the subsequent clinical cases.

SELECTING MASKING AGENTS

These initial laboratory studies suggested that the argon fluoride excimer laser could be used to smooth irregular corneal surfaces with a high degree of precision and with relative ease. It was hypothesized that, where the aim was removal of a uniform, diffuse, superficial corneal opacity, the precision of the techniques described would be entirely suited to the task. However, excimer laser photoablation is a surface phenomenon and, therefore, irregular surfaces cannot be levelled as a single-stage procedure by irradiation. If a rough surface of homogeneous tissue is irradiated, then a uniform layer of tissue will be removed with each laser pulse (Fig. 21.4) and, in order to produce a smooth surface, a masking agent with a similar ablation rate to that of the target material must be used (Fig. 21.5).

For masking purposes, a liquid more easily ablated than the surrounding tissue would have to be constantly reapplied in order not to perpetuate surface perturbations deeper in the tissue. If the ablation rate were less than the surrounding tissue, less frequent applications would be required and flow of the liquid between laser pulses would ensure that smoothing still occurred. The viscosity and the surface tension of the masking agent are also of importance. If liquids have high viscosity or surface tension they may form droplets and, on irradiation, contribute to further surface disturbances rather than smoothing. Surface tension and surface adhesion may also create problems in relation to filling relatively deep excavations, that is, those with low aspect ratios in terms of width and depth. The wetting agents selected in these early studies were those in clinical use and have a relatively prolonged contact with the corneal surface. All agents used were adequate for smoothing, but polyvinyl alcohol and HPMC 2% were too viscous and did not have good 'surface contour-following' properties. However, HPMC 1% was found to have ideal viscosity and was also convenient to apply and remove.

In these early laboratory investigations it was possible only to produce models of uneven surfaces that consisted of tissue with uniform ablation rate. While these models were identical to some surfaces encountered clinically (e.g. during lamellar keratoplasty or following removal of pterygia), a special case is encountered where surface projections are formed by

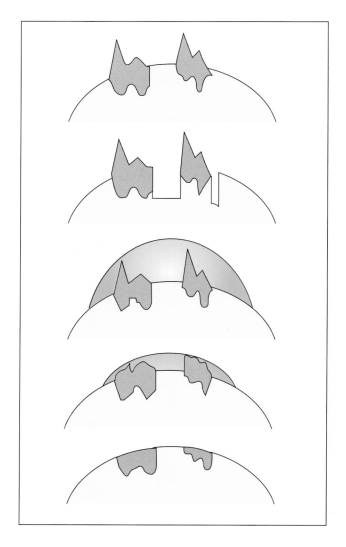

Figure 21.6 *Ablation of dense calcium deposits embedded within the stroma and projecting from the surface. (a) Initial surface. Calcium deposits are shaded. (b) After excimer laser irradiation without masking. The calcium deposits, having a lower ablation rate per pulse, are barely altered from their original heights (dotted line) while the intervening exposed stroma which has a higher ablation rate, has been unnecessarily excavated. (c) The same surface shielded with a masking liquid. (d) During ablation only exposed peaks and masking liquids are removed. (e) At the end of the procedure the surface has been smoothed. To remove the remaining calcium deposits embedded in the stroma normal corneal stroma will, of necessity, have to be removed but its rate of removal can be regulated by further applications of masking liquid. (Courtesy of* The British Journal of Ophthalmology *(1991)* **75***:258–69 and DS Gartry, MG Kerr Muir and J Marshall.)*

inclusions (e.g. calcium) with a much lower ablation rate than that of intervening tissue troughs (Fig. 21.6). Surface smoothing in this case requires an adjustable 'shield' through which the calcium peaks protrude and are ablated while the troughs are protected. The shield may then be lowered in order to complete the smoothing process. An ablation fluid with a slow ablation rate would obviously be preferable for such shielding. In practice, although HPMC 1% was not optimal for this purpose it was certainly adequate as a shielding agent.

The control of the distribution of HPMC 1% during photoablation is an interactive process between manual application and removal. The closed tip size and curvature of Colibri forceps, or similar, facilitates delivery of small quantities of HPMC without impairing the surgeon's view. Cellulose (Weck-cell) sponges applied to the edge of the target zone can be used to remove excess liquid; however, the fluid movement thus created by capillarity was found to be too rapid for accurate adjustment. It can be hypothesized that new sponge materials whose capillarity engenders less rapid fluid uptake would be more suited to the techniques described.

SECONDARY FLUORESCENCE

All three masking agents fluoresced when irradiated and the difference in the intensity and wavelength of fluorescence between the masking agent and the corneal substrate was helpful in monitoring the ablation process. The difference in fluorescence was best appreciated when viewing ablation of masked patterns of regular geometry. However, discrimination became more difficult during the ablation of masked, irregular, shallow surface perturbations. As a result of this target fluorescence, longer wavelength photons are generated, which may have deeper penetration and potential for DNA damage. The fluence associated with such secondary radiation at sites remote from the ablation surface, however, is low and as the fluorescence of the masking agent is primarily in the short wavelength (visible) portion of the electromagnetic spectrum, the predominant wavelengths produced are likely to be too long to be a secondary hazard of clinical significance.[1,2]

MORPHOLOGICAL ASSESSMENT

The use of masking agents did not seem to affect the nature of the ablated surface, in comparison with excimer laser ablation without masking agents, since it was uniform in the pattern experiments. Although chemical analysis of the resultant surface after ablation was not pursued, the homogeneity seen in these early morphological studies indicated that no chemical interactions had occurred between the masking liquid and adjacent biological tissues. All surfaces were sealed with a 'pseudomembrane'[3–6] as shown by wrinkling, and previous studies had shown that, whatever the nature of the pseudomembrane, it is transitory and does not interfere with subsequent healing processes.[7]

CONCLUSIONS BASED ON LABORATORY STUDIES

The conclusions from these early laboratory studies suggested that the excimer laser could be used to remove tissue from the corneal surface with a high degree of precision, leaving a smooth surface that was likely to be of good optical quality.

INITIAL PHOTOTHERAPEUTIC KERATECTOMY STUDY AT ST. THOMAS' HOSPITAL, LONDON

OUTLINE OF THE STUDY

The aim of this study was to evaluate the safety and efficacy of excimer laser treatment (PTK) in a series of patients with various forms of superficial corneal pathology. A UV200 Excimed excimer laser (Summit Technology, Waltham, Massachusetts, USA), with an emission wavelength of 193 nm, a fixed pulse repetition rate of 10 Hz and a fixed radiant exposure of 180 mJ/cm^2 at the corneal plane, was used.

The initial study comprised 25 patients who volunteered to undergo excimer laser superficial keratectomy to remove band keratopathy or to smooth a roughened corneal surface arising from some other pathology (Tables 21.1–21.6). Amethocaine 1% eyedrops were instilled, a speculum inserted (Fig. 21.7a) and the patient taught to fixate the center of a ring of fiber optic lights located around the laser aperture (Fig. 21.7b). A beam diameter was selected to match the areas to be treated and, in some cases, this was altered at different stages in the procedure. The effects of photoablation were assessed with the integral binocular operating microscope positioned alongside the laser aperture. Once steady fixation was achieved, masking liquid was applied to the corneal surface and photoablation commenced. During the process the surgeon could vary the site of ablation by making small movements of the patient's head (Fig. 21.7c). Following the procedure, which

lasted about 15 minutes, a mydriatic (homatropine 2% eyedrops) and antibiotic (chloramphenical 1% ointment) were instilled and the eye padded for 24 hours. For the first month, chloramphenicol 0.5% eyedrops were used four times a day. The team

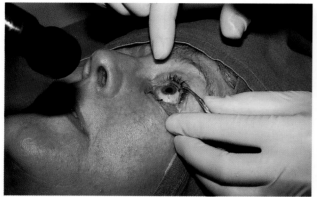

(a)

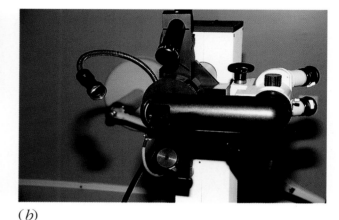

(b)

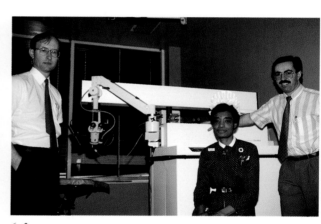

(d)

(c)

Figure 21.7 (a) After careful preoperative draping the patient is positioned supine with the eye to be treated directly beneath the laser aperture. Topical anesthetic is instilled and a lid speculum is inserted by the surgeon (Mr David S Gartry MD,FRCS, Moorfields Eye Hospital, London). (b) A patient's eye view of the laser aperture. The patient is encouraged to fixate on a central target within the aperture while the surgeon utilizes the geometry of the intersecting beams from the two helium neon lasers at each side of the main aperture to position the patient precisely. (c) The alignment of the patient is more critical when performing photorefractive keratectomy (PRK) and is facilitated by small corrective movements of the patient's head made by the surgeon throughout the procedure. (d) The members of the first UK team to perform PTK and PRK. From left to right: Mr Malcolm Kerr Muir FRCS, Sister Anne Welch SRN, and David Gartry MD,FRCS. (Note: there appears to be a 66% myopia prevalence!)

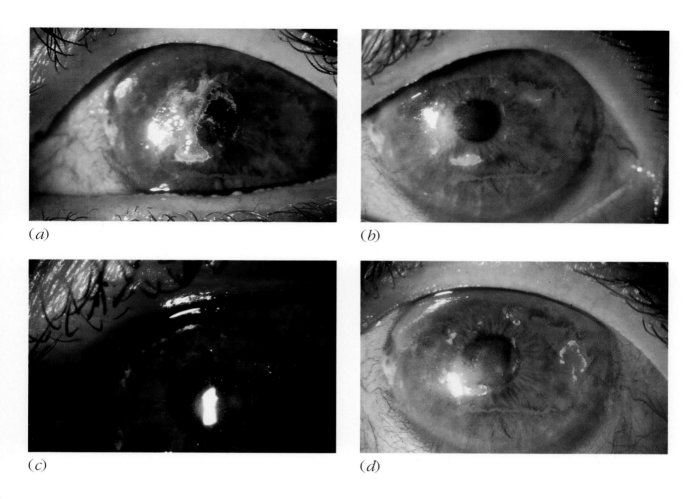

(a)　(b)　(c)　(d)

Figure 21.8　*Case 1. Rough band keratopathy. (a) Preoperative appearance. Extensive calcium deposition is present producing a grossly uneven surface. (b) Immediate postoperative appearance. The majority of the calcium has been ablated leaving a smooth surface. (c) Appearance 5 months after treatment with the excimer laser. (d) Appearance 18 months after ablation. The treated areas remain clear; however, recurrence of band keratopathy has resulted in some loss of corneal transparency. (Courtesy of* The British Journal of Ophthalmology *(1991)* **75***:258–69 and DS Gartry, MG Kerr Muir and J Marshall.)*

members from the original study are shown in Figure 21.7d.

The corneal surface characteristics of selected patients were examined and recorded with a prototype photokeratoscope.[8] In addition, while it was impossible in the majority of cases to comment on the preoperative status of the corneal endothelium due to superficial opacification, it was examined postoperatively at intervals via specular reflection with the slit lamp. Refraction was carried out where possible. Although the morphology of band keratopathy varied considerably, patients were subdi-vided into two broad categories. The first had rough, craggy deposits with varying degrees of discomfort, the second smooth even deposits with little or no discomfort and a healthy corneal epithelium.

Two treatment regimes were undertaken. Either a single 4 mm diameter ablation zone or a series of partially overlapping 4 mm diameter zones were used. The single area technique was most commonly used for smooth bands causing impaired vision and glare, and the multiple zone technique for rough, painful band keratopathy. The following 3 cases represent the spectrum of pathology created.

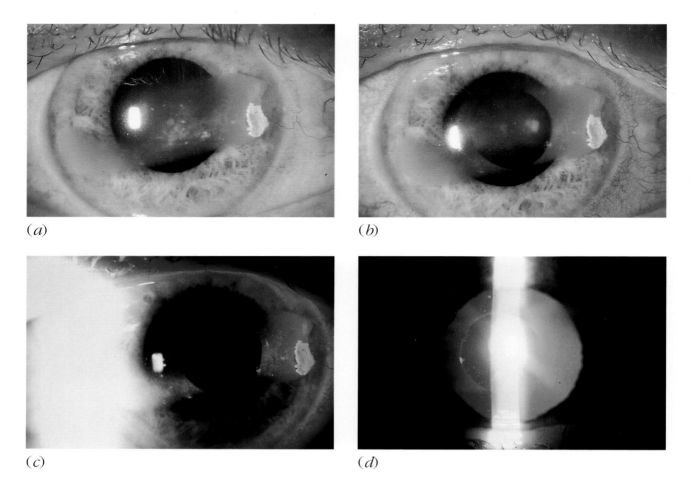

(a) (b)

(c) (d)

Figure 21.9 *Case 2. Even, diffuse band keratopathy. (a) Preoperative appearance showing an even, diffuse band keratopathy—granular in places. (b) The appearance 3 months after excimer ablation of a single, central 'on axis' zone to clear the visual axis. The increased clarity of the central ablated zone is evident and the slight central haze represents lenticular opacity. (c) Postoperative appearance at 3 months utilizing sclerotic scatter to highlight the clarity of the treated area. Note the remarkable clarity of this central zone (underlying lenticular opacities now being excluded). (d) Appearance 4 months after ablation by retroillumination, which confirms the enhanced transparency of the central cornea. (Courtesy of The British Journal of Ophthalmology (1991) **75**:258–69 and DS Gartry, MG Kerr Muir and J Marshall.)*

SELECTED CASE STUDIES

Group 1 Rough symptomatic (uncomfortable/painful) band keratopathy

Case 1

A 49-year-old female with systemic lupus erythematosus, who had been undergoing renal dialysis since 1981 and who had undergone parathyroidectomy in 1984 for primary hyperparathyroidism. Her left eye had been painful since 1974 and the mainstay of her treatment was topical lubricants. In 1987 she had undergone removal of band keratopathy with the aid of a chelating agent, EDTA. In spite of this, she still had severe pain in the left eye, aggravated by blinking, which disrupted sleep. She exhibited an extensive irregular, thickened band keratopathy with a best corrected visual acuity of 6/36. Islands of calcium protruded through unstable epithelium (Fig. 21.8a). The right eye was normal.

In February 1988 she became the first sighted patient in the UK to undergo excimer laser PTK. She had multiple overlapping zones located in the central

6 mm of the cornea (Fig. 21.8b). Approximately 300–400 pulses were delivered to each site of ablation. The procedure was pain free. One hour later, however, she complained of some discomfort, which resolved over 36 hours when the cornea had re-epithelialized. One week later she was entirely asymptomatic. At this stage the area of photoablation was smooth with minimal central thinning and a faint anterior stromal haze. The acuity was 6/24, improving to 6/12 with pinhole. At 5 months post-treatment there was early recurrence of band keratopathy (Fig. 21.8c) and by 18 months this began to cause discomfort. A small central epithelial erosion and faint central stromal haze were noted at this time, with the zone of ablation remaining markedly clearer than the surrounding area (Fig. 21.8d).

Group 2 Smooth (glare-inducing) band keratopathy

Case 2

A 72-year-old male had bilateral, evenly distributed idiopathic band keratopathy (Fig. 21.9a). He had no discomfort but complained of glare and impaired vision: 6/24 right and 6/18 left. He had a right 4 mm axial PTK without 1% HPMC masking, and the appearance at 3–4 months is shown in Figures 21.9b–d. Figure 21.9c, using sclerotic scatter, highlights the clarity of the central cornea compared to the adjacent band keratopathy against the background of the dilated pupil. Visual acuity in the right eye improved to 6/12 but 'veiling' glare was subjectively unchanged.

Case 3

A 67-year-old male developed a dense, evenly distributed band keratopathy in his right eye after retinal detachment surgery, which had included injection of silicone oil (Fig. 21.10a). He had also undergone right extracapsular cataract extraction. Before PTK there was only a limited view into the anterior chamber, which was full of silicone oil. Vision was restricted to hand movements in the inferior field only. Phototherapeutic keratectomy was undertaken primarily for cosmetic reasons and to improve the view of the posterior segment. Overlapping ablation zones were used to clear the cornea of band keratopathy and 1% HPMC was used to mask previously ablated areas. At 3 months the cornea was clear with an optically smooth surface (Fig. 21.10b). A good view of the anterior chamber, intraocular lens and retina was obtained. As expected there was no significant improvement in vision.

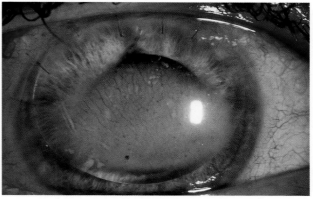

(a)

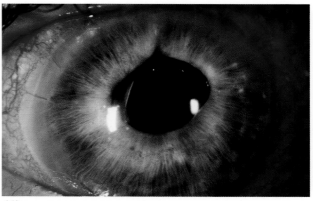

(b)

Figure 21.10 *Case 3. Dense, even band keratopathy treated with overlapping ablation zones in order to clear the entire corneal surface. (a) Preoperative appearance. A dense, even band keratopathy extends across most of the cornea. Silicone oil was present in the anterior chamber, shown by the reflex which delineates its margin underlying the 10/0 nylon sutures from previous cataract surgery. (b) Appearance 3 months following excimer laser ablation utilizing overlapping and contiguous zones. There has been total clearance of the calcium leaving a smooth, clear cornea. Slight residual haze represents deep, pre-existing, stromal scarring. (Courtesy of* The British Journal of Ophthalmology *(1991)* **75***:258–69 and DS Gartry, MG Kerr Muir and J Marshall.)*

GENERAL CONSIDERATIONS

No patients reported discomfort during the excimer laser PTK procedure; however, postoperatively the majority of patients experienced some discomfort for 24–48 hours. The intensity and duration of discomfort appeared to be related to the area of ablation.

Table 21.1
Rough band keratopathy treated by several overlapping ablation zones

Number	Sex	Age (years)	Band type	Etiology	Preoperative symptoms	Visual acuity (pre-operative)	Postoperative symptoms	Visual acuity (post-operative)	Follow-up (months)	Comment
1	F	49	rough surface, very irregular	increased serum Ca^{++}	pain, photophobia, reduced visual acuity	6/36	asymptomatic	6/12	30	band recurrence after 18 months
2	M	45	rough, very irregular	trauma	pain	PL	asymptomatic	PL	30	stable
3	M	50	rough, raised, thick band	trauma	pain	NPL	asymptomatic	NPL	30	stable
4	M	34	rough, irregular, disorganized anterior segment	high myope, failed retinal detachment surgery	irritable, red, pain on blinking	PL	asymptomatic, pleased with cosmesis	PL	14	stable
5	F	66	central, proud, Ca^{++} plaque	HSV keratitis	pain, reduced visual acuity	CF	asymptomatic, (occasional ache)	6/36	14	stable
6	F	72	classic band	herpes zoster	pain, epiphora, reduced visual acuity	6/24	asymptomatic	6/18	12	stable
7	F	33	islands of Ca^{++} (previous EDTA treatment)	uveitis in childhood	poor cosmesis, minimal discomfort	NPL	unchanged	NPL	10	highly mobile eye during treatment (surgery abandoned)
8	F	78	central Ca^{++} area and diffuse Ca^{++} surround	HSV keratitis	pain, epiphora, reduced visual acuity	CF	asymptomatic, slight increase in VA	4/60	10	stable

PL = perception of light
NPL = No perception of light
CF = Counting finger vision

Table 21.2
Rough band keratopathy treated with single 'on axis' ablation zones

Number	Sex	Age (years)	Band type	Etiology	Preoperative symptoms	Visual acuity (pre-operative)	Postoperative symptoms	Visual acuity (post-operative)	Follow-up (months)	Comment
9	F	20	central Ca++ plaque	uveitis in childhood	poor cosmesis	NPL	improved cosmesis	NPL	10	epithelial ablation only required
10	F	80	rough, central, Ca++ deposit	interstitial keratitis	pain, epiphora	2/60	marked improvement	2/60	12	stable

Table 21.3
Other disorders resulting in rough corneal surfaces treated by excimer ablation

Number	Sex	Age (years)	Band type	Etiology	Preoperative symptoms	Visual acuity (pre-operative)	Postoperative symptoms	Visual acuity (post-operative)	Follow-up (months)	Comment
11	M	27	mucus plaque	atopic, vernal eye disease	pain, photophobia, reduced visual acuity	6/60	asymptomatic	6/18	14	re-epithelialized, no plaque recurrence
12	F	45	rough, raised, granular dystrophy	recurrent granular dystrophy in a grafted (PK) eye	soreness, photophobia, reduced visual acuity	6/24	asymptomatic	6/18	30	no recurrence
13	F	46	extensive lattice dystrophy	lattice dystrophy	glare, photophobia, reduced visual acuity	6/60	asymptomatic, marked increase in visual acuity	6/9	6	no recurrence, no glare hyperopic shift
14	F	46	central raised nodules	Salzmann's degeneration	discomfort, reduced visual acuity	6/18	asymptomatic	6/12	10	stable
15	F	82	anterior stromal scarring	Cogan's epithelial dystrophy	reduced visual acuity, recurrent erosion	4/60	asymptomatic improved visual acuity	6/12	10	stable, central area treated

Table 21.4
Smooth surface band keratopathy treated with multiple overlapping ablation zones

Number	Sex	Age (years)	Band type	Etiology	Preoperative symptoms	Visual acuity (pre-operative)	Postoperative symptoms	Visual acuity (post-operative)	Follow-up (months)	Comment
16	F	32	even, inferior cornea	trauma in childhood	discomfort	NPL	asymptomatic	NPL	30	stable but recurrence after 18/12 (slight)
17	M	67	even, dense, thick band	failed RD, surgery, silicon oil in AC	glare, reduced visual acuity poor cosmesis	HM	glare unchanged good cosmesis	CF	12	recurrence after 6/12
18	F	81	even, moderately dense	idiopathic	glare, reduced visual acuity	6/18	reduced glare	6/18	12	change in refraction (hyperopic shift)
19	F	45	even	uveitis glaucoma surgery	glare, reduced visual acuity	6/9	glare greatly improved but reduced visual acuity	6/18	12	change in refraction (hyperopic shift) and induced astigmatism
20	F	70	even, fine	idiopathic	reduced visual acuity, Rx to improve view for cataract surgery	6/36	improved visual acuity	6/12	10	cataract surgery facilitated

Table 21.5
Smooth surface band keratopathy treated with 'on axis' single ablation zones

Number	Sex	Age (years)	Band type	Etiology	Preoperative symptoms	Visual acuity (pre-operative)	Postoperative symptoms	Visual acuity (post-operative)	Follow-up (months)	Comment
21	M	23	even, fine	uveitis	reduced visual acuity	6/36	improved visual acuity	6/9	30	cornea remained clear, refraction change (hyper-opic shift)
22	M	84	even, fine	idiopathic	glare, reduced visual acuity	6/24	glare improved and improved visual acuity	6/12	14	refraction change (hyper-opic shift)
23	F	73	even, fine	idiopathic	reduced visual acuity	6/36	improved visual acuity	6/18	14	change in refraction (hyperopic shift)
24	F	82	even, fine	idiopathic	glare, reduced visual acuity	6/36	glare improved and improved visual acuity	6/18	6	cornea remained clear
25	F	14	even, fine	idiopathic	glare, reduced visual acuity	3/60	glare improved and improved visual acuity	6/60	12	cornea remained clear

Table 21.6
Refraction results before and after ablation (where applicable)

Number	Preoperative symptoms	Preoperative refraction	Postoperative visual acuity	Postoperative refraction
18	6/18	+3.00 D	6/18	+5.50 DS
19	6/9	plano	6/18	+4.00 DS/−2.50 DC ×85
21	6/36	plano	6/9	+1.50 DS
22	6/24	+1.00 DS	6/12	+4.50 DS
23	6/36	+0.50 DS	6/18	+5.00 DS/−1.75 DC × 35

Oral analgesics were required for 24 hours in all patients but in all cases re-epithelialization was complete by 48 hours. Sixteen of the 25 patients had an improvement in visual acuity (Tables 21.1–21.6). The 13 patients with uneven, symptomatic (painful) band keratopathy were greatly improved and five became symptom-free.

THERAPEUTIC OUTCOME

These early studies did not identify any complications or undesirable findings that would have precluded further investigations of the clinical use of excimer lasers in ophthalmic surgical practice. Although preoperative visual acuity was poor in a large proportion of patients, all except four were able to fixate with the eye undergoing treatment. In these four patients adequate alignment was achieved, with the normal eye fixating an adjustable target at one side of the laser aperture. In only one patient was it impossible to treat the band keratopathy because of eye movement. None of the patients detected the induced fluorescence during ablation in spite of this being clearly visible to all observers. It is of interest that some of the patients in a group undergoing PRK subsequently were aware of a faint blue haze with each pulse. In contrast to the lack of visual stimulation, auditory and olfactory sensations were notable. The patients were warned about the noise and the smell of burning, which were demonstrated prior to the procedure by ablating paper.

Tables 21.1–21.5 show that postoperative progress was related to the extent of the initial pathology. Systematic analysis of the patient subsets was difficult because there were, by definition, significant variations in pathology. However, all patients with rough band keratopathy who had experienced pain preoperatively became asymptomatic (Tables 21.1 and 21.2). Most were treated with several overlapping ablation zones in order to smooth the cornea completely (Table 21.1). Table 21.2, however, includes those patients who had a relatively small rough central area of band, which was successfully treated with a single central ablation. In four patients visual acuity improved. Those with no improvement had extensive pathology of which the band formed only one part. Four of the five patients with allied disorders that resulted in a rough corneal surface showed an improvement in visual acuity. Those with symptoms of soreness, pain and photophobia were rendered asymptomatic (Tables 21.1–21.3).

Smooth-surfaced band deposition was treated with either several overlapping ablation zones (Table 21.4) or a single 'on-axis' ablation zone, 4 mm in diameter (Table 21.5). The principal indications were reduced visual acuity and glare. Those patients suffering glare disability had a marked improvement, which was sustained throughout the follow-up period (6–30 months). In the group treated with overlapping zones, one patient showed an increase in visual acuity, one a reduced visual acuity and the other three no significant difference. In case 19, glare was markedly improved but acuity decreased. This reduction was due to irregular astigmatism because of the faceted surface generated by overlapping ablation zones. In contrast, in the group in which a central 'on-axis' was ablated (Table 21.5), visual acuity was improved in each case and glare reduced.

THE 'HYPEROPIC SHIFT'

Where refraction results could be obtained, a 'plus shift' (i.e. towards hypermetropia) was noted. Those patients in whom accurate subjective refraction was possible are listed in Table 21.6. The mean hyperopic shift for this group was 2.85 diopters.

This hyperopic shift (which is equivalent to a myopic correction) was an unexpected finding as the smoothing procedure is not analogous to PRK in which a deliberate attempt is made to reprofile the anterior corneal surface in order to effect a change in refraction. This flattening of the cornea implies that some form of differential ablation must have occurred.[5,9–12]

There are several potential mechanisms that could account for this hyperopic shift:

- If a band progressively thins towards the visual axis then constant irradiance from the laser will effect greater ablation centrally and induce a hyperopic shift. This effect would be enhanced if the ablation rate of the band was less than stroma.
- Although excimer laser radiation will remove an even layer of tissue, regardless of the curvature of the surface, the subsurface structure of the cornea is laminated. Removal of central portions of corneal lamellae could, theoretically, cause centrifugal differential contraction and central flattening.
- The centrifugal spray of particles of debris and ablation products might be expected to shield the stroma and could, theoretically, provide progressively greater shielding towards the edge of the ablated zone.
- Increased obliquity of incident radiation falling upon more peripheral cornea might result in a relative decrease in energy density as the edge of the ablation zone is approached. It is unlikely, however, that the degree of differential ablation encountered could arise from inhomogeneities in the excimer beam.
- The maximum diameter of the ablation zone used in these early studies was limited to only 4 mm, in part due to the conservative approach that was adopted in these early cases (larger ablation zones would, by definition, remove a greater volume of corneal tissue) but mainly due to technical constraints with the Summit laser. It is possible that a relative surface flattening could have occurred if the new corneal epithelium thinned towards the center of the treated area. Conversely, the new epithelium could conceiv-

ably have become slightly 'heaped up' or hyperplastic at the edge of the ablation zone due to the relatively sharp change in contour that occurred in this region. This would have the same relative effects as central epithelial thinning. We therefore hypothesized that the hyperopic shift may be considerably reduced if larger diameter ablation zones are used, and this would seem to be borne out by our subsequent longer-term studies in which the mean hyperopic shift was approximately 1.4 D.

CONCLUSIONS AND PATIENT SELECTION GUIDELINES FOR PTK

From these studies, which included the first series of patients with corneal pathology treated with an excimer laser worldwide, it was possible to put forward recommendations for patient selection:

- For patients with rough band keratopathy the excimer laser is a successful treatment. All patients with pain and photophobia became asymptomatic (these eyes will usually have limited visual potential).
- Where pathology is limited to the anterior stroma, pain relief is likely to be accompanied by an improvement in visual acuity.
- In eyes with good visual potential it is best not to clear all of the band keratopathy by using overlapping ablation zones since, although glare will be markedly reduced, irregular astigmatism may result, which could lead to reduced visual acuity.

Thus, a single, axial zone of ablation should be employed. We also demonstrated that a hyperopic shift occurs when the central cornea is ablated and patients should be warned about the possibility of anisometropia. In conclusion, given the encouraging results, the ease with which the procedure can be performed, the patient acceptance of the procedure, and the fact that all cases in these early studies were treated on an outpatient basis, PTK would seem to be an excellent alternative treatment modality for these cases.

REFERENCES

1. Sliney DH, Krueger RR, Trokel SL, Rappaport KD, Photokeratitis from 193 nm argon-fluoride laser radiation, *Photochem Photobiol* (1991) **53**:739–44.
2. Muller-Stolzenburg NW, Muller GJ, Buchwald HJ, et al, UV exposure of the lens during 193 nm excimer laser corneal surgery, *Arch Ophthalmol* (1990) **108**:915–6.
3. Marshall J, Trokel S, Rothery S, Schubert H, An ultrastructural study of corneal incisions induced by an excimer laser at 193 nm, *Ophthalmology* (1985) **92**:749–58.
4. Marshall J, Trokel S, Rothery S, Krueger RR, A comparative study of corneal incisions induced by diamond and steel knives and two ultraviolet radiations from an excimer laser, *Br J Ophthalmol* (1986) **70**:482–501.
5. Marshall J, Trokel S, Rothery S, Krueger RR, Photoablative reprofiling of the cornea using an excimer laser: Photorefractive keratectomy, *Lasers in Ophthalmol* (1986) **1**:21–48.
6. Kerr Muir MG, Trokel SL, Marshall J, Rothery S, Ultrastructural comparison of conventional surgical and Argon Fluoride excimer laser keratectomy, *Am J Ophthalmol* (1987) **103**:448–53.
7. Marshall J, Trokel S, Rothery S, Krueger RR, Long-term healing of the central cornea after photorefractive keratectomy using an excimer laser, *Ophthalmology* (1988) **95**:1411–21.
8. Zabel RW, Tuft SJ, Fitzke FW, Marshall J, Corneal topography: A new photokeratoscope, *Eye* (1989) **3**:198–301.
9. Munnerlyn CR, Koons SJ, Marshall J, Photorefractive keratectomy: A technique for laser refractive surgery, *J Cataract Ref Surg* (1988) **14**:46–52.
10. Seiler T, Kahle G, Kriegerowski M, Bende T, Myopic excimer laser (193 nm) keratomileusis in sighted and blind human eyes, *Refract Corneal Surg* (1990) **6**:165–73.
11. McDonald MB, Frantz M, Klyce SD et al, Central photorefractive keratectomy for myopia: The blind eye study, *Arch Ophthalmol* (1990) **108**:799–808.
12. Taylor DM, L'Esperance FA, Del Pero RA, Human excimer laser lamellar keratectomy: A clinical study, *Ophthalmology* (1989) **96**:654–64.

Chapter 22 Phototherapeutic keratectomy: clinical studies

Christine R Ellerton and Charles N J McGhee

THE DEVELOPMENT OF PHOTOTHERAPEUTIC KERATECTOMY (PTK)

The use of excimer lasers in ophthalmic surgery was first suggested in 1983 by Trokel et al[1] after its successful industrial application in etching precise patterns in plastics. Indeed, excimer laser enables the removal of superficial corneal tissue with great precision and the resulting excisional cuts are highly accurate in terms of the intended depth, length and reproducibility.[2,3] Ultimately this has led to 'sculpting' of the healthy corneal surface to produce refractive change—photorefractive keratectomy (PRK)—the most popular and widespread use of the excimer laser. However, due to its potential for accurate ablation of anterior stromal corneal lesions, without significant damage to adjacent non-ablated tissue, the initial clinical utilization for this laser was removal of diseased corneal tissue—phototherapeutic keratectomy (PTK).

In 1985 Serdaveric et al[4] proposed the first therapeutic use of the excimer laser to treat an experimental Candida infectious keratitis. Concerns about ablating an already thinned, ulcerated cornea leading to inadvertent perforation, the uncertainty surrounding the effectiveness of treating organisms in adjacent intact stroma by excimer laser (due to poor corneal penetration at 193 mm), and possible risk of spreading micro-organisms during the treatment, subsequently resulted in limited interest in this technique.[5] Thereafter, clinical interest in PTK turned to the possibility of excising superficial corneal stromal opacities and to smoothing irregular surface abnormalities.

The Food and Drug Administration (FDA) sponsored multicentred trials in the USA investigating the safety and effectiveness of PTK in humans using the Visx[6] and the Summit[7] excimer lasers commencing in 1989. The initial inclusion criteria required the patients to have significant functional impairment and to be candidates for conventional invasive corneal surgery. Patients fell into several categories:

- Visual impairment due to opacities in the anterior third of the cornea.
- Visual impairment due to fine corneal surface irregularities.
- Superficial infectious keratitis resistant to medical treatment.
- Significant functional impairment due to pathologic or postsurgical refractive abnormalities of the eye.
- Significant recurrent corneal epithelial breakdown.

FDA exclusion criteria included immunocompromised patients, uncontrolled uveitis, severe blepharitis, lagophthalmos, or dry eye. The immediate (residual) postoperative corneal thickness had to be not less than 250 μm, with the maximum of one-third corneal depth ablation.

INITIAL VISX FDA STUDIES

In the Visx laser group, the patients received preoperative oral analgesia and sedation. The procedure was then performed under topical anaesthesia (0.5% proparacaine drops). Typical treatment parameters included laser fluence of 160 ±10 mJ/cm², repetition rate of 10 Hz, giving an ablation rate of 0.20–0.35 μm per pulse, and an ablation zone of 5.5–6.0 mm diameter. The epithelium was manually removed in cases where the anterior stromal surface was judged to be smooth, otherwise it was ablated with the laser allowing the epithelium to act as a smoothing agent. Masking agents were used if required to help produce an even surface. Postoperatively the patients were reviewed every 24–48 hours until re-epithelialization had occurred and thereafter at 1, 3, 6, 12 and 24 months from treatment.

Initial FDA results of 271 consecutive PTK cases carried out by the Visx laser[6] found 55% of patients had corneal scars or leukomas, 39% had corneal dystrophies, and 5% had corneal surface irregularities. The postoperative best corrected visual acuity (BCVA) improved by two or more lines compared to the preoperative level in 45% of patients; and worsened to the same degree in 10% of cases. Unaided visual acuity increased by two or more lines in 42–44% and deteriorated in 18–19%.

INITIAL SUMMIT FDA STUDIES

In the Summit laser group, initial assessment of 67 procedures with an average follow-up of 8.2 months were analyzed[7] according to the indication for treatment: corneal opacity, irregular surface, or epithelial breakdown. The unaided visual acuity improved by at least one line in 64–69%; whilst BCVA improved by this degree in 77% of corneal opacity cases, 70% of the irregular surface group and 36% in recurrent erosion patients. Deterioration in vision occurred in approximately 20% of all the groups, the exception being only 9% of epithelial breakdown subjects suffering a reduction of their unaided vision.

DEVELOPMENT OF PTK

Early PTK reports documented significant induced hyperopic shift in refraction following treatment; however, the FDA-sponsored studies demonstrated that adaptation of the laser technique can help reduce this complication. The encouraging results from these initial studies led to FDA conditional approval for PTK (March 1994)[8] prior to its approval of PRK in the USA (1995). In the UK, the first Ethics Committee approval was given to treat overt corneal lesions by excimer laser in February 1988 and the first PTK to be performed upon a sighted eye was carried out by Mr David Gartry MD in February 1988.[2]

CURRENT INDICATIONS FOR PTK

The current clinical practice of excimer laser PTK has expanded to include a wide diversity of corneal disorders. These may be considered in broad terms to fall into the following five overlapping categories:

1. To remove superficial corneal stromal opacities, such as post-infectious, traumatic scarring and anterior stromal dystrophies. The aims of treatment are to improve visual acuity and relieve symptoms of glare or monocular secondary images.
2. To treat or smooth irregular surface disorders, for example post-inflammatory, traumatic or degenerative corneal nodules as seen in Salzmann's nodules and keratoconic patients. Here the goal of treatment is to improve visual acuity, often by allowing contact lens wear.
3. To treat epithelial instability and failure of re-epithelization, for instance in recurrent corneal erosion syndrome, and vernal keratoconjunctivitis. Relief of ocular discomfort and the re-establishment of an intact, healthy epithelial surface is the major indication for treatment in this group of patients.
4. To reduce iatrogenically produced refractive errors, including induced astigmatism, irregular astigmatism and myopic anisometropia following cataract surgery, penetrating keratoplasty or other ophthalmic procedures.
5. Other miscellaneous uses of PTK include treatment to improve cosmesis and as an aid in the surgical treatment of pterygia.

The diagnostic indication for PTK may fall into several of these categories, one such example being rough band keratopathy, which may present both with visual symptoms and ocular pain. Careful assessment of the patient's requirements and their comprehension of the treatment goals are essential for appropriate patient selection (see Table 22.1 for important preoperative parameters to consider). The

Table 22.1

Important parameters to consider in the preoperative assessment of the PTK patient.

Patient symptoms and expectations
The type of corneal pathology
The depth of the pathology
Potential visual acuity
The proximity to the visual axis
Irregular astigmatism
Preoperative refraction

Table 22.2
The common indications for PTK.

Recurrent corneal epithelium erosions
Band keratopathy
Post-infectious corneal scars
Corneal dystrophies
Traumatic scars
Post-inflammatory corneal nodules

most commonly reported indication for PTK over the last few years is recurrent corneal erosion syndrome, followed by band keratopathy. The common indications for PTK treatment as cited from recent studies in Table 22.2.

DEVELOPMENTS IN PTK TECHNIQUE

Corneal epithelium, Bowman's layer and corneal stroma are ablated at different rates by the 193 nm excimer laser.[9] Pathological tissue also responds at varying rates: Campos et al[10] found longstanding scar tissue to be difficult to treat and had to abandon the procedure in one case of corneal calcification, after a total ablation depth of 140 µm failed to show increasing smoothness of the corneal surface, with regions of the scar being resistant to ablation. With increasing experience, it has become apparent that not all anterior stromal pathologies will yield to excimer laser PTK.

In patients with good visual potential in the eye particular care must be taken to avoid excessive refractive changes and irregular astigmatism. Initial PTK studies were performed with the eye kept stationary.[11] This led to sharply demarcated ablation zones with a high incidence of induced hyperopia. Early techniques utilizing relatively small ablation zone diameters, with overlapping treatment areas, resulted in high degrees of irregular astigmatism in some cases, especially if the anterior stroma was significantly ablated. Attempts to avoid these problems have included: utilizing a larger ablation zone size (5–6 mm); tapering the contour of the junction between the ablated and non-ablated region by moving the eye in a circular fashion under the laser; and applying 2 mm diameter 20 µm deep laser spots to the circumference of the ablation zone.[12]

Currently, many surgeons are employing manual movement of the patient's head during the procedure, in very small circular excursions, to smooth out the edge effects.

During the laser treatment of the corneal pathology, care must be taken to prevent ablation beyond the base of the lesion or of the adjacent healthy stroma. If this occurs the resultant corneal thinning can compromise the ocular integrity[13] and give rise to increased stromal remodelling. An induced hyperopic shift and irregular astigmatism can ensue. In general terms, to remove the irregularity whilst limiting the ablation of deeper tissues, several strategies may be applied:

- Frequent slit-lamp examination during the procedure to assess treatment progress.
- Restrict the laser ablation beam diameter to the zone of pathology. This option may not be suitable in regions adjacent to the visual axis in potentially seeing eyes, as irregular astigmatism caused at the junction of ablated to non-ablated tissues can limit the surgical success.
- Use a masking fluid or utilize the epithelium to shield adjacent healthy tissue and protect depressions between irregularities from excessive ablation.

MASKING AGENTS

Unlike many clinical laser systems, which focus their energy into a concentrated spot, the excimer laser beam has a large cross-sectional area and photoablation can therefore potentially take place over the entire region exposed. Assuming even rates of ablation across the zone, the original surface contour will be reproduced in the base of the treated area. Masking agents are used to smooth out any such surface irregularities by shielding the troughs from ablation. Different histological and pathological tissues have varying rates of ablation, therefore tissue surrounding opacities of relatively lower ablation rates, such as calcium in band keratopathy, require shielding from excessive ablation. A fluid can be used to mask deeper structures whilst leaving exposed protruding irregularities for laser ablation. The important properties of a masking agent have already been outlined in section one of this chapter.

Masking fluids of varying viscosities have been investigated. Kornmehl et al[14] in 1991 reported a comparative study of various masking agents: Hydroxypropylmethylcellulose (HPMC) 0.3% with Dextran 70 0.1%, carboxymethylcellulose 1% and saline 0.9%. A control group treated without masking fluid was established and assessment of the ability of each masking fluid to produce a smooth surface in an irregular anterior corneal model was made. Twenty-eight de-epithelialized fresh calf eyes were abraded with sandpaper and then subjected to excimer laser (Summit 2000; 180 mJ/cm² 10 Hz; nominally removing 0.24 µm per pulse, 4 mm ablation zone, 500 pulses). Immediately before the procedure the masking agent under investigation was applied with a cellulose microsurgical sponge. Intermittently during the laser treatment, if the surface appeared to be drying or bubbles developed in the masking agent, more fluid was applied by a single unidirectional wipe of the sponge across the surface. The globes were then promptly fixed and examined with the scanning electron microscope. The residual irregularity was independently graded as mild, moderate or severe. Seven eyes were examined in each group. Without masking fluid, the authors detected the most severe surface irregularity of undulating ripples and waves (a finding perhaps partly related to the processing method used for the electron microscope). Saline 0.9% produced a similar but less severe picture; whilst HPMC with Dextran 70 resulted in a smooth granular surface. Carboxymethylcellulose gave an intermediate pattern. These findings supported the use of a masking agent in clinical practice.

A similar study using a wire screen to create the initial irregular surface was performed by Fasano et al.[15] They assessed the benefits of HPMC 0.3% (n=12) against no masking agent (n=12), as well as investigating the effect of altering the ablation rate. They concluded that this masking agent provided a smooth surface, especially at an ablation rate of 2 Hz compared to 10 Hz, and conjectured that the slower ablation rate may allow the masking agent time to flow over the corneal surface filling in depressions. Gartry et al.[2] testing the relative merits of HPMC 1%, HPMC 2%, and polyvinyl alcohol, suggested that 1% solution of HPMC is the most suitable general purpose masking agent.

Clinical studies have utilized a variety of masking agents including a combination of methylcellulose and Dextran 70,[12] tetracaine eye drops,[16] sodium hyaluronate;[16,17] polyvinyl alcohol[2,10] and a range of HPMC concentrations from 0.25 to 2.5%.[2,16,18–21] The most popularly used masking fluid at present appears to be HPMC, a 1% solution used at the commencement of lasering, with different concentrations subse-quently being utilized if varying viscosity properties are required. To prevent a meniscus effect of the masking agent within surface depressions blotting the edges with cellulose sponges or spotting the masking fluid on using microcollibri forceps is recommended.[2,20] It should always be remembered that the use of a masking agent may result in the true depth of tissue ablation being significantly less than indicated by the laser settings, since considerable laser energy is dissipated ablating the fluid. Of course the use of fluid shielding agents is not routine in every instance of PTK, e.g. in the treatment of recurrent epithelial erosions masking of the surface of Bowman's layer is rarely required.

In PRK the epithelium is usually removed mechanically for a variety of reasons, including the concern that irregular epithelial thickness and the differential ablation rates of epithelial nuclei and cytoplasm may lead to uneven stromal ablation. However, for PTK the smooth epithelium can be utilized to act as a natural masking agent for the underlying stroma. In cases of smooth band keratopathy (intact epithelium, opacity at the level of Bowman's layer) and superficial corneal opacities, the epithelium has been used as a template for the excimer laser.[16,19,20,22,23] Hersh et al[19] denuded the epithelium over focal corneal excrescences whilst leaving it in situ over the adjacent tissues to help prevent excessive ablation around the lesions. O'Brart et al[20] and others have proposed that the good results achieved in PTK following transepithelial ablation may have implications for the current practice of mechanical epithelial removal in PRK (see Chapter 9).

PTK INDUCED HYPEROPIA

Early studies of PTK soon highlighted an induced hyperopia shift as a frequent complication of the treatment. Great variations in the incidence and degree of this problem appear in the literature. This variation may in part be due to the multiple pathologies involved in addition to the varied ablation zone diameter and treatment depths employed (Table 22.3). The potential mechanisms which may create this hyperopic shift have already been outlined in section one of this chapter.

The first published series of 25 cases of corneal disease undergoing PTK, reported by Gartry et al[2] in 1991, identified five patients with increased hypermetropia amongst those subjects in whom pre- and

Table 22.3

Hyperopic shift following PTK.

Study (Year)	Diagnosis	No. cases with refraction (n)	Hyperopic shift (Spherical equivalent (D)) (%) of n	Mean	Range	Ablation Zone diameter (mm)	Follow-up (months)
Gartry[2] (1991)	sBK^	5	100	2.85	1.5–4.13	various	12–30
Hersh[19] (1993)	mixed	12	67	5.40	—	1.5–5.0	1–4
O'Brart[20] (1993)	sBK	32	100	1.4	0–4.25	4.0–5.0	6
Campos[10] (1993)	mixed	18	56	6.4	—	5.3–6.0	3*
O'Brart[26] (1994)	RES	16	0	—	—	various	6–24
Claoue[21] (1995)	BK	9	100	2.4	1.25–5.25	6.0	7.5 (mean)

•Data for 3 months follow-up; see text.

post-operative refraction was available. They noted this complication in patients treated with multiple overlapping ablation zones as well as single 'on-axis' zones for smooth band keratopathy. The mean hyperopic change was +2.85 D.

Fagerholm et al[16] carried out PTK on 166 eyes of mixed pathology, in 28 of whom sufficient refractive data was available to allow analysis at 6 months. They reported significant hyperopia correlating to the number of stromal pulses used during the PTK. Another study of PTK for mixed diagnoses, with a limited follow-up of 1–4 months, reported by Hersh et al,[19] noted a refractive change in all patients. Eight out of the 12 eyes showed a hyperopic shift with a mean of +5.40 D spherical equivalent, whereas three eyes actually exhibited a mean myopic shift of –1.6 D. This study included off-axis peripheral treatments and ablation zones of varied diameter.

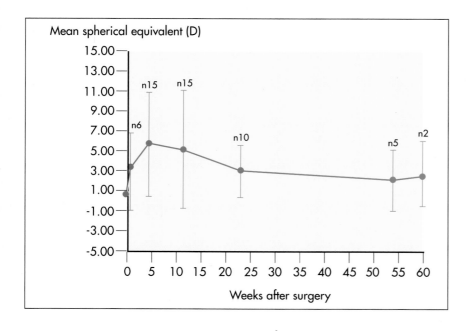

Figure 22.1 *Hyperopic shift post phototherapeutic keratectomy shown against time. In this early series a very dramatic induced hyperopia was noted in the first three months, although this diminished with time from procedure (Adapted from Campos et al 1993[10]).*

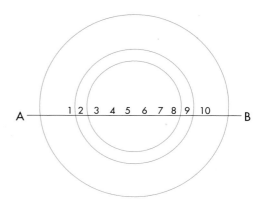

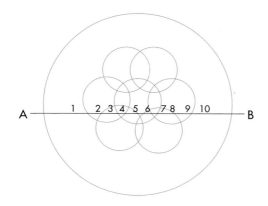

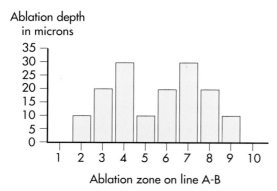

Ablation zone on line A-B

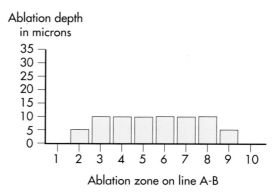

Ablation zone on line A-B

Figure 22.2 *Prior to the availability of wider ablation zones, if PTK was required over an area greater than the laser beam width this was performed using a series of overlapping zones. In this illustrative case a series of 7 overlapping 3 mm diameter ablation zones, each of 10 µm depth, shown being utilized to treat a central 8 mm diameter region of the cornea. Consideration of the variable depth of ablation across the treated zone (line A-B) highlights the manner in which unwanted refractive effects, such as induced hyperopia and irregular astigmatism could be produced by this technique.*

Figure 22.3 *Using a 6 mm diameter PTK ablation zone coupled with small oscillatory movements of the head produces an even ablation depth without a stepped interface between treated and untreated cornea. Compare the theoretical ablation depths along line A-B for this single wide zone PTK of 10 µm to the variable depths created by multiple overlapping smaller zones (Fig. 22.2).*

The initial hyperopic shift tends to regress after treatment. Campos and colleagues[10] reported their findings of 18 eyes undergoing PTK for various corneal opacities with a follow-up of 2–18 months. They utilized a centrally aligned ablation zone of 5.3–6.0 mm diameter to a depth of 80–200 µm. Ten eyes (55.6%) exhibited a hyperopic shift post-operatively. In terms of the mean spherical equivalent of the group, a gradual decrease in the hyperopia occurred with time which was reflected by a rise in mean keratometry measurements (Fig. 22.1).

MINIMIZING AND PREVENTING UNWANTED REFRACTIVE CHANGES POST PTK

Measures to avoid significant refractive change include (Figs 22.2 and 22.3):

- Limiting the depth of corneal stromal ablation
- Preventing a sharp junction between the ablated and non-ablated zone by smoothing techniques such as head rotation during the laser procedure

- Avoiding the overlap of zone margins near the visual axis
- Avoiding eccentrically placed ablation zones which may produce astigmatism.

Knowledge of the preoperative refraction status in a potentially sighted eye is essential wherever possible and the induced hyperopic change may be utilized in myopic patients. Indeed, one patient treated for Reis–Buckler's corneal dystrophy reported by Hersh[19] improved from a preoperative myopic correction of $-7.00/-2.00 \times 90°$ to -1.00 D at three months. However, in the emmetropic or presbyopic eye such changes may result in undesirable hyperopia/anisometropia. Patients must be fully informed and adequately consented preoperatively in respect of the risks of refractive change.

TREATMENT OF POST-PTK INDUCED HYPEROPIA BY CONTACT LENS

Hyperopia and induced irregular astigmatism following PTK can be difficult to manage. Contact lens fitting based on the central keratometric readings is virtually impossible.[23] Campos et al[10,24] believe that the possibility of induced refractive change must be carefully considered by the patient preoperatively; treatment should not be carried out if a contact lens alone will improve the visual acuity and it should be ensured that the patient will be able to wear a contact lens postoperatively if necessary.

However, Eggink and Beekhuis[23] report the successful contact lens correction of both eyes of a patient with granular dystrophy following a 5.0 mm diameter ablation zone PTK. At 1 week high oxygen-transmissible, aspheric, rigid contact lenses were used successfully to correct the +3.5 D hyperopic shift and central irregular astigmatism. The pericentral corneal region outside the ablation zone was used to bear the contact lenses and a 10.2 mm diameter lens riding under the upper lid was used to facilitate lens movement and tear film exchange. The authors compared the corneal topography maps at 1 week and 4 months after PTK and contact lens fitting, concluding that the change in corneal surface profile demonstrated represented epithelial hyperplasia or possibly stromal remodelling, modifying the refractive power of the cornea. There was no change in the corrected visual acuity over this period. The authors acknowledged the concerns of applying a contact lens at 1 week post-PTK, at a time when epithelial thickness and hemidesmosome numbers may not have not returned to preoperative levels. Other methods considered in the management of hyperopia following excimer laser photoablation are discussed in Chapter 17.

CLINICAL RESULTS OF PTK FOR INDIVIDUAL PATHOLOGIES

RECURRENT CORNEAL EROSION SYNDROME

First described by Hansen in 1872, recurrent corneal epithelial erosion typically causes episodes of acute pain, lacrimation and photophobia on waking. There may be a history of previous ocular trauma, or it may occur spontaneously – probably in association with epithelial basement membrane degeneration or Cogan's dystrophy. Phototherapeutic keratectomy has been reserved for patients in whom conventional medical treatments, including topical lubricants and hyperosmotic solutions, mechanical debridement, and soft contact lenses, have all failed.

Dausch et al[25] in 1988 treated the first patient with recalcitrant recurrent corneal erosion syndrome by PTK, having observed the apparently increased re-epithelialization rate produced after PTK of a corneal tumour. The first case responded favorably and the group went on to treat other patients, reporting their findings of 74 eyes. Subsequently several other authors have reported series of PTK for recurrent corneal erosion after failed medical treatment.[18,26–30] Dausch[25] employed the MEL 50 Aesculap Meditec laser in spot mode with a high radiant exposure at the cornea of 800 mJ/cm², repetition rate 2 Hz, and pulse duration of 20 ns. Thomann[28] used the MEL 60 Aesculap Meditec laser with similar parameters in both spot mode and scanning mode. However, most authors have reported PTK treatment carried out with the Summit UV200, ExciMed, or OmniMed lasers – with radiant exposure at the cornea of 180 mJ/cm²; repetition rate 10 Hz; ablation depth per pulse 0.25 µm; and ablation zone diameters of 1–6.5 mm depending on the area involved.

A large, single central zone of ablation (5.0–6.5 mm) is recommended for paracentral or axial epithelial abnormalities to avoid possible irregular astigmatism. The size of a peripherally placed lesion determines the treatment spot size. O'Brart et al[26] purposefully left the paralimbal areas untreated in cases in which there was virtually complete corneal

Table 22.4

Results of PTK for recurrent corneal epithelial erosions (RCEE).

Study	No. of cases	Age mean (years)	Follow-up mean (months)	Follow-up range (months)	Recurrence RCEE (%)	Repeat PTK (%)	Haze at 3 months (%)
Dausch[25]	74	39	21	6–50	25.7	0	1.4
Fagerholm[16]	37*	47	12	6–28	16.2	16.2	—
O'Brart[26]	17	43	11	6–28	23.5	11.7	5.9A
Algawi[27]	15	41	9	2–16	0	0	0
Thomann[28]	13	62	14	1–28	—	38.5	***
Forster[18]	9*	—	—	6–?	11.1	0	—
John[29]	2	37	18	18	0	0	—

*cases of RES as part of a multipathology PTK study
**resolved by 6 months
***cases of bullous keratopathy secondary to endothelial failure

epithelial disturbance. The depth of ablation is restricted to within Bowman's membrane (12 µm); with Fagerholm,[16] Foster,[18] and Hersh[19] aiming to remove less than 4 µm; whilst Algawi[27] and O'Brart[26] suggest deeper ablation to 5–12.5 µm. Treatment is restricted only to affected areas of the cornea which may be highlighted by areas of microcystic change, irregular fluorescein staining or corneal topographic changes.[31]

Mechanical removal of the loose or abnormal epithelium identified by slit-lamp examination, using a cellulose sponge or surgical blade, is usually carried out at the commencement of the procedure. However, Dausch et al[25] have avoided mechanical debridement and used the excimer laser to ablate the abnormal epithelium with projected depths of 30–40 µm, smoothing out the ablation margins in an attempt to aid epithelial cell migration. The denuded areas are then ablated to a projected depth of 1–3 µm. Mechanical removal was only used in this particular study when the loose epithelium appeared 'bleb-like'.

Most investigators report rapid re-epithelialization, with the vast majority of cases healing within 4–6 days.[18,25,26] Patients may experience moderate ocular pain, usually over the initial 24 hour post-PTK period; however, the majority of patients become symptom-free within the first few days after treatment. Some patients are rendered recurrence-free but still report minor symptoms of dry eye and discomfort requiring the occasional use of topical lubricants,[25] but these symptoms are at a much reduced intensity and

frequency relative to their preoperative state.[16,25,27] (Results of representative clinical studies are highlighted in Table 22.4).

Recurrence rate following PTK for recurrent corneal erosions

Of 74 eyes reported by Dausch et al[25] following PTK for recurrent epithelial erosion 55 eyes (74.3%) remained symptom-free of recurrences over a follow-up period of 6 to 50 months, 19 eyes (25.6%) experienced recurrent episodes, with multiple attacks in approximately 40% of this latter group. These recurrent symptoms occurred 1 to 22 months post-treatment (mean 8.4 months). O'Brart[26] also identified recurrent episodes in 23.5% of eyes at 3–6 months post PTK. Further PTK was performed in two cases, rendering both asymptomatic. Algawi[27] found no objective evidence of recurrences, although 13% of subjects noted mild symptoms of foreign body sensation. Fagerholm[16] reported PTK retreatment in 6 of 37 patients (16.2%), in 2 eyes within the previously treated corneal area, and in a further four cases additional PTK was applied to adjacent regions.

Post-PTK corneal haze and visual acuity

The presence of a persistent corneal haze after PTK for recurrent corneal erosion syndrome is rare due to the shallow ablation depth. Dausch[25] reported one patient with a superficial haze (grade 1) present 9 months post-treatment, which was ascribed to a postoperative infection and did not affect the visual acuity. In the study's remaining 73 eyes no slit-lamp evidence of the laser treatment was visible. Although O'Brart[26] identified five cases (29%) with faint subepithelial haze at 3 months, all cases of haze had cleared by 6 months, leaving only one patient with pre-existing anterior stromal scars. In contrast, Algawi[27] reported grade 0.5 haze in all eyes within the initial 4 weeks postoperatively; however, these cases of minor haze resolved completely over several months. Corneal topography has demonstrated no evidence of surface irregularities or the ablation zones.[27]

Most investigators[18,26–29] have found no adverse effects on the unaided and best corrected visual acuities (BCVA) following PTK for recurrent epithelial erosions. Indeed, 47% of cases reported by O'Brart actually had improved by at least one Snellen line 6 months postoperatively.[26]

Post PTK refractive change

Although it has been shown that subjective refraction after PTK for recurrent erosion syndrome appears unchanged,[27,29] others,[26] although demonstrating no statistical difference between the preoperative and 6 month post-operative manifest refraction, have noted a myopic shift, greater than –0.5 D persisting at 6 months post laser. This has not been associated with central corneal steepening on topography and may reflect a change in epithelial thickness or stability.

Comparison with anterior stromal puncture

Anterior stromal puncture with a hypodermic needle or a Nd:YAG laser has been advocated for the treatment of difficult recurrent corneal erosion cases.[32,33] Table 22.5 outlines a comparison between these two surgical treatment methods—it appears excimer PTK may be a better clinical option, especially in cases involving the axial cornea.

PTK for recurrent erosions associated with bullous keratopathy

Most of the studies to date have involved patients with recurrent corneal epithelial erosions related to

Table 22.5

Comparison of anterior stromal puncture and PTK for recurrent corneal epithelial erosions.

Feature	Anterior stromal puncture	Excimer PTK
Availability	Widespread	Restricted
Cost	Inexpensive	Expensive
Success rate	High	High
Postoperative stromal scars	Yes	No
Visual acuity worsened	Yes, if axial treatment	No
Risk of corneal perforation	Yes, especially with small gauge needles	No

trauma or underlying epithelial basement membrane disorders; however, recently PTK has been investigated for epithelial erosions occurring in bullous keratopathy. Thomann et al[28] have reported PTK on 13 eyes of such patients who were unsuitable candidates for penetrating keratoplasty—too unfit for surgery, or with no visual potential due to other ocular morbidity. Their goal was to relieve ocular pain and reduce the risk of secondary infectious keratitis. In all cases the initial laser therapy considerably reduced the symptom of pain; 4 patients were pain free over the follow-up interval of 1–28 (mean of 14.1) months; 4 patients had mild symptoms; and in the remaining 5 cases repeat PTK was performed at the patients' request for persistent irritation. Bullae rarely persisted after 1–2 months following the treatment.

Summary: PTK for recurrent corneal erosion

Excimer laser PTK appears to offer a safe and successful means of treating recurrent painful corneal erosions which are resistant to conventional medical therapy. The overall success rate is 74–89%.[18,25,26] Probably because of the limited ablation depths required, restricted to within Bowman's membrane, complications are minimal. A transient corneal haze may occur in the first few months following treatment. Visual acuity appears to be unaffected or

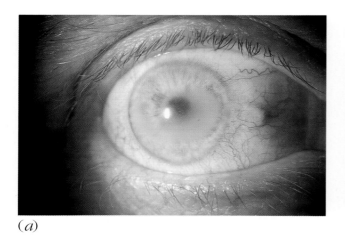

(a)

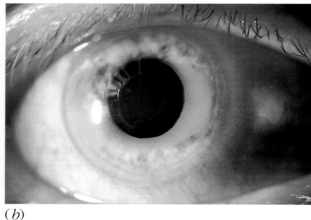

(b)

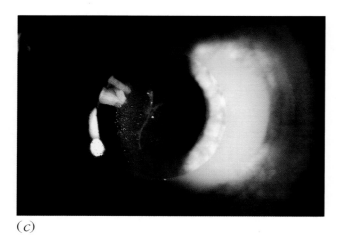

(c)

Figure 22.4 *(a) Demonstrates an eye with smooth band keratopathy, intact epithelium and a BSCVA of 6/9 associated with severe glare symptoms. (b) One day after a 6 mm diameter transepithelial PTK the eye demonstrates complete clearance of calcium in the central cornea and the epithelial defect has healed more than 50%. (c) On the third postoperative day the epithelial defect was fully closed with a vertical epithelial healing line. The sharply demarcated edge of the PTK ablation zone can clearly be seen in retro-illumination. Pre-operatively the eye exhibited −0.75 D of myopia. Six months post-operatively all symptoms of glare and decreased contrast had dissipated, the eye obtained 6/6 unaided acuity and corrected to 6/5 with a +0.50 D correction.*

improved. No significant manifest refractive change occurs; however, there may be a tendency to slight myopia. Slit-lamp and corneal topography reveal no abnormalities. Promising initial results have been reported for recurrent erosions secondary to bullous keratopathy.

PHOTOTHERAPEUTIC KERATECTOMY FOR BAND KERATOPATHY

In band keratopathy there is extracellular deposition of granular material in the epithelial basement membrane, Bowman's layer and anterior stroma. This usually consists of calcium phosphate and carbonate salts. Traditional treatments for this condition include chelating agents such as ethylene-diamine-tetra-acetic acid (EDTA), and mechanical keratectomy. In some cases the opacification represents elastotic degeneration of collagen and may explain why chelating agents are not always an effective mode of therapy.[20] Patients with band keratopathy may be subdivided into two broad groups: those with a smooth surface of intact epithelium, with calcified material lying at Bowman's membrane, who experience symptoms of glare and disturbed vision when the visual axis is involved; the remaining patients have a rough band keratopathy where the overlying epithelium is unstable. In the latter group pain may occur and the eye often has poor visual potential due to coexisting ocular pathology.

Table 22.6
Indications for PTK in band keratopathy.

Study	No. of cases	Pain (%)	Glare (%)	Reduced VA (%)	Other (%)
O'Brart[20]	122 total	30	39	63	5.7
	78 smooth	—	62	87	3.8*
	44 rough	84	—	20	9**
Claoue[21]	21 total	33	—	67	29***
	8 smooth	—	—	100	—
	13 rough	46	—	46	—

Several indications for treatment may occur in one eye.
*three eyes treated to improve perop. view for cataract surgery.
**four eyes treated to allow cosmetic contact lens wear.
*** six eyes treated for poor cosmesis.

Indications and technique

As in all cases considered for PTK, careful preoperative evaluation of the patient is essential. In one of the largest published series, O'Brart[20] stresses that the presence of ocular pain, other than foreign body sensation, and the absence of subtarsal inflammation in rough band keratopathy suggest the eye is unlikely to benefit from PTK, and other explanations for the pain should be sought. Assessment of the presenting symptoms and the potential for good vision is required to plan the most appropriate ablation technique. Single axial ablation zones restricted to the anterior 100 µm of the stroma for sighted eyes reduces the complications of induced irregular astigmatism and hyperopic shift (Fig. 22.4). Whereas in blind eyes the emphasis is on pain relief and multiple overlapping ablation zones extending deeper into the stroma may therefore be indicated. Table 22.6 summarizes the indications for PTK from two recent

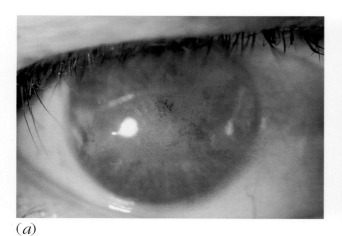

(a)

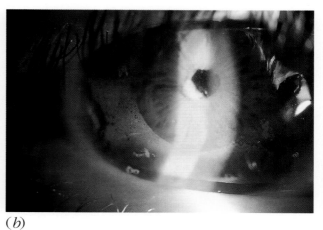

(b)

Figure 22.5 (a) The cornea of a patient with chronic rheumatoid arthritis and recurrent uveitis which exhibited a granular, smooth band shaped keratopathy with BSCVA of 6/18. (b) One month after a 6 mm diameter, transepithelial PTK the axial cornea is free from calcium and only trace subepithelial haze can be seen (BSCVA 6/9). Corneal topography was regular with less than +0.50 D of induced hyperopia.

studies reporting exclusively on PTK for band keratopathy.

Unlike PTK for recurrent erosion, masking fluids are commonly employed in the treatment of band keratopathy. The epithelium may also be used as a smoothing template (Fig. 22.5) in smooth band keratopathy and therefore is not debrided mechanically in these cases.[20,21] In contrast, in cases of rough band keratopathy large calcified plaques should be removed mechanically prior to lasering, with the advantages of: enabling the PTK to be performed more quickly; reducing the need for multiple applications of masking fluid; and achieving a smoother ocular surface.[20]

Results and complications of PTK for band keratopathy

Subsequent to Gartry's[2] initial investigation of PTK including 20 cases of band keratopathy (outlined in the earlier section of this chapter), several authors have reported the results of large series (Table 22.7 summarizes this data).

O'Brart[20] in a large study of 122 eyes reported rapid recovery in all 78 eyes treated for smooth band keratopathy. Comparing each category of preoperative symptom, the postoperative results demonstrated: 88% improved visual acuity; and 88% reduction in glare. Complications in this group included: one case of recurrent epithelial erosions (which resolved after

3 months), minimal subepithelial haze which was insignificant compared to the preoperative band opacity, and a universally induced hyperopic shift—with a mean of 1.4 D at 6 months. In the 44 eyes with rough band keratopathy ocular discomfort lessened in 95% of patients, and the mean visual acuity improved, but did not reach statistically significant levels. In three eyes undergoing PTK to facilitate cataract surgery success was achieved in all cases and a further three eyes treated to allow a cosmetic contact lens fitment responded successfully. One case of transient recurrent erosions occurred and one patient suffered a reduction in Snellen acuity due to induced irregular astigmatism. Recurrence of band keratopathy occurred in nine eyes (7.4%) and three underwent repeat PTK. Five of these cases were associated with silicone oil within the anterior chamber.

Claoue,[21] reporting on 21 cases, noted improved Snellen acuity in 53% of eyes judged to have good visual potential. In six (35%) patients the postoperative visual acuity was unchanged following PTK. Pain was reduced or absent in all patients. Some patients exhibited stromal haze but in all cases the cornea clarity was improved compared to pretreatment. Refractive data was available in 9 patients and showed a hyperopic shift in 100%, with a mean of 2.4 D (range 1.25–5.25 D). Induced astigmatic change occurred in 35%, increasing by a mean of 1.3 D. One patient developed delayed re-epithelialization, requiring a bandage contact lens and preservative-free drops for 3 weeks.

Table 22.7
Results of PTK in band keratopathy.

Study	No. of cases	Mean follow-up (months)	Range follow-up (months)	BCVA* improved	Hyperopic shift**	Pain relief
O'Brart[20]	78s	10	3–54	88%	100% mean 1.4 D	—
O'Brart[20]	44r	16	3–60	Not stated		95%
Claoue[21]	21	7.5	–	53%	100% mean 2.4 D	100%

*of eyes with potentially good visual acuity.

**of eyes with sufficient refraction data.

s = smooth band keratopathy.

r = rough band keratopathy.

Tununanen and Tervo[17] treated 9 cases of band keratopathy by a combination of EDTA, manual debridement and PTK. A resultant improvement of corneal clarity occurred in 100%; transient corneal decompensation was noted in two eyes—one was a corneal graft after ocular trauma and the other was a case of uveitis with secondary glaucoma.

Other authors commenting on smaller numbers of eyes have achieved similar results for pain relief, and improved corneal clarity with few complications,[10,16,18,19] confirming the initial promising results reported by Gartry.[2]

Post PTK morphology

The histology of one patient who underwent PTK for smooth band keratopathy secondary to intraocular silicone oil, and who subsequently had a penetrating keratoplasty for corneal decompensation 1 year later, has been reported by O'Brart.[20] In the area corresponding to previous laser ablation the epithelium showed normal anatomy, whereas, in the untreated regions, the cellular layers were attenuated and disrupted with loss of the basal columnar layer. This suggests epithelial cell maturation and function is adversely affected by the underlying granular deposits. PTK and other forms of surgical treatment appear to allow the epithelium to re-establish its normal characteristics by removing the deposits. Binder et al[34] reporting on the histopathology of 12 eyes previously treated with PTK include one case of herpes zoster keratitis with band keratopathy who underwent corneal transplantation after 9 months for persistent scarring and recurrent erosions. The epithelium was absent over the ablated zone probably reflecting a change in the epithelial attachment to the underlying substrata, and a heavy band of keratocytes was found in the mid-stromal region localized deep to the ablated zone. The authors could not determine whether the scar tissue was related to the laser or the primary disease process.

Summary: PTK for band keratopathy

Excimer PTK appears to be a very successful out-patient treatment option for band keratopathy both to relieve the associated pain and to improve the corneal clarity, and hence visual acuity in potentially sighted eyes. It is well tolerated by the patients and has a rapid rehabilitation time with minimal complications, other than the induced hyperopic shift, reported to date.

PHOTOTHERAPEUTIC KERATECTOMY FOR CORNEAL DYSTROPHIES

The clinical use of PTK for corneal dystrophies is less well documented than that for recurrent corneal erosions or band keratopathy. Most cases in the literature are included in studies involving various other corneal disorders. Statistically significant results are therefore limited by the small case numbers available. A wide range of dystrophies have undergone PTK.[2,10,16,17,19,22,23,35]

The objectives of excimer PTK in the treatment of corneal dystrophies overlap with those for other corneal pathologies: painful recurrent corneal erosions may be prominent in Cogan's and Reis–Buckler's dystrophies, whereas reduced vision secondary to the subepithelial opacities of Reis–Buckler's and loss of stromal clarity in granular and lattice dystrophies provide optical indications for treatment (Figs 22.6 and 22.7). In those conditions where the corneal opacities are anteriorly placed, PTK appears to be becoming a promising alternative to lamellar or penetrating keratoplasty.

Fagerholm et al[16] included 27 patients with a corneal dystrophy in their long-term results of 166 eyes, but unfortunately did not analyse the various

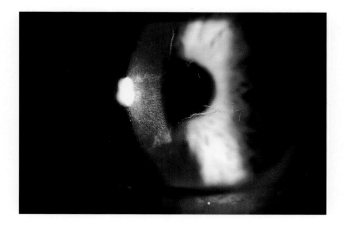

Figure 22.6 *The cornea of a subject with lattice dystrophy and painful recurrent corneal erosion syndrome. Following a small zone focal PTK in the region of the recurrent epithelial defect all corneal symptoms resolved but the cornea developed focal grade I subepithelial corneal haze which did not affect BSCVA. (Courtesy of Mr Stephen Morgan MD.)*

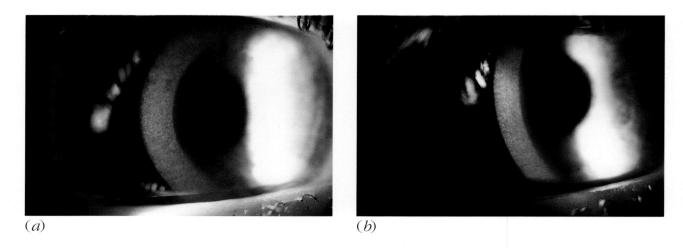

(*a*)   (*b*)

Figure 22.7 (*a*) *Pre-operative appearance of a subject with Reis Bucklers corneal dystrophy associated with very severe recurrent corneal erosion syndrome. (b) Corneal appearance of the same eye six weeks after a superficial PTK. The eye became entirely asymptomatic with a healthy epithelium and a modest decrease in the corneal opacity. (Courtesy of Mr Stephen Morgan MD.)*

dystrophies (Fuch's, granular, lattice, Schnyder's, Meesman's and anterior basement membrane) independently. As expected from the range of diagnoses, there were several treatment goals: to improve visual acuity in 22 cases; to increase visual acuity and wound healing in three cases; and to stabilize the refraction of two cases. Reported as one group, 21 of the 27 patients (77.8%) achieved the therapeutic goal. Tuunanen and Tervo[17] also achieved an improved best corrected visual acuity in four of five cases of corneal dystrophy, the exception being a macular dystrophy which lost one line of Snellen acuity due to irregular astigmatism.

Ablation of the epithelium overlying irregular anterior stromal opacities in certain cases of corneal dystrophy may be beneficial.[22] PTK also appears to be developing as an attractive alternative treatment modality for cases of recurrent corneal dystrophies (such as lattice[19] and granular[35]) following penetrating keratoplasty, when the alternative is repeat keratoplasty. John[35] reported a case of recurrent granular dystrophy in which the eye underwent PTK for a combination of symptomatic stromal opacification and post-keratoplasty myopia of –6.00 D. Both symptomatic relief and visual improvement were achieved postoperatively; however, after 8 months there were signs of recurrence of the dystrophy within the treated eye.

The complications following PTK for corneal dystrophies, as might be anticipated, are similar to those previously documented following PTK for band keratopathy and recurrent corneal erosion. In two eyes with lattice dystrophy reported by Campos,[10] in which a large ablation zone of 5.5–6.0 mm diameter was employed, each case resulted in a marked improvement of best corrected visual acuity from 20/200 to 20/30 or better, although a significant hyperopic shift occurred.

PHOTOTHERAPEUTIC KERATECTOMY FOR CORNEAL SCARS

PTK has been used to treat anterior stromal corneal scars secondary to various etiologies including post-infectious keratitis and following trauma. The technique of PTK for corneal scars follows the general principles outlined earlier in this chapter. Assessment of the depth to which the scar extends can be made by slit-lamp examination with an optical pachymeter. Masking agents are employed during the procedure and frequent slit-lamp biomicroscopic evaluation is undertaken to gauge treatment progress.

Fagerholm et al[16] treated 30 eyes with post-infectious scars (excluding herpes simplex) with a maximum ablation depth of 75 mm to the stroma: 73% achieved their treatment goal; 50% of the failures were scheduled for penetrating keratoplasty for residual deep corneal opacification. Campos[10] noted a 50% improved visual acuity result for six cases of post-infective scarring.

Trachoma resulting in diffuse superficial corneal scarring is a major cause of blindness in the world. Corneal transplantation might normally be considered in superficial corneal scarring; however, post-infectious trachomatous scarring of the conjunctiva and lids, coupled with corneal vascularization, provides a very poor environment for penetrating keratoplasty survival. Goldstein et al[36] have reported three patients in whom excimer phototherapeutic keratectomy was performed; the visual acuity was significantly increased in two of the cases, although a hyperopic shift was present. The remaining patient had no postoperative improvement and subsequently underwent penetrating keratoplasty. The authors suggest survival of the graft should not be compromised.

PTK has been effectively performed for post-herpes simplex corneal scarring. Fagerholm[16] reported 15 such patients including two children under general anesthesia; with a mean follow-up period of 15.7 months. Eighty per cent achieved the goal of three or more Snellen lines of improved visual acuity. Hersh[19] treated a central Herpes simplex scar which resulted in a drop of unaided visual acuity from 20/70 to 20/320 due to postoperative irregular astigmatism; however, the contact lens corrected vision was improved to 20/50, and the authors felt this was acceptable as the alternative to PTK had been a penetrating keratoplasty.

Herpes simplex virus can be reactivated by excimer laser treatment (Fig. 22.8). One patient in Fagerholm's study[16] had three attacks of recurrent keratitis during the 28 month post-operative period. Campos et al[10] used prophylactic systemic acyclovir (200 mg orally, four times a day preoperatively and for 10 days postoperative) in a patient with a post-herpetic scar and lattice dystrophy. No recurrence of herpetic keratitis occurred during the 15 months follow-up. Hersh[19] also prescribed oral Acyclovir and topical antiviral agents perioperatively in one case treated for post-herpetic scarring. Talamo[37] pretreated a patient with trifluoro-thymadine daily for several days prior to PTK for a herpes simplex scar which had shown no clinical signs of active keratitis for more than one year. This treatment was continued along with fluorometholone 0.25% postoperatively. No reactivation of the keratitis was recorded.

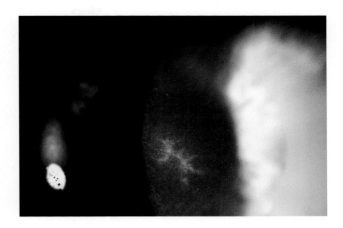

Figure 22.8 *A cornea one week post phototherapeutic keratectomy for band shaped keratopathy, demonstrating reactivation of Herpes Simplex keratitis. This reactivation responded rapidly, without sequelae, to the institution of topical acyclovir.*

Relatively small numbers of post-traumatic scars treated by PTK[10,16–18] have been published. The results however appear to be favorable.

PHOTOTHERAPEUTIC KERATECTOMY FOR IATROGENIC REFRACTIVE DISORDERS

An increasing use of the excimer laser is to correct iatrogenically-induced myopia or astigmatism. PARK programs designed to remove the toric surface of regular astigmatism have been used in the management of cases of astigmatism secondary to cataract surgery,[38] penetrating keratoplasty,[35,38,39] and epikeratoplasty.[40]

Campos et al[39] performed cylindrical ablations with the excimer laser in 12 patients with contact lens intolerant severe post-keratoplasty astigmatism. Follow-up ranged from 6 to 14 months (mean of 8 months). Unaided VA improved in 75%, was unchanged in 16.7%, and decreased in 8.3%; the corresponding values for spectacle-corrected vision being 58%, 33.3%, and 8.3%. Although the mean preoperative refractive cylinder of 7.0±3.6 D had reduced at 1 month to 3.1±0.7 D, regression of effect resulted in a mean 'final' cylinder of 4.3±2.9 D at the last follow-up (i.e. overall a mean decrease of 39%)

with a mean axis shift of 58±62°. Four patients were overcorrected. Pachymetry showed a substantial thinning of 0.09±0.05 mm in corneal thickness. Re-epithelialization after the PTK was not prolonged except in one patient who had a penetrating kerato-plasty after a chemical injury to the eye. No case of clinically significant corneal haze or graft rejection occurred.

In contrast John et al[35] reported that one eye, out of three cases of PTK for residual myopia after penetrating keratoplasty, who developed a moderate degree (3+) of corneal haze reducing the vision at 3 months. Campos et al[39] acknowledge that their small series of patients does not demonstrate that PTK is a superior technique over other surgical methods for dealing with the difficult clinical problem of post-keratoplasty astigmatism.

Rapuano and Laibson[38] report the results of four patients with surgically induced myopia and/or astig-matism who were contact lens intolerant and demon-strated stable refractions at least 1 year post-surgery. Corneal transplantation had resulted in astigmatism in two cases and myopia in one case. Cataract surgery causing high astigmatism accounted for the remaining patient. Follow-up data was limited to a mean of 4 months (range 1–6 months). A mild post-PTK reticular haze occurred in all eyes but was not associated with symptoms of glare nor was it thought to account for decreased vision. Three eyes showed increased unaided VA. Best corrected visual acuity improved in one patient by four Snellen lines, remained unchanged in two cases, and decreased in one eye at 1 month – possibly related to new macular edema from an old branch retinal vein occlusion. Mean keratometric readings reduced by 2.4 D (range 1.5–3.25 D) and in the astigmatic cases the keratometric cylinder decreased by an average of 2.5 D (range 0.5–5.5 D). No episode of graft rejection or failure occurred.

The authors have treated a small series of subjects with post cataract and post keratoplasty myopic/astigmatic refractive errors and whilst the initial 2–3 month results for both groups look promising, longer term results have been disappointing in the kerato-plasty group. Both haze and significant regression are more common in the post-keratoplasty group compared to other causes of iatrogenic refractive disorder, and it may transpire that transplanted corneal tissue heals in a distinctly different way from normal healthy cornea (Figs 22.9–22.11).

To date the reported results of PTK/PARK for iatro-genic refractive disorders involve small series with very short-term results. Further follow-up and greater numbers are required before its usefulness can be

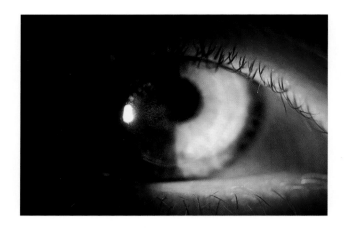

Figure 22.9 *A cornea one year after a –5.00 D PRK to correct induced myopic anisometropia following penetrating keratoplasty. Trace subepithelial corneal haze can be seen within the corneal graft, but this did not affect BSCVA at any point post operatively.*

assessed. Regression of the initial improved refraction obtained by PTK appears to be a limiting factor for its application.[35,39]

Combining PTK and PRK

In some circumstances a combination of phototherapeutic and photorefractive ablation patterns is more appropriate. The PTK may be indicated for an associated corneal opacity, such as recurrent dystrophies in penetrating keratoplasty,[19,35] or to treat irregular astigmatism (Fig. 22.12).

Gibralter and Trokel[41] have described a method of incorporating PTK and PRK. A topographic map was used to identify 'steep' areas of the cornea which were then lasered by focal small-diameter PTK ablations, employing Dextran 70 as a masking agent following mechanical epithelial removal. A guide to the ablation depth required for localized irregular areas of corneal steepness was based on an approx-imation relating the thickness of a solid spherical element to its diameter for each diopter of power shown on the topographic map:

Depth in μm = 1/3 diameter^2 × Diopters

This calculation is limited by the smoothing functions of the topographic software. Once the differences between 'steeper' and 'flatter' geographic areas within the optical zone had been treated, PRK

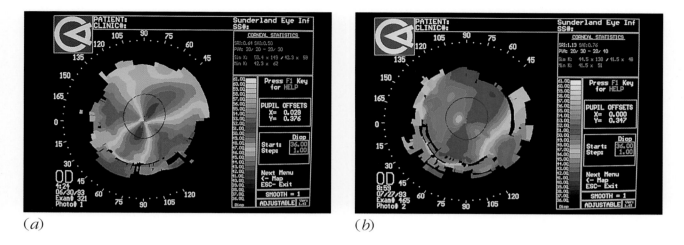

(*a*)   (*b*)

Figure 22.10 *Computerised corneal topography of an eye with post penetrating keratoplasty myopic astigmatism. (a) Pre-PARK topographic appearance demonstrating 8.1 D of keratometric astigmatism. (b) Four weeks after a PARK of −2.00/−8.00 at 60° demonstrating a reduction in manifest and keratometric astigmatism by approximately 5.00 D.*

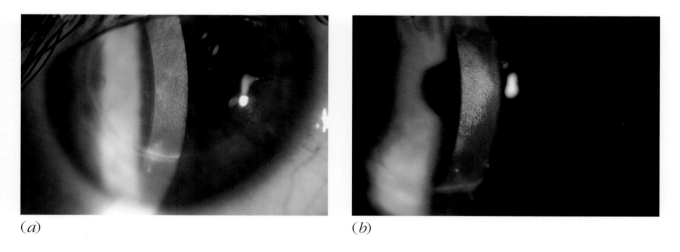

(*a*)   (*b*)

Figure 22.11 *Clinical slit-lamp photographs of the eye illustrated by corneal topography Fig. 22.10b. (a) Six months post-PARK. Diffuse grade I haze with focal areas of reticular grade II within the ablation zone. (b) The eye was retreated one year after the initial PARK because of regression and corneal haze but, despite an entirely clear cornea and 6/9 unaided visual acuity for several months post retreatment, severe corneal haze recurred between 6 and 9 months and persists at 18 months post retreatment.*

was then performed centered over the entrance pupil to correct residual myopia. Two patients with high degrees of irregular astigmatism intolerant of contact lenses (following myopic keratomileusis, and penetrating keratoplasty for keratoconus) were treated in this fashion. The unaided visual acuities improved from preoperative values. In one patient the PRK component was intentionally adjusted for an undercorrection of −2.25 D due to concern that the peripherally placed PTK focal treatments might contribute to the overall corneal flattening. A residual myopia of −2.75 D resulted.

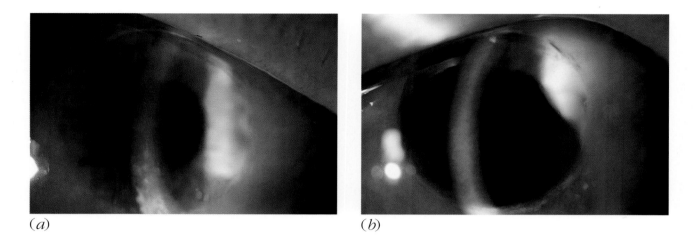

(a)

(b)

Figure 22.12 *(a) Pre-operative appearance of an eye that had undergone a 6 mm penetrating keratoplasty for corneal macular dystrophy several years earlier. Recurrence of the dystrophy can readily be seen in the superficial graft inferiorly accompanied by axial deposition of iron. (b) Three months after PRK for post keratoplasty induced myopic anisometropia the graft is entirely clear and free of clinically visible macular dystrophy.*

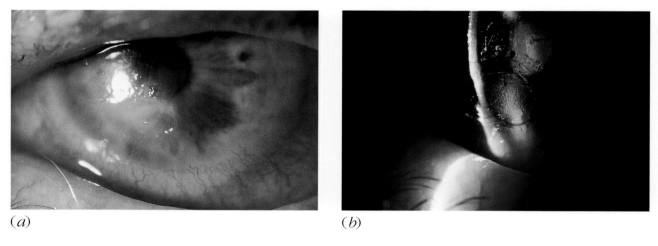

(a)

(b)

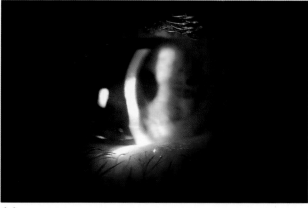

(c)

Figure 22.13 *PTK treatment of a longstanding, non-healing, sterile epithelial trophic ulcer recalcitrant to conventional management. (a) Pre-operative appearance with grey lustreless epithelium surrounding a central defect just inferior to the visual axis. (b) Immediately post photatherapeutic keratectomy following debridement of loose epithelium and a very superficial PTK to the ulcer base. (c) The epithelial defect healed within three days of PTK and the epithelium remained stable—as demonstrated six weeks post PTK (subepithelial haze subjacent to the area of the ulcer was present prior to PTK). (Courtesy of Mr Stephen Morgan MD.)*

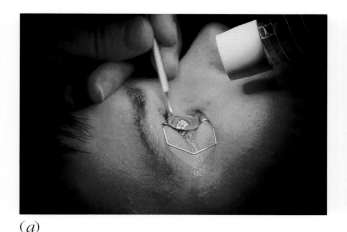

(*a*)

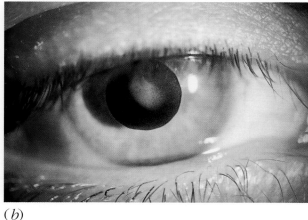

(*b*)

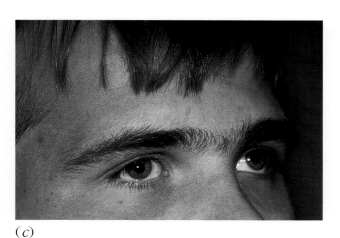

(*c*)

Figure 22.14 *A very unusual indication for PTK— excimer laser assisted corneal tattooing in a young man with a (painless) blind right eye and a densely white cataract unsuitable for intraocular surgery. (a) The right eye is fixated by a Thornton ring intra-operatively as a 5 mm transepithelial superficial central PTK is performed prior to staining the lasered bed with platinum. (b) A slit lamp phototgraph of the corneal appearance four weeks after laser assisted tattooing. (c) Clinical appearance of the right eye four months after PTK and platinum tattooing. The patient, who had previously requested enucleation of the blind eye because of its poor cosmetic appearance, was delighted with the result. (Courtesy of the Australian and New Zealand Journal of Ophthalmology)*

Lawless et al[42] reported 14 eyes that required a dual PTK and PRK treatment for manifest scarring and regression unresponsive to topical corticosteroids after an initial myopic PRK. A 5.0 mm trans-epithelial PTK ablation zone was employed and then a subsequent PRK was performed. The amount of PRK was generally set at the pretreatment refraction plus −1.00 D to allow for remaining central epithelium; however, the authors varied this depending on the pretreatment refraction and scar depth. The follow-up period was short, ranging from 1 to 9 months; however, within this time no scarring redeveloped nor did significant refractive regression occur. The eyes appeared to stabilize more rapidly than after the primary PRK.

These promising initial results suggest a future role for PTK combined with PRK in the management of the challenging problem of iatrogenically induced refractive astigmatism.

PHOTOTHERAPEUTIC KERATECTOMY FOR PTERYGIUM

The use of PTK in the management of pterygia has been explored, both in the treatment of post-excisional scarring[16,19,43] and during surgical removal to smooth the wound bed.[17,44] Seiler et al[44] studied 31 eyes with primary pterygium and 24 eyes with recurrent pterygium undergoing surgical excision with PTK to the wound bed followed postoperatively with topical Mitomycin C. No recurrences in the primary group occurred whilst 12.5% recurred in the recurrent subgroup. 16.4% of cases gained at least two lines of visual acuity by 1 year.

Tuunanen and Tervo[17] report 11 eyes with primary or recurrent pterygium who underwent PTK with the aim of preventing recurrences. Surgical excision of the lesion was immediately followed by excimer laser PTK. Overlapping ablation zones of 3–6 mm diameters were employed to smooth the wound bed. In two of the six patients with reduced visual acuity, PTK resulted in an improvement in visual acuity. Recurrences occurred in four cases (36%) leading the authors to question the ability of PTK to decrease the recurrence rate. The role of PTK in this clinical setting obviously requires further investigation.

PHOTOTHERAPEUTIC KERATECTOMY FOR MISCELLANEOUS CONDITIONS

The number of single case reports and small series of PTK performed for various miscellaneous anterior ocular disorders continues to expand. The published literature covers a wide diversity of conditions including proud corneal nebulae in keratoconus leading to contact lens intolerance;[45] shield ulcers and corneal plaques in vernal keratoconjunctivitis;[46] refractive errors related to keratoconus;[47] and benign conjunctival lesions.[48] It is likely this list will continue to increase due to the high success rates and patient acceptance, with few complications compared to current alternative surgical treatments. Long-term analyses of the effectiveness of PTK in these areas are awaited.

CONCLUSIONS

Despite the use of the 193 mm excimer laser in the management of anterior corneal disorders for almost 8 years, PTK is, in many respects, still in the early stages of investigation and development. However, the initial medium-term results confirm that PTK is well tolerated with significant and varied clinical applications. The clinical results of PTK, as outlined in this chapter, suggest the most suitable diagnoses for treatment include recurrent corneal epithelial erosions, band keratopathy, and corneal dystrophies with opacities confined to the anterior stroma.

Table 22.8
Comparison of PTK with lamellar keratoplasty. (Adapted from Talamo et al.[37])

	PTK	*Lamellar keratoplasty*
Treatment:		
a. location	Laser suite	Operating theatre
b. duration	15–30 minutes	45–90 minutes
c. anesthetic	Topical	peri/retrobulbar/GA
Costs:	Savings on facility, anesthesia, donor tissue	More expensive procedure
Pathology limitations:	Anterior 50–100 µm	Healthy endothelium
Immediate postoperative pain:	Moderate	Mild
Visual recovery:	1–2 months	3–6 months
Induced optical change:	Hyperopia, induced astigmatism	Hyperopia, myopia, induced astigmatism
Activity restriction:	None/minimal	Mild
Follow-up procedure for failures (s):	Lamellar/penetrating keratoplasty	Repeat lamellar/penetrating keratoplasty

Corneal scarring tends to require deeper stromal ablation, with an attendant increase in the postoperative complication rate ultimately limiting success; however, for many of these patients a lamellar or penetrating keratoplasty are the only alternative management options currently available. In such circumstances, PTK has the advantage of allowing an outpatient procedure which is simpler and less invasive, with fewer potentially blinding complications. It allows the treatment of patients unable to withstand grafting and has no requirement of donor tissue. See Table 22.8 for a comparison of PTK with lamellar keratoplasty.[37] The results of PTK/PARK in the management of iatrogenic induced refractive disorders, particularly post keratoplasty myopic astigmatism, although encouraging, require further research before its role is conclusively established.

There are, as yet, several issues unresolved: the possible role of postoperative pharmacological modulation of wound healing, the chronic tissue response to laser treatment including epithelium, stroma, endothelium, keratoconic corneas and grafted tissue, and recurrence rates of the primary pathology following PTK. Further investigation into the accurate determination of the differences in ablation rates for various abnormal corneal constituents is required. Future avenues of inquiry include the selection of the optimal materials to assist in ablation such as viscous masking agents and ablatable solids such as collagen or plastic shields. Refinement of the technique of PTK might include the development of a (scanning) laser delivery system to slowly oscillate the laser beam, rather than the patient's head, to achieve smoothing of the edge effect between ablated and non-ablated zones, thus limiting the induced refractive changes presently encountered with broad beam systems. Although some time away, several companies, especially those with a scanning option, are presently working towards the incorporation of corneal topographic data, or real time corneal shape, into the final laser treatment plan—perhaps the ultimate control in PTK.

The concerns of the FDA panel considering the approval of the excimer laser phototherapeutic keratectomy[8]—the need for long term results, exact criteria for suitability for PTK, induced refractive errors including the impact of induced anisometropia; and unanticipated longterm complications—have largely been answered in the medium longterm. However, unlike PRK, no generalized or generic surgical plan can be employed to cater for the myriad corneal disorders which have yielded, or may yet yield, to the precision of excimer laser PTK. Therefore it remains the paramount responsibility of the ophthalmic surgeon to carefully chose, and fully counsel, subjects suitable for PTK treatment and to tailor the subsequent PTK strategy on an individual basis.

REFERENCES

1. Trokel SL, Srinivasan R, Braren B, Excimer laser surgery of the cornea, *Am J Ophthalmol* (1983) **96**: 710–15.
2. Gartry D, Kerr Muir M, Marshall J, Excimer laser treatment of corneal surface pathology a laboratory and clinical study, *Br J Ophthalmol* (1991) **75**: 258–69.
3. Kerr Muir MG, Trokel SL, Marshall J, Rothery S, Ultrastructural comparison conventional surgical and argon fluoride excimer laser keratectomy, *Am J Ophthalmol* (1987) **103**: 448–53.
4. Serdaveric O, Darrel RW, Krueger RR, et al, Excimer laser therapy for experimental Candida keratitis, *Am J Ophthalmol* (1985) **99**: 534–8.
5. Gottsch JD, Gilbert ML, Goodman DF, et al, Excimer laser ablative treatment of microbial keratitis, *Ophthalmology* (1991) **98**: 146–9.
6. Azar DT, Jain S, Woods K, et al, Phototherapeutic Keratectomy: The VISX Experience. In: Salz JJ, ed, *Corneal Laser Surgery* (Mosby: St Louis, 1995)
7. Durrie DS, Schumer DJ, Cavanaugh T, Phototherapeutic Keratectomy: The Summit Experience. In: Salz JJ, ed, *Corneal Laser Surgery* (Mosby: St Louis, 1995)
8. Waring GO, FDA Panel recommends conditional approval of excimer laser phototherapeutic keratectomy (PTK), *J Refract Corneal Surg* (1994) **10**: 77–78.
9. Seiler T, Bende T, Wollensak J, Ablation rate of human corneal epithelium and Bowman's layer with the excimer laser (193 nm), *Refract Corneal Surg* (1990) **6**: 99–102.
10. Campos M, Neilson S, Szerenyi K, Garbus JJ, McDonnell PJ, Clinical follow-up of phototherapeutic keratectomy for treatment of corneal opacities, *Am J Ophthalmol* (1993) **115**: 433–40.
11. Stark WJ, Chamon W, Azar D et al, Phototherapeutic keratectomy: Corneal opacities. In: Thompson FB, McDonnell PJ, ed, *Excimer laser surgery of the cornea* (Igaku–Shoin: Tokyo, 1983).
12. Stark WJ, Chamon W, Kamp MT et al, Clinical follow-up of 193 nm ArF excimer laser photokeratectomy, *Ophthalmology* (1992) **99**: 805–12.
13. Campos M, Lee M, McDonnell PJ, Ocular integrity after refractive surgery: Effects of photorefractive keratectomy, phototherapeutic keratectomy, and radial keratotomy, *Ophthalmic Surgery* (1992) **23**: 598–602.

14. Kornmehl EW, Steinert RF, Puliafito CA, A comparative study of masking fluids for excimer laser phototherapeutic keratectomy, *Arch Ophthalmol* (1991) **109**: 860–86.

15. Fasano AP, Moreira H, McDonnell PJ, Sinbawy A, Excimer laser smoothing of a reproducible model of anterior corneal surface irregularity, *Ophthalmology* (1991) **98**: 1782–5.

16. Fagerholm P, Fitzsimmons TD, Orndahl M, et al, Phototherapeutic keratectomy: long-term results in 166 eyes, *J Refract Corneal Surg* (1993) **9**: S76–S81.

17. Tunnanen TH, Tervo TM, Excimer laser phototherapeutic keratectomy for corneal diseases: A follow-up study, *CLAO Journal* (1995) **21**: 67–72.

18. Foster W, Grewe S, Atzler U, Lunecke C, Busse H, Phototherapeutic keratectomy in corneal diseases, *Refract Corneal Surg* (1993) **9**: S85–S90.

19. Hersh PS, Spinak A, Garrana R, Mayer M, Phototherapeutic keratectomy: strategies and results in 12 eyes, *Refract Corneal Surg* (1993) **9**: S90–S95.

20. O'Brart DP, Garty DS, Lohmann CP, et al, Treatment of band keratopathy by excimer laser phototherapeutic keratectomy: surgical techniques and long term follow up, *Br J Ophthalmol* (1993) **77**: 702–8.

21. Claoué C, Stevens J, Steele A, Band keratopathy and excimer laser phototherapeutic keratectomy, *Eur J Implant Ref Surg* (1995) **7**: 260–5.

22. McDonnell PJ, Seiler T, Phototherapeutic keratectomy with excimer laser for Reis–Buckler's corneal dystrophy, *Refract Corneal Surg* (1992) **8**: 306–10.

23. Eggink FA, Beekhuis WH, Granular dystrophy of the cornea. Contact lens fitting after phototherapeutic keratectomy, *Cornea* (1995) **14**: 217–22.

24. Koenig SB, Clinical follow-up of phototherapeutic keratectomy for treatment of corneal opacities, *Am J Ophthalmol* (1993) **116**: 256 (lett).

25. Dausch D, Landesz M, Klein R, Schroder E, Phototherapeutic keratectomy in recurrent corneal epithelial erosion, *Refract Corneal Surg* (1993) **9**: 419–24.

26. O'Brart DP, Muir MG, Marshall J, Phototherapeutic keratectomy for recurrent corneal erosions, *Eye* (1994) **8**: 378–83.

27. Algawi K, Goggin M, O'Keefe M, 193 nm excimer laser phototherapeutic keratectomy for recurrent corneal erosions, *Eur J Implant Ref Surg* (1995) **7**: 11–13.

28. Thomann U, Meier-Gibbons F, Schipper I, Phototherapeutic keratectomy for bullous keratopathy, *Br J Ophthalmol* (1995) **79**: 335–8.

29. John ME, Van der Karr MA, Noblitt RL, Boleyn KL, Excimer laser phototherapeutic keratectomy for treatment of recurrent corneal erosion, *J Cataract Refract Surg* (1994) **20**: 179–81.

30. Thompson V, Durrie DS, Cavanaugh TB, Philosophy and technique for excimer laser phototherapeutic keratectomy (Review) *Refract Corneal Surg* (1993) **9**: S81–S85.

31. McGhee CNJ, Bryce IG, Anastas CN, et al, Corneal topographic lagoons: a potential new marker for post-traumatic recurrent corneal erosion syndrome, *Australian and New Zealand J Ophthalmol* (1996) **24**.

32. McLean N, MacRea S, Rich L, Recurrent erosion. Treatment by anterior stromal puncture, *Ophthalmology* (1986) **93**: 784–8.

33. Geggel HS, Successful treatment of recurrent corneal erosions with Nd:YAG anterior stromal puncture, *Am J Ophthalmol* (1990) **110**: 404–7.

34. Binder PS, Anderson JA, Rock ME, Vrabec MP, Human excimer laser keratectomy clinical and histopathological correlations, *Ophthalmology* (1994) **101**: 979–89.

35. John ME, Martines E, Cvintal T et al, Phototherapeutic keratectomy following penetrating keratoplasty, *J Refract Corneal Surg* (1994) **10**: S296–S10.

36. Goldstein M, Loewenstein A, Rosner M, et al, Phototherapeutic keratectomy in the treatment of corneal scarring from trachoma, *J Refract Corneal Surg* (1994) **10**: S290–S92.

37. Talamo JH, Steinert RF, Puliafito CA, Clinical strategies for excimer laser therapeutic keratectomy, *Refract Corneal Surg* (1992) **8**: 319–24.

38. Rapuano CJ, Laibson PR, Excimer laser phototherapeutic keratectomy, *CLAO Journal* (1993) **19**: 235–40.

39. Campos M, Hertzog L, Garbus J, Lee J, McDonnell PJ, Photorefractive keratectomy for severe postkeratoplasty astigmatism, *Am J Ophthalmol* (1992) **114**: 429–36.

40. Loewenstein A, Lipshitz I, Lazar M, Photorefractive keratectomy for the treatment of myopia after epikeratoplasty: a case report, *J Refract Corneal Surg* (1994) **10**: S285–S86.

41. Gibralter R, Trokel SL, Correction of irregular astigmatism with the excimer laser, *Ophthalmology* (1994) **101**: 1310–4.

42. Lawless MA, Cohen PR, Rogers CM, Retreatment of undercorrected photorefractive keratectomy for myopia, *J Refract Corneal Surg* (1994) **10**: S174–S77.

43. Rapuano CJ, Laibson PR, Excimer laser phototherapeutic keratectomy for anterior corneal pathology, *CLAO Journal* (1994) **20**: 253–7.

44. Seiler T, Schnelle B, Wollensak J, Pterygium excision using 193-nm excimer laser smoothing and topical mitomycin C, *German Journal of Ophthalmology* (1992) **1**: 429–31.

45. Moodaley L, Liu C, Woodward EG, et al, Excimer laser superficial keratectomy for proud nedulae in keratoconus, *Br J Ophthalmol* (1994) **78**: 454–7.

46. Cameron JA, Antonios SR, Badr IA, Excimer laser phototherapeutic keratectomy for shield ulcers and corneal plaques in vernal keratoconjunctivitis, *J Refract Surg* (1995) **11**: 31–35.

47. Mortensen J, Ohrstrom A, Excimer laser photorefractive keratectomy for the treatment of keratoconus, *J Refract Corneal Surg* (1994) **10**: 368–72.

48. Kim JH, Hahn TW, Excimer laser ablation of conjunctival epithelial melanosis. *J Cataract Refract Surg* (1993) **19**: 309–11.

Chapter 23 Complications of excimer laser photorefractive surgery

Charles N J McGhee and Christine R Ellerton

INTRODUCTION

Excimer laser photorefractive surgery, heralded in the late 1980s as computer-controlled precision surgery, with submicron ablative steps, has in most respects lived up to its initial promise. Certainly, in the treatment of myopia up to −10.00 D and in the correction of low levels of astigmatism, recent studies have produced enviable outcome results which are highlighted in Chapters 11–16. However, no surgical technique, regardless of refinement, is without complication and the addition of a computerized element to the surgery does not abrogate the essential responsibility of the surgeon to control the proper execution of the procedure. Indeed, the sophistication of the excimer laser adds components to refractive surgery which make the learning process more complex and require a structured and rigorous approach to each photorefractive procedure.

The reported incidence of complications varies from less than 1% to 40%[1-11] depending upon (a) the era of PRK development that a particular study reviews, (b) the criteria used to define complications and (c) the time-point post-PRK at which complications were recorded. Some complications, such as halo formation, were much more common with earlier machines using 3.4–4.5 mm diameter treatment zones than with current lasers using 6.0–7.0 mm zones.[5,12] Defining a complication is particularly difficult; for example, is grade II haze which does not compromise Snellen visual-acuity and which settles spontaneously within 12 months of PRK a normal healing phenomenon in higher attempted refractions, or is this a genuine complication? With respect to the chronological occurrence of complications and their identification, it must always be noted that some complications, such as central islands, may be transient phenomena present only in the first few weeks post-PRK, whereas others, such as severe corneal haze, may not occur for several months post-surgery. In general, the complication rate will appear greater at 6 months than 12 months, and should be least in those studies presenting 18–24-month review data. In many respects it is therefore difficult to provide absolute data for the incidence of specific complications; however, this chapter attempts to crystallize the available scientific data on complications in the widest sense, whilst highlighting key points by clinical illustration.

AVOIDING COMPLICATIONS – PREOPERATIVELY

There are several relative, and absolute, contraindications to PRK and these have been highlighted in an earlier section (Chapter 8). Undoubtedly there is a learning curve in PRK surgery, as in any surgical procedure, and PRK is much more than 'simply wiping off the epithelium and asking the patient to stare at a target while the laser fires'. The practical aspects of PRK have already been discussed (Chapter 9) but it is worth reiterating the importance of adequate training, since some complications, such as ablation zone decentration, appear to be more common and of greater magnitude during the learning period. The authors' suggested two-day training course incorporates a review of relevant training and background literature; a practice PRK session on synthetic or porcine eyes; observation of 5–10 treatments performed by an experienced PRK surgeon; and supervision, by an experienced PRK training surgeon, of the first treatment session performed by the beginning PRK surgeon.

DEFINING COMPLICATIONS

Several methods can be applied to rationalize post-PRK complications, such as classification on the basis of chronological occurrence; by severity, for example, non-sight-threatening or sight-threatening; whether refractive or nonrefractive complications; likelihood of resolution without further intervention or long-term sequelae; frequency, in terms of whether common or rare; or on a purely anatomical basis. No classification is all-encompassing and all produce grey areas of overlap. In an attempt to provide a logical and relatively simple classification the authors have organized complications temporally in relation to the PRK procedure.

INTRAOPERATIVE COMPLICATIONS

Table 23.1
Intraoperative complications.

1 Failure to adequately remove epithelium
2 Decentration of ablation zone
3 Input of incorrect refractive error
4 Laser failure of ablation
5 Laser mechanical failure

There are only two groups of complication that should be encountered intraoperatively: those related to the surgical procedure and those related to laser operation (Table 23.1).

In relation to surgical complications, removal of the healthy corneal epithelium in a period of a minute or two is more difficult than many imagine prior to actually performing the procedure. The beginning PRK surgeon, due to tentative technique, is more likely to inadequately remove the epithelium than to cause damage to underlying Bowman's owing to an overenthusiastic epithelial debridement. Inadequate removal may induce undercorrection, irregular ablation, or even central island formation. Some of the caution inherent in the use of a sharp implement on the corneal surface can be obviated by employing a blunt spatulate instrument to remove epithelium in initial cases (Chapter 9).

The second important aspect of surgical technique which can lead to significant complication is that of

proper centering of the ablation zone. The intraoperative aspects of this complication are covered in detail in Chapter 9 and assessment and management of decentration is discussed later in this chapter.

Presuming that a laser has been properly calibrated and serviced to produce an homogenous and centered beam, only three laser-related complications are likely to occur: input of an incorrect refractive correction; complete failure of the laser to fire; and mechanical failure of an iris or scanning element producing either an inappropriate ablation profile or deposition of excessive ablation at one point on the cornea. Techniques to avoid and manage these complications are highlighted in Chapter 9.

IMMEDIATE POSTOPERATIVE COMPLICATIONS

Table 23.2
Immediate postoperative complications.

Related to the surgical procedure
1   Delayed epithelial healing
2   Sterile corneal infiltrates
3   Bacterial keratitis
4   Reactivation of herpes simplex keratitis
5   Mucus plaques or tags
6   Corneal edema
7   Anterior uveitis
8   Lid edema and ptosis

Related to topical medication
9   Drug toxicity
10 Drug hypersensitivity

DELAYED EPITHELIAL HEALING

The cause of delayed epithelial healing beyond 4–5 days post-PRK is multifactorial. Most studies report complete epithelial healing within 3–4 days and delay beyond 7 days is uncommon.[1–3,5,11–13] Local environmental factors that might contribute to delayed epithelial closure include epithelial toxicity from topical drugs, or accompanying preservatives, particularly such drugs as local anesthetics, nonsteroidal anti-inflammatory drugs (NSAIDS), aminoglycoside antibiotics and corticosteroids. Subjects with clinical dry eye syndrome or keratoconjunctivitis sicca are more likely to exhibit delayed healing and also have

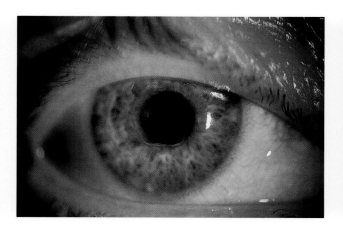

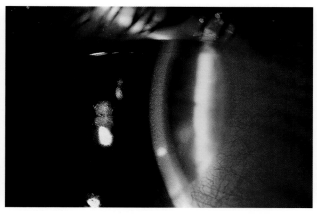

Figure 23.1 *The right cornea of an eye five days after an uncomplicated PRK of −11.50 D correction. A large epithelial defect of approximately 3.5–4.0 mm diameter with grey, rather heaped, epithelial margins is evidence of delayed healing. Prescribed topical antibiotics and non-steroidal drugs were stopped at this point and the eye treated solely with preservative free lubricant drops every two hours. The defect healed fully, without sequelae, by day 10 post PRK.*

Figure 23.2 *Two sterile infiltrates noted in an eye 36 hours post PRK. Neither NSAID nor corticosteroid were prescribed prior to development of these infiltrates. Both infiltrates were at the periphery of the debridement zone (one highlighted in the slit beam, the other a little right and superior to the first), and were covered by healing epithelium and did not stain with fluorescein.*

a predisposition to the toxic effects of topical preparations. Persisting epithelial defects prolong the risk period for infective keratitis and anecdotal reports suggest that delayed healing is associated with increased subepithelial haze.

Limiting the diameter of the epithelial debridement zone to the minimum required to accommodate the excimer ablation should, theoretically, result in more rapid healing. However, comparing laser transepithelial ablation with manual debridement in one study demonstrated no statistical difference between the groups, although manual epithelial debridement usually produces a larger epithelial defect than a laser transepithelial approach.[14]

Standard management of persistent corneal epithelial defects is to remove all potentially toxic drugs and preservatives and treat with copious preservative-free lubricants or tear substitutes. Although topical sodium hyaluronate and a variety of growth factors have been employed to encourage epithelial healing (Chapter 25), the addition of topical sodium hyaluronate has not been shown to speed epithelial healing or reduce pain post-PRK.[15]

Although Seiler and McDonnell[1] have reported one case of delayed epithelial healing, in a case of previously undiagnosed systemic lupus erythematosus

which progressed to a central corneal melt and perforation, persisting epithelial defects have rarely been reported in the scientific literature. In the authors' personal series of more than 350 consecutive cases in the Sunderland Eye Infirmary (SEI) prospective PRK study, only two cases of defect persisting beyond 6 days have been encountered, suggesting an incidence of approximately 0.5% (Fig. 23.1). Other studies have noted delayed epithelial healing beyond 4 days post-PRK in 1.5–9.4% of eyes.[1,16]

STERILE CORNEAL INFILTRATES

Sterile infiltrates fall into two categories which may overlap, both in clinical appearance and etiology. Peripheral, noninfectious sterile infiltrates are an uncommon and usually non-sight-threatening complication of PRK, frequently associated with pre-existing staphylococcal blepharitis which may be very mild in many cases. However, in contrast, a more severe paracentral form of sterile infiltrate, associated with the use of bandage contact lenses and topical diclofenac has been reported in North American meetings, but little has been published specifically on this subject.

Management of these infiltrates depends to a large extent on the clinician's certainty of diagnosis and accepted local practice. Those infiltrates associated with blepharitis and staphylococcal toxins are usually small, near to the limbus but often separated by a clear zone, frequently multiple, and have an intact overlying epithelium which does not stain with fluorescein (Fig. 23.2). Mild mixed blepharitis is usually present in both eyes if examined carefully. These small peripheral infiltrates, with intact overlying epithelium, do not usually require scrape and culture and will usually respond within 24 hours to the addition of a mild topical corticosteroid such as fluorometholone 0.1% four to six times per day. The subject should be continued on the standard postoperative topical antibiotic, although the frequency might be increased to six or eight times per day. The eye must be reviewed 24 hours later. At review, if there has not been an improvement, or if there is any suggestion of deterioration, the diagnosis must be reassessed and the lesion investigated and treated as a potential microbial keratitis. In the SEI study, in which bandage contact lenses were not used postoperatively and patients received no steroids until epithelial closure had occurred, peripheral sterile infiltrates were noted at an incidence of 4% in the first 100 eyes treated. Subsequently, even the mildest forms of blepharitis were treated aggressively prior to PRK and the incidence of small peripheral sterile infiltrates fell to less than 1%.

In contrast, infiltrates associated with NSAIDs and bandage contact lenses are more extensive, often paracentral, and annular or ring-like in appearance. Teal et al[17] surveyed the incidence of stromal opacification occurring within 72 hours of PRK in eyes treated postoperatively with topical NSAIDs and bandage contact lenses. Of 50 Canadian ophthalmologists contacted in the study, 17 surgeons replied, reporting 30 such cases. Typically, after uncomplicated PRK, acute pain, redness and lacrimation developed on the second postoperative day. The most frequent clinical pattern was of an inferiorly-placed large opacity, often in the shape of an immune ring with one or two round peripheral opacities. Two of the cases had an associated stromal melt. Microbiological cultures were negative. Various treatments were used including intensive topical antibiotics, topical steroid, and patching. Regardless of the therapy the pattern of resolution was the same. Permanent scarring accompanied by reduced vision was the commonest outcome, with 80% of eyes exhibiting loss of best spectacle-corrected visual acuity (BSCVA) at 3 months. Possible causes

suggested by the authors included anoxic contact lens occlusion, immune reaction, and a toxic reaction to the combination of contact lens and NSAIDs.

Sher et al,[18] reporting on a prospective randomized study comparing diclofenac with placebo vehicle, identified three cases of corneal infiltrate in a series of 32 eyes, one case in the placebo group and two in the diclofenac group. In this series all eyes were treated with a bandage contact lens postoperatively. All three eyes with infiltrate healed with a degree of corneal scarring and a BSCVA of 20/25 or less. The use of topical NSAIDs and contact lenses without the concurrent use of topical corticosteroid might, theoretically, predispose the post-PRK cornea to inflammatory infiltrates[19] by cyclo-oxygenase inhibition, which may lead to increased amounts of arachidonic acid and increased formation of leukotrienes, the latter being strongly chemotactic for polymorphonuclear leucocytes (PMNs) (Chapter 25).

In contrast to the high incidence of corneal infiltrates (9%) reported by Sher et al,[18] reporting on a three-year experience of PRK in 240 eyes, Maguen et al[3] noted only one case of a paracentral corneal infiltrate within the ablation zone. This occurred in an eye treated postoperatively with a bandage contact lens, diclofenac and topical ciprofloxacin. Removal of the contact lens and intensive antibiotic therapy settled this culture-negative case without long-term sequelae.

Teichmann et al[20] described a Wessely-type immune ring in a 25-year-old man who underwent phototherapeutic keratectomy (PTK) for childhood opacities of unknown etiology. A bandage contact lens was applied postoperatively. On the fourth day an incomplete dense white ring formed in the corneal periphery, separated from the limbus by a clear zone. Corneal scrapes were culture-negative, whereas corneal biopsy demonstrated a focal keratocyte depopulation, occasional polymorphonuclear leucocytes and active fibroblasts. No lymphocytes or plasma cells were detected. The authors suggested that this reaction might be related to the photoradiation at the margin of the ablation zone. They speculated that an antigen–antibody complex reaction, involving locally produced corneal heat shock protein (HSP) might cross-react with pre-existing circulating antibodies against bacterial HSPs. The immune ring gradually faded without impairing visual acuity.

Sher et al[19] have suggested that these NSAID-related sterile infiltrates might be largely avoided by commencing a topical corticosteroid at the same time as NSAID application post-PRK. It is also worth noting that in the UK, where bandage contact lenses are seldom used post-PRK, these worrying paracentral, annular or ring infiltrates have not been reported at keratorefractive conferences or in the scientific literature.

MICROBIAL KERATITIS

Fortunately, in contrast to sterile corneal infiltrates, bacterial keratitis appears to be very rare indeed in the postoperative period. Seiler and McDonnell, in a recent major review,[1] document only six published cases of bacterial keratitis, all of which were associated with the wearing of a bandage contact lens in the postoperative period. Interestingly, in one of the series cited, Faschinger et al,[21] in a series of 161 eyes, actually report four severe cases of fungal keratitis, one of which was associated with endophthalmitis. The authors postulated that renovations of buildings in the clinic area had led to a higher concentration of *Aspergillus* in the air and that this, coupled with the overnight wearing of disposable contact lenses, may have predisposed the post-PRK eyes to infection.

In the UK and Australia, clinical trends, and the theoretically increased risk of keratitis of either a sterile or infective nature associated with the use of bandage contact lenses post-PRK, has led to a very limited use of this modality. The only case of bacterial keratitis with hypopyon in the Melbourne excimer laser study group of more than 3800 eyes was associated with bandage contact lens wear (Hugh Taylor, personal communication, 1996).

Obviously, not all cases of bacterial keratitis will be published and the temporal relationship to PRK may be remote. Indeed, the authors are aware of one case of bacterial keratitis occurring more than 6 months after PRK, and several months after cessation of all topical medication, in the SEI series. This bacterial keratitis occurred within the ablation area in an eye which had apparently been stable from a refractive and clinical standpoint for several months post-PRK. The patient did have local predisposing factors to keratitis in the form of blepharitis, dry eye disease and acne rosacea. Whether this keratitis was entirely coincidental in a patient with several risk factors or causally related to the removal of Bowman's layer by PRK is entirely open to conjecture.

A case of severe keratitis caused by *Streptococcus pneumoniae* 9 weeks after PRK was identified by Sampath et al.[22] The patient, who had been applying topical corticosteroids four times per day since the PRK procedure, presented with a large central corneal abscess in his only seeing eye. Although this responded to appropriate antibiotic therapy the subsequent scar reduced the patient's BSCVA to counting fingers. The authors postulated that this late post-PRK keratitis might be related to pre-existing blepharitis, possible ocular surface abnormality secondary to PRK and prolonged use of topical corticosteroids.

REACTIVATION OF HERPES SIMPLEX KERATITIS

Pepose et al[23] demonstrated in a mouse model that 193 nm excimer laser ablation can reactivate latent herpes simplex. Subsequently, Vrabec et al[24] reported three cases of recurrent herpes simplex keratitis following (PTK) treatment of herpetic corneal scars. Failure to provide adequate topical or systemic antiviral coverage when corticosteroids are used in the post PTK/PRK period can lead to the development of geographic and stromal keratitis. Unfortunately, a past history of herpetic disease is not always elicited, but the surgeon should always be wary of this possibility in eyes demonstrating unexplained subepithelial scarring. The authors encountered a case of dendritiform keratitis one week after an uncomplicated PTK for band-shaped keratopathy in an eye with a history of recurrent, apparently idiopathic, anterior uveitis. Fortunately, this responded very rapidly to topical acyclovir and the eye achieved a BSCVA of 6/6 (Fig. 23.3).

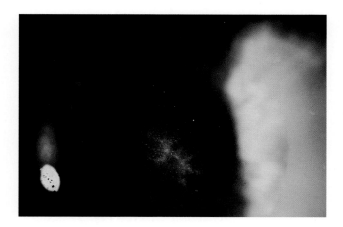

Figure 23.3 *Re-activation of herpes simplex keratitis within the PTK zone one week after treatment of a band keratopathy. The keratitis responded very rapidly to topical oc. acyclovir without stromal involvement.*

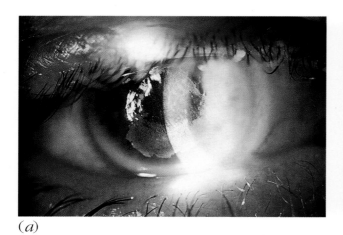

(a)

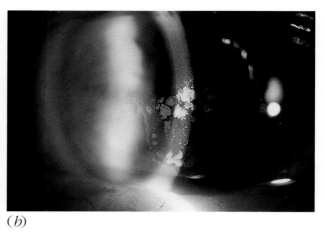

(b)

Figure 23.4 (a) A large plaque, presumed to be composed of mucus and proteinaceous material, occupying the area of epithelial debridement 24 hours post PRK. This plaque was simply wiped off gently with a sterile cellulose sponge. (b) The contralateral eye of the patient shown in Fig. 23.4a also developed a similar mucus plaque following PARK six months later. No intervention was undertaken in this eye and healing was complete by day three post PARK with no adverse healing phenomena.

A past history of herpes simplex keratitis (HSK) should be considered a contraindication for PRK and possibly a relative contraindication for PTK. Seiler and McDonnell[1] have suggested that oral acyclovir should be utilized for 2 weeks after surgery where a preoperative history of HSK is elicited. If corticosteroids are employed following PTK for herpetic scarring, their use should also be accompanied by antiviral cover in the form of a topical agent such as acyclovir.

TRANSIENT MINOR POST-PRK COMPLICATIONS

The stromal surface underlying the post-PRK epithelial defect may be the focus for mucus and cellular debris forming mucus tags or plaques in 14% of eyes.[25] While large mucus plaques can have a dramatic appearance (Fig. 23.4) when they occur on day 1 or 2 post-treatment, they can be readily removed with a sterile swab or by the application of topical acetyl cysteine. However, since these plaques do not appear to slow epithelial healing or adversely affect anterior stromal haze, they may simply be observed.

During the postoperative period while an epithelial defect is present, a mild to moderate degree of stromal edema is often observed, associated with

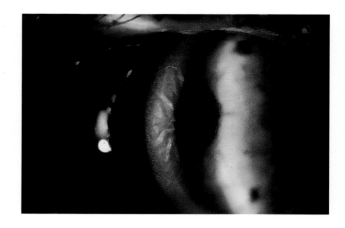

Figure 23.5 Mild to moderate corneal stromal edema with folds in Descemet's membrane is not uncommonly seen on the first day post PRK. However, this edema usually resolves by day 2 as the exposed stroma is re-epithelialized.

mild folds in Descemet's membrane (Fig. 23.5). Clinically, such edema appears to be greater with higher ablations but no publications have addressed this transient phenomenon directly. This mild corneal edema rapidly resolves as the epithelial defect begins

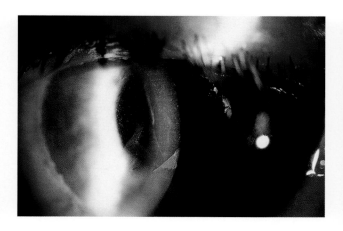

Figure 23.6 *Loose epithelial tags, such as the area illustrated in the lower third of the slit beam, that are attached to the periphery of the epithelial debridement, may occasionally be observed on day one post PRK. Since these may be associated with increased discomfort on blinking they are best removed with a sterile cellulose sponge or sterile instrument.*

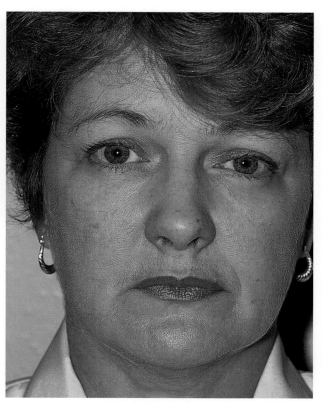

Figure 23.7 *Blepharoptosis is evident in the left upper lid of a patient four weeks after uncomplicated left PRK. The ptosis fully resolved without intervention over the following eight weeks.*

to close and is barely discernible in most cases by day 2 or 3 postoperatively.

Occasionally, flaps or tags of loosened epithelium may be detected at the edge of the epithelial debridement zone on the first postoperative day. While these tags do not appear to overtly affect the rate or manner of epithelial closure, they can be associated with increased patient discomfort on blinking, and if troublesome are best removed using a sterile spatula or sterile pledget (Fig. 23.6).

Following PRK it is not uncommon to see occasional cells and a hint of aqueous flare in the anterior chamber by high-power slit lamp microscopy. However, anterior uveitis is very uncommon and the authors have identified only one case in the SEI series (0.25%). This subject had no prior history or signs of uveitis but evidenced flare, 5–10 cells per beam, and a scattered fine endothelial dusting of white cells on day 1. The uveitis settled completely within 72 hours following the instigation of topical fluorometholone four times per day.

LID EDEMA AND BLEPHAROPTOSIS

Mild to moderate lid edema associated with a degree of mechanical blepharoptosis is not uncommon in the first few days after PRK. The origin of this lid swelling is open to conjecture but may be related to local release of prostaglandins and other inflammatory mediators following the PRK procedure, coupled with the orthostatic effect of eye-patching. Fortunately the lid edema and ptosis normally resolves within the first few days. However, in some cases the ptosis, which is generally mild (1–2 mm), persists for weeks or even months (Fig. 23.7). In the SEI series approximately 6% of eyes demonstrated a clinical ptosis obvious to the clinician and the patient between 1 and 3 months post-PRK.[25] Fortunately only one case in a series of more than 350 treatments has persisted beyond one year. Therefore, while self-limiting ptosis is relatively common, permanent blepharoptosis must be considered a relatively rare phenomenon. Nonetheless, all prospective PRK candidates should be advised of this risk.

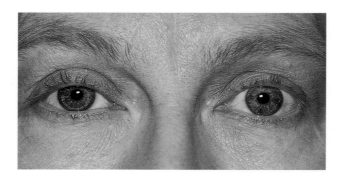

Figure 23.8 *Pseudoptosis of the right contact lens wearing eye, compared to the left eye that had recently undergone PRK. Removal of the right contact lens relieved the right pseudoptosis.*

Others have reported an approximate 1% incidence of unilateral ptosis at 1 month post-PRK and one case of surgical correction of a ptosis utilizing a Muller's muscle–conjunctival resection has been reported in the Cedars Sinai series.[26] Genuine ptosis should not be confused with contact-lens-related pseudoptosis in subjects wearing a contact lens in the untreated eye after PRK in the contralateral eye (Fig. 23.8).

The origin of this self-limiting ptosis is uncertain, with possibilities including the following: (1) a corticosteroid myopathic effect upon Muller's muscle (since topical ocular corticosteroid will readily penetrate the overlying conjunctiva this might most readily explain the limited time course of the ptosis and ultimate resolution); (2) a direct mechanical injury of Muller's muscle by the lid speculum has also been postulated; (3) a bystander inflammatory response, with edema secondary to inflammatory mediators, released in response to the PRK, temporarily compromising Muller's muscle function; (4) prolonged or severe upper lid swelling might lead to partial aponeurotic disinsertion leading to a more permanent ptosis. Goggin et al[13] have reported a single case in a large series (0.6%), that exhibited a 3 mm ptosis that subsequently required surgical correction.

COMPLICATIONS RELATED TO TOPICAL MEDICATION

Hypersensitivity to the active ingredient of topical preparations is not uncommon and has been reported in as many as 17% of eyes post-PRK.[25] Conjunctival injection, burning or smarting of the eye associated with lid erythema, should immediately alert the surgeon to this possibility. Removal of the responsible drug, or drugs, and, if necessary, substitution with alternative, preferably preservative-free topical agents, is usually sufficient to settle mild hypersensitivity reactions. If the hypersensitivity is more marked a topical corticosteroid drug might be added if not already included in the postoperative management regimen.

Epithelial toxicity can be induced by excessive application of any topical agent which contains preservatives or epithelial toxic active ingredients in sufficient dose, for example, aminoglycoside antibiotics. This is most likely to manifest with a punctate epitheliopathy or delayed epithelial closure. Management of this complication has been discussed in an earlier section.

INTERMEDIATE TO LONG-TERM COMPLICATIONS

Table 23.3
Intermediate to long-term complications.

Primary refractive complications

1. Overcorrection
2. Undercorrection
3. Induced astigmatism
4. Irregular astigmatism
5. Ablation zone decentration
6. Central islands
7. Permanent anisometropia
8. Reduced best-spectacle-corrected visual acuity

Complications related to the PRK procedure or abnormal healing

1. Corneal haze or scar
2. Recurrent corneal erosion syndrome
3. Recurrent corneal microerosion syndrome
4. Steroid-related elevation of intraocular pressure
5. Apparent reduction in intraocular pressure (IOP) as measured by Goldmann tonometry
6. Corneal hypoesthesia
7. Corneal endothelial damage
8. Epithelial iron lines
9. Inability to properly fit contact lenses

PRIMARILY REFRACTIVE COMPLICATIONS

Overcorrection, undercorrection/regression and induced astigmatism

As excimer laser PRK has matured refractive results have generally improved, although with each major change in algorithm or technique, such as from single to multizone ablation, results are likely to show a slightly greater variability until the algorithm is refined. Predictability of refractive and visual outcome has increased both for low and high myopia, although despite continuing refinements in technique, myopia greater than –10.00 D is likely to come under the domain of LASIK rather than surface-based PRK in the long-term.

Reviewing a representative selection of PRK/PARK papers with greater than one-year follow-up data published in the last three years, it is notable that in attempted correction of myopia up to –7.50 D, 71–93% of eyes are within ±1.00 D of intended final refraction and 91–95% of eyes obtain 20/40 or better unaided vision.[2,3,13,27,28] Recent studies have shown similar results up to –10.00 D correction and greater (Chapter 16). Indeed, in the SEI prospective PRK study, 12-month follow-up results on 255 eyes demonstrated that 89% of eyes with preoperative myopia up to –5.00 D and 87% of eyes with preoperative myopia between –5.25 D and –10.00 D obtained 20/40 or better vision without correction.[29] However, despite these encouraging results there continue to be cases of over- and undercorrection of myopia by PRK. Interestingly, in a recently reported study[30] of 341 patients receiving PRK, 14.9% of subjects had not undergone treatment of the second eye at the completion of the study (mean follow-up 31 months). A statistically greater number of eyes in this group (33.3%) were overcorrected to hyperopia compared with eyes of patients who progressed to PRK in the second eye (3.5%), and almost half of those who did not undergo treatment of the second eye due to dissatisfaction with refractive outcome experienced symptoms related to hyperopia (42%). Schallhorn et al,[31] reporting the one-year results of active-duty navy personnel who had undergone attempted corrections of –2.00 D to –5.50 D with a Summit Omnimed (Summit Technology International Inc., Waltham, MA) utilizing a 6.0 mm ablation zone, noted that, while all eyes achieved 20/20 or better unaided vision, 13% of eyes exhibited more than one diopter of hyperopic overcorrection.

Durrie et al[32] retrospectively classified 116 eyes treated with a Summit laser using a 4.5 or 5.0 mm diameter ablation zone for attempted myopic correction up to –7.0 D. They classified eyes into three subgroups on the basis of six-month refraction: normal healers (type I), achieving final refraction within 1.00 D of the attempted correction: inadequate responders or type II healers that remained overcorrected; and aggressive responders or type III healers that were undercorrected by more than –1.00 D. This natural variation in healing may be the root cause of many cases of under- and overcorrection and as such is not predictable, although a correction factor might usefully be employed in the subsequent treatment of the contralateral eye. Overcorrection may also occur in prolonged epithelial debridement with stromal dehydration and consequent overablation, and undercorrection may be observed with inadequate removal or increased stromal hydration following topical application of fluid to the exposed stroma prior to ablation (Chapter 9).

Table 23.4

Mean refractive error in diopters (D) following surface-based PRK. Aggressive responders demonstrated a statistically significant increased postoperative haze. The inadequate responders were more likely to have a clear cornea at 1 month relative to the normal group. The authors suggest that inadequate responders do not mount the usual healing response to the laser and early reduction of steroids postoperatively might be of benefit (after Durrie et al[32]).

	Normal healers	*Inadequate healers*	*Aggressive healers*
No. of eyes	98	13	5
Preoperative mean refraction (D)	–4.58	–4.85	–6.28
1 month post-PRK mean refraction (D)	+0.90	+2.58	+1.53
3 months post-PRK mean refraction (D)	+0.23	+1.78	+1.53
6 months post-PRK mean refraction (D)	+0.03	+1.78	–2.25

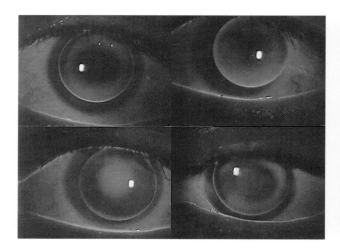

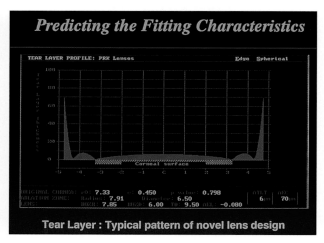

Figure 23.9 *Contact lens fitting post PRK. Upper left: a specially designed PRK lens demonstrates good centration without apical pooling of fluorescein. Upper right: in contrast a contact lens fitted in respect to post PRK central K readings demonstrates a poor, tight fit with temporal displacement. Lower left: a contact lens based on pre-operative K values demonstrates marked fluorescein pooling over the ablation zone. Lower right: a contact lens designed to accommodate both central and peripheral corneal contour post PRK demonstrates good centration, no apical pooling of fluorescein and a fine annular fluorescein pattern. (Courtesy of Mr Keith Edwards, Bausch and Lomb, UK).*

Figure 23.10 *Tear layer profile of the PRK lens illustrated in Fig. 23.9. (Courtesy of Mr Keith Edwards, Bausch and Lomb, UK.)*

Primary undercorrection, or myopic regression without significant haze development should respond to PRK retreatment 6–12 months after primary treatment (Chapter 24) and mild, induced hyperopia may yield to laser thermokeratoplasty (LTK) or hypermetropic PRK (Chapter 17). Unfortunately those eyes which exhibit severe haze and 50% or greater myopic regression are unlikely to respond well to repeat PRK. However, patients who do not wish to undergo, or who are unsuitable for, a secondary procedure, may be left unacceptably hyperopic or anisometropic, and therefore may be considered for refitting of contact lenses (Chapter 8). Contact lenses specifically designed for the post-PRK eye are beginning to appear on the market and offer less stagnation of tear fluid over the apex of the ablation zone than a normally vaulted contact lens (Figs 23.9 and 23.10).

Kim et al[33] report that regression can occur up to three years after PRK using a 5.0 mm zone and a maximum correction of −6.0 D. The formula calcu-

lated by this group for myopic regression over three years was $Y=3.679-0.6876 \log(X)$ (where Y is the expected manifest refraction and X is the number of days after PRK). Reviewing 35 consecutive eyes with a minimum follow-up of three years the following mean refractive errors were noted: −4.71 D preoperatively; −0.45 D at one year; −0.48 D at two years; and −1.14 D at three years. Presuming a constant regression rate, the authors suggest that the mean refraction at five years would be −1.48 D.

In a subsequent study, Kim et al[34] noted in a retrospective review of 228 eyes treated by a Summit laser with a 5 mm zone that the amount of myopic regression was statistically correlated with the amount of attempted correction. Interestingly, Epstein et al,[28] using a Summit laser and a 4.3 or 4.5 mm diameter ablation zone, also noted a significant difference in mean myopia at 12 and 24 months post-PRK, being −0.01±0.78 D and −0.27±0.74 D respectively.

However, in a prospective randomized trial[12] comparing 5.00 mm and 6.00 mm ablation zones, predictability of outcome was greater in the 6.00 mm group, and the authors suggested that problems with long-term refractive stability should not occur, although longer follow-up studies were required. Snibson et al[35] have subsequently published one-year follow-up data on 150 procedures performed using a Visx 20/20 laser (Visx, Sunnyvale, CA) employing a 6.00 mm ablation zone. Attempted PRK and PARK up to a mean spherical equivalent of −10.00 D demonstrated remarkable stability of refractive outcome between 6 and 12 months post-treatment, with 79% of eyes achieving uncorrected visual acuity of 20/40 or better at 12 months.

Regression of myopic effect can be very marked, especially in high myopic corrections,[36-38] and has also been correlated with the presence of significant corneal haze and the intraoperative use of nitrogen.[32,36] Krueger et al[36] report one case of myopic regression of greater than −20.0 D which left the eye more myopic 6 months after PRK than before; a similar result occurred after retreatment.

Induced astigmatism is relatively uncommon and theoretically may be due to decentered ablation zones, asymmetric corneal healing, or gross inhomogeneity across the laser beam. The prevalence of induced astigmatism of greater than 0.75 D has been reported to be as low as 2.5% of eyes at 12 months post-PRK, reducing to 0.5% at two years post-treatment.[39] Waring et al[16] noted that induced astigmatism at one year post-PRK had increased in 6% of cases by 0.5–2.0 D. In contrast, in extreme myopia[36] an induced astigmatism of greater than 1.00 D was identified in 33% of eyes at some point during the postoperative period (see Chapter 15).

Goggin et al[40] noted that 60% of patients had a change in the astigmatic element of their refraction at 6 months after PRK. The commonest change encountered was the development of a new cylindrical element in a previously spherical eye, and a decrease in a pre-existing cylinder. The mean cylindrical power change was 0.75 D and approximately one-fifth of cases had a change in the axis of their cylinder only. No statistically significant relationship to degree of preoperative myopia, mean laser correction, postoperative haze, or regression was found in respect of these astigmatic changes. Maguen et al[3] found that new astigmatism axes were generally within 20° of the preoperative cylindrical axis, whereas Taylor et al[41] noted that, following PARK, the postoperative axis of astigmatism was within ±−10° of the preoperative axis in most cases. However, using vector analysis, no consistent error in the application of astigmatism correction was noted with a mean angle of error of −1.1±−23.9° (mean ± standard deviation) at 6 months postoperatively.[41] (See Chapter 23).

Ablation zone decentration

Methods of ablation zone centration have previously been discussed (Chapter 9), as have aspects of

Table 23.5
Clinical effects of decentration.

Decreased BSCVA
Less predictable refractive outcome
Induced corneal astigmatism
Monocular diplopia
Glare and halo
Decreased patient satisfaction

computerized videokeratographic analysis (Chapter 7). Therefore this section will concentrate on the incidence of significant decentration and associated side-effects.

Several factors may contribute to decentration, including poor patient fixation; poor or improper alignment of the ablation zone relative to the center of the pupil by the operating surgeon; and misalignment of centering aids or laser optics in the laser delivery system. Significant decentration of the ablation zone may result in: reduced best corrected visual acuity; induced or irregular astigmatism; and halo, glare or edge effects. Unsurprisingly, some authors have reported a decreasing rate of decentration with increasing PRK experience.[8,42,43]

Although several large studies demonstrate a mean ablation zone decentration of less than 0.7 mm,[2,3,8,35,43-48] with the majority reporting decentration of approximately 0.3–0.6 mm, up to 32% of eyes[8] have been noted to exhibit decentration greater than 1.0 mm (Table 23.5). While the mean and standard deviation of decentration in these studies provide a good indication of the reproducibility of the centration technique, it is the upper range of decentration which is more likely to be associated with clinical symptoms. Surprisingly, decentrations greater than 2.0 mm have not infrequently been reported[2,3,8] and to put such decentrations in perspective, it should be noted that, in a cornea of 11.0 mm diameter, a 2.6 mm decentration[2] of a 6.00 mm ablation zone places the periphery of the ablation at the corneoscleral limbus.

Centration may be more crucial in smaller ablation diameters, and it has been calculated that a 1.0 mm decentration of a 4.00 mm ablation zone results in almost one-third of the light rays falling on the retina passing through untreated cornea, possibly resulting in a defocused, secondary, ghost image and monocular diplopia.[49] However, decentration of up to 1.5 mm, in one small series using a 5.0 mm ablation

Table 23.6

Mean, standard deviation and range of decentration of excimer laser ablation zones for several large PRK series are highlighted. Although the mean and standard deviation are indicative of the accuracy and reproducibility of centration techniques, the upper limit of the range of decentration, and the percentage of cases with decentration greater than 1.0 mm, are equally important in terms of symptomatic decentration.

Study (authors, year)	No, of eyes	Sphere equiv. (D)	Zone (mm)	Laser	Mean decentration (mm)	Range	Decentered >1 mm
Talley et al 1994[2]	91	1.00–7.50	6.0–7.0	Visx 2015	0.57±0.44	0.1–2.6	20%
Maguen et al 1994[3]	50	1.00–6.00	–	Visx 2020	0.62±0.47	0.0–2.1	16%
Sher et al 1994[8]	48	8.00–15.00	5.5–6.2	Visx 2015	0.70±0.50	0.1–2.4	32%
Amano et al 1994[44]	60	1.75–12.50	4.5	ExciMed	0.51±0.31	0.06–1.64	6.7%
Lin, 1994[43]	502	1.00–24.00	5.0–6.0	Visx 2020	0.34±0.23	0.0–1.50	–
Shimizu et al 1994[45]	60	1.00–15.00	4.5	ExciMed	0.51±0.31	–	5%
Schwartz–Goldstein et al 1995[47]	185	1.50–6.00	4.5–5.0	Omni/ ExciMed	0.46±0.26	0.0–1.44	2.9%
Doane et al 1994[2]	38	2.00–6.00	5.0	ExciMed	0.40±0.19	0.12–0.89	0%
Webber et al 1996[48]	53	1.25–12.00	6.0	Visx 2020	0.46±0.27	0.0–1.1	4%

zone, was associated with unaided vision better than 20/40, with only one of five subjects complaining of visual aberration.[50]

Although decentrations of up to 1.5 mm may still be associated with good unaided visual acuity[50] many workers have logically presumed, from basic optical principles, that significant ablation zone decentration is likely to be associated with a poorer outcome for the patient (Table 23.5). However, Doane et al,[46] reporting a multivariate analysis of two subgroups, one with decentration less than 0.5 mm and the other with decentration greater than 0.5 mm, failed to show any statistical significance between the groups in terms of halo, glare and problems with night-driving. Nonetheless, comparing the individual patient ratings within each group did show a statistically significant worsening of halo symptoms postoperatively in the latter group. The authors concluded that decentrations of less than 0.89 mm from the pupillary center were unlikely to produce significant visual symptoms.

Halos are among the most commonly reported subjective complications after PRK and have been related to ablation zone size as well as decentration. A high incidence of symptomatic halos under night-driving conditions occurred with the smaller diameter ablation zones utilized in early studies.[1,51,52] O'Brart et

al[53] recorded fewer night-time halos in eyes treated with 5.00 mm diameter zones compared with 4.00 mm zones, and a reduction in the severity of halos with time from surgery has also been described.[4,51,54] Kim et al[4] reported marked halos in 30% of patients within 3 months of treatment, compared with only 9% at one year. O'Brart et al[12] further considered halo symptoms after a spherical correction of –3.00 D or –6.00 D PRK employing either a 5.0 or 6.0 mm ablation zone. The authors noted a greater magnitude of halo in the –6.00 D groups, and significantly greater halos in the smaller ablation groups. In contrast, Rogers et al[55] found postoperative halos rarely a problem in myopes with corrections greater than –10.00 D and speculated that the image outside the 5 mm treatment zone in such cases was so defocused, relative to the primary image, that it was not troublesome.

In a study of 185 patients,[47] decentration was noted to be associated with higher attempted myopic corrections, with five of the six eyes evidencing more than 1.0 mm decentration, having undergone a correction greater than –5.00 D. Although not statistically associated with induced refractive astigmatism, 66% of eyes with more than 1.00 D of induced keratometric astigmatism had greater than 0.5 mm decentration and a negative correlation was identified

Table 23.7

The percentage of eyes losing two lines of Snellen BSCVA is illustrated for series dealing with low to moderate myopic corrections up to –7.50 D (0–8.9%), and for series correcting high and extreme myopia (6–40%).

Study (authors, year)	Laser	Myopic sphere Equiv. (diopters)	Ablation zone diameter (mm)	Total no. of eyes	% loss two lines BSCVA
Seiler et al, 1991[51]	ExciMed	1.40–7.25	3.5	26	0
Gartry et al, 1992[5]	ExciMed	1.50–7.00	4.0	120	3.3
Salz et al, 1993[58]	Visx 2020	1.25–7.50	5.0–5.5	71	1.0
Kim et al, 1993[54]	ExciMed	2.00–6.00	5.0	135	8.1
Brancato et al, 1993[27]	ExciMed	0.80–6.00	–	146	1.4
Talley et al, 1994[2]	Visx 2015	1.00–7.50	6.0–7.0	85	3.5
Maguen et al, 1994[3]	Visx 2020	1.00–6.00	–	149	4
Dutt et al, 1994[11]	ExciMed	1.50–6.10	5.0	47	0
Waring et al, 1995[51]	ExciMed	2.20–6.90	4.5	80	8.9
Kwitco et al, 1996[66]	ExciMed	1.00–6.00	5.0	106	0
Schallhorn et al, 1996[31]	OmniMed	2.00–5.00	6.0	30	0
Snibson et al, 1995[35]	Visx 2020	1.25–15.00	4.5/5.0/6.0	150	6
Buratto et al, 1993[9]	Summit	6.00–10.00	4.3–4.5	40	40
Sher et al, 1994[8]	Visx 2020/15	8.00–15.25	5.5–6.2	40	15
Carson et al, 1995[10]	Visx 2020	5.10–9.90	5.0/6.0	194	12.9
		10.20–21.00	4.5/5.0/6.0	53	13.0

between magnitude of decentration and patient satisfaction. While there was a trend towards worse uncorrected vision with increasing decentration, there was no statistically significant correlation with BSCVA, predictability of refractive outcome or glare/halo symptoms.

Although a number of studies have looked specifically at decentration, due to the relatively small numbers of eyes with large decentrations larger prospective studies are still required to clearly delineate highlighted trends and associations. The management of decentration is discussed elsewhere (Chapters 7, 24).

Central topographic islands

Central islands of greater than 3.0 D central power are relatively common with wider ablation zones and may occur in almost one-third of eyes analyzed by computerized videokeratography within the first 6 months post-PRK.[56] Fortunately the majority of such islands resolve spontaneously without further intervention. An extensive discussion of the etiology, natural history and visual associations of central islands is provided in Chapter 7.

Permanent anisometropia

Although failure to have the second eye treated has been reported to be as high as 14.9% in one series,[30] little has been published on patients who chose to remain untreated in the second eye due to dissatisfaction with the refractive result, or complications such as severe haze or decreased BSCVA in the first eye. These subjects, and those who have asymmetry of refractive outcome (for example, hyperopic overcorrection), may be left with troublesome permanent anisometropia and aneisokonia if they are unable to comfortably wear contact lenses. In the authors' personal series only 1.4% of subjects remained uniocularly treated, and significantly anisometropic, due to complications or dissatisfaction with initial PRK, and all these eyes had a preoperative myopia greater than –7.00 D. Therefore, although this problem may be less common with newer lasers and wider ablation zones, all prospective PRK candidates should be warned of the possibility of anisometropia and uniocular treatment by default.

Loss of best corrected visual acuity

Although many authors have utilized the loss of two lines of corrected Snellen acuity as the reporting

Table 23.8

Three studies illustrate the changing prevalence of loss of two lines or more of BSCVA post-PRK. The percentage of eyes with loss of two lines or more BSCVA is greatest in the first month post-treatment and improves dramatically by 6 months or one year postoperatively, although some patients may exhibit this loss of corrected vision for two years or more. (*n* = total number of patients reviewed at each time-point.)

Study (authors, year)	1 month	3 months	6 months	12 months	24 months	36 months
Salz et al 1993[58]	22.3%	6.5%	1.6%	1.4%	0%	
	n=152	n=139	n=124	n=71	n=12	
Maguen et al 1994[3]	20%	10%	7%	4%	5%	0%
	n=206	n=177	n=189	n=149	n=59	n=10
Schallhorn et al 1996[31]	17%		0%	0%		
	n=30		n=30	n=30		

threshold for visual loss, others have noted that Snellen charts are not sensitive enough in assessing the visual function postoperatively, suggesting that LogMAR charts and measurement of contrast sensitivity, glare and forward light scatter are more appropriate tests of visual function.[57] However, at the present time the majority of reports remain based upon Snellen acuity. In low to moderate myopia, usually less than 4% of eyes lose two lines of BSCVA at one year,[2,3,5,11,27,51,58] although this has been reported to be as high as 8.9%.[16,54] Loss of BSCVA has generally been greater with attempted corrections of high or extreme myopia, with most studies reporting 10% or more of eyes losing at least two lines of BSCVA (Table 23.7).

The cause of this loss of BSCVA may be multifactorial and authors have variously cited corneal haze or scar,[2,3,5,8,16,35,54] irregular astigmatism,[3,8,54,59] central islands,[10] and ablation zone decentration.[16] In the case of irregular astigmatism lines of BSCVA may be regained with an appropriately fitted contact lens.

Loss of BSCVA generally has a temporal relationship, being most common in the first 6 months post-PRK and progressively less common at one year and thereafter (Table 23.8 and Fig. 23.11). Kim et al[33] report that 94% of patients followed for three years after PRK for low to moderate myopia (<6.0 D) achieved a BSCVA equal to, or better than, BSCVA preoperatively. Hamberg–Nystrom et al[60] in a 36-month follow-up report of excimer laser for less than –7.25 D of myopia, noted that less than 0.5% of 456 eyes had lost one Snellen line of BSCVA.

Since most reports concentrate on visual results in terms of Snellen acuity and loss, relatively few studies

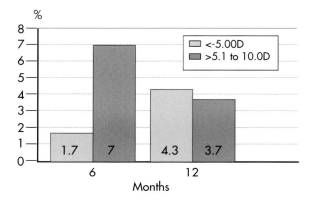

Figure 23.11 *Loss of two lines or more of best spectacle corrected visual acuity (BSCVA) in the Sunderland Eye Infirmary prospective PRK study, in subjects with more than 12 months follow-up (n=179). At six months 7% of those with attempted correction of between 5.1 D and 10.0 D of myopia had lost two lines of Snellen visual acuity or more compared to only 1.7% of those with lesser attempted corrections. However, at twelve months there was no statistical difference between the two refractive groups with approximately 4% of eyes in each group losing two lines of BSCVA. No eye had lost more than two lines and all had corrected acuity of 6/9 (20/30) or better.*

have reported other aspects of visual function. However, reduced contrast sensitivity in the early post-PRK period has been documented,[45,61,62] even in the presence of unimpaired Snellen acuity. In low myopic corrections return to baseline values are approached 3–6 months after surgery,[61,62] whereas both static and dynamic contrast sensitivity functions may remain abnormal at 6 months in high myopes.[61] An association between loss of contrast sensitivity and the presence of corneal haze post-PRK has been identified in some studies.[45,62]

Gartry et al[63] note in an early study that 10% of excimer patients declined treatment of the second eye because of disturbances in their night vision in the treated eye. Dutt et al[11] measured contrast sensitivity in dilated and undilated pupil states in pre- and post-PRK eyes treated with a 5 mm ablation, noting a significant reduction in contrast sensitivity for virtually all frequencies tested. The contrast sensitivity reached its lowest levels in the dilated pupil state, which the authors suggested might contribute to complaints of poorer night vision. However, Lohmann et al[64] investigated contrast sensitivity and forward scatter in myopic patients corrected by spectacles, hard contact lenses and one year after excimer PRK and noted that these corrective modalities all proved to be superior to soft contact lens correction in terms of reduced contrast sensitivity.

Waring et al[16] reported reduced BSCVA under glare conditions in 9.7% of patients one year after a 4.5 mm ablation zone PRK, and other studies[57] have noted that, compared with a control group, approximately one year after PRK 22–28% of eyes fall outwith the 95% confidence limits for high and low contrast Bailey–Lovie visual acuities, Pelli–Robson contrast sensitivity and forward light scatter measured by a van den Berg stray light meter. However, Harrison et al,[65] studying the effect of a 6.0 mm ablation zone PRK on the forward scatter of light 1 month after PRK, found no significant increase, tending to support the theoretical use of larger ablation zones to decrease visual disability.

COMPLICATION RELATED TO THE PRK PROCEDURE OR ABNORMAL HEALING

Corneal haze or scar

Most reports have used a subjective assessment of the slit-lamp appearance of haze post-PRK with several different scales (Chapter 8). However, others have utilized a variety of objective techniques including quantification of haze objectively utilizing a charge-coupled device camera system which analyzes a gray-scale disturbance caused by the combined signal of light reflected and scattered back from the cornea;[12,67] high-frequency ultrasound biomicroscopy;[68–70] and opacity lensometers.[71] Nonetheless, at the time of writing no objective technique is in widespread use.

Unfortunately there are a large number of subjective classifications of haze, with between four and seven categories, which are not directly comparable. In order to allow an approximate comparison between studies the authors have tried to correlate these studies by assuming that significant haze, which we have classified as greater than Grade II, is considered usually of sufficient magnitude to result in loss of BSCVA. However, any simple grading system has difficulty in classifying certain cases, for example, focal scattered Grade III curvilinear haze on a generally homogeneous Grade I background haze,[72] and too coarse a grading system may limit the physician's ability to accurately record subtle changes.[72]

The etiology of haze is probably multifactorial with few absolute correlates other than association with increasing myopia,[6,10,12,35,72,74] higher attempted myopic correction[6,10,72] and the use of an intraoperative nitrogen blower.[75] Surprisingly, a direct positive association of haze with absolute ablation depth is debatable.[5,12,44,76] Early studies suggested an increased level of haze post-PRK in patients who exhibited noncompliance with steroid regimens;[1,74] however, controlled studies have failed to demonstrate a beneficial effect of topical corticosteroids in the prevention or management of haze (Chapter 25). A variety of topical medications have been suggested to be used in the prevention of haze in animal models and preliminary human trials but at the present time no single agent is in general clinical use (Chapter 25).

Corneal haze is typically time-dependent, being most marked between 1 and 6 months post-PRK,[5,6,10,16,45,72] with most studies reporting progressive clearing of haze toward 12 and 18 months (Fig. 23.12). However, rarely severe haze may persist for two years or more (Figs 23.13–23.16). Severe haze is frequently associated with myopic regression[5,32,36,37,55,74] and loss of BSCVA.[35,36,55] Rogers et al.[55] noted in a series of high myopic corrections a strong tendency for significant scarring and regression to occur in the second eye treated if it had occurred in the first eye. This symmetry of outcome was also noted by Loewenstein et al.[77] in low and moderate myopes.

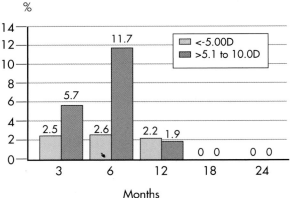

Figure 23.12 *Eyes exhibiting grade 2 or greater corneal haze in the Sunderland Eye Infirmary prospective PRK study. In attempted corrections up to −5.00 D the prevalence of grade 2 or greater haze was never higher than 2.6% of eyes. In contrast, in higher attempted PRK corrections of −5.10 D to −10.0 D, the prevalence of grade 2 or greater haze reached 11.7% six months post PRK, although in common with those eyes that had undergone corrections less than −5.10 D, no eyes were noted to exhibit grade 2 haze at the 18 or 24 month post operative intervals.*

Recurrent corneal erosion syndrome

Post-PRK, true recurrent corneal erosion syndrome (RCES), with recurrent early-morning severe ocular pain and epiphora lasting up to several hours associated with areas of epithelial erosion, appears to be very rare. Indeed, excimer PTK has become the gold-standard treatment for recurrent corneal erosion syndrome (Chapter 21). In an early study, Gartry et al[63] reported symptoms suggestive of a mild form of recurrent erosion in 18% of patients, although these symptoms tended to resolve by 6–9 months post-PRK. Seiler and McDonnell noted only one symptomatic case in more than 600 treatments.[1] Although others have noted changes which might predispose to erosive symptoms, such as dot-like epithelial changes[78] or asymptomatic thickening of the anterior basement membrane at the edge of the ablation zone,[2] it does appear that true RCES is not a frequent post-PRK complication. While other studies[3,5,13,16] have reported the incidence of symptoms and signs of recurrent corneal erosion post-PRK in the region of 1.2–2.5%, milder symptoms, such as a transient sensation of corneal foreign body upon awakening, have been reported by up to 20–30% of subjects in the postoperative period.[5,13]

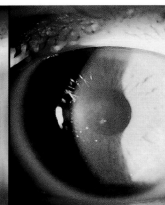

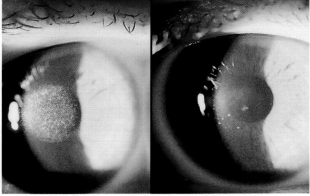

Figure 23.13 *Identification and photographic documentation of post PRK haze is very dependent on slit lamp illumination. An intense, narrow beam, oblique illumination readily highlights reticular grade 2 haze in an eye six months after a −7.00 D PRK correction (right), whereas, diffuse illumination of the same eye (left) fails to clearly demonstrate the severity of the haze.*

Figure 23.14 *Confluent grade 2 haze demonstrated in an eye 4 months after a −5.00 D correction (left) has almost fully resolved by 12 months post PRK leaving trace haze and an epithelial iron line (right).*

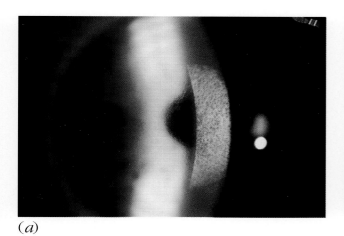

(a)

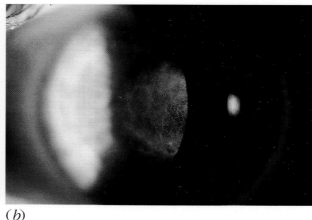

(b)

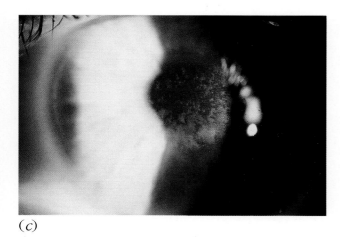

(c)

Figure 23.15 *a–c. Variants of corneal haze within one classification group: Grade 2 haze. (a) Grade 2 confluent haze with a regular reticular pattern five months after a −6.50 D PRK correction. Despite apparent severity of haze, unaided vision was 6/9 correcting to 6/6 with −0.50 D, and the patient asymptomatic other than minor glare in scotopic conditions. The haze had fully resolved by eleven months with final unaided vision of 6/9. (b) Grade 2 haze with an irregular pattern and variable density 6 months after a −6.50 D PRK correction. The irregular haze was associated with irregular astigmatism and loss of two lines of BSCVA. The patient was very aware of decreased quality of vision and moderate scotopic symptoms. Unlike the case illustrated in Fig. 23.15a this haze was slow to resolve over a two year period with preoperative BSCVA only being regained 18 months post PRK. (c) Small scattered 'snowflake' foci of grade 2 haze twelve months after a −3.00 D PRK. Unaided acuity was 6/5 and the patient was completely asymptomatic throughout the postoperative period.*

Recurrent corneal microerosion syndrome

It is surprising that RCES is so uncommon when one considers that the area of corneal epithelial debridement which lies outwith the PRK ablation zone, presuming a mechanical epithelial debridement 0.5–1.0 mm greater than ablation zone diameter, is essentially an annular epithelial abrasion. In a prospective analysis of 306 consecutive eyes treated by the authors, minor symptoms suggestive of a mild variant of RCES were reported in 1.3% of patients at one year post-PRK but only persisted beyond 18 months in one subject. These symptoms were generally described as discomfort or mild smarting pain on first eye opening after a night's sleep. The pain typically lasted between a few and 30 seconds with momentary watering of the eye; thereafter the eyes were comfortable for the remainder of the day. Such symptoms were more common in the first 6 months after PRK and patients with these symptoms frequently were aware of a sensation that the lid was adherent to the eye on awakening and that, by gently moving the eyes around under closed lids, or gently massaging the ocular surface through closed lids, the symptoms could be averted. Careful examination of

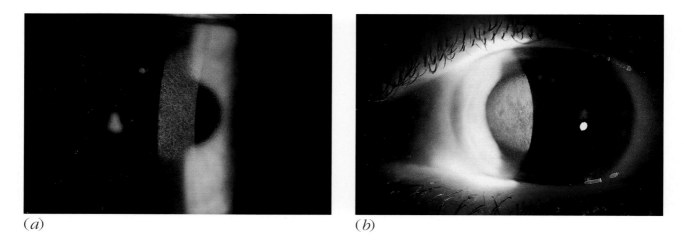

(a)   (b)

Figure 23.16 *Recurrence of haze following excimer laser retreatment. One year after a −14.00 D PRK correction this eye demonstrated a BSCVA of 6/9 with an even grade 2 haze and a residual −6.50 D correction (a). The patient underwent a −6.50 D PRK retreatment and initially enjoyed 6/9 unaided vision and 6/6 corrected acuity over a six month period, however, by eight months post PRK the eye exhibited severe, confluent grade 3 haze with loss of four lines of BSCVA and a refraction of −3.50 D (b).*

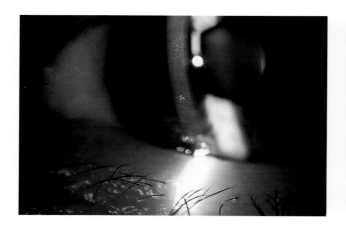

Figure 23.17 *Microcystic change in the corneal epithelium post PRK associated with putty-like grey dots highlighted by the slit beam.*

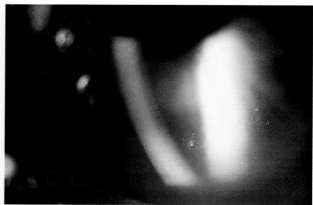

Figure 23.18 *Asymptomatic microcystic changes in the epithelium highlighted by retroillumination are demonstrated to the right of the primary slit lamp beam and to the right of the beam striking the iris. These microcystic changes are within the area of epithelial debridement but outside the PRK ablation zone.*

all eyes in this study demonstrated that 2.9% of eyes exhibited epithelial microcysts at 3 months post-PRK and this had reduced to 1.6% of eyes by 12 months postoperatively. However, the majority of the eyes with microcysts were asymptomatic, and few patients with recurrent corneal microerosion syndrome (RCMES) actually exhibited microcysts (Figs 23.17 and 23.18). In all cases these microcysts were seen outside the ablation zone in areas which had previously been debrided of epithelium.

Steroid-related elevation of intraocular pressure

Corticosteroid-related elevation of intraocular pressure (IOP) has been commonly documented in early series utilizing regimens of topical dexamethasone, betamethasone or prednisolone for 3–6 months post-PRK. Moderate elevation of IOP has been noted in these series in 8.6–24% of eyes, whereas elevation of IOP greater than 30 mmHg is less common, being cited in 1.0–8.2% of eyes.[5,7,51,54,59] The more common current practice of utilizing steroids such as fluorometholone, which have a lesser propensity to produce ocular hypertension, has been associated with a much lower incidence of moderate elevation of IOP in the region of 1.7–10.6% of eyes in recent PRK studies.[2,3,11,35,41] Elevation of IOP greater than 30 mmHg has rarely been reported in those studies utilizing fluorometholone.[2,3,11,35,42] Steroid-related ocular hypertension usually resolves quickly upon cessation of topical corticosteroids although, where IOP is 30 mmHg or greater, a short course of topical antihypertensive medication may be required to reduce IOP until the hypertensive effect of the steroid has been eliminated. Generally no long-term problems associated with such IOP elevation have been reported, with the exception of a study by Kim et al[59] who reported a severe steroid-induced intraocular pressure rise in 0.14% of subjects, which represented four eyes of three patients in a review of 2920 eyes. Visual field defects and glaucomatous optic disk cupping developed in all four eyes, the bilateral case requiring trabeculectomies. Corticosteroids and their use in the post-PRK eye are discussed in depth in Chapter 25.

Apparent reduction in IOP as measured by Goldmann tonometry

Sustained undermeasurement of IOP by applanation tonometry after refractive surgery (radial keratotomy) was noted by Mendez in 1989,[79] and it was suggested that, by steepening the peripheral cornea and flattening the central cornea, increased outflow might be responsible. However, analysis of the PERK study data in 1993 suggested that radial keratotomy did not affect IOP in any meaningful way.[80] In November 1993, at the Annual Congress of the Australian College of Ophthalmologists, the Lawless and Rogers group from Sydney noted that, following PRK, a statistically significant mean drop in measured IOP of 0.9 mmHg was detectable. The following year this group recorded a significant apparent decrease in IOP in subjects following PRK for extreme myopia.[55] In the same year a prospective analysis by the authors demonstrated that, despite the concurrent application of topical corticosteroids, IOP post-PRK was statistically lower than pre-PRK as measured by Goldmann applanation tonometry ($P < 0.001$).[81] Recently, McGhee et al.[82] updated this preliminary study and noted that 6 months after PRK, and 3 months after cessation of all topical steroids, the mean measured IOP in 86 consecutive eyes was 2.7 mmHg lower than pre-PRK recordings ($P < 0.001$).

Postulated reasons for this apparent undermeasurement of IOP post-PRK include change in corneal thickness and corneal curvature which increase the inherent inaccuracies of Goldmann applanation tonometry. It has previously been noted that true intraocular pressure may be underestimated in thinner corneas, and Ehlers et al[83] demonstrated that, at a true intraocular manometric reading of 20 mmHg, a cornea of 0.45 mm thickness recorded an IOP of 14.8 mmHg, whereas a cornea of 0.59 mm thickness recorded an applanation IOP of 24.7 mmHg. Recently, in a study comparing corneal thickness in 36 subjects with ocular hypertension (OHT) to similar size control and glaucoma groups, mean corneal thickness was noted to be significantly greater in the OHT group (0.610 mm) than the glaucoma group (0.557 mm) or the control group (0.567 mm).[84] The authors concluded that a significant number of patients with OHT would actually have normal IOP if corneal thickness was taken into account. Similarly, subjects with ocular hypertension have been shown to have thicker corneas – Tomlinson et al reported that patients with so-called 'low tension glaucoma' tend to have flatter corneas than patients with chronic open-angle glaucoma (COAG) or control populations, while the corneas of subjects with COAG have corneal curvature similar to the control population.[85] In a group of 400 eyes the mean IOP was noted to increase with increasing corneal curvature at a rate of approximately 0.34 mmHg per diopter of corneal power in the range 40–49 D; thus steepening or flattening of the cornea in this range might account for approximately 3.0 mmHg change in measured IOP.[86]

Subsequently, Schipper et al, measuring IOP by applanating the central and temporal cornea before and after PRK, noted that IOP measured in the temporal cornea was identical before and after PRK, whereas readings in the central cornea were 2–3 mmHg lower using Goldmann tonometry, and about 2 mm lower using the Tonopen (Mentor,

Norwell, MA) post-PRK.[87] Recently, an analysis of IOP in 1320 eyes before and after PRK demonstrated a statistically significant mean drop in apparent IOP of 3.1 mmHg following PRK. The authors suggest that a linear relationship exists between the apparent reduction in IOP and the magnitude of attempted myopic correction and devised a correction equation for the estimate of IOP post-PRK:

undercorrection (mmHg) = (0.4 × treatment spherical equivalent in diopters).[88]

In light of the foregoing data the authors suggest that glaucoma and ocular hypertension are relative contraindications to PRK since one of the commonly measured variables, IOP, assessed in the management of glaucoma, is no longer reliable.

Decreased corneal sensation

Although rapid recovery of epithelial innervation has been demonstrated after PRK in rabbits, stromal nerves may show prolonged abnormalities for 12 months or more.[89] Ishikawa et al[90] have also demonstrated differences in epithelial reinnervation dependent upon whether laser or manual removal of the epithelium was employed. In a rabbit model it was noted that in laser-ablated epithelium return to normal corneal sensitivity occurred within 5 days, but thereafter increased corneal sensitivity was noted for several months before returning to normal preoperative levels at approximately 7 months post-treatment. The relative density of intraepithelial innervation was significantly greater in eyes with laser epithelial removal compared with eyes with mechanical epithelial debridement, and corneal sensitivity was greater in the laser-treated eyes throughout the study period. The authors suggest that manual debridement might therefore engender a quicker recovery route to normal corneal sensitivity.[91]

The clinical significance of these findings is uncertain. Sher et al.[92] found no significant difference in corneal sensation pre- and post-PRK at 3 months in 31 patients. However, a persisting reduction in corneal sensation has been detected in some eyes at 6 months post-PRK.[90] In a small study of 14 consecutive adults, Campos et al. demonstrated decreased corneal sensation in the first 6 weeks post-PRK that had returned to within normal limits by 3 months post-treatment, although there was a trend towards slightly delayed recovery in deeper ablations.[93] The significance, if any, of transient alteration in corneal

sensitivity is unknown; however, it must be recalled that these sensory nerves have a trophic effect on corneal epithelium and may affect corneal metabolic activity post-PRK.

Corneal endothelial damage

Maintenance of the integrity of the corneal endothelium is a paramount consideration in any form of ocular surgery involving the cornea and anterior segment. Early studies utilizing a 193 nm excimer laser beam to create central linear corneal incisions found endothelial changes to be similar to those created when a diamond micrometer knife was used to incise to the same depth.[94] However, such endothelial cell loss, only associated with laser incisions within 40 microns of Descemet's membrane,[95] are not analogous to current PRK techniques restricted to the anterior one-third of the cornea. Indeed, central PTK procedures in porcine eyes with ablation depths to 200, or even 400, microns, failed to show any significant endothelial change compared with controls.[96] In a human study involving myopic corrections between −1.75 D and −13.50 D (maximum ablation depth of 113 microns), no changes in endothelial cell density were revealed when preoperative and 3- and 12-month postoperative endothelial analyses were compared in 76 eyes.[97] In a human study with a longer mean post-PRK follow-up of 33 months, no damage to central corneal endothelium was detected.[98] It therefore appears that surface-based PRK, within the anterior one-third of the cornea, has no long-term detrimental effects upon the corneal endothelium; however, deeper ablations associated with LASIK correction of extreme myopia have yet to be fully assessed in relation to endothelial changes.

Epithelial iron lines

Epithelial iron lines are very common following PRK, and Seiler and Holshbach have noted these in more than 80% of eyes.[99] In the authors' own series, epithelial iron lines, or dots, were the rule rather than the exception post-PRK. The prevalence of iron deposition increased with time from treatment, being present in 1.7, 9.3, 29 and 55% of eyes at 3,6,12 and 24 months post-PRK, respectively (Fig. 23.19). These iron deposits may be related to altered tear flow across the ablation zone due to changes in corneal curvature, but were not associated with any visual impairment or disturbance.

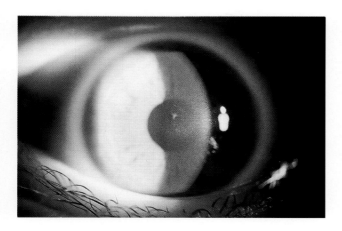

Figure 23.19 *An epithelial iron line or dot twelve months after PRK.*

Table 23.9
Rare and theoretical complications.

Rare and theoretical complications
1. Cystoid macular edema
2. Decompensated phoria
3. Steroid-induced cataract
4. Corneal graft rejection
5. Miscalculation of IOL power in the PRK eye
6. Mechanical predisposition to bursting injuries
7. DNA damage due to ultraviolet radiation
8. Cataractogenesis due to 193 nm irradiation
9. Retinal hemorrhage
10. Effect of pregnancy

Fitting of contact lenses

At the present time no publications have dealt extensively with the problems of fitting contact lenses post-PRK, although this has been discussed in a previous section (Chapter 8). Contact lens manufacturers, aware that a number of highly myopic individuals are unlikely to be fully emmetropized by excimer laser refractive surgery and may continue to require contact lens provisions, have begun to produce contact lenses specifically for the post-PRK cornea.

RARE AND THEORETICAL COMPLICATIONS

A small number of rare or uncommon complications related to excimer laser PRK have occasionally been reported, including cystoid macular edema;[100] decompensated esophoria producing manifest and symptomatic esotropia (Suzanne Webber FRCOphth, personal communication, 1995); corneal graft rejection;[101] and corticosteroid-induced cataract.

Theoretical complications of PRK include difficulty in accurately calculating IOL power;[102] a predisposition to corneal bursting injury – although experimental evidence suggests that mechanical integrity of the cornea is unaffected by PRK;[103] DNA damage due to ultraviolet irradiation (Chapter 3); and cataractogenesis due to secondary irradiation (Chapter 3). Retinal hemorrhage at the macula has been reported in the follow-up period of PRK in high myopia[27] but while this might theoretically be related to the acoustic shock wave generated by ablation this phenomenon is more likely to be related to the natural history of macular pathology in these eyes. Changes in corneal physiology have been related to the menstrual cycle[104] and the hormonal changes of pregnancy or hormone replacement therapy might therefore theoretically affect the outcome of PRK surgery; however, a recent preliminary report of nine eyes of eight women who became pregnant within 1–5 months post-PRK suggests that pregnancy does not influence the refractive outcome.[105]

CONCLUSION

The safety and predictability of excimer laser photorefractive keratectomy has improved dramatically over the last six years; however, despite refinement, no surgical intervention upon the cornea is without risk of complication. Nonetheless, surface-based PRK/PARK, utilizing 6.00 mm or greater ablation zones in the treatment of myopia up to 7.50 D, is currently associated with less than a 4% risk of significant complications that might adversely affect vision at one year. Further refinements in excimer laser technology and software algorithms, coupled with ongoing attempts to identify those patients likely to produce aggressive healing responses, will ensure that the risk of complication is constantly eroded.

REFERENCES

1. Seiler T, McDonnell PJ, Excimer laser photorefractive keratectomy, *Surv Ophthalmol* (1995) **40**: 89–118.

2. Talley AR, Hardten DR, Sher NA, et al, Results one year after using the 193 nm excimer laser for photorefractive keratectomy in mild to moderate myopia, *Am J Ophthalmol* (1994) **118**: 304–11.

3. Maguen E, Salz JJ, Nesburn AB, et al., Results of excimer laser photorefractive keratectomy for the correction of myopia, *Ophthalmology* (1994) **101**: 1548–57.

4. Kim JH, Hahn TW, Lee YC, Sah WJ, Excimer laser photorefractive keratectomy for myopia: two-year follow-up, *J Cataract Refract Surg* (1994) **20 (suppl)**: 229–33.

5. Gartry DS, Kerr Muir MG, Marshall J, Excimer laser photorefractive keratectomy, *Ophthalmology* (1992) **99**: 1209–19.

6. Leroux les Jardins S, Auclin F, Roman S, et al, Results of photorefractive keratectomy on 63 myopic eyes with six months minimum follow-up, *J Cataract Refract Surg* (1994) **20 (suppl)**: 223–8.

7. Machet JJ, Tayfour F, Photorefractive keratectomy for myopia: preliminary results in 147 eyes, *Refract Corneal Surg* (1993) **9 (suppl)**: 16–19.

8. Sher NA, Hardten DR, Fundingsland B, et al, 193 nm excimer photorefractive keratectomy in high myopia, *Ophthalmology* (1994) **101**: 1575–82.

9. Buratto L, Ferrari M, Photorefractive keratectomy for myopia from 6.00 D to 10.00 D, *Refract Corneal Surg* (1993) **9**: S34–S36.

10. Carson CA, Taylor HR, Excimer laser treatment for high and extreme myopia, *Arch Ophthalmol* (1995) **113**: 431–6.

11. Dutt S, Steinert RF, Raizman MB, Puliafito CA, One year results of excimer laser photorefractive keratectomy for low to moderate myopia, *Arch Ophthalmol* (1994) **112**: 1427–36.

12. O'Brart DPS, Corbett MC, Lohmann CP, et al. The effects of ablation diameter on the outcome of excimer laser photorefractive keratectomy, *Arch Ophthalmol* (1995) **113**: 438–43.

13. Goggin M, Algawi K, O'Keefe M, The complications of excimer photorefractive keratectomy for myopia in the first year, *Eur J Implant Ref Surg* (1995) **7**: 154–9.

14. Gimbel HV, DeBroff BM, Beldavs RA, van Westenbrugge JA, Ferensowicz M, Comparison of laser and manual removal of corneal epithelium for photorefractive keratectomy, *J Refract Surg* (1995) **11**: 36–41.

15. Algawi K, Agrell B, Goggin M, O'Keefe M, Randomized clinical trial of topical sodium hyaluronate after excimer laser photorefractive keratectomy, *J Refract Surg* (1995) **11**: 42–4.

16. Waring GO, O'Connell MA, RK, et al, Photorefractive keratectomy for myopia using a 4.5-millimeter ablation zone, *J Refract Surg* (1995) **11**: 170–80.

17. Teal P, Brelin C, Arshinoff S, Edmison D, Corneal subepithelial infiltrates following excimer laser photorefractive keratectomy, *J Cataract Refract Surg* (1995) **21**: 516–18.

18. Sher NA, Frantz JM, Talley A, et al, Topical diclofenac in the treatment of ocular pain after excimer photorefractive keratectomy, *Refract Corneal Surg* (1993) **9**: 425–36.

19. Sher NA, Krueger RR, Teal P, Jans RG, Edmison D, Role of topical corticosteroids and nonsteroidal antiinflammatory drugs in the etiology of stromal infiltrates after excimer laser photorefractive keratectomy, *J Refract Corneal Surg* (1994) **10**: 587–8 (letter).

20. Teichmann KD, Cameron J, Huaman A, Rahi AHS, Bahr I, Wessely-type immune ring following photorefractive keratectomy, *J Cataract Refract Surg* (1996) **22**: 142–6.

21. Faschinger C, Faulborn J, Ganser K, Infectious corneal ulcers – once with endophthalmitis – after photorefractive keratectomy with disposable contact lens, *Klin Monatsbl Augenheilkd* (1995) **206**: 96–102.

22. Sampath R, Ridgway AEA, Leatherbarrow B, Bacterial keratitis following excimer laser photorefractive keratectomy: a case report, *Eye* (1994) **8**: 481–2.

23. Pepose JS, Laycock KA, Miller JK, et al, Reactivation of latent herpes simplex virus by excimer laser photokeratectomy, *Am J Ophthalmol* (1992) **114**: 45–50.

24. Vrabec MP, Anderson JA, Rock ME, et al, Electron microscopic findings in a cornea with recurrence of herpes simplex keratitis after excimer laser phototherapeutic keratectomy, *CLAO Journal* (1994) **20**: 41–4.

25. McGhee CNJ, Weed KH, Bryce IG, A prospective analysis of minor and major complications of excimer laser PRK and PARK, *Proc Int Soc Refract Surg: midsummer symposium* (1995): 93–4.

26. Seiler T, Schmidt-Petersen H, Wollensak J, Complications after myopic photorefractive keratectomy, primarily with the Summit excimer laser. In: Salz JJ, ed, *Corneal Laser Surgery* (Mosby: St Louis, PA, 1995) 131–42.

27. Brancato R, Tavola A, Carones F, et al. Excimer laser photorefractive keratectomy for myopia: results in 1165 eyes, *Refract Corneal Surg* (1993) **9**: S95–S104.

28. Epstein D, Fagerholm P, Hamberg-Nystrom H, Tengroth B, Twenty-four months' follow-up of excimer laser photorefractive keratectomy for myopia. Refractive and visual acuity results, *Ophthalmology* (1994) **101**: 1558–63.

29. McGhee CNJ, Weed KH, Bryce I, Anastas CN, Steele CF, A three-year experience of excimer laser multizone PRK and PARK in a UK National Health Service setting, *Proc Int Soc Refract Surg: midsummer symposium* (1996): 39–40.

30. Quah BL, Wong EYM, Tseng PSF, et al, Analysis of photo-refractive keratectomy patients who have not had PRK in their second eye, *Ophthalmic Surg Lasers* (1996) **27**: S429–S434.

31. Schallhorn SC, Blanton Cl, Kaupp SE, et al, Preliminary results of photorefractive keratectomy in active-duty United States navy personnel, *Ophthalmology* (1996) **103**: 5–22.

32. Durrie DS, Lesher MP, Cavanaugh TB, Classification of variable clinical response after photorefractive keratectomy for myopia, *J Refract Surg* (1995) **11**: 341–7.

33. Kim JH, Sah WJ, Kim MS, Lee YC, Park Ck, Three-year results of photorefractive keratectomy for myopia, *J Refract Surg* (1995) **11**: S248–S252.

34. Kim JH, Sah WJ, Park CK, Hahn TW, Kim MS, Myopic regression after photorefractive keratectomy, *Ophthalmic Surg Lasers* (1996) **27**: S435–S439.

35. Snibson GR, Carson CA, Aldred GF, Taylor HR, One-year evaluation of excimer laser photorefractive keratectomy for myopia and myopic astigmatism, *Arch Ophthalmol* (1995) **113**: 994–1000.

36. Krueger RR, Talamo JH, McDonald MB, Varnell RJ,

Wagoner MD, McDonnell PJ, Clinical analysis of excimer laser using a multiple zone technique for severe myopia, *Am J Ophthalmol* (1995) **119**: 263–74.

37. Amano S, Shimizu K, Excimer laser photorefractive keratectomy for myopia: two-year follow-up, *J Refract Surg* (1995) **11**: S253–S260.

38. Menezo JL, Martinez-Costa R, Navea A, Roig V, Cisneros A, Excimer laser photorefractive keratectomy for high myopia, *J Cataract Refract Surg* (1995) **21**: 393–7.

39. Seiler T, Holschbach A, Derse M, et al, Complications of myopic photorefractive keratectomy with the excimer laser, *Ophthalmology* (1994) **101**: 153–60.

40. Goggin M, Algawi K, O'Keefe M, Astigmatism following photorefractive keratectomy for myopia, *J Refract Corneal Surg* (1994) **10**: 540–4.

41. Taylor HR, Guest CS, Kelly P, Alpins N, Comparison of excimer laser treatment of astigmatism and myopia, *Arch Ophthalmol* (1993) **111**: 1621–6.

42. Tavola A, Carones F, Galli L, Fontanella G, Brancato R, The learning curve in myopic photorefractive keratectomy, *Refract Corneal Surg* (1994) **10**: S188–S193.

43. Lin DTC, Corneal topographic analysis after excimer laser photorefractive keratectomy, *Ophthalmology* (1994) **101**: 1432–9.

44. Amano S, Tanaka S, Shimizu K, Topographical evaluation of centration of excimer laser myopic photorefractive keratectomy, *J Cataract Refract Surg* (1988) **14**: 46–52.

45. Shimizu K, Amano S, Tanaka S, Photorefractive keratectomy for myopia: one-year follow-up in 97 eyes, *Refract Corneal Surg* (1994) **10**: S178–S187.

46. Doane JF, Cavanaugh TB, Durrie DS, Hassanein KM, Relation of visual symptoms to topographic ablation zone decentration after excimer laser photorefractive keratectomy, *Ophthalmology* (1995) **102**: 42–7.

47. Schwartz-Goldstein BH, Hersh PS, Corneal topography of phase III excimer laser photorefractive keratectomy: optical zone centration analysis, *Ophthalmology* (1995) **102**: 951–62.

48. Webber SK, McGhee CNJ, Bryce IG, Decentration of photorefractive keratectomy ablation zones after excimer laser surgery for myopia, *J Cataract Refract Surg* (1996) **22**: 299–303.

49. Maloney RK, Corneal topography and optical zone location in photorefractive keratectomy, *Refract Corneal Surg* (1990) **6**: 363–71.

50. Maguire LJ, Zabel RW, Parker P, Lindstrom RL, Topography and raytracing analysis of patients with excellent visual acuity 3 months after excimer laser photorefractive keratectomy, *Refract Corneal Surg* (1991) **7**: 122–8.

51. Seiler T, Wollensak J, Myopic photorefractive keratectomy with the excimer laser. One-year follow-up, *Ophthalmology* (1991) **98**: 1156–63.

52. Hamberg-Nystrom H, Tengroth B, Fagerholm P, Epstein D, van der Kwast E, Patient satisfaction following photorefractive keratectomy for myopia, *J Refract Surg* (1995) **11**: S335–S336.

53. O'Brart DPS, Gartry DS, Lohmann CP, Kerr Muir MG, Marshall J, Excimer laser photorefractive keratectomy for myopia: comparison of 4.00 and 5.00 millimeter ablation zones, *J Refract Corneal Surg* (1994) **10**: 87–94.

54. Kim JO, Hahn TW, Lee YC, Joo CK, Sah WJ, Photorefractive keratectomy in 202 myopic eyes: one-year results, *Refract Corneal Surg* (1993) **9**: S11–S16.

55. Rogers CM, Lawless MA, Cohen PR, Photorefractive keratectomy for myopia of more than –10 diopters, *Refract Corneal Surg* (1994) **10**: S171–S173.

56. Levin S, Carson CA, Garrett SK, Taylor HR, Prevalence of central islands after excimer laser refractive surgery, *J Cataract Refract Surg* (1995) **21**: 21–26.

57. Butuner Z, Elliot DB, Gimbel HV, Slimmon S, Visual function one year after excimer laser photorefractive keratectomy, *J Refract Corneal Surg* (1994) **10**: 625–30.

58. Salz JJ, Maguen E, Nesburn AB, et al, A two-year experience with the excimer laser photorefractive keratectomy for myopia, *Ophthalmology* (1993) **100**: 873–82.

59. Kim JH, Sah WJ, Hahn TW, Lee YC, Some problems after photorefractive keratectomy, *Refract Corneal Surg* (1994) **10**: S226–S230.

60. Hamberg-Nystrom H, Fagerholm P, Tengroth B, Sjoholm C, Thirty-six month follow-up of excimer laser photorefractive keratectomy for myopia, *Ophthalmic Surg Lasers* (1996) **27**: S418–S420.

61. Ambrosio G, Cennamo G, De Marco R, Loffredo L, Rosa N, Sebastiani A, Visual function before and after photorefractive keratectomy for myopia, *J Refract Corneal Surg* (1994) **10**: 129–36.

62. Esente S, Passarelli N, Falco L, Passani F, Guidi D, Contrast sensitivity under photopic conditions in photorefractive keratectomy: a preliminary report, *Refract Corneal Surg* (1993) **9**: S70–S72.

63. Gartry DS, Kerr-Muir MG, Marshall J, Photorefractive keratectomy with an argon fluoride excimer laser: a clinical study, *Refract Corneal Surg* (1991) **7**: 420–35.

64. Lohmann CP, Fitzke F, O'Brart D, et al, Corneal light scattering and visual performance in myopic individuals with spectacles, contact lenses, or excimer photorefractive keratectomy, *Am J Ophthalmol* (1993) **115**: 444–53.

65. Harrison JM, Tennant TB, Gwin MC, et al, Forward light scatter at one month after photorefractive keratectomy, *J Refract Surg* (1995) **11**: 83–8.

66. Kwitco ML, Gow J, Bellavance F, Wu JW, Excimer laser photorefractive keratectomy: one-year follow-up, *Ophthalmic Surg Lasers* (1996) **27**: S454–S447.

67. Lohmann CP, Timberlake GT, Fitzke FW, Gartry DS, Kerr-Muir MG, Marshall J, Corneal light scattering after excimer laser photorefractive keratectomy: the objective measurements of haze, *Refract Corneal Surg* (1992) **8**: 114–21.

68. Alleman N, Chamon W, Silverman RH, et al, High frequency ultrasound quantitative analyses of corneal scarring following excimer laser photorefractive keratectomy, *Arch Ophthalmol* (1993) **111**: 968–73.

69. McWhae J, Willerscheidt A, Gimbel H, Freese M, Ultrasound biomicroscopy in refractive surgery, *J Cataract Refract Surg* (1994) **20**: 493–7.

70. Pavlin CJ, Harasiewicz K, Foster SF, Ultrasound biomicroscopic assessment of the cornea following excimer laser photokeratectomy, *J Cataract Refract Surg* (1994) **20**: 206–10.

71. Andrade HA, McDonald MB, Liu JC, Abdelmegeed M, Evaluation of an opacity lensometer for determining corneal clarity following excimer laser photoablation, *Refract Corneal Surg* (1990) **6**: 346–51.

72. Caubert E, Cause of subepithelial corneal haze over 18 months after photorefractive keratectomy for myopia, *Refract Corneal Surg* (1993) **9**: S65–S70.

73. Bailey IL, Bullimore MA, Raasch TW HR, Clinical grading and the effects of scaling, *Invest Ophthalmol Vis Sci* (1991) **32**: 422–32.

74. Orssaud C, Ganem S, Binaghi M, et al, Photorefractive keratectomy in 176 eyes one-year follow-up, *Refract Corneal Surg* (1994) **10**: S199–S205.

75. Campos M, Cuevas K, Garbus J, Lee M, McDonnell PJ, Corneal wound healing after excimer laser ablation: effects of nitrogen gas blower, *Ophthalmology* (1992) **99**: 893–7.

76. Ditzen K, Anschuetz T, Shroeder E, Photorefractive keratectomy to treat low, medium and high myopia: a multicenter study, *J Cataract Refract Surg* (1994) **20**: 234–8.

77. Loewenstein A, Lipshitz I, Ben-Shirah A, Barak V, Lazar M, Symmetry of outcome after photorefractive keratectomy for myopia, *J Refract Surg* (1995) **11**: S268–S269.

78. Busin M, Meller D, Corneal epithelial dots following excimer laser photorefractive keratectomy, *J Refract Corneal Surg* (1994) **10**: 357–9.

79. Mendez A, Radial keratotomy in myopic patients with glaucoma, *Refract Corneal Surg* (1989) **5**: 327–9.

80. Sastry S, Sperdut RD, Waring GO, et al, Radial keratotomy does not affect intraocular pressure, *Refract Corneal Surg* (1993) **9**: 459–64.

81. Phelan PS, McGhee CN, Bryce IG, Excimer laser PRK and corticosteroid induced IOP elevation: the tip of an emerging iceberg? *Br J Ophthalmol* (1994) **78**: 802–3.

82. McGhee CNJ, Anastas CN, Bryce IG, Allen W, Phelan PS, Implications of sustained undermeasurement of IOP by Goldmann applanation tonometry after excimer laser PRK, *Proc Int Soc Refract Surg: midsummer symposium* (1996): 42.

83. Ehlers N, Bramsen T, Sperling S, Applanation tonometry and central corneal thickness, *Arch Ophthalmol* (1975) **53**: 34–43.

84. Argus WA, Ocular hypertension and central corneal thickness, *Ophthalmology* (1995) **102**: 1810–12.

85. Tomlinson A, Leighton DA, Ocular dimensions in low tension glaucoma compared with open-angle glaucoma and the normal population, *Br J Ophthalmol* (1972) **56**: 97–103.

86. Mark HH, Corneal curvature in applanation tonometry, *Am J Ophthalmol* (1973) **76**: 223–4.

87. Schipper I, Senn P, Niessen U, Are we measuring the right intraocular pressure after excimer laser photorefractive keratoplasty in myopia, *Klin Monatsbl Augenheilkd* (1995) **206**: 322–4.

88. Chaterjee A, Shah S, Bessant SA, et al, Reduction in ocular pressure after excimer laser photorefractive keratectomy: correlation with pre-treatment myopia. The third annual UK international ophthalmic excimer laser congress, *Eye News (suppl)* (1996) **3**: S18.

89. Tervo K, Latvala TM, Tervo MT, Recovery of innervation following photorefractive keratoablation, *Arch Ophthalmol* (1994) **112**: 1466–70.

90. Ishikawa T, Park SB, Cox C, del Cerro M, Aquavella JV, Corneal sensation following excimer laser photorefractive keratectomy in humans, *J Refract Corneal Surg* (1994) **10**: 417–22.

91. Ishikawa T, del Cerro M, Liang FQ, Loya N, Aquavella JV, Corneal sensitivity and regeneration after excimer laser ablation, *Cornea* (1994) **13**: 225–31.

92. Sher NA, Chen V, Bowers RA, et al, The use of the 193-nm excimer laser for myopic photorefractive keratectomy in sighted eyes, *Arch Ophthalmol* (1991) **109**: 1525–30.

93. Campos M, Hertzog L, Garbus JJ, McDonnell PJ, Corneal sensitivity after photorefractive keratectomy, *Am J Ophthalmol* (1992) **114**: 51–54.

94. Dehm EJ, Puliafito CA, Adler CM, Steinert RF, Corneal endothelial injury in rabbits following excimer laser ablation at 193 and 248 nm, *Arch Ophthalmol* (1986) **104**: 1364–8.

95. Marshall J, Trokel S, Rothery S, Krueger RR, A comparative study of corneal incisions induced by diamond and steel knives and two ultraviolet radiations from an excimer laser, *Br J Ophthalmol* (1986) **70**: 482–501.

96. Frueh BE, Bohnke M, Endothelial cell morphology after phototherapeutic keratectomy, *German J Ophthalmol* (1995) **4**: 86–9.

97. Carones F, Brancato R, Venturi E, Morico A. The corneal endothelium after myopic excimer laser photorefractive keratectomy, *Arch Ophthalmol* (1994) **112**: 920–24.

98. Mardelli PG, Peibenga LA, Matta CS, Hyde LL, Gira J. Corneal endothelial status 12 to 55 months after excimer laser photorefractive keratectomy, *Ophthalmology* (1995) **102**: 544–9.

99. Seiler T, Holshbach A, Central corneal iron deposit after photorefractive keratectomy, *German J Ophthalmol* (1993) **2**: 143–5.

100. Janknetcht P, Soriano JM, Hansen LL, Cystoid macular oedema after excimer laser photorefractive keratectomy, *Br J Ophthalmol* (1993) **77**: 681 (letter).

101. Hersh PS, Jordan AJ, Mayers M, Corneal graft rejection episode after excimer laser photorefractive keratectomy, *Arch Ophthalmol* (1993) **111**: 735–6.

102. Lesher MP, Schumer DJ, Hunkeler JD, Durrie DS, McKee FE, Phacoemulsification with intraocular lens implantation after excimer photorefractive keratectomy: a case report, *J Cataract Refract Surg* (1994) **20**: S265–S267.

103. Burnstein Y, Klapper D, Hersh PS, Experimental globe rupture after excimer laser photorefractive keratectomy, *Arch Ophthalmol* (1995) **113**: 1056–9.

104. Guttridge NM, Changes in ocular and visual variables during the menstrual cycle, *Ophthalmic Physiol Opt* (1994) **14**: 38–48.

105. Hefetz L, Gershevich D, Haviv D, et al, Influence of pregnancy and labor on outcome of photorefractive keratectomy, *J Refract Surg* (1996) **12**: 511–12.

Chapter 24 **Regression and retreatment**

Grant R Snibson

BACKGROUND

The effectiveness of the excimer laser in the correction of low and moderate degrees of myopia is now well established. In this group of patients the predictability of photorefractive keratectomy (PRK) is good and, in most cases, the resultant refraction stabilizes within 6 months with little loss of effect with the passage of time. There are, however, patients for whom treatment does not fully correct their myopia. Analysis of these cases offers some insight into the factors that predispose to regression and undercorrection and an assessment of the effectiveness of repeat ablations.

DEFINITION

It is now apparent that the refractive response to surgery varies to some degree according to the laser used and the treatment algorithms employed, as well as the magnitude of the myopic correction attempted. Early treatment paradigms involving small diameter ablation zones produced immediate overcorrections followed by early regression, bringing the refraction close to emmetropia.[1] This form of regression is obviously desirable but, for the purposes of this chapter, regression may be defined as a myopic shift in the manifest and cycloplegic refractions following PRK resulting in the recurrence of clinically significant myopia. Regression in this context represents the loss of effect following PRK of a degree greater than might be expected after a given treatment at a specific time point postoperatively.

It is convenient to consider regression with respect to its timing in relation to the treatment. Early regression occurs within 6 months of PRK, whilst late regression refers to changes occurring during the balance of the first year. Long-term regression may actually be observed after the first year.[2] Although a stable refraction should be a prerequisite in the preoperative consideration of refractive surgery, it is inevitable that a proportion of patients will experience some 'natural' increase in their myopia in the medium- to long-term, whether or not PRK is performed. This change, which is frequently bilateral, should be viewed as progression of the myopia rather than regression of effect.

Undercorrection evident in the immediate postoperative period results from an ineffective ablation. This may be due to calibration or programming errors, beam inhomogeneity or a number of other technical faults in the laser or its delivery system. The surgeon may produce undercorrection by incomplete epithelial removal or by permitting overhydration of the cornea during treatment.

RISK FACTORS

HIGH MYOPIA

The major risk factor for regression and undercorrection is the degree of preoperative myopia. In a multicenter study using the Aesculap-Meditec MEL60 excimer laser (Heroldsberg, Germany), Ditzen et al.[3] demonstrated a clear relationship between preoperative myopia and residual myopia at 12 months after PRK (Table 24.1). The variation in the degree of regression (reflected in the standard deviation of spherical equivalent at 12 months) also increased with increasing myopia. This trend has also been reported from studies of treatments performed with Summit[4] and Visx[5,6] lasers. For a more complete review of the results of the treatment of high myopia, see Chapter 10.

Table 24.1
Changes in refraction following PRK for varying degrees of myopia. (Modified after Ditzen et al., 1994[3])

Group (n=325 eyes)	Myopia range (D)	Mean spherical equivalent (D)	Postoperative mean spherical equivalent (standard deviation)			
			1 month	3 months	6 months	12 months
1 n=93	0.00 to −6.00	−4.1	+0.4 (1.4)	0.0 (1.1)	−0.5 (1.0)	−0.8 (0.8)
2 n=97	−6.25 to −10.00	−8.3	+0.5 (2.3)	−0.3 (1.8)	−0.7 (2.0)	−1.7 (2.3)
3 n=87	−10.25 to −15.00	−12.5	0.0 (2.8)	−1.4 (2.6)	−1.9 (2.9)	−2.0 (2.8)
4 n=48	−15.25 or more	−19.9	−4.2 (3.7)	−5.2 (4.0)	−6.5 (3.6)	−9.9 (6.5)

The cause of more pronounced regression that frequently occurs after PRK for high myopia has not been determined with any certainty. We do know that, in general, regression increases with increasing depth of the stromal ablation. Epithelial hyperplasia may be promoted by deeper and steeper ablations; or it may be that the stimulation of, or damage to, deeper stromal keratocytes results in an exaggerated fibroblastic response with enhanced collagen production and stromal remodelling. Alternatively, there could be something qualitatively different about the cornea itself and, therefore, its response to photoablation, in high myopia. In order to minimize the depth required in higher degrees of myopia, algorithms employing multiple ablation zones have been adopted (Fig. 24.1). However, this strategy has not eliminated the problem of regression in high myopia.[6,7]

Occasionally, highly myopic patients will experience marked regression such that their final refraction approaches their preoperative spherical equivalent. This dramatic, idiosyncratic form of regression is most frequently seen after treatments for myopia of more than 8 D and is commonly associated with corneal haze.[1,7]

Case Report
A 40-year-old woman underwent left photoastigmatic keratectomy (PARK) for extreme myopia and astigmatism using the Visx 20/20 laser and a multizone treatment algorithm. This was followed by regression to approximately 50% of her preoperative spherical

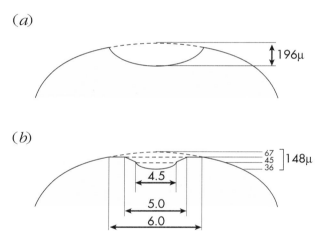

Figure 24.1 *Comparison of a single ablation zone and a multizone approach to correct 15 D of myopia. The multizone approach results in a 25% reduction in the depth of the ablation (based on Visx version 2.7 software) and an aspheric refracting surface. Greater reduction in depth can be achieved by increasing the proportion of the total correction allocated to the smaller zones. The diagrams are not drawn to scale and dimensions have been exaggerated for illustrative purposes. (a) Single 6.0 mm ablation zone. (b) Multiple (6.0 mm, 5.0 mm and 4.5 mm) ablation zones with the spherical correction evenly divided between zones.*

Table 24.2

The results of PRK and retreatment of the left eye of a 40-year-old female with high myopia and astigmatism (see case report).

Examination	Subjective refraction	Maximum power change in difference map	Corneal haze score
Preoperative	−13.75/−2.75 × 165	–	0.0
Initial PRK Intended correction	−13.75/−2.75 × 165		
1 month	−1.25/−0.25 × 135	13.6 D	1.0
3 months	−1.50/−0.50 × 15	13.1 D	1.0
6 months	−4.00/−0.50 × 180	10.2 D	2.0
9 months	−6.75/−0.75 × 175	8.4 D	3.0
Retreatment Intended correction	−6.75/−0.75 × 175		
1 month	+1.00/−2.00 × 10	–	1.0
3 months	+0.75	–	1.5
6 months	+0.75/−0.50 × 180	–	2.0
12 months	−1.25/−0.50 × 170	–	1.5

equivalent. Retreatment was performed after 9 months and, although again followed by regression, the outcome was regarded as satisfactory (Table 24.2). Her right eye (−14.00/−2.25 × 172) behaved similarly, regressing to −9.00/−1.00 × 10 by 12 months after PRK. Corneal topography at 1 month using the Tomey TMS-1 videokeratoscope demonstrates a well-centered ablation with more than 13 D of power change evident when compared with the preoperative study (Fig. 24.2a) using a difference map (Fig. 24.2b). By 6 months, more than 3 D of steepening (regression) had occurred with increased surface irregularity (Fig. 24.2c). Regression continued to almost 50% of the original refraction and was accompanied by significant haze.

The long-term stability of the refraction following PRK is yet to be established. Epstein et al.[8] have documented stability from 18 months after PRK and an early report of a series with 3 year follow-up did not describe regression during the third postoperative year.[9] Kim et al.,[2] however, did observe regression between 12 and 36 months after PRK with a 5.0 mm ablation zone. Longer periods of follow-up of larger numbers of eyes are required before this question can be answered with confidence.

LASER CHARACTERISTICS AND TREATMENT PARAMETERS

Ablation zone diameter

The central depth of a spherical ablation increases exponentially with the diameter of the ablation zone:

$$d = \frac{D \times AZ^2}{3}$$

d = central ablation depth (μm)
D = dioptric correction (D)
AZ = ablation zone diameter (mm)

Small ablation zones were used by early investigators so that the depth of the ablation could be minimized. This was based on evidence that the degree of postoperative corneal opacification is related to ablation depth.[10,11] However, ablation zone diameter also appears to be a major factor determining the

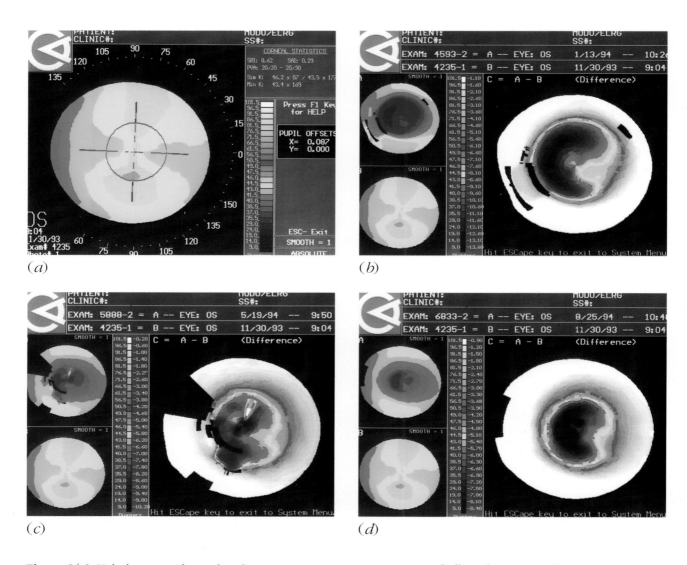

Figure 24.2 *Videokeratography studies demonstrating progressive regression of effect of a PARK performed for high myopia (see case report and Table 24.2). (a) Preoperative corneal topography. (b) Difference map showing the initial refractive change evident at 1 month. (c) Difference map showing the refractive change evident at 6 months. (d) Difference map showing the refractive change evident at 9 months (preretreatment). (Courtesy of Hugh Taylor MD.)*

degree of early regression. The smaller the ablation zone, the greater the early regression that is seen. When 4 and 5 mm ablation zones were compared in a series of patients undergoing bilateral treatment of similar magnitude, a significantly greater refractive change (i.e. less regression) was observed in the eyes treated with the larger ablation zone.[12] A prospective, randomized study comparing 5.0 and 6.0 mm zones has also demonstrated less regression (and less haze) with the larger ablation zone diameter.[13] With smaller ablation zone diameters, the effect of epithelial

hyperplasia, which seems to occur in an attempt to restore the previous surface contour, is more pronounced (see below) (Fig. 24.3).

Beam profile

In addition, beam inhomogeneity may explain some of the differences observed between lasers. The energy distribution across the beam produced by high-powered excimer lasers is far from uniform (Fig.

(*a*)

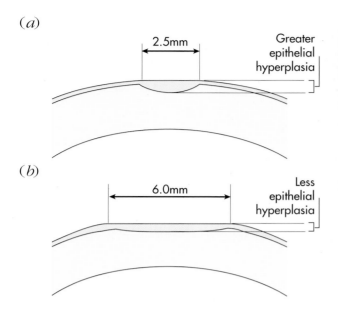

(*b*)

Figure 24.3 *Epithelial hyperplasia following PRK. Filling in of the stromal ablation leads to regression of effect. The smaller and deeper the ablation zone, the greater the refractive regression attributable to epithelial hyperplasia.*

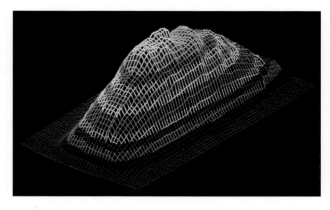

Figure 24.4 *The energy profile that is typically produced by a high-powered excimer laser. The base corresponds to the beam's cross-section and the height corresponds to the energy at that point. (Courtesy of Paul van Saarloos, Lions Eye Institute, Perth, Australia.)*

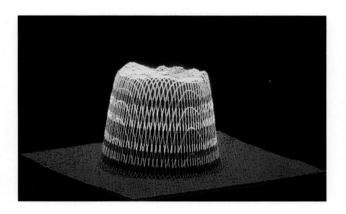

Figure 24.5 *The energy profile after the excimer laser beam has passed through the delivery system of a TELCO (The Excimer Laser Company, Perth) excimer laser. (Courtesy of Paul van Saarloos, Lions Eye Institute, Perth, Australia.)*

24.4). The beam is then 'smoothed' by a number of the optical elements in the delivery system (Fig. 24.5). Despite manufacturers' attempts to produce an even distribution of energy across the beam, there are differences between lasers in this respect. Beams with a 'hot center' (i.e. greater concentration of energy at the center of the beam) may be more likely to be associated with early regression than those that are more homogenous or those that have 'cold centers' (Fig. 24.6).

Fluence

The energy density of the laser pulse, or fluence, may be a factor in the development of haze and regression. The acoustic shock wave generated by the laser pulse is approximately proportional to the fluence of the laser output for large area ablations.[14] The greater acoustic shock waves associated with higher fluences may cause deeper and more widespread stimulation of keratocytes, with a resultant increase in haze and regression.[15] There is currently little evidence to support this theory.

Treatment algorithm

The characteristic pattern of regression seen with a particular laser is a result not only of the ablation zone diameters used and the nature of the beam, but also of the treatment algorithm with which it is programmed. Controlling software will take these

(a)

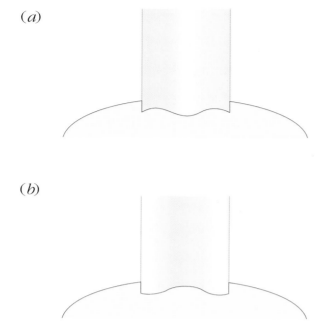

(b)

Figure 24.6 *Energy profiles of excimer laser beams. (a) A beam with greater energy density centrally ('hot center') may produce early overcorrections. (b) A beam with a lower density centrally ('cold center') may produce undercorrections and/or central islands.*

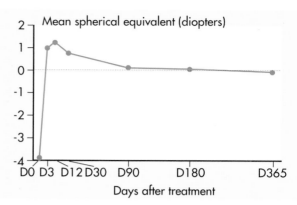

(a)

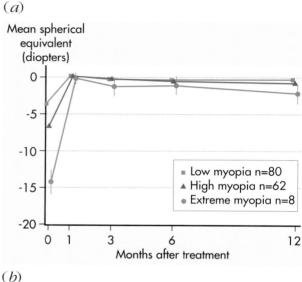

(b)

Figure 24.7 *Regression of refractive effect over time following PRK with two laser systems. (a) Change in spherical equivalent (D) with time (days) after PRK with the Summit Excimed UV200 LA excimer laser (Orssaud et al., 1994).[75] (b) Change in spherical equivalent following PRK with the Visx 20/20 excimer laser. (Snibson et al., 1995).[5]*

properties into account to produce an ablation that will hopefully result in a refraction close to emmetropia. With the benefit of clinical experience, correction factors can be applied to address under-correction (or overcorrection), which may then be incorporated into the controlling software. For example, we understand that early Visx software was written to produce a small undercorrection of approximately −0.3 D in order to reduce the frequency and severity of overcorrection, whilst more recent software targets an emmetropic endpoint.

For these reasons, different excimer laser systems are unlikely to produce identical results and the early changes in refraction that occur following PRK are often characteristic of the type of laser used. The Summit Technology Excimed UV200 (Waltham, MA) laser can be expected to produce an overcorrection within the first month after treatment and early regression is relied upon to bring the refraction close to that intended by the third month (Fig. 24.7a). The Visx 20/20 laser, with larger treatment zones (6.0 mm), produces less early overcorrection and corre-

spondingly less regression (Fig. 24.7b). The more recent Summit Omnimed and Apogee lasers, like other wide area ablation lasers employing larger ablation zone diameters, are also producing less early overcorrection and regression.

Miscellaneous

Comparisons of astigmatic treatments with purely spherical ablations have suggested that regression and subsequent retreatment may be more common after PARK. This observation may be explained, to some extent, by the association of significant astigmatism with higher degrees of myopia. However, when appropriate statistical analyses are applied that control for the degree of preoperative myopia, PARK would still seem to be associated with a greater likelihood of retreatment.[16] Further studies are needed to confirm this finding.

Age, gender and race have not been shown to be major risk factors for regression.

MECHANISMS OF REGRESSION

EPITHELIAL HYPERPLASIA

Epithelial healing commences within 4–6 hours of completion of the procedure.[17] The epithelial defect has usually closed by the third postoperative day and rarely persists beyond 7 days. Initially, the ablated cornea is surfaced by a single layer of epithelial cells. During the ensuing weeks the epithelium increases in thickness. Frequently this thickening is non-uniform, resulting in the variable topographic disturbances that may be observed during the early postoperative period. Ultimately, the central epithelium becomes thickest, usually thicker than the epithelium over the untreated cornea, in an attempt to restore the original contour of the corneal surface.[18,19] This epithelial hyperplasia is observable clinically and has been shown histologically.[20,21] The effect of this hyperplasia is to reduce the change in surface curvature produced by the treatment and shift the refraction in the direction of myopia (see Fig. 24.3).

There is histological evidence that, at least in the cynomolgus monkey, the epithelium attains normal thickness by 6 months.[22] However, this may not be the case in human eyes that have undergone significant refractive regression. When a uniform ablation with the excimer laser is used to remove the epithelium in eyes undergoing retreatment, it is usual to observe the loss of fluorescence first in the periphery of the treatment area, with the appearance of a dark ring as the basal epithelium is removed. Residual epithelium in the center requires further ablation, suggesting that the epithelial layer is substantially thicker centrally. Epithelial thickness has been measured following unilateral PRK, using a modified optical pachymeter, and shown to be increased in comparison with the untreated eye. Epithelial thickness may continue to increase beyond the second postoperative year.[23,24]

EXTRACELLULAR MATRIX

Scrapings taken at the time of retreatment have revealed an increase in extracellular material in the majority of specimens studied.[25] Hyaluronic acid has been identified as one component of this matrix and has been nominated as a possible contributing factor in the development of myopic regression after PRK (see below). A histopathologic examination of human corneal tissue from eyes exhibiting haze and regression has shown excessive, newly synthesized, extracellular matrix with virtually no new collagen evident. This subepithelial material was much less evident in the single overcorrected (hypermetropic) eye studied.[26]

COLLAGEN SYNTHESIS AND STROMAL REMODELLING

Collagen expression in the rat cornea has been detected as early as 30 minutes after PRK, reaching a peak 1–2 weeks after injury.[27] Activated corneal fibroblasts (keratocytes) with prominent, dilated, rough endoplasmic reticulum have been observed in the ablated monkey cornea, surrounded by disorganized collagen fibrils.[22] Similar changes have been observed in the human cornea.[28] This would suggest that new collagen synthesis is occurring during the months after PRK. This new collagen (type III)[29] is deposited over the ablated stromal surface and its thickness increases with the depth of the ablation.[21]

Clinically, new collagen formation may be visible as a diffuse or reticular, subepithelial opacity or 'haze' and may result in some filling in of the stromal ablation and alteration in the curvature of the corneal surface. Asymmetric collagen deposition may also contribute to topographic disturbances, regression of astigmatic ablations[21] and irregular astigmatism. Nonetheless, the ability to observe the concentric ablation rings on the corneal stromal surface after epithelial removal some months (or even years) after PRK would suggest that stromal remodelling does not play a major role in all cases of regression leading to retreatment.

CORNEAL HAZE

The production of new and disorganized collagen fibrils is regarded by some as the major cause of corneal haze after excimer laser ablation, but the extent to which altered extracellular matrix and other factors contribute to the corneal opacity is unknown.

Both regression[30] and the degree of postoperative haze[4] appear to be related to the degree of preoperative myopia (and ablation depth) and are commonly seen together. The precise relationship between haze and regression is not clear; regression may occur in the absence of haze and prominent haze may be seen without regression. It is likely, though, that both haze and regression are the result of an exaggerated healing response to the stimulus of excimer laser photoablation.

TREATMENT OF REGRESSION

CORTICOSTEROIDS

In most centers, topical corticosteroids have been routinely used for periods of weeks to several months after PRK. This treatment is based on the assumption that postoperative corneal haze and regression are decreased by the corticosteroids by means of an inhibitory effect on DNA synthesis within keratocytes[31] and, consequently, collagen synthesis.[32–35] It would be expected that any such effect would be maximal during the first few months after surgery, when keratocyte activity and stromal remodelling are maximal.[22]

Initial support for the use of topical steroids derived from rabbit studies in which some effect was noted on postoperative haze[36,37] and the inflammatory response.[38] Steroids have also been shown, in this model, to reduce the cellular density and activity within the stroma underlying the ablated surface.[39] A number of clinical studies have also suggested a role for corticosteroids in modulating the refractive outcome of PRK.[40–43]

In a prospective, randomized, placebo-controlled trial, Gartry et al.[44,45] did demonstrate less regression in a topical dexamethasone 0.1% treated group 6 weeks after PRK compared to placebo controls, but this effect was not sustained after withdrawal of the corticosteroids. No effect on haze was detected. Because of the hazards of topical corticosteroid therapy and the lack of a demonstrable long-term benefit, the authors of this report recommended that corticosteroids should not be used after PRK. Another randomized study (using a Visx 20/20 laser) involving 214 eyes failed to demonstrate any benefit of 6

months of topical dexamethasone compared to a 3-week course of the same steroid.[46]

In contrast, Fagerholm et al.[47] concluded from a larger, but non-randomized study (using the Summit ExciMed laser) that postoperative topical dexamethasone does reduce the regression observed at the 6 month follow-up visit. A supplementary retrospective study comparing 40 patients who did not receive postoperative topical steroids with another two groups of 40 patients with topical dexamethasone drops for 5 weeks or 3 months also revealed a difference in refraction 9 months after surgery. The same authors reported a consistent beneficial effect of corticosteroids on corneal haze

A more recent prospective study[48] has supported Gartry's original findings by demonstrating that corticosteroids were able to maintain a hyperopic shift during their administration, with loss of this effect following their withdrawal. It should be noted, however, that the difference in refractive change observed at 12 months for ablations of −6.00 D was of borderline statistical significance and a role for corticosteroids in the postoperative management of highly myopic patients remains undetermined.

Although there is some controversy regarding the routine use of topical corticosteroids during the early postoperative period, the anecdotal experiences of excimer laser surgeons would suggest that some patients do exhibit delayed regression, which is quite clearly steroid responsive.[49,50] In these patients, the corticosteroids may inhibit the expression of hyaluronan by keratocytes and epithelial cells. Hyaluronan is a high molecular weight disaccharide polymer capable of binding large quantities of water. It is not normally found in the epithelium or corneal stroma but is produced in variable quantities following excimer laser stromal ablation[51] as well as in a range of other corneal disorders.[52] Whilst this may represent a non-specific response to corneal injury, hyaluronan production would lead to an increase in corneal hydration and thickness. The resultant changes in refractive index and/or corneal curvature would impact on the refractive power of the cornea. The modification of hyaluronan expression by topical corticosteroids, for which there is some experimental evidence,[53] might be consistent with the rapid response (change in refraction) following the initiation or withdrawal of topical steroid treatment noted in some patients (see Chapter 25).

Clearly more long-term studies of the effect of topical corticosteroids on refractive outcome after PRK are needed. The benefit, if any, of topical steroids also needs to be demonstrated for the different laser systems and the larger treatment zones now employed, as well as in the treatment of low myopia where regression and haze are less problematic. The role of topical corticosteroids following PRK has been reviewed recently by Corbett, O'Brart and Marshall.[54]

NON-STEROIDAL ANTI-INFLAMMATORY AGENTS

In many centers, topical non-steroidal anti-inflammatory (NSAID) agents are used during the early postoperative period to minimize the pain associated with the healing epithelial defect.[55,56] Although randomized controlled trials are lacking, a reduction in myopic regression has also been attributed to flurbiprofen, and to a lesser extent diclofenac, when used in conjunction with topical corticosteroids.[57] Further studies are necessary to determine if NSAID agents have a genuine role to play in modulating the refractive results of PRK (see Chapter 25).

PLASMIN INHIBITORS

It has been suggested that inhibitors of the plasminogen-activator/plasmin system may have a role in improving the outcome of photorefractive surgery.[58] However, topical aprotinin, an inhibitor of both plasmin and plasminogen activator,[59] produced no beneficial effect when compared with placebo in a prospective randomized trial.[48]

CONTACT LENS FITTING

Some patients who experience regression and undercorrection following PRK may elect to resume contact lens wear rather than undergo retreatment. Others will be reliant on contact lenses until their refraction stabilizes sufficiently to consider a second procedure. Rigid contact lenses may be the only effective means of dealing with irregular astigmatism due to decentration or irregularity of the postablation corneal surface, important causes of loss of best corrected visual acuity following PRK. To date, little has been published on the subject of contact lens fitting after excimer laser surgery.[60,61]

In most cases, fitting is based on preoperative keratometry readings. The area of central corneal flattening is vaulted by rigid lenses (producing a thick tear lens) and powers approaching the preoperative spectacle prescription may be required.[61] Reduced

tear exchange and some bubble trapping may result. Modification of the central back surface curvature to improve alignment with the central cornea may help alleviate these problems. Soft lenses will generally conform to some degree to the new surface curvature but frequently more minus power is required than expected from the spectacle refraction, suggesting that some vaulting is occurring. Disposable soft lenses are a convenient and inexpensive means of dealing with undercorrection whilst waiting for the refraction to stabilize prior to retreatment.

EPITHELIAL DEBRIDEMENT

Manual scraping of the epithelium has been claimed to produce a modest improvement in patients with myopic regression after PRK.[26,62] This treatment is based on the assumption that regression results predominantly from epithelial hyperplasia, with or without subjacent extracellular matrix deposition, and that these changes will not recur to the same extent following the debridement. Fagerholm et al.[63] found that only six eyes (30%) of 20 treated in this way actually improved by more than 0.50 D whereas five eyes (25%) deteriorated by a similar amount. In nine eyes (45%) the refraction was unchanged. Although this treatment may be appropriate for the correction of persistent topographic abnormalities, it is not generally sufficient to deal with significant undercorrection or regression.

RETREATMENT

Patients who find themselves undercorrected in one or both eyes after PRK may elect to undergo a second procedure. Some will have exaggerated corneal haze or topographic abnormalities, with or without undercorrection, which would lead the excimer laser surgeon to offer retreatment. In counselling these patients, an understanding of the likely outcome and potential risks of retreatment is important.

RETREATMENT RATES

The incidence or rate of retreatment will be dependent on a number of variables, including the proportion of highly myopic eyes in a given series, the

Table 24.3
Retreatment rates following PRK for myopia.

Author	Number of primary procedures	Mean preoperative refraction (D)	Range of myopia treated (D)	Number of eyes retreated	Retreatment rate (%)
Sutton et al.[70]	285	ns	ns	19	7
Snibson et al.[16]	645	−5.94	−0.88 to −18.20	58	9
Sher et al.[74]	48	−11.20	−8.00 to −15.25	11	23

minimum duration of follow-up, the proportion of the initial ametropia targeted with the first treatment, and the criteria on which the decision to retreat is based. As retreatment is deferred until refractive stability has been established, the second procedure is frequently performed late in the first year or during the second year of follow-up. For this reason, retreatment rates should be estimated from the experience with cohorts of patients who have been followed at least two years after PRK. Currently available data based on shorter periods of follow-up provide some indication, but probably underestimate the likelihood of retreatment (Table 24.3).

As might be expected, in view of the relationship between high myopia and regression, retreatment rates appear to increase with increasing mean preoperative myopia. In a series of 58 retreatment procedures, we have shown that the likelihood of retreatment increases substantially with increasing myopia (Table 24.4).[16]

INDICATIONS FOR RETREATMENT

Primary undercorrection

Primary undercorrection is an uncommon indication for retreatment. Refractive stability is often achieved quickly and early retreatment is possible.

Regression

Loss of the effect of the initial procedure with regression to an unacceptable degree of residual myopia is the most common reason for contemplating retreatment. Some eyes will also have significant haze or topographical abnormalities.

Corneal haze

Retreatment in the form of phototherapeutic keratectomy (PTK) is sometimes performed for persistent

Table 24.4
Estimated retreatment rates following PRK for different degrees of myopia (Snibson et al., 1995).[16]

Spherical equivalent (at corneal plane) prior to initial treatment	Number of patients treated and followed 12 months	Number of patients retreated (approximate retreatment rate)
0.00 to −5.00 D	347 (54%)	17 (5%)
−5.01 to −10.00 D	240 (37%)	30 (13%)
−10.01 to −15.00 D	58 (9%)	11 (19%)

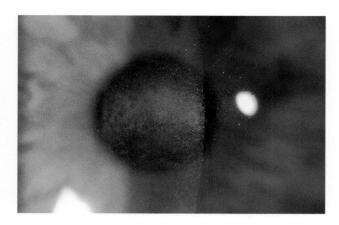

Figure 24.8 *Clinical photograph of moderately severe corneal haze 6 months after PRK for high myopia (–8.75 D).*

corneal opacity in eyes without significant residual refractive error (Fig. 24.8). Frequently, the development of more marked corneal haze is accompanied by regression and a refractive retreatment procedure may adequately deal with both problems. A plano ablation (PTK) may also be combined with a refractive procedure (PRK) when haze is prominent and the required correction small.[64,65] However, because the natural history of corneal haze is one of gradual and often complete resolution over 1–3 years, it is generally inappropriate to offer retreatment for corneal haze alone within the first year or two (see Chapter 23).

Central islands

Central islands may also be effectively treated by a second ablation placed at the location of the island. However, central islands are frequently transient or will flatten with the passage of time,[66,67] making retreatment unnecessary. Furthermore, it is often difficult to obtain accurate refractions in the presence of a central island, making the planning of the refractive (non-island) component of the retreatment difficult.

Decentration

Minor degrees of decentration are frequently asymptomatic. However, if the ablation zone is decentered

by several millimeters, disabling visual symptoms may result, with reduction in best corrected visual acuity. Using the modulating effect of the corneal epithelium, the topographic appearance and symptoms of decentration may be ameliorated by retreatment.

Relative contraindications

Retreatment should be performed with caution in the following situations:

- unstable refraction
- unaided vision better than 6/12
- haze in the absence of undercorrection
- central islands followed less than 12 months
- predicted residual stromal thickness of less than 300 μm after retreatment.

PREOPERATIVE ASSESSMENT

Retreatment should not be performed within 6 months of the primary procedure as refractive stability cannot be expected during this period. It is also essential to demonstrate at least 3 months' stability after cessation of topical steroids before proceeding to retreatment.

Stability may be assumed under the following conditions:

- a minimum of 6 months have passed after the initial treatment and
- a minimum of 3 months have passed after withdrawal of topical steroid therapy, and
- a minimum of three refractions have been performed over at least a 3-month period, demonstrating change in the spherical equivalent of not more than 0.50 D.

Corneal topography is crucial to the planning of appropriate retreatment. Identification of asymmetric healing, decentration, central islands and other surface irregularities is vital and often assisted by subtraction or differential studies comparing the current map with the study performed prior to the initial surgery.

Ultrasonic pachymetry should be performed when retreatment is considered in the setting of high myopia since significant amounts of stromal tissue are removed in high myopic corrections and the magnitude of retreatments in this group can also be quite large. A 'safe depth' has not been determined for excimer laser surgery but it would seem prudent to limit treatments so that the remaining central stroma is at least 300 µm thick. The thickness of the epithelium after PRK is variable and cannot be easily measured, but preoperatively the epithelial thickness can be assumed to be approximately 45–55 µm. The following formula can then be used to determine the estimated residual stromal thickness and plan a safe ablation depth for the second procedure:

Preoperative central corneal thickness (ultrasonic pachymetry)
– estimated epithelial thickness (55 µm)
= estimated central stromal thickness

Estimated central stromal thickness
– stromal ablation depth (initial PRK)
= postoperative central stromal thickness

Postoperative central stromal thickness
– stromal ablation depth (retreatment)
= residual central stromal thickness (minimum: 300 µm)

Example:
520 µm (central corneal thickness)
– 55 µm (estimated epithelial thickness)
= 465 µm (estimated central stromal thickness)

465 µm (estimated central stromal thickness)
– 120 µm (stromal ablation depth)
= 345 µm (residual corneal stromal thickness)

Thus, the maximum depth permissible for the second stromal ablation would be 45 µm.

METHODS

Epithelial removal

Epithelial removal can be performed without difficulty in most cases using a blunt spatula or a dulled blade. It is not uncommon, after the epithelium is removed, to see the concentric rings of the initial ablation, indicating that minimal stromal remodelling has occurred. However, in eyes with significant haze the anterior stroma may appear to have widespread irregular ridges and valleys, which correspond with the haze pattern seen preoperatively. Removal of the epithelium using the laser (transepithelial ablation) may offer some advantages over the mechanical

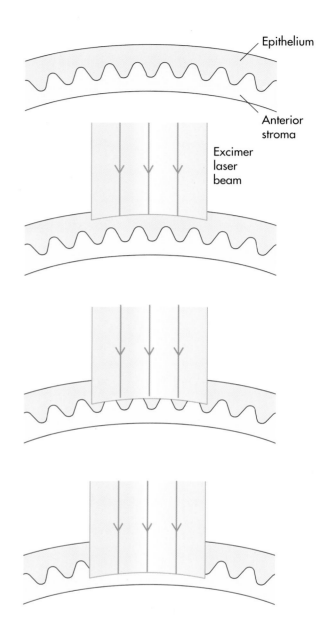

Figure 24.9 *Smoothing effect of the epithelium during transepithelial ablation.*

method in eyes that have undergone previous photorefractive surgery, particularly when haze is prominent. The epithelium acts as a smoothing agent and will help reduce any stromal surface irregularity that may be present (Fig. 24.9). In addition, healing of the epithelial defect may be slightly more rapid after transepithelial ablation. A different ablation rate applies to epithelium[68] and the ablation depth must be sufficient to remove the central epithelium, which is usually thicker than the peripheral epithelium. This can be monitored by dimming the microscope illumination and observing the fluorescence of the epithelium with each laser pulse against the darker background of the stroma. If the entire epithelium is removed using the excimer laser in PTK mode (i.e. a large diameter, plano ablation) some peripheral stroma will be exposed whilst the central epithelium is being ablated. This can result in an inadvertent steepening of the stromal surface and lead to undercorrection.

Ablation parameters

In most cases, the same treatment algorithm is used in retreatments as is currently recommended for initial procedures. The manifest subjective refraction is usually targeted if emmetropia is the goal. An additional 'correction factor' may be incorporated to compensate for the undercorrection that can result from transepithelial ablation (see above).

Caution should be exercised in planning the magnitude of the retreatment in cases where marked regression has occurred. Although a healing response similar to that following the primary procedure may be anticipated, overcorrection can result from retreatment if the full refraction is targeted and the subsequent epithelial hyperplasia and other tissue responses are less marked. In such cases, it may be prudent to attempt a lesser correction (e.g. 75% of the manifest refraction) to minimize this risk. If a small ablation zone was used for the first PRK, a larger diameter (6.0 or 6.5 mm) should be used for the retreatment. For larger corrections, a multizone approach should be employed (see Chapter 10).

Retreatment for haze

When retreatment is performed for corneal haze alone, a uniform (plano) ablation beam is used (PTK) with a large ablation zone diameter. Patients should be warned of the loud sound of the large area ablation, which may be startling if not expected. Once the epithelium is removed, a 10–15 μm ablation is performed, which may be sufficient to remove the bulk of the opacity. Further ablations of 5–10 μm are then performed if significant haze is still evident on slit-lamp examination. It is not essential to remove all

of the visible haze, and the depth of the stromal ablation should be kept to a minimum to avoid excessive hyperopic shift and minimize the stimulus for aggressive healing and further haze formation. A transition zone should be used to prevent the formation of a step at the edge of the ablation. A modulating agent, such as methylcellulose, can be helpful during PTK for asymmetric haze to smooth the final ablated surface and minimize topographic disturbances once the epithelium is healed.

Occasionally, it is possible to identify an edge of what appears to be a formed plaque of collagen or scar after manual removal of the epithelium. Rarely, this can then actually be peeled off with the assistance of some blunt dissection.[65] The underlying stromal surface can then be smoothed with a few laser pulses. This procedure alone can be sufficient to deal with much of the associated undercorrection, and subsequent PRK may not be necessary.

Retreatment for central islands

Several strategies have been suggested for the correction of central islands but the results of these treatments have not been adequately assessed. A reasonable approach is to perform an ablation of a depth and diameter that correspond with the dioptric power ('height') and approximate diameter of the island evident on videokeratoscopy. Any undercorrection may then be addressed using larger ablation zones.

Retreatment for decentration

There is currently no satisfactory treatment for decentration, which remains one of the complications most feared by excimer laser surgeons. Flattening may be extended centrally using a centered ablation following partial epithelial removal.[69] This technique employs epithelium as a masking agent to restrict the stromal ablation to the steeper areas evident on the topographic map. This kind of approach is very dependent on careful attention to the videokeratoscopy difference (subtraction) maps, which provide an indication of the changes induced by the initial treatment. Unfortunately this method is unlikely to produce a regular spherocylindrical refracting surface. In the future, it may be possible to treat decentration with a scanning beam excimer laser specifically directed to correct individual topographic abnormalities using data derived from the videokeratoscopic image (see Chapter 7).

Table 24.5

Published results of retreatment with 6 months minimum follow-up. (SE= spherical equivalent; SD = standard deviation; UCVA = uncorrected visual acuity)

Author	Number of eyes studied	Duration of follow-up (months)	Mean SE prior to retreatment (SD)	Mean SE after retreatment (SD)	Within 1 D of intended refraction (%)	UCVA 6/12 or better (%)
Epstein et al.[72]	17	6	−2.91 D (0.86)	−0.97 D (2.10)	59	65
Sutton et al.[70]	18	6	−6.05 D (3.91)	−2.07 D (4.60)	50	50
Seiler et al.[73]	30	6	−3.45 D (3.0)	−0.29 D (2.37)	63	NS
Snibson et al.[16]	39	12	−2.88 D (1.49)	−1.13 D (1.38)	69	64

POSTOPERATIVE CARE

Postoperative care after retreatment differs little from that used after the initial procedure except, perhaps, in the use of topical corticosteroids. If an eye exhibits an exaggerated healing response after PRK, with pronounced corneal haze and regression, it is likely that the same response will be seen after retreatment and more intensive use of corticosteroids may be appropriate. An agent such as dexamethasone 0.1% or prednisolone acetate 1% may be used at least four times daily for 2–4 weeks and the healing response assessed. The dose is then titrated at regular reviews according to the refraction and corneal clarity. Whilst there is some rationale for this approach, its effectiveness is thus far unproven and the surgeon must be aware of the increased risk of steroid-induced glaucoma.

RESULTS OF RETREATMENT

Retreatment is capable of bringing about a significant reduction in the residual myopia of eyes that are undercorrected following PRK, with a corresponding improvement in unaided vision.

When the results of retreatment are viewed in terms of the proportion of eyes within 1 D of the intended refraction and with unaided vision of at least 6/12, the results are not as good as we have come to expect from primary procedures for the correction of comparable degrees of myopia (Table 24.5). This may reflect the predisposition of patients who require retreatment to again undergo regression with the development of haze.[70] However, as yet, the series reported to date are small and there are few publications describing the outcome of retreatment beyond 6 months.[70,16]

Corneal haze frequently accompanies regression and may be a major consideration in the decision to offer retreatment. Therefore, the effect of reablation on corneal clarity is an outcome of some significance. Given the evidence that would suggest that haze increases with increasing depth of the stromal ablation and the fact that reablation inevitably results in removal of deeper stromal tissue, it would be reasonable to expect haze to increase following retreatment. Hanna et al.[71] reported an increased wound-healing response and exaggerated haze in rabbits after repeated ablation but, fortunately, this has not been a common finding in humans undergoing retreatment. In a series of 17 eyes, Epstein et al.[72] noted an increase in the haze score in six eyes, whilst in the remainder haze either improved (two eyes) or remained unchanged (nine eyes). The mean haze score was not significantly different at 6 months from mean haze prior to retreatment. Seiler et al.[73] were able to demonstrate improvements in mean haze scores at both 3 and 6 months after retreatment, with an associated improvement in visual acuity in the presence of a glare source. We have noted reduction in haze in those eyes with haze scores of 2.0 or greater prior to retreatment, but mean haze scores (which were less than 1.0 at all time points after retreatment) were not significantly different from those observed after initial ablations.[16]

Although a small proportion of eyes undergoing retreatment will experience some loss of best corrected visual acuity, improvement is more often observed,[73,64] particularly in those patients with prominent haze before retreatment. Other adverse reactions would seem no more common after retreatment than after the initial procedure, except in those high myopes with aggressive healing, severe haze and regression after primary PRK.[16,76]

SUMMARY

Refractive regression following excimer laser PRK does lead to unsatisfactory outcomes in a significant minority of patients. Changes in delivery systems and treatment algorithms have gone some way towards minimizing this complication but regression remains a problem, particularly in severely myopic eyes. Topical corticosteroids have at least some short-term effect on regression but their place in the routine management of patients after PRK continues to be controversial.

For most patients with persistent undercorrection, reablation is an effective intervention. Although the clinical course after retreatment may resemble that after the primary procedure, with a tendency towards the recurrence of haze and regression, retreatment for low or moderate regression does not appear to be associated with greater risks than does the initial procedure. However, larger studies with longer periods of follow-up are required. All patients, particularly those with higher degrees of myopia, should be advised preoperatively of the risk of regression after PRK and that retreatment may be necessary.

REFERENCES

1. Gartry DS, Kerr Muir MG, Marshall J, Photorefractive keratectomy with an argon fluoride excimer laser: a clinical study, *J Refract Corneal Surg* (1991) **7**: 420–35.
2. Kim JH, Sah WJ, Kim MS, et al, Three-year results of photorefractive keratectomy for myopia, *J Refract Surg* (1995) **11(suppl):** S248–S252.
3. Ditzen K, Anschutz T, Schröder E, Photorefractive keratectomy to treat low, medium and high myopia: a multicenter study, *J Cataract Refract Surg* (1994) **20(suppl):** 234–8.
4. Gartry DS, Kerr Muir MG, Marshall J, Excimer laser photorefractive keratectomy: 18 month follow-up, *Ophthalmology* (1992) **99**: 1209–19.
5. Snibson GR, Carson CA, Aldred GF, et al, One-year evaluation of excimer laser photorefractive keratectomy for myopia and myopic astigmatism, *Arch Ophthalmol* (1995) **113**: 994–1000.
6. Carson CA, Taylor HR, Excimer laser treatment for high and extreme myopia, *Arch Ophthalmol* (1995) **113**: 431–6.
7. Krueger RR, Talamo JH, McDonald MB, et al, Clinical analysis of excimer laser photorefractive keratectomy using a multiple zone technique for severe myopia, *Am J Ophthalmol* (1995) **119**: 263–74.
8. Epstein D, Fagerholm P, Hamberg-Nyström H, Twenty-four-month follow-up of excimer laser photorefractive keratectomy for myopia, *Ophthalmology* (1994) **101**: 1558–63.
9. Epstein D, Hamberg-Nyström H, Fagerholm P, et al, Three-year follow-up of excimer laser photorefractive keratectomy for myopia, *Invest Ophthalmol Vis Sci* (1994) **35(suppl):** 1650 (abst).
10. Marshall J, Trokel SL, Rothery S, et al, Long-term healing of the central cornea after photorefractive keratectomy using an excimer laser, *Ophthalmology* (1988) **95**: 1411–21.
11. Goodman GL, Trokel SL, Stark WJ, et al, Corneal healing following laser refractive keratectomy, *Arch Ophthalmol* (1989) **107**: 1799–803.
12. O'Brart DPS, Gartry DS, Lohmann CP, et al, Excimer laser photorefractive keratectomy for myopia: comparison of 4.00- and 5.00-millimetre ablation zones, *J Refract Corneal Surg* (1994) **10**: 87–94.
13. O'Brart DPS, Corbett MC, Lohmann CP, et al, The effects of ablation diameter on the outcome of excimer laser photorefractive keratectomy. A prospective, randomised, double-blind study, *Arch Ophthalmol* (1995) **113**: 438–43.
14. Kermani O, Lubatschowski H, Structure and dynamics of photo-acoustic shock-waves in 193 nm excimer laser photo-ablation of the cornea, *Fortschr Ophthalmol* (1991) **88**: 748–53.
15. Lindstrom RL, Sher NA, Barak M, et al, Excimer laser photorefractive keratectomy in high myopia: a multicentre study, *Tr Am Ophth Soc* (1992) **90**: 277–96.
16. Snibson GR, Carson CA, Aldred GF, et al, Retreatment following excimer laser photorefractive keratectomy, *Am J Ophthalmol* (1996) **121**: 250–7.
17. Dua HS, Gomes JAP, Singh A, Corneal wound healing, *Br J Ophthalmol* (1994) **78**: 401–8.
18. Tuft SJ, Zabel RW, Marshall J, Corneal repair following keratectomy. A comparison between conventional surgery and laser photoablation, *Invest Ophthalmol Vis Sci* (1989) **30**: 1769–77.
19. Dillon EC, Eagle RC Jr, Laibson PR, Compensatory epithelial hyperplasia in human corneal disease, *Ophthalmic Surg* (1992) **23**: 729–32.
20. Fagerholm P, Hamberg-Nyström H, Tengroth B, Wound healing and myopic regression following photorefractive keratectomy, *ACTA Ophthalmol* (1994) **72**: 229–34.
21. Shieh E, Morieira H, D'Arcy J, Quantitative analysis of wound healing after cylindrical and spherical excimer laser ablations, *Ophthalmology* (1992) **99**: 1050–5.

22. Del Pero RA, Gigstad JE, Roberts AD, A refractive and histologic study of excimer laser keratectomy in primates, *Am J Ophthalmol* (1990) **109:** 419–29.

23. Gauthier CA, Holden BA, Epstein D, et al, Corneal thickness following photorefractive keratectomy for myopia, *Invest Ophthalmol Vis Sci* (1994) **35(suppl):** 2014 (abst).

24. Gauthier CA, Epstein D, Holden BA, et al, Epithelial alterations following photorefractive keratectomy for myopia, *J Refract Surg* (1995) **11:** 113–18.

25. Fagerholm P, Hamberg-Nyström H, Tengroth B, Wound healing and myopic regression following photorefractive keratectomy, *ACTA Ophthalmol* (1994) **72:** 229–34.

26. Lohmann CP, MacRobert I, Patmore A, et al, A histopathological study of photorefractive keratectomy, *Lasers and Light in Ophthalmology* (1994) **6:** 149–58.

27. Power WJ, Kaufman AH, Arrunategui-Correa V, et al, Expression of collagen types I, III, IV and V in rat cornea following excimer laser keratectomy: analysis by semi-quantitative PCR, *Invest Ophthalmol Vis Sci* (1994) **35(suppl):** 1724 (abst).

28. Wu WCS, Stark W, Green R, Corneal wound healing after 193-nm excimer laser keratectomy, *Arch Ophthalmol* (1991) **109:** 1426–32.

29. Malley DS, Steinert RF, Puliafito CA, Immunofluorescence study of corneal wound healing after excimer laser anterior keratectomy in the monkey eye, *Arch Ophthalmol* (1990) **108:** 1316–22.

30. Carson CA, Snibson GR, Taylor HR, An analysis of clinical correlations one, three, six and 12 months after excimer laser photorefractive keratectomy, *Lasers and Light in Ophthalmology* (1995) **6:** 249–57.

31. Polack FM, Rosen PN, Topical steroids and tritiated thymidine uptake: effect on corneal healing, *Arch Ophthalmol* (1967) **77:** 400–12.

32. Gassett PR, Lorenzetti DWC, Ellison EM, et al, Quantitative corticosteroid effect on corneal wound healing, *Arch Ophthalmol* (1969) **81:** 589–91.

33. Sugar J, Chandler JW, Experimental corneal wound strength: effect of topically applied corticosteroids, *Arch Ophthalmol* (1974) **92:** 248–9.

34. McDonald TO, Borgmann AR, Roberts MD, et al, Corneal wound healing, I: inhibition of stromal healing by three dexamethasone derivatives, *Invest Ophthalmol Vis Sci* (1970) **9:** 703–9.

35. Phillips K, Arffa R, Cintron C, et al, Effects of prednisolone and medroxyprogesterone on corneal wound healing, ulceration, and neovascularisation, *Arch Ophthalmol* (1983) **101:** 640–3.

36. Tuft SJ, Zabel RW, Marshall J, Corneal repair following keratectomy. A comparison between conventional surgery and laser photoablation, *Invest Ophthalmol Vis Sci* (1989) **30:** 1769–77.

37. Talamo JH, Gollamudi S, Green WR, et al, Modulation of corneal wound healing after excimer laser keratomileusis using topical mitomycin C and steroids, *Arch Ophthalmol* (1991) **109:** 1141–6.

38. Campos M, Abed HM, McDonnell PJ, Topical fluoro-metholone reduces stromal inflammation after photo-refractive keratectomy, *Ophthalmic Surg* (1993) **24:** 654–7.

39. You X, Zheng X, Bergmanson JPG, et al, Manipulation of post-PRK stromal remodelling in rabbit corneas with corticosteroids, *Invest Ophthalmol Vis Sci* (1994) **35(suppl):** 2015 (abst).

40. Tengroth B, Epstein D, Fagerholm P, et al, Excimer laser photorefractive keratectomy for myopia. Clinical results in sighted eyes, *Ophthalmology* (1993) **100:** 739–45.

41. Cerruti S, Traverso CE, Murialdo U, et al, The efficacy of topical corticosteroids in reversing the regression of refractive effect after myopic photorefractive keratectomy (PRK), *Invest Ophthalmol Vis Sci* (1994) **35(suppl):** 2019 (abst).

42. Tengroth B, Fagerholm MD, Söderberg P, et al, Effect of corticosteroids in postoperative care following photorefractive keratectomies, *Refract Corneal Surg* (1993) **9(suppl):** S61–S64.

43. Marques EF, Leite EB, Cunha-Vaz JG, Corticosteroids for reversal of myopic regression after photorefractive keratectomy, *J Refract Surg* (1995) **11(suppl):** S302–S308.

44. Gartry DS, Kerr Muir MG, Lohmann CP, Marshall J, The effect of topical corticosteroids on refractive outcome and corneal haze after photorefractive keratectomy, *Arch Ophthalmol* (1992) **110:** 944–52.

45. Gartry DS, Kerr-Muir M, Marshall J, The effect of topical corticosteroids on refraction and corneal haze following excimer laser treatment of myopia: an update. A prospective, randomised, double-masked study, *Eye* (1993) **7:** 584–90.

46. Stevens JD, Steele ADMcG, Ficker LA, et al, Prospective randomised study of two topical steroid regimes after excimer laser PRK, *Invest Ophthalmol Vis Sci* (1994) **35(suppl):** 1651 (abst).

47. Fagerholm P, Hamberg-Nyström H, Tengroth BE, et al, Effect of postoperative steroids on the refractive outcome of photorefractive keratectomy for myopia with the Summit excimer laser, *J Cataract Refract Surg* (1994) **20(suppl):** 212–15.

48. O'Brart DPS, Lohmann CP, Klonos G, et al, The effects of topical corticosteroids and plasmin inhibitors on refractive outcome, haze, and visual performance after photorefractive keratectomy. A prospective, randomised, observer-masked study, *Ophthalmology* (1994) **101:** 1565–74.

49. Carones F, Brancato R, Venturi E, et al, Efficacy of corticosteroids in reversing regression after myopic photorefractive keratectomy, *Refract Corneal Surg* (1993) **9(suppl):** S52–S56.

50. Fitzsimmons TD, Fagerholm P, Tengroth B, Steroid treatment of myopic regression: acute refractive and topographic changes in excimer photorefractive keratectomy patients, *Cornea* (1993) **12:** 358–361.

51. Fitzsimmons TD, Fagerholm P, Harfstrand A, et al, Hyaluronic acid in the rabbit cornea after excimer laser superficial keratectomy, *Invest Ophthalmol Vis Sci* (1992) **33:** 3011–16.

52. Fitzsimmons TD, Molander N, Stenevi U, et al, Endogenous hyaluronan in corneal disease, *Invest Ophthalmol Vis Sci* (1994) **35:** 277–82.

53. Fitzsimmons T, Fagerholm P, Härfstrad A, et al, Steroids after excimer laser surgery decrease corneal hyaluronic acid content, *Invest Ophthalmol Vis Sci* (1992) **33(suppl):** 766 (abst).

54. Corbett MC, O'Brart DPS, Marshall J, Do topical corticosteroids have a role following excimer laser photorefractive keratectomy? *J Refract Surg* (1995) **11:** 380–7.

55. Sher NA, Frantz JM, Talley A, et al, Topical diclofenac in the treatment of ocular pain after excimer photorefractive keratectomy, *Refract Corneal Surg* (1993) **9:** 425–36.

56. Richard Ch, Assouline M, Renard G, et al, Prospective randomised trial of topical soluble 0.1% indomethacin for the control of pain following excimer photoablation of the cornea, *Invest Ophthalmol Vis Sci* (1994) **35(suppl):** 1672 (abst).

57. Arshinoff S, Addario D, Sadler C, et al, Use of topical nonsteroidal anti-inflammatory drugs in excimer laser photorefractive keratectomy, *J Cataract Refract Surg* (1994) **20(suppl):** 216–22.

58. Lohmann CP, Marshall J, Plasmin- and plasminogen-activator inhibitors after excimer laser photorefractive keratectomy: new concept in prevention of postoperative myopic regression and haze, *Refract Corneal Surg* (1993) **9:** 300–2.

59. Bowman WC, Rand MJ, *Textbook of pharmacology, 2nd edn* (Blackwell Scientific Publications: Oxford, 1980) p. 21.20.

60. Shoulin JP, The anterior segment: a comparison between patients wearing contact lenses following radial keratotomy and myopic photorefractive keratectomy with excimer laser, *ICLC* (1992) **19:** 141–2.

61. Schipper I, Businger V, Pfarrer R, Fitting contact lenses after excimer laser photorefractive keratectomy for myopia, *CLAOJ* (1995) **21:** 281–4.

62. Loewenstein A, Lipschitz I, Lazar M, Scraping of epithelium for treatment of undercorrection and haze after photorefractive keratectomy, *J Refract Corneal Surg* (1994) **10(suppl):** S274–S276.

63. Fagerholm PP, Epstein D, Tengroth BM, et al, Refractive outcome following epithelial abrasion in eyes with regression after photorefractive keratectomy for myopia, *Invest Ophthalmol Vis Sci* (1994) **35(suppl):** 1724 (abst).

64. Lawless MA, Cohen PR, Rogers CM, Retreatment of undercorrected photorefractive keratectomy for myopia, *Refract Corneal Surg* (1994) **10(suppl):** S174–S177.

65. Carr JD, Patel R, Hersh PS, Management of late corneal haze following photorefractive keratectomy, *J Refract Surg* (1995) **11(suppl):** S309–S313.

66. Lin DT, Corneal topographic analysis after excimer laser photorefractive keratectomy, *Ophthalmology* (1994) **101:** 1432–9.

67. Krueger RR, Saedy NF, McDonnell PJ, Clinical analysis of topographic steep central islands following excimer photorefractive keratectomy (PRK), *Invest Ophthalmol Vis Sci* (1994) **35(suppl):** 1740 (abst).

68. Seiler T, Kriegerowski M, Schnoy N, Ablation rate of human corneal epithelial and Bowman's layer with the excimer laser, *Refract Corneal Surg* (1990) **6:** 99–102.

69. Talamo JH, Wagoner MD, Lee SY, Management of ablation decentration following excimer photorefractive keratectomy, *Arch Ophthalmol* (1995) **113:** 706–7.

70. Sutton G, Kalski RS, Lawless MA, et al, Excimer retreatment for scarring and regression after photorefractive keratectomy for myopia, *Br J Ophthalmol* (1995) **79:** 756–9.

71. Hanna KD, Pouliquen YM, Waring GO, Corneal wound healing in monkeys after repeated excimer laser photorefractive keratectomy, *Arch Ophthalmol* (1992) **110:** 1286–91.

72. Epstein D, Tengroth B, Fagerholm P, et al, Excimer retreatment of regression after photorefractive keratectomy, *Am J Ophthalmol* (1994) **117:** 456–61.

73. Seiler T, Derse M, Pham T, Repeated excimer laser treatment after photorefractive keratectomy, *Arch Ophthalmol* (1992) **110:** 1230–3.

74. Sher NA, Hardten DR, Fundingsland B, et al, 193-nm excimer photorefractive keratectomy in high myopia, *Ophthalmology* (1994) **101:** 157–82.

75. Orssaud C, Binaghi M, Patarin D, et al, Photorefractive keratectomy in 176 eyes: one year follow-up, *J Refract Corneal Surg* (1994) **10(suppl):** S199–S205.

76. Gartry DS et al, Retreatment for significant regression following excimer laser photorefractive keratectomy (PRK)—a randomised double-masked trial, *Invest Ophthalmol Vis Sci* (1995) **36:** S190 (Abst).

Chapter 25 Essential pharmacology for photorefractive surgery

Charles N J McGhee and Peter Koay

The use of corticosteroids following PRK

INTRODUCTION

Over the last 30 years, corticosteroids have become one of the most widely used groups of topical ophthalmic drugs and their role in the postoperative management of intraocular surgery is well established. It is, therefore, unsurprising that routine post-photorefractive keratectomy (PRK) application of topical corticosteroid has become widespread policy. Early studies by Seiler[1] suggested an important role for corticosteroids in the modulation of both postoperative haze and refraction. However, currently available data suggest that there is still substantial controversy in respect of the beneficial effect, if any, associated with the routine use of topical steroids following photorefractive surgery.[2–4]

OPHTHALMIC CORTICOSTEROIDS

The greatest barrier to penetration of topical corticosteroids is the lipid-rich corneal epithelium, which retards the ingress of polar compounds, such as prednisolone phosphate,[5] whilst allowing rapid penetration of lipophilic preparations, such as prednisolone acetate and dexamethasone alcohol.[6,7] Although initial PRK studies frequently utilized dexamethasone, more recently fluorometholone preparations have become standard in postoperative regimes. Fluorometholone has the benefit of being as equipotent an anti-inflammatory as dexamethasone on a gram for gram basis,[8] but it penetrates the anterior chamber in much lower concentrations[9,10]

and is therefore associated with a lower incidence of steroid-induced glaucoma[11,12] and lesser potential to produce steroid-induced cataract. It therefore seems logical, when the greatest effect is required in the anterior one-third of the cornea and the beneficial effects are inconclusive, that a compound with the least risk of serious side-effects should be used.

Because of the high steroid concentrations obtained in the cornea following topical administration of corticosteroids,[10] there is no role for systemic or subconjunctival administration of steroids in the postoperative management of the post-PRK eye.

BENEFITS AND RISKS ASSOCIATED WITH THE USE OF CORTICOSTEROIDS

The postulated benefits associated with post-PRK administration of corticosteroids are:

- Decreased local inflammation
- Decreased corneal haze
- Decreased refractive regression
- Reversal of 'late' myopic regression.

The risks of prolonged topical steroids include:

- Steroid-induced glaucoma
- Steroid-induced cataract
- Increased susceptibility to ocular infection
- Decreased tensile strength of ocular incisions
- Corticosteroid-related ptosis.

The risks associated with prolonged corticosteroid therapy are discussed more fully in Chapter 23.

POSTULATED BENEFICIAL EFFECTS OF CORTICOSTEROIDS IN THE POST-PRK EYE

Decreased local inflammation

The inflammatory reaction in humans following PRK is mild and responds rapidly to mild topical corticosteroids. Therefore, although in the rabbit model a significant increase in polymorphonuclear leucocytes (PMNs), which rapidly responds to fluorometholone treatment, has been identified,[13] it is debatable whether corticosteroids should be considered for this purpose alone in humans. If steroids are utilized solely to combat local inflammation they should probably be commenced on day 1 and are likely to be required for less than 2 weeks. Commencing corticosteroids in the presence of a large epithelial defect might obviously be associated with delayed epithelial healing[14] and, in order to avoid delayed healing, many practitioners do not commence corticosteroids until epithelial closure has occurred.

Corticosteroids and post-PRK corneal haze

Early animal studies demonstrated the development of corneal haze with deeper ablations in the rabbit cornea[15,16] and in the non-human primate cornea,[17] although paradoxically, in one primate study, greater haze was identified in the more shallow ablations.[18] Early[19,20] and later studies[21–23] in the rabbit model indicated that the development of postoperative subepithelial haze or scar could be modified by the topical application of corticosteroids.

Initial studies suggested that this beneficial effect of corticosteroids also occurred in human corneas post-PRK, and non-compliance with the corticosteroid regime was a risk factor for corneal haze development.[1,24] However, although anecdotal reports continue to support the thesis that topical corticosteroids reduce corneal haze formation, and early clinical trials suggested that steroids might modulate the severity of haze,[1,25] prospective controlled studies have failed to conclusively support this hypothesis.[26–27] Indeed, since the natural history of corneal haze is one of progressive resolution with time, and several other variables in technique may predispose to the development of haze, any beneficial effect of topical steroids upon haze development or resolution is difficult to prove (see Chapter 23). Currently, there appears to be no role for the application of corticosteroids purely in relation to post-PRK corneal haze.

Routine use of corticosteroids and effect on refractive outcome

During the American phase of radial keratotomy (RK) development, many workers believed that by modulating wound healing by the topical application of corticosteroids, the final refractive outcome of RK could be manipulated. Ultimately it has been demonstrated that corticosteroids do not have a useful role in altering the refractive outcome of incisional refractive surgery.[28] A similar evolution of clinical thought may well be slowly developing amongst clinicians practising PRK surgery.

In initial European,[1,24,25] UK[30,31] and USA FDA trials[32,33] post operative application of corticosteroids was a routine part of the PRK procedure. Whilst the relative importance of the steroid regime attributed to final refractive result varied between groups, many of these early studies concluded that steroids were important in terms of refractive outcome and haze.[1,24,25,32] However, none of these studies were particularly designed to assess the efficacy of corticosteroids in improving PRK outcome and few subsequent studies have addressed this specific question prospectively[26–28,33] or retrospectively.[3]

A series of papers from the St Thomas' Hospital group in London, utilizing a prospective, randomized, double masked approach to assess the importance of corticosteroids in relation to refractive outcome post PRK, represent the core of our knowledge on this subject.[26–28] All three studies have demonstrated no statistically significant lasting beneficial effect of steroids upon the development of corneal haze or refractive outcome, although in the larger studies[26,27] refractive results were significantly better in the steroid group compared to the placebo group in the early post-operative period (while topical steroids were being applied). In the group of 50 eyes completing one year follow up after a −3.00 D correction, using a Summit UV200 excimer laser and a single zone 4 mm diameter ablation, the placebo group demonstrated a mean change in refraction of 2.05 D and the dexamethasone (0.1%) treated group demonstrated a mean change of 2.33 D—the difference of 0.28 D (14%) between the placebo and treated groups not reaching statistical significance.[27] Similarly, in a randomized group of 52 eyes completing one year follow-up of a −6.00 D attempted correction, at 6 and 12 weeks post PRK the dexamethasone treated group demonstrated a statistically significant greater mean refractive change at these time points of 2.16 D and 1.43 D respectively, compared to the placebo group (Table 25.1). However, although a greater mean

Table 25.1a

The chronological refractive changes (induced mean refractive change ± standard deviation) in a group of patients with an attempted correction of −3.00 D is demonstrated. Although a statistically significant difference is noted in favour of greater refractive effect in the steroid-treated group at 6 weeks, there is no statistically significant difference between the groups thereafter, although at 1 year the steroid-treated group demonstrates a 0.28 D (14%) greater refractive effect than the placebo group. (Adapted from Gartry et al. (1993).[2]

	−3.00 D placebo (Group A)	−3.00 D steroid (Group B)	Difference in refractive change (B–A)	p-value
Eyes completing study	23	27	–	–
PRK performed	−3.00 D	−3.00 D	0.00 D	N/A
Preoperative refraction	−2.82 ± 0.36 D	−2.94 ± 0.38 D	0.12	N/A
6 weeks post-PRK	2.17 ± 0.82 D	2.93 ± 0.77 D	0.76	0.0015
3 months post-PRK	1.68 ± 1.03 D	2.14 ± 0.89 D	0.46	0.1
6 months post-PRK	2.14 ± 0.95 D	2.28 ± 0.96 D	0.14	0.62
1 year post-PRK	2.05 ± 0.84 D	2.33 ± 0.85 D	0.28	0.45

Table 25.1b

The chronological refractive changes (induced mean refractive change ± standard deviation) in a group of patients with an attempted correction of −6.00 D is demonstrated. Although a statistically significant difference is noted in favour of greater refractive effect in the steroid-treated group up to 12 weeks (during the period of topical steroid application), there is no statistically significant difference between the groups thereafter, although at 1 year the steroid-treated group demonstrates a +0.78 D (24%) greater refractive effect than the placebo group, which may be clinically significant. (Adapted from Gartry et al (1993).[2]

	−6.00 D placebo (Group A)	−6.00 D steroid (Group B)	Difference in refractive change (B–A)	p-value
Eyes completing study	25	27	–	–
PRK performed	−6.00 D	−6.00 D	0.00 D	N/A
Preoperative refraction	−6.02 ± 0.51 D	−5.90 ± 0.54 D	−0.12	N/A
6 weeks post-PRK	4.56 ± 1.29 D	6.72 ± 1.87 D	2.16	0.001
3 months post-PRK	2.76 ± 1.83 D	4.19 ± 2.14 D	1.43	0.013
6 months post-PRK	2.93 ± 1.78 D	3.72 ± 2.45 D	0.79	0.2
1 year post-PRK	3.22 ± 1.72 D	4.00 ± 2.31 D	0.78	0.2

refractive correction was still evident in the steroid treated group following cessation of topical dexamethasone, both at 6 (0.79 D) and 12 months (0.78 D) post treatment, neither figure reached statistical significance.[26,27]

It is worth noting in this study that a 4 mm ablation was utilized, wide standard deviations were encountered, and a dramatic myopic regression occurred in all groups between two weeks and one year post-PRK. In the −6.00 D group, mean myopic regression was 4.71 D (with a final refractive change of 3.22 ±

1.72 D) in the placebo group and 5.29 D (with a final refractive change of 4.00 ± 2.3 D) in the steroid-treated group.

In a subsequent study[27] by the same group on a smaller number of eyes, 59 eyes were randomized once more into −3.00 D and −6.00 D attempted corrections; however, a larger 5 mm ablation zone was utilized. Using fluorometholone versus placebo, a statistically significant greater refractive effect was noted in both the −3.00 D and −6.00 D steroid-treated groups whilst steroids were being applied. Following cessation of fluorometholone at 6 months, no significant refractive differences were noted between the groups at periods greater than 9 months after PRK. The authors concluded that routine application of corticosteroids was not advantageous but there might be a role in selected patients. Interestingly, at 1 year the –6.00 D fluorometholone-treated group exhibited a mean 1.00 D greater refractive effect than the corresponding placebo group.

In a recent study[33] of two prospectively randomized steroid regimes following excimer laser PRK with a Visx 20/20 excimer laser using a 6 mm ablation zone, no statistically significant beneficial effect was identified in the group receiving dexamethasone 0.1% for 6 months postoperatively (n = 111) compared to the group receiving dexamethasone 0.1% for 3 weeks (n = 103). Assessed at 6 months, the group undergoing the 3-week regime showed a mean residual refractive error of –1.03 ± 1.38 D compared to –0.91 ± 1.31 D in the group on prolonged steroid treatment.

Although some authors have questioned the statistical analysis[3] or the small numbers[34] of the St Thomas' studies, they have yet to be bettered in prospective design or execution. Tengroth, partly in response to the Gartry et al. studies, constructed two retrospective studies.[3] In a paired design study, one eye of each patient (n = 26) was treated with corticosteroids, the other without. Both eyes of each patient were treated within a 6-month period. Eyes treated with steroid were prescribed dexamethasone 0.1% five times per day in month 1, three times per day in the second month and once per day in the third month. At 3 months post-PRK, a significant statistical difference in refractive error was noted between those eyes receiving steroids (+1.28 ± 0.30 D, mean ± SD) compared to those eyes not receiving steroids (–0.53 ± 0.53). However, it must be noted that this difference was noted 3 months post-PRK, when the steroid-treated eyes were still receiving topical dexamethasone— therefore, these data merely echo the London studies, which demonstrated a statistically significant, greater refractive effect whilst steroids were applied, but this effect waned once steroids were discontinued.[26,27]

In a second retrospective study by this Scandinavian group, 30 subjects were matched for preoperative myopia and age, and 15 eyes from 15 individuals that had received the aforementioned dexamethasone regime postoperatively were compared to 15 matched eyes that received no topical steroid. Although statistically greater refractive effect was noted in the steroid-treated eyes at 3 months, once more no data were provided for refractive differences once the topical steroids had been discontinued.[3]

Although many of the earlier studies utilized dexamethasone postoperatively, since it appears to confer little benefit over fluorometholone in the postoperative period, fluorometholone has largely superceded dexamethasone in the management of the post-PRK eye. In a unique prospective PRK case report, Machat[35] reported on a comparison of two steroid regimes, fluorometholone 0.1% compared to dexamethasone 0.1% over a 3-month period, in the left eyes of two identical twins with identical preoperative refractions. Both 31-year-old brothers exhibited an identical unaided visual acuity and refractive error of +0.75 D at 6 months post-PRK. No differences were identified between the eyes receiving differing regimes in this case study.

Viewed in the context of contemporary wider zone ablations and newer algorithms, some reservations must be made in respect of the initial St Thomas' studies, particularly in regard to the 4 mm zone and dramatic myopic regression in all groups. Nonetheless, it would appear from the preceding data that routine application of corticosteroids in the postoperative period, at least in low myopia, is unlikely to produce any lasting benefits in terms of greater refractive effect or decreased corneal haze. This conclusion has not been seriously challenged by subsequent publications.[36] One might still debate, as others have done,[34] despite the lack of supporting statistically significant data, whether there is still a role for routine topical corticosteroids in higher levels of attempted correction. Indeed, Gartry et al. succinctly expressed this sentiment in the discussion of their studies – "while these differences, particularly in the –6.00 D group, would appear to be beneficial they are not statistically significant".[2] As previously highlighted, this *statistically non-significant difference* represented a mean 0.78 D (24%) greater refractive effect in the steroid-treated eyes compared to the placebo-treated eyes at 1 year post-PRK. In practice, this might represent a *clinically significant difference* in refractive outcome of –0.25 D rather than –1.00 D.

In the light of the foregoing evidence, and the inability to specifically identify patients or eyes preoperatively which might benefit from topical corticosteroids, many practitioners, including the authors, have come to abandon the routine use of corticosteroids in PRK for pre-operative myopia of –5.00 D or less, reserving the use of corticosteroids – in the form of topical fluorometholone – to short courses of 6–12 weeks in corrections of high and extreme myopia.

Tables 25.2a and b

The effect of reinstitution of corticosteroids in 29 consecutive eyes with myopic regression is highlighted in this table. Columns B and C highlight the preoperative and 3-month refractive data for each subgroup of attempted myopic correction (*In 25 eyes emmetropia was the intended correction and in four eyes, residual myopia of greater than −1.50 D was the intended preoperative correction). All patients routinely received topical guttae fluorometholone 0.25%, four times daily, from 3 days post-PRK until the 3 month review (column C) at which point the mean refractive outcome for all three groups was ±0.50 D of emmetropia and only four of the 29 eyes (13.7%) demonstrated a myopia of greater than −1.00 D (column D). However, following cessation of fluorometholone, myopic regression occurred in all eyes (column E) and topical fluorometholone, four times daily, was reinstituted at a mean time of 6.2 (range 4–9) months post-PRK for 1 month and reduced stepwise and stopped over a further period of 1–2 months. Column F shows refractive outcome 3 months after cessation of this reinstituted steroid regime (**a minimum of 12 months post-PRK). Columns G and H show the percentage of eyes with a refractive error of less than −1.00 D and the percentage obtaining unaided visual acuity of 6/12(20/40) or better. Of 20 eyes with a preoperative myopia of less than −10.00, in which emmetropia had been the intended outcome, prior to reintroduction of topical steroids all eyes exhibited greater than −1.00 D of myopia. Nine of these 20 eyes demonstrated no significant reversal of myopic regression in response to topical fluorometholone and went on to repeat PRK (column I); however, 11 eyes (55%) demonstrated a significant reversal of myopia, which was maintained on cessation of topical steroids.

Table 25.2a

Myopia	A No eyes	B Preoperative myopia (mean ± SD)	C Refraction at 3 months (mean ± SD)	D Range	<−1.00 D %
0.00 to −5.0 D	8	−3.98 ± 0.95	−0.25 ± 0.54	+0.25 to −1.50	25
−5.10 to −10.0 D	12	−6.79 ± 1.24	+0.10 ± 0.99	+2.87 to −2.00	8.3
−10.10 to −15.0 D	9	−12.10 ± 1.06	+0.47 ± 0.89	+2.50 to −1.12	11.1
0.00 to −15.0 D*	29	−7.65 ± 3.36	+0.29 ± 0.88	+2.87 to −2.00	13.7

Table 25.2b

Myopia	E Post cessation of steroids Number of eyes	F Post-reinstitution of steroids Spherical equivalent at ≥12 Months** Mean ± SD	Range (D)	G Refraction (< −1.00)	H Unaided va ⩾ 6/12	I Repeat PRK
0.00 to −5.0 D	8 (100%)	-0.73 ± 0.38	0.00 to −1.12	5 (62%)	4(50%)	25%
−5.10 to −10.0 D	12(100%)	−0.30 ± 0.22	+0.25 to −0.75	4(33%)	5(42%)	58%
−10.10 to −15.0 D	9(100%)	−0.88 ± 0.55	−0.25 to −1.75	4 (44%)	4(44%)	0%
0.00 to −15.0 D	29(100%)+	−0.60 ± 0.49	+0.25 to −1.75	13(52%)+	9(36%)+	31%

Reversal of 'late' myopic regression

Following cessation of topical steroids, some eyes demonstrate a significant regression of refractive effect within weeks or months. This effect can occasionally occur over several days or a few weeks, which, due to its rapidity, is more likely to be related to corneal hydration and relative concentrations of glycosaminoglycans than corneal healing or deposition of collagen per se[36] (see Chapter 4). Many clinicians who have recommenced topical corticosteroids in such cases have reported dramatic, and often rapid (in terms of days rather than weeks), reversal of this myopic regression[37] in at least a subgroup of eyes. Unfortunately, such widely discussed cases have occasionally led to scientifically unsubstantiated claims in response to time scale for intervention[3] and few papers deal specifically with this reversal effect.[37–39]

An early report from Fitzsimmons et al. demonstrated remarkable reversal of myopic regression (+0.75 to +3.00 D) and associated changes in computerized videokeratography upon the reinstitution of corticosteroids 3–8 months after initial cessation.[37] However, two of the five eyes reported subsequently demonstrated further myopic regression and some eyes were still receiving topical steroids at the time of final refraction.

Carones et al reported one study on six eyes treated for –6.00 to –8.00 D of myopia using a 5 mm diameter ablation zone.[38] All six eyes received dexamethasone drops for 2 months or more post-PRK but after cessation of topical steroid all six eyes demonstrated myopic regression between 1.00 D and 3.00 D (mean 2.00 D). Following reinstitution of corticosteroids, all eyes demonstrated a reversal of myopic regression greater than 1.00 D (range 1.00–3.50 D) and five of the six eyes regained the attempted correction. Reversal of refractive and topographic regression was identified within days of commencing topical dexamethasone, which the authors postulated might relate to reduction of stromal hyaluronic acid and corneal hydration. The mean period of follow-up, following cessation of the reinstituted dexamethasone, was longer than 12 weeks and greater than 8 weeks in all but one case. Reversal of myopic regression was maintained in this follow-up period.

Utilizing a short 'pulsed' treatment regime of dexamethasone eight times per day tapered over 2 weeks, Ceruti et al[39] reinstituted topical steroid therapy in patients who showed a myopic regression of 0.75 D or greater. Of 11 eyes, with a median follow up of 7 months, five (45%) regained attempted correction and maintained this recovery after steroids were discontinued. The authors concluded that, since 45% of regressions in the series had responded to topical corticosteroids, a trial of topical corticosteroids should be attempted before further surgery is considered.

The rapidity of refractive change highlighted in studies in which corticosteroids have been reintroduced does indicate that a rapid change in hydration, possibly related to glycosaminoglycan production or

distribution,[36] is likely to be at the root of changes in corneal thickness and refraction. However, in the normal healthy, unoperated, cornea, 4 weeks of topical dexamethasone 0.1% has been associated with a small but statistically significant increase, rather than decrease, in corneal thickness in approximately 35% of eyes.[40]

In a large prospective study of PRK and photoastigmatic refractive keratectomy (PARK), the authors have followed a policy of reinstituting steroids, in the form of guttae fluorometholone 0.1% four times daily, for a 1-month trial period in all eyes developing –0.75 D or greater regression. In eyes with no significant improvement in unaided visual acuity (one line of Snellen acuity or greater) or reversal of myopic regression (+0.50 D or greater), topical steroids were discontinued at the end of this 4-week period. In those eyes demonstrating a significant improvement in refraction or unaided visual acuity, the fluorometholone was tapered and stopped over an 8-week period. At a minimum of 1 year post-PRK, of 29 eyes in which fluorometholone had been reintroduced for myopic regression but had been discontinued for a minimum of 3 months, only nine (31%) eyes received repeat PRK. The average time from PRK to recommencement of corticosteroids (N.B. all eyes routinely received guttae fluorometholone 0.1% four times daily for 3 months post-PRK) for myopic regression was 6.2 ± 1.6 months (range 4–9 months) (Table 25.2).

In this study, nine eyes exhibited a preoperative myopia of greater than –10.00 D and emmetropia was not the refractive aim in four cases. However, of 20 eyes with a preoperative myopia of less than –10.00 D, in which emmetropia had been the intended outcome, prior to reintroduction of topical steroids all eyes exhibited greater than –1.00 D of myopia. Nine of these 20 eyes demonstrated no significant reversal of myopic regression in response to topical fluorometholone and went on to repeat PRK; however, 11 eyes (55%) demonstrated a significant reversal of myopia, which was maintained on cessation of topical steroids. Of these 11 eyes, nine exhibited a final refractive error of less than –1.00 D, and 10 (90%) obtained an unaided visual acuity of 6/12 (20/40) or better, with eight eyes achieving 6/9 (20/25) or better.

Overall, 20 of 29 eyes demonstrated a positive reversal of myopic regression greater than +0.50 D and 11 eyes (38%) demonstrated a hyperopic shift greater than +0.75 D (range +0.75 to +7.25 D, mean +1.62 ± 2.13 D standard deviation), which was maintained after cessation of corticosteroids.

CONCLUSIONS

As the risks of prolonged topical corticosteroids, including steroid-induced glaucoma, cataract and predisposition to ocular infection are well known, the use of topical corticosteroids, without substantive evidence of benefit, in the post-PRK eye is controversial. There appears to be little indication for the routine use of topical corticosteroids in the treatment of low myopia and debatable long-term benefit in higher levels of treated myopia.

There is compelling evidence that steroids do exert a beneficial refractive effect whilst being administered, and whilst this effect is no longer statistically significant once steroids have been stopped, arguably there is a clinically significant benefit in the treatment of high myopia. Unfortunately, subjects or individual eyes that will respond beneficially to the application of corticosteroids cannot be specifically identified at the present time. Certainly a subgroup of eyes do appear to respond to the application of corticosteroids in the circumstance of myopic regression and a short trial period of topical corticosteroid should always be considered prior to embarking upon excimer laser retreatment.

Although central corneal thickness is reduced, epithelial attachments diminished and stromal constituents altered in the post-PRK eye, topical steroids do not appear to penetrate into the anterior chamber in greater quantities.[41] Nonetheless, sensible clinical practice dictates that the mildest corticosteroid with the least propensity to elicit side-effects should always be employed for the shortest period.

REFERENCES

1   Seiler T, Kahle G, Kriegerowski M, Bende T, Myopic excimer laser keratomileusis in sighted and blind human eyes, *Refract Corneal Surg* (1990) **6**: 165–73.

2.   Gartry DS, Kerr Muir MG, Marshall J, The effect of topical corticosteroids on refraction and corneal haze following excimer laser treatment of myopia: an update. A prospective, randomised, double masked study, *Eye* (1993) **7**: 584–90.

3.   Tengroth B, Fagerholm P, Soderberg P, Hamberg-Nystrom H, Epstein D, Effect of corticosteroid in post-operative care following photorefractive keratectomies, *Refract Corneal Surg* (1993) **9**: S61–S64.

4.   Corbett MC, O'Brart DPS, Marshall J, Do topical steroids have a role following excimer laser photorefractive keratectomy? *J Refrac Surg* (1995) **11**: 380–7.

5.   McGhee CNJ, Noble MJ, Watson DG, et al, Penetration of topically applied prednisolone sodium phosphate into human aqueous humor, *Eye* (1989) **3**: 463–7.

6.   McGhee CNJ, Watson DG, Midgley JM, et al, Penetration of synthetic corticosteroids into human aqueous humour, *Eye* (1990) **4**: 526–30.

7.   Watson DG, Noble MJ, Dutton GN, et al, Penetration of topically applied dexamethasone into human aqueous humour, *Arch Ophthalmol* (1988) **106**: 686–7.

8.   Kupferman A, Leibowitz HM, Therapeutic effectiveness of fluorometholone in inflammatory keratitis, *Arch Ophthalmol* (1975) **93**: 1011–4.

9.   Iqbal Z, Watson DG, Midgley JM, Dennison PR, McGhee CNJ, The metabolism of fluorometholone by bovine cornea, *J Pharmaceutical Biomedical Analysis* (1993) **11**: 1115–20.

10.   McGhee CNJ, Pharmacokinetics of ophthalmic corticosteroids, *Br J Ophthalmol* (1992) **11**: 681–4.

11.   Morrison E, Archer DB, Effect of Fluorometholone (FML) on the intraocular pressure of corticosteroid responders, *Br J Ophthalmol* (1984) **68**: 581–4.

12.   Mindel JS, Tavitian HO, Smith H, Walker EC, Comparative ocular pressure elevation by medrysone, fluorometholone and dexamethasone phosphate, *Arch Ophthalmol* (1980) **98**: 1577–8.

13.   Campos M, Abed HM, McDonnell PJ, Topical fluorometholone reduces stromal inflammation after photorefractive keratectomy, *Ophthalmic Surgery* (1993) **24**: 654–7.

14.   Petroutsos G, Guimaraes R, Giraud I, Pouliquen Y, Corticosteroids and corneal epithelial wound healing, *Br J Ophthalmol* (1982) **66**: 705–8.

15.   Hanna KD, Pouliquen Y, Waring GO, Salvodelli M, et al, Corneal stromal wound healing in rabbits after 193 nm excimer laser surface ablation, *Arch Ophthalmol* (1989) **107**: 895–901.

16.   Goodman Gerri L, Trokel SL, Stark WJ, Munnerlyn CR, Green RW, Corneal healing following laser refractive keratectomy, *Arch Ophthalmol* (1989) **107**: 1799–803.

17.   Marshall J, Trokel SL, Rothery S, Krueger RR, Long-term healing of the central cornea after photorefractive keratectomy using an excimer laser, *Ophthalmology* (1988) **95**: 1411–21.

18.   Fantes FE, Hanna KD, Waring GO, et al, Wound healing after excimer laser keratomileusis (Photorefractive keratectomy) in monkeys, *Arch Ophthalmol* (1990) **108**: 665–75.

19.   Tuft SJ, Zabel RW, Marshall J, Corneal repair following keratectomy. A comparison between conventional surgery and laser photoablation, *Invest Ophthalmol Vis Sci* (1989) **30**: 1770–7.

20.   Talamo JH, Gollamudi S, Green WR, et al, Modulation of corneal wound healing after excimer laser keratomileusis using topical mitomycin C and steroids, *Arch Ophthalmol* (1991) **109**: 1141–6.

21.   You X, Bergmanson JPG, Zheng XM, et al, Effect of corticosteroids on rabbit corneal keratocytes after photorefractive keratectomy, *J Refract Surg* (1995) **11**: 460–7.

22. Rawe IM, Zabel RW, Tuft SJ, Chen V, Meek KM, A morphological study of rabbit corneas after laser keratectomy, *Eye* (1992) **6**: 637–42.

23. Nassaralla BA, Szerenyi K, Wang XW, Reaves T, McDonnell PJ, Effect of diclofenac on corneal haze after photorefractive keratectomy in rabbits, *Ophthalmology* (1995) **102**: 469–74.

24. Tengroth B, Epstein D, Fagerholm P, Hamberg-Nystrom H, Fitzsimmons TD, Excimer laser photorefractive keratectomy for myopia: clinical results in sighted eyes, *Ophthalmology* (1993) **100**: 739–45.

25. Seiler T, Wollensak J, Myopic photorefractive keratectomy with the excimer laser: 1 year follow-up, *Ophthalmology* (1991) **98**: 1156–63.

26. Gartry DS, Kerr-Muir MG, Lohmann CP, Marshall J, The effect of topical corticosteroids on the refractive outcome and corneal haze after photorefractive keratectomy, *Arch Ophthalmol* (1992) **110**: 944–52.

27. O'Brart DP, Lohmann CP, Klonos G, et al, The effects of topical corticosteroids and plasmin inhibitors on refractive outcome, haze, and visual performance after photorefractive keratectomy: a prospective randomised observer masked study, *Ophthalmology* (1994) **101**: 1565–74.

28. Haverbeke L, Assessing the efficacy of topical corticosteroids following radial keratotomy, *Refract Corneal Surg* (1993) **9**: 379–82.

29. Gartry DS, Kerr Muir MG, Marshall J, Photorefractive keratectomy with an argon-fluoride excimer laser: a clinical study, *Refract Corneal Surg* (1991) **7**: 420–35.

30. Gartry DS, Kerr Muir MG, Marshall J, Excimer laser photorefractive keratectomy: 18 months follow-up, *Ophthalmology* (1992) **99**: 1209–19.

31. Sher NA, Barak M, Daya S, et al, Excimer laser photorefractive keratectomy in high myopia. A multicenter study, *Arch Ophthalmol* (1992) **110**: 935–43.

32. Salz JJ, Maguen E, Macy JI, et al, One year results of excimer laser photorefractive keratectomy for myopia, *Refract Corneal Surg* (1992) **8**: 269–73.

33. Stevens JD, Steele AD McG, Ficker LA, et al, Prospective randomised study of two topical steroid regimes after excimer laser PRK, *Invest Ophthalmol Vis Sci* (1994) **35**: 1839.

34. Seiler T, McDonnell PJ, Excimer laser photorefractive keratectomy (Review), *Surv Ophthalmol* (1995) **40**: 89–118.

35. Machat JJ, Double blind corticosteroid trial in identical twins following photorefractive keratectomy, *Refract Corneal Surg* (1993) **9**: S105–S107.

36. Corbett MC, O'Brart DPS, Marshall J, Do topical corticosteroids have a role following excimer laser photorefractive keratectomy? *J Refract Surg* (1995) **11**: 380–7.

37. Fitzsimmons TD, Fagerholm P, Tengroth B, Steroid treatment of myopic regression: acute refractive and topographic changes in excimer laser photorefractive keratectomy patients, *Cornea* (1993) **12**: 358–61.

38. Carones F, Brancato R, Venturi E, Scialdone A, Bertuzzi A, Tavola A, Efficacy of corticosteroids in reversing regression after myopic photorefractive keratectomy, *Refract Corneal Surg* (1993) **9**: S52–S56.

39. Cerruti S, Traverso CE, Munaldo U, et al, The efficacy of corticosteroids in reversing the regression of refractive effect after myopic photorefractive keratectomy, *Invest Ophthalmol Vis Sci* (1994) **35**: 3533–52.

40. Baum JL, Levene RZ, Corneal thickness after topical corticosteroid therapy, *Arch Ophthalmol* (1968) **79**: 366–9.

41. McDermott ML, Wang J, Cowden JW, Brine BJ, Tayfour F, Intraocular steroid penetration after photorefractive keratectomy, *Invest Ophthalmol Vis Sci* (1994) **35**: 3512–31.

Corneal healing, growth factors, NSAIDs and anesthetics

THE INITIAL HEALING PROCESS

The normal corneal healing process is extensively covered in Chapter 4 and this section will only highlight aspects of post-PRK healing, particularly those relevant to pharmacological manipulation. As previously noted, within a few hours following corneal wounding, epithelial cells at the wound edges begin to slide centrally, augmented by proliferation of adjacent epithelial cells,[1] to cover the wound edges with a thin layer of epithelial cells. The corneal wound becomes coated with fibronectin, an extracellular structural glycoprotein with the ability to bind both cells and collagen, and the concentration of fibronectin excreted in tears is increased following PRK.[2] Fibronectin appears within 8 hours of corneal wounding, promotes healing[3] and probably forms a matrix that provides a platform for the sliding of epithelial cells.[4] Sliding epithelial cells undergo intracellular reorganization to allow them to move over the fibronectin-coated surface. Actin is a protein involved in cell-substrate adhesion, cell motility and constitutes about 4–6% of the total cellular protein of the human corneal epithelium.[5] In normal corneal epithelium, intracytoplasmic actin filaments are most dense beneath the microplicae of the superficial corneal epithelial cells. After corneal wounding, actin filaments are present in the leading edges of the sliding epithelial cells.[6] During the healing process, regenerating epithelial cells synthesize a basement membrane assisting cohesion between epithelium and underlying stroma.[7] The epithelium surrounding the corneal wound begins to replicate within 24 hours and eventually restores the initial epithelial layer to its normal thickness.

Examination of the central cornea in primates after excimer PRK subsequently shows normal epithelial morphology except at the wound edge where there are more cell layers. The epithelium appears to be thickest in the central treated area.[8] In one study, regenerated basal lamina averaged 86% intact over ablated areas with normal thickness and with no duplications; however, overall, the density of hemidesmosomes was significantly less in the ablated areas compared to unablated areas.[9] By 6 months after excimer laser ablation, in the primate model, almost all vacuolation has disappeared and the increase in keratocytes returns to normal. Indeed, corneal morphology is near normal by 8 months with the exception that Bowman's layer is absent, and there is still some disorder in the immediate subepithelial stromal fibers.[10] Exposure to ablative and subablative excimer laser beams has not been shown to cause oncogenic transformation of corneal cells.[11]

CORNEAL HAZE

A mild, transient corneal haze usually appears in treated areas 3–4 weeks after PRK. This may be followed by the development of a dense haze beginning 6–12 weeks post-PRK.[12] Corneal haze grading is covered in detail in Chapter 8. These areas of anterior stromal fibrosis show extracellular matrix deposition in the subepithelial stroma,[13–16] collagen production and an increase in fibroblastic keratocytes. The keratocyte density in the anterior 17 μm of stroma peaks at 4 months and haze generally improves when stromal reorganization is complete, with associated keratocyte reduction to normal levels.[9,17] Fortunately, there appears to be no significant differences in forward light scatter secondary to haze 1 month after PRK with a 6 mm ablation zone.[18]

Interestingly, in the primate model, excimer laser PRK repeated 3 months after an initial ablation that produced only mild subepithelial haze, results in dense subepithelial opacity and a thickened epithelium.[19] The clinical aspects of corneal haze are covered in Chapter 23.

PHARMACOLOGIC INTERVENTION IN THE PRK EYE

There are four classes of pharmaceutical agents that can be used in the PRK eye:

- Factors which affect corneal healing, e.g. growth factors, plasmin inhibitors
- Anti-inflammatory agents, e.g. corticosteroids, NSAIDs
- Anesthetic and analgesic agents
- Miscellaneous agents that might reduce corneal haze.

FACTORS TO PROMOTE RAPID CORNEAL EPITHELIAL HEALING

Growth factors

Although minimal stromal healing is the ultimate objective of excimer laser PRK, a rapid and uncomplicated healing of the epithelial defect is desirable. Factors involved in corneal wound healing after PRK include the level of inflammatory response, growth factors, sensory innervation and infection.[20] Growth factors, or mitogens, are a heterogenous group of proteins capable of stimulating growth and multiplication of various cell types. These substances exert their activity at nanomolar concentrations by binding to specific high-affinity receptor sites localized in the plasma membrane of the target cells. The biologic action of a growth factor is dependent on the nature of the target cell. Growth factors that involve corneal tissue or have an effect on the cornea include epidermal growth factor (EGF), fibroblast growth factor (FGF), epithelial neuronotrophic factor (ENF), mesodermal growth factor (MGF), angiogenic growth factor and somatomedin-C (Sm-C) or insulin-like growth factor I (IGF-I).[21] (Also see Chapter 4.)

Epidermal growth factor and FGF stimulate the proliferation of corneal epithelium, keratocytes and endothelium. Expression of EGF receptors is initially at the limbal area near the epithelial defect. After covering the defect with several layers of regenerating epithelium, the main site of the expression of EGF and proliferating cell nuclear antigen moves to the basal layer of regenerated epithelium.[22] Epidermal growth factor can be demonstrated in vitro and in vivo to accelerate the process of epithelial healing,[23–27] increase the fibroblastic response and enhance wound strength when optimal doses are used.[28,29] Topical EGF has been shown to be effective and safe in the treatment of traumatic corneal ulcers in human subjects.[30] Mesodermal growth factor appears to stimulate cell proliferation and hasten wound healing in experimental corneal stromal wounds.[31] However, currently these growth factors remain potential ophthalmic pharmaceuticals and are undergoing investigations.

MODULATION OF THE PLASMIN SYSTEM

Theoretically, an alternative approach to improve healing is to modulate the plasminogen-activator/plasmin system, which regulates wound healing. Plasminogen is activated to plasmin by plasminogen activators, which are found in the cornea following PRK. Plasmin degrades matrix proteins such as fibronectin and laminin within the extracellular matrix. It has been postulated that inhibition of plasmin may facilitate epithelial regeneration and stromal removal. However, one study involving the use of the plasmin inhibitor, aprotonin, following PRK did not demonstrate any beneficial effects.[32]

MISCELLANEOUS TECHNIQUES TO PROMOTE EPITHELIAL HEALING

Topical administration of sodium hyaluronate appears to accelerate the healing of epithelial defects in rabbit epithelium removed surgically or with n-heptanol. It has been postulated that larger amounts of fibronectin production or retention of larger amounts by sodium hyaluronate may assist in the healing process.[33] Unfortunately, the effect of improved corneal healing following topical sodium hyaluronate has not been demonstrated in human subjects.[34]

Collagen shields speed re-epithelialization of keratectomy wounds in animal models and appear to be most effective during the first 8 hours after wounding.[35,36] The use of collagen shields post-radial keratotomy has been suggested to result in more

patient comfort as well as accelerating epithelial and stromal healing.[37] The promotion of epithelial healing by preservative-free artificial tears is uncertain. However, preservatives such as benzalkonium and thiomersal are known to be toxic and are best avoided in topical medications during the healing process.[38,39]

ANTI-INFLAMMATORY AGENTS

PRK, prostaglandins and non-steroidal anti-inflammatory drugs

Corticosteroids have been used for some time, with debatable efficacy, to modulate post-PRK corneal healing (see the earlier part of this chapter). Because of the associated risks of corticosteroids, suitable alternative topical ophthalmic drugs have been sought in many spheres of ophthalmology, including the photorefractive arena, for many years. Non-steroidal anti-inflammatory drugs (NSAIDs), as a group, may influence corneal wound healing after excimer laser PRK. In a recent laboratory study involving excimer laser PRK to correct 5D, there was less corneal haze in rabbit eyes treated with topical diclofenac 0.1% or fluorometholone 0.1% compared to control eyes; however, the results were statistically significant only in the diclofenac-treated group. Combination treatment with both diclofenac and fluorometholone did not result in a further decrease in haze. These results, albeit in a rabbit model, continue to suggest a potential role of the use of topical NSAIDs in the prevention or modulation of excessive corneal haze after excimer laser surgery.[40]

Prostaglandins (PG) are biologically active derivatives of unsaturated fatty acids present everywhere in human and animal organisms. They are important as mediators or modulators of inflammatory reactions. Prostaglandins are formed mainly from arachidonic acid and are produced in response to tissue insults. Since inflammation is a complicated process, involving a large number of mediators and products, and interpretation of animal studies may be complicated by the specific nature of the experimental insults, or the timing of measurements and the animal model used, results of animal studies might not be readily extrapolated to the human situation. The points of action and the effect on specific inflammation parameters change not only from medicament to medicament but also in some cases from patient to patient, depending perhaps upon genetic and constitutional factors. This may explain the occurrence of different

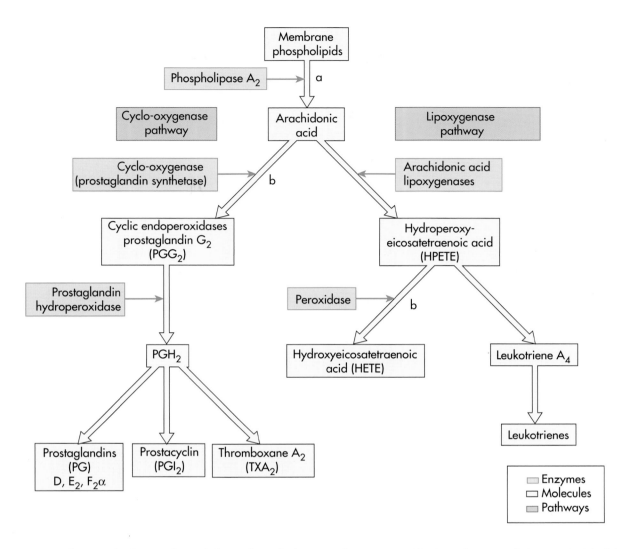

Figure 25.1 *Schematic pathway of metabolism of arachidonic acid to eicosanoids. Site of action of glucocorticoids (a) and NSAIDs (b).*

types of activity and in some cases poorly interpretable, unexpected and deviant results during treatment with different anti-inflammatory drugs, particularly by the NSAIDs.[41]

The cornea has a lesser capacity to synthesize cyclo-oxygenase and lipoxygenase products from arachidonic acid when compared to the conjunctiva and anterior uvea. Nevertheless, following 193 nm excimer laser on rabbit corneas, prostaglandin E_2 (PGE_2) production (mediated by the cyclo-oxygenase pathway) has been noted to be rapid and sustained with leukocyte infiltration in the cornea, whereas no significant changes in the levels of leukotriene B_4 (mediated by the lipoxygenase pathway) are identified.[42] In another experiment, 193 nm excimer laser irradiation caused a greater increase of PGE_2 production in rabbit corneal tissue than did keratectomy with a microkeratome to the same depth. There was an 8.6-fold increase in PGE_2 compared to unoperated cornea.[43] These observations suggest that the inflammatory response following excimer laser irradiation is mediated primarily by prostaglandins.

In mammalian cell cultures, ultraviolet A light stimulates cyclo-oxygenase metabolism and produces high levels of PGE_2 that acts as a chemoattractant for polymorphonuclear leukocytes (PMNs). Topical

Table 25.1

Commercially available topical ophthalmic NSAIDs

Chemical class	Generic name	Trade name (Manufacturer)
Indoles	indomethacin	Indomethacin 0.5% & 1% in castor oil eye drops (Moorfields Eye Hospital)
		Indocid Ophthalmic Suspension (Merck Sharp and Dohme)
Phenylalkanoic acids	flurbiprofen	Ocufen (Allergan)
	ketorolac	Acular (Allergan)
	suprofen	Profenal (Alcon)
Phenylacetic acids	diclofenac	Voltaren/Voltarol (Ciba Vision Ophthalmics)
Pyrazolons	oxyphenbutazone	Tanderil 10% (Geigy)

diclofenac sodium 0.1% reduces the local release of PGE_2 and the migration of PMNs in the rabbit cornea after 193 nm excimer laser ablation.[44] Diclofenac was also shown to inhibit the chemokinetic activity (speed of PMN locomotion) of human PMNs elicited in vitro.[45,46] Polymorphonuclear leukocytes in tear fluid of rabbits subjected to corneal de-epithelialization were also inhibited by topically applied diclofenac 0.1%,[47] flurbiprofen 0.01%, indomethacin 0.5% and aspirin 0.5%.[48]

This significant decrease in prostaglandin E_2 levels following topical diclofenac sodium treatment was confirmed in another study that noted a significant increase in corneal leukocytes at 10 hours. Treatment with fluorometholone, a corticosteroid, did not significantly alter prostaglandin E_2 levels but depressed leukocyte ingress.[41]

Classification of NSAIDs

Non-steroidal anti-inflammatory drugs are chemically heterogeneous compounds that do not include in their chemical structures a steroid nucleus derived biosynthetically from cholesterol. They are referred to as cyclo-oxygenase inhibitors (COI) and inhibit the biosynthesis of prostaglandins (PGs). Although NSAIDs inhibit the formation of PGs, they are not capable of inhibiting the actions of PGs once formed. The sites of action of NSAIDs and corticosteroids are indicated in Figure 25.1.

Non-steroidal anti-inflammatory drugs are a group of compounds, that in chemical terms belong to different structural classes. These include salicylates (aspirin), fenamates, indoles (indomethacin), pyrazolons (oxyphenbutazone), phenylalkanoic acids (flurbiprofen, suprofen, ketorolac) and phenylacetic-

acids (diclofenac) (Table 25.1). Indomethacin was the first topically administered COI and has been shown to significantly decrease levels of prostaglandin E_2 in the cornea.[49] Phenylalkanoic acids are water soluble and are readily formulated as ophthalmic solutions. These include flurbiprofen 0.03% and suprofen 1%. The main phenylacetic acid derivative is diclofenac 1%.

Advantages of NSAIDs

Topical ophthalmic NSAIDs avoid the undesirable effects of topical corticosteroids, which include decreased immunological response to infection,[50] cataract formation and steroid-induced raised intraocular pressure.[51,52] Corticosteroids may also retard the formation of fibrinous coagulum, cellular infiltration, fibroblastic repair, epithelial and endothelial regeneration.[53] Furthermore, the use of NSAIDs, such as flurbiprofen sodium or diclofenac sodium, unlike corticosteroids, does not exacerbate acute herpetic keratitis or prolong shedding of virus.[54]

Effect of NSAIDs on epithelial healing and corneal wound strength

Non-steroidal anti-inflammatory drugs (indomethacin 0.5% and flurbiprofen 0.01%) can inhibit PMN arrival in tear fluid but do not inhibit the re-epithelialization by either corneal or conjunctival epithelial cells. Topical diclofenac sodium 0.1% does not delay corneal re-epithelialization following excimer laser treatment in rabbits.[55] These findings in rabbits suggest topical NSAIDs have less adverse effects on epithelial wound healing when compared to topical corticosteroids.[56] In contrast, in one study, corneal scrape wounds of rabbits treated with flurbiprofen sodium 0.03%, diclofenac sodium 0.1% and prednisolone acetate 1%, demonstrated delayed epithelial healing rates in all groups compared to placebo.[57] However, in a clinical study, McDonald et al. did not find any significant difference in the rate of re-epithelialization, manifest refractions, visual acuities or central corneal clarity in eyes treated with diclofenac compared to fluorometholone.[58]

Although one study in rabbits with full-thickness corneal wounds showed treatment with flurbiprofen or diclofenac actually resulted in stronger wounds than untreated controls, which were stronger in turn than corneal wounds treated with prednisolone acetate.[59] In contrast, another rabbit study comparing the effect of equipotent anti-inflammatory doses of flurbiprofen and prednisolone upon the wound bursting pressure of 4 mm corneal incisions, suggested that flurbiprofen and prednisolone did not differ in their effect on corneal wound healing.[60]

The advantage of NSAIDs on epithelial healing and corneal wound strength is, for the moment, far from conclusive. Interpretation of studies needs to take into account the animal model used, the drug dose and the time of application of drugs following experimental wounding.

NSAID use without corticosteroids

The use of NSAIDs without corticosteroids following excimer PRK has resulted in cases of corneal infiltrates with or without associated use of occlusive contact lens.[61] Theoretical inhibition of the cyclooxygenase pathway for prostaglandin generation may result in increased formation of leukotrienes[62] recognized as chemotactic[63,64] and this may possibly encourage PMN infiltrate formation in the earlier healing stage. Patients on NSAID alone have also been reported to have more corneal haze and regression of effect.[65] However, in a small study involving 20 eyes (4–9 D myopia intended correction), comparing the use of topical diclofenac sodium 0.1% and dexamethasone 0.1%, no significant difference in haze or regression effect was demonstrated.[66]

Concurrent use of NSAIDs and corticosteroids

Polymorphonuclear leukocytes play a central role in the inflammatory process. In a study involving experimental keratitis, the ability of an NSAID (suprofen) and a corticosteroid (prednisolone acetate) to suppress PMN invasion of the rabbit cornea was evaluated. Suprofen therapy, initiated immediately after induction of inflammation, was ineffective and was only efficacious if therapy was started 48 hours prior to corneal insults. In contrast, prednisolone acetate therapy was effective when initiated immediately after induction of inflammation and, additionally, produced a marked increase in therapeutic effect when started 48 hours earlier. Combined treatment was significantly more effective than with either drug alone.[67] In a small clinical trial, concurrent use of corticosteroids and NSAIDs appeared to reduce myopic regression for 1 year post-PRK and the effect was more pronounced with flurbiprofen sodium than diclofenac sodium.[68]

Analgesic effects of NSAIDs following PRK

Following excimer PRK, patients may experience significant ocular pain and discomfort until corneal re-epithelialization. Hypersensitivity may occur following excimer laser ablation.[69] Studies on topical diclofenac sodium show that it reduces corneal sensitivity,[70] has an anesthetic effect[71] and decreases post-excimer laser treatment discomfort.[71–74] Sher et al have reported, in a clinical series of 16 diclofenac-treated patients and 16 placebo-treated patients, that topical diclofenac appears to significantly reduce the ocular pain following excimer PRK and the diclofenac-treated patients rarely experience the early post-PRK peak in pain and have less pain overall until 72 hours postoperatively. In addition, such patients have significantly less post laser photophobia, burning and stinging symptoms. Significantly fewer patients prescribed topical diclofenac required oral narcotics. There was no difference in epithelial healing times between the diclofenac-treated and untreated eyes.[75] Topical ketorolac tromethamine 0.5% has also been reported as an analgesic[76,77] and as effective as topical diclofenac.[78] Topical indomethacin does not appear to have any significant analgesic activity.[79] Non-steroidal anti-inflammatory drugs may be used systemically, utilizing their central and peripheral analgesic properties.[81–82] Piroxicam is an NSAID with a potent analgesic action that is centrally acting and independent of the opioid system.[83]

Table 25.2
Commercially available topical anesthetics

Trade name	Active agent	Preservatives	Adverse reactions
Minims® Benoxinate 0.4%	oxybuprocaine 0.4%	chlorhexidine acetate 0.01%	Epithelial keratitis.
Minims® Amethocaine 0.5%, 1%	amethocaine 0.5%, 1%	phenylmercuric nitrate 0.002%	Contraindicated in patients treated with sulphonamides. Dermatitis in hypersensitive patients. Initial burning sensation on instillation. Epithelial and stromal keratitis.
Ophthaine 0.5%	proxymetacaine 0.5%	chlorbutol 0.2% and benzalkonium chloride 0.01%	Pupillary dilatation. Cycloplegic effects. Irritation of conjunctiva. Severe immediate-type hyperallergic corneal reaction. Acute, intense and diffuse epithelial keratitis. Epithelial necrosis. Corneal filaments. Iritis with descemetitis.
	cocaine 4%		Toxic effects to epithelium and corneal stroma. Mydriasis, which may cause secondary glaucoma.

Complications and contraindications associated with the use of NSAIDs

The most frequent reported adverse reactions are transient burning, stinging on instillation and minor signs of ocular irritation. Hypersensitivity reactions with itching, reddening, photosensitivity and keratitis punctata may occur, especially in patients in whom attacks of asthma,[84] urticaria, or acute rhinitis are precipitated by drugs with prostaglandin synthetase inhibiting activity (e.g. acetylsalicylic acid). Although topical NSAIDs are safer than corticosteroids, they are generally contraindicated in epithelial herpes simplex keratitis (dendritic keratitis) and patients with a history of herpes simplex keratitis should be monitored closely. Post-PRK sterile infiltrates have already been discussed.

Topical NSAIDs can reach the systemic circulation by way of absorption from the nasolacrimal outflow system. Non-steroidal anti-inflammatory drugs may increase the risk of bleeding (including hyphemas) and are contraindicated in patients with known hemostatic defects or on medications that may prolong bleeding time. As there are no adequate and well-controlled studies in pregnant women, topical NSAIDs should be avoided in these patients.

TOPICAL ANESTHETICS

Topical anesthetics act by stabilizing cell membranes and preventing nerve impulse transmission. All topical anesthetic agents in commercial use appear to be toxic to corneal epithelium. The mechanism for this toxicity is unclear and may be due to a direct effect of the anesthetic agent on epithelium or an impairment of the trophic action of the corneal nerve fibers.[85] Most topical anesthetic agents cause stinging and irritation. Experiments on the healing of rat corneal epithelial defects using clinical concentrations of topical anesthetics applied at 15 minute intervals over a 3-hour period showed that only topical piperocaine 2% and lidocaine 2% allowed for the normal regeneration of the epithelium. Tetracaine 0.5% delayed healing slightly. Oxybuprocaine hydrochloride 0.4%, naepaine 2%, butacaine sulphate 2%, cocaine 4%, phenacaine 1%, dibucaine 0.1% and proxymetacaine 0.5% all impaired healing of the corneal epithelium.[86]

Repeated instillation of benoxinate, lidocaine, or tetracaine results in loss of microvilli and disruption of plasma membranes, with stippling on slit lamp examination.[87] Proxymetacaine hydrochloride is a rapidly acting local anesthetic but may cause possible irritation to the conjunctiva, with severe immediate-type hyperallergic corneal reactions, with acute, intense, diffuse epithelial keratitis.[88] Amethocaine and cocaine are considered longer acting than benoxinate and proxymetacaine. However, benoxinate and proxymetacaine are less toxic, producing less corneal disturbance.[89,90] Topical anesthetics may affect the blink reflex and it is recommended that the anesthetized eye should be protected from dust and bacterial contamination in the postoperative period. Commercially available topical anaesthetics are listed in Table 25.2.

There is evidence to suggest that opiate agonists exhibit peripheral analgesic effects in inflamed tissue of animals which contain opiate receptors[91,92] that mediate anti-nociception in inflammatory and/or stress situations.[93,94] Topical morphine sulphate 0.5% has an analgesic effect on eyes with corneal abrasions but not on intact corneas. The fast analgesic response suggests that topical morphine sulphate exerts its effects locally, primarily through opioid receptor-mediated mechanisms.[95] Topical morphine sulphate 0.5% showed no adverse effects on corneal wound closure in animal studies[96] and may be an ideal topical analgesic, with re-establishment of corneal sensitivity when corneal epithelial healing is completed.

EFFECTS OF TOPICAL OPHTHALMIC DRUGS ON CORNEAL HAZE

Several drugs have demonstrated an effect on post-PRK haze in animal models; however, convincing efficacy in the human eye has yet to be demonstrated. Topical prednisolone acetate, 5-fluorouracil, heparin, prednisolone/heparin combination and prednisolone/5-fluorouracil combination provided only a transient benefit in rabbits at 2 weeks in reducing corneal haze. The control corneas cleared to an equivalent haze by 6 weeks.[97]

In another rabbit study, although less haze was observed 3 weeks following PRK in the group treated with prednisolone 1% compared with flurbiprofen 0.03%, the difference was not significant.[98] In rabbits, corticosteroids apparently reduce haze by limiting the synthesis of subepithelial collagen, but in humans corticosteroids do not appear to have a lasting effect on either haze or regression.[99] Corneal haze after PRK varies considerably from patient to patient using identical corticosteroid regimes.[100–103]

Topical interferon-alpha 2b appears to reduce corneal haze produced by excimer laser PRK in rabbits.[104] Notably, though not a topical agent per se, nitrogen gas blown over the cornea during PRK in rabbits results in a rougher corneal surface, greater corneal haze[105] and less rapid epithelial healing.[106]

REFERENCES

1. Haskjold E, Bjerknes R, Refsum SB, Cell kinetics during healing of corneal epithelial wounds, *Acta Ophthalmol* (1989) **67**: 174–80.

2. Virtanen T, Ylatupa S, Mertaniemi P, et al, Tear fluid fibronectin levels after photorefractive keratectomy. *J Refract Surg* (1995) **11**: 106–12.

3. Ding M, Burstein NL, Fibronectin in corneal wound healing (Review), *J Ocular Pharmacol* (1988) **4**: 75–91.

4. Nishida T, Nakagawa S, Awata T, et al, Fibronectin promotes epithelial migration of cultured rabbit cornea in situ. *J Cell Biology* (1983) **97**: 1683–87.

5. Soong HK, Fairley JA, Actin in human corneal epithelium, *Arch Ophthalmol* (1985) **103**: 565–8.

6. Gipson IK, Keezer L, Effects of cytochalasins and colchicine on the ultrastructure of migrating corneal epithelium, *Invest Ophthalmol Vis Sci* (1982) **22**: 643–50.

7. Leuenberger PM, Functional morphology of the cornea, *Advances in Ophthalmology* (1978) **35**: 94–166.

8. Gauthier CA, Epstein D, Holden BA, et al, Epithelial alterations following photorefractive keratectomy for myopia, *J Refract Surg* (1995) **11**: 113–18.

9. Beuerman RW, McDonald MB, Shofner RS, Quantitative histological studies of primate corneas after excimer laser photorefractive keratectomy, *Arch Ophthalmol* (1994) **112**: 1103–10.

10. Marshall J, Trokel SL, Rothery S, et al, Long term healing of the central cornea after photorefractive keratectomy using an excimer laser, *Ophthalmology* (1988) **95**: 1411–21.

11. Gebhardt BM, Salmeron B, McDonald MB, Effect of excimer laser energy on the growth potential of corneal keratocytes, *Cornea* (1990) **9**: 205–10.

12. Sher NA, Barak M, Daya S, et al, Excimer laser photorefractive keratectomy in high myopia, *Arch Ophthalmol* (1992) **110**: 925–43.

13. Lohmann C, Gartry D, Muir MK, et al, 'Haze' in

photorefractive keratectomy: its origins and consequences, *Laser Light Ophthalmol* (1991) **4**: 15–34.

14. Hanna KD, Pouliquen YM, Waring GO, et al, Corneal wound healing in monkeys after repeated excimer laser photorefractive keratectomy, *Arch Ophthalmol* (1992) **110**: 1286–91.

15. Hanna KD, Pouliquen YM, Savoldelli M, et al, Corneal wound healing in monkeys 18 months after excimer laser photorefractive keratectomy, *Refract Corneal Surg* (1990) **6**: 340–45.

16. Alleman N, Chamon W, Silverman RH, et al, High-frequency ultrasound quantitative analyses of corneal scarring following excimer laser keratectomy, *Arch Ophthalmol* (1993) **111**: 968–73.

17. McDonald MB, Frantz JM, Klyce SD, et al, One-year refractive results of central photorefractive keratectomy for myopia in the non-human primate cornea. *Arch Ophthalmol* (1990) **108**: 40–47.

18. Harrison JM, Tennant TB, Gwin MC, et al, Forward light scatter at one month after photorefractive keratectomy, *J Refract Surg* (1995) **11**: 83–88.

19. Hanna KD, Pouliquen YM, Waring GO, et al, Corneal wound healing in monkeys after repeated excimer laser photorefractive keratectomy, *Arch Ophthalmol* (1992) **110**: 1286–91.

20. Parrish CM, Chandler JW, Corneal trauma. In: McDonald MB, Waltman SR, Barron BA, Kaufman HE, eds, *The Cornea*, 1st edn (Churchill Livingstone: New York, 1988) 599–605.

21. Tripathi BJ, Kwait PS, Tripathi RC, Corneal growth factors: a new generation of ophthalmic pharmaceuticals, *Cornea* (1990) **9**: 2–9.

22. Murata T, Ishibashi T, Inomata H, Localizations of epidermal growth factor receptor and proliferating cell nuclear antigen during corneal wound healing, *Graefes Archive for Clinical & Experimental Ophthalmology* (1993) **231**: 104–8.

23. Daniele S, Frati L, Fiore C, et al, The effect of the epidermal growth factor (EGF) on the corneal epithelium in humans, *Albrecht Von Graefes Archiv fur Kinische und Experimentelle Ophthalmologie* (1974) **210**: 159–65.

24. Petroutsos G, Jacomini C, Patey A, et al, PHZ-102 (epidermal growth factor) and cicatrization of the corneal epithelium, *Journal Francais D'Ophthalmologie* (1983) **6**: 959–62.

25. Petroutsos G, Courty J, Guimaraes R, et al, Comparison of the effects of EGF, pFGF and EDGF on corneal epithelium wound healing, *Curr Eye Res* (1984) **3**: 593–8.

26. Artuson G, Epidermal growth factor in the healing of corneal wounds, epidermal wounds and partial-thickness scalds. A controlled animal study, *Scandinavian Journal of Plastic & Reconstructive Surgery* (1984) **18**: 33–7.

27. Beaubien J, Boisjoly HM, Gagnon P, et al, Mechanical properties of the rabbit cornea during wound healing after treatment with epidermal growth factor, *Can J Ophthalmol* (1994) **29**: 61–5.

28. Mathers WD, Sherman M, Fryczkowski A, et al, Dose-dependent effects of epidermal growth factor on corneal wound healing, *Invest Ophthalmol Vis Sci* (1989) **30**: 2403–6.

29. Petroutsos G, Sebag J, Courtois Y, Epidermal growth factor increases tensile strength during wound healing, *Ophthalmic Research* (1986) **18**: 299–300.

30. Scardovi C, De Felice GP, Gazzaniga A, Epidermal growth factor in the topical treatment of traumatic corneal ulcers, *Ophthalmologica* (1993) **206**: 119–24.

31. Smith RS, Smith LS, Rich L, et al, Effects of growth factors on corneal wound healing, *Invest Ophthalmol Vis Sci* (1981) **20**: 222–29.

32. O'Brart DPS, Lohmann CP, Klonos G, et al, The effect of topical corticosteroids and plasmin inhibitors on refractive outcome, haze, and visual performance after photorefractive keratectomy, *Ophthalmology* (1994) **101**: 1565–74.

33. Sugiyama T, Miyauchi S, Machida A, et al, The effect of sodium hyaluronate on the migration of rabbit corneal epithelium. The effect of topical administration, *J Ocular Pharmacol* (1991) **7**: 53–64.

34. Algawi K, Agrell B, Goggin M, et al, Randomized clinical trial of topical sodium hyaluronte after excimer laser photorefractive keratectomy, *Refract Surg* (1995) **11**: 42–4.

35. Frantz JM, Dupuy BM, Kaufman HE, et al, The effect of collagen shields on epithelial wound healing in rabbits, *Am J Ophthalmol* (1989) **108**: 524–8.

36. Shaker GJ, Ueda S, LoCascio JA, et al, The effect of a collagen shield on cat corneal epithelial wound healing, *Invest Ophthalmol Vis Sci* (1989) **30**: 1565–8.

37. Marmer RH, Therapeutic and protective properties of the corneal collagen shield, *J Cataract Refract Surg* (1988) **14**: 496–9.

38. Garner A, Corneal wound healing. In: Casey TA, Mayer DJ, eds, *Corneal grafting* (WB Saunders: Philadelphia, 1984) 28–29, 40.

39. Collin HB, Grabsch BE, The effect of ophthalmic preservatives on the healing rate of the rabbit corneal epithelium after keratectomy, *Am J Optometry & Physiological Optics* (1982) **59**: 215–22.

40. Nassaralla BA, Szerenyi K, Wang XW, et al, Effect of diclofenac on corneal haze after photorefractive keratectomy in rabbits, *Ophthalmology* (1995) **102**: 469–74.

41. Van Husen H, Topical treatment of anterior ocular diseases with diclofenac Na eye drops, *Klin Mbl Augenheill* (1986) **188**: 615–9.

42. Phillips AF, Szerenyi K, Campos M, et al, Arachidonic acid metabolites after excimer laser corneal surgery, *Arch Ophthalmol* (1993) **111**: 1273–8.

43. Szerenyi KD, Campos M, McDonnell PJ, Prostaglandin E2 production after lamellar keratectomy and photorefractive keratectomy, *J Refract Corneal Surg* (1994) **10**: 413–6.

44. Szerenyi K, Wang XW, Lee M, et al, Topical diclofenac treatment prior to excimer laser photorefractive keratectomy in rabbits, *Refract Corneal Surg* (1993) **9**: 437–42.

45. Perianin A, Gougerot-Pocidalo ME, Giroud JP, et al, Diclofenac sodium, a negative chemokinetic factor for neutrophil locomotion, *Biochem Pharmacol* (1985) **34**: 3433–8.

46. Perianin A, Giroud JP, Hajim J, Stimulation of human polymorphonuclear leukocytes potentiates the uptake of diclofenac and inhibition of chemotaxis, *Biochem Pharmacol* (1990) **40**: 2039–45.

47. Kulkarni P, Srinivasan BD, Diclofenac and enolicam as ocular anti-inflammatory drugs in rabbit corneal wound model, *J Ocular Pharmacol* (1986) **2**: 171–5.

48. Srinivasan BD, Kulkarni PS, Polymorphonuclear leukocyte response. Inhibition following corneal epithelial denudation

by steroidal and non-steroidal anti-inflammatory agents, *Arch Ophthalmol* (1981) **99:** 1085–9.

49. Frucht-Pery J, Zauberman H, The effect of indomethacin on prostaglandin E2 in human cornea and conjunctiva, *Arch Ophthalmol* (1992) **110:** 343–5.

50. Fraser-Smith EB, Matthews TR, Effect of ketorolac on *Pseudomonas aeruginosa* ocular infection in rabbits, *J Ocular Pharmacol* (1988) **4:** 101–9.

51. Hic J, Gigon S, Leuenberger PM, Comparison of the anti-inflammatory effect of dexamethasone and diclofenac ophthalmic preparations, *Klin Mbl Augenheilk* (1984) **184:** 494–8.

52. Geiser DK, Hoda PPE, Goldberg I, et al, Flurbiprofen and intraocular pressure, *Ann Ophthalmol* (1981) **13:** 831–3.

53. Ashton N, Cook C, Effect of cortisone on healing of corneal wounds, *Br J Ophthalmol* (1951) **35:** 708–18.

54. Trousdale MD, Barlow WE, McGuigan LJB, Assessment of diclofenac on herpes keratitis in rabbit eyes, *Arch Ophthalmol* (1989) **107:** 1664–6.

55. Loya N, Bassage S, Vyas S, et al, Topical Diclofenac following excimer laser: effects on corneal sensitivity and wound healing in rabbits, *J Refract Corneal Surg* (1994) **10:** 423–7.

56. Srinivasan BD, Corneal reepithelialization and anti-inflammatory agents (Review), *Transactions of the American Ophthalmological Society* (1982) **80:** 758–822.

57. Hersh PS, Rice BA, Baer JC, et al, Topical nonsteroidal agents and corneal wound healing, *Arch Ophthalmol* (1990) **108:** 577–83.

58. McDonald MB, Herschel MK, Ahmed RJ, et al, Effects of Voltaren and FML drops in post-excimer laser photorefractive keratectomy therapy, *Invest Ophthalmol Vis Sci* (1993) **34:** 803.

59. McCarey BE, Napalkov JA, Pippen PA, et al, Corneal wound healing strength with topical anti-inflammatory drugs, *Invest Ophthalmol Vis Sic* (1993) **34:** 1321.

60. Miller D, Gruenberg P, Miller P, et al, Topical flurbiprofen or prednisolone. Effect on corneal wound healing in rabbits, *Arch Ophthalmol* (1981) **99:** 681–2.

61. Teal P, Breslin C, Arshinoff S, Edmison D, Corneal subepithelial infiltrates following excimer laser photorefractive keratectomy, *J Cataract Refract Surg* (1995) **21:** 516–8.

62. Moreira H, McDonnell PJ, Fasano AP, et al, Treatment of experimental Pseudomonas keratitis with cyclo-oxygenase and lipoxygenase inhibitors, *Ophthalmology* (1991) **98:** 1693–7.

63. Napoli SA, Helm C, Inslar MS, et al, External ocular inflammatory effects of lipoxygenase enzyme products, *Ann Ophthalmol* (1990) **22:** 30–34.

64. Palmer RMJ, Stepney RJ, Higgs GA, et al, Chemokinetic activity of arachidonic acid lipoxygenase products on leukocytes of different species, *Prostaglandins* (1980) **20:** 411–8.

65. Johnson D, Aston J, Issues and answers in Excimer Laser PRK, *Review Ophthalmol* (1994) **7:** 84–93.

66. Ferrari M, Use of topical nonsteroidal anti-inflammatory drugs after photorefractive keratectomy, *J Refract Corneal Surg* (1994) **10(Suppl):** 287–9.

67. Leibowitz HM, Ryan WJ, Kupferman A, et al, Effect of concurrent topical corticosteroid and NSAID therapy of experimental keratitis, *Invest Ophthalmol Vis Sci* (1986) **27:** 1226–9.

68. Arshinoff S, D'Addario D, Sadler C, et al, Use of topical nonsteroidal anti-inflammatory drugs in excimer laser photorefractive keratectomy, *J Cataract Refract Surg* (1994) **20(Suppl):** 216–22.

69. Ishikawa T, del Cerro M, Liang FQ, et al, Hypersensitivity following excimer laser ablation through the corneal epithelium, *Refract Corneal Surg* (1992) **8:** 466–74.

70. Szerenyi K, Sorken K, Garbus JJ, et al, Decrease in normal human corneal sensitivity with topical diclofenac sodium, *Am J Ophthalmol* (1994) **118:** 312–5.

71. Zaidman GW, Diclofenac and its effect on corneal sensation, *Arch Ophthalmol* (1995) **113:** 262.

72. Herschel MK, McDonald MB, Ahmed SD, et al, Voltaren for treatment of discomfort after excimer ablation, *Invest Ophthalmol Vis Sci* (1993) **34(Suppl):** 893.

73. Lipner M, NSAIDs shown to dramatically cut post-PRK pain, *Ocular Surgery News* (1994) **12:** 58, 61.

74. Harr D, PRK: No pain, major gain, *Ocular Surgery News* (1992) **21:** 73, 74.

75. Sher NA, Frantz JM, Talley A, et al, Topical diclofenac in the treatment of ocular pain after excimer photorefractive keratectomy, *Refract Corneal Surg* (1993) **9:** 425–36.

76. Ekdahl J, Promising use of non-steroidals with PRK, *Eyecare Technology* (1994) **4:** 58–9, 62, 105.

77. Stein R, Stein HA, Cheskes A, et al, Photorefractive keratectomy and post-operative pain, *Am J Ophthalmol* (1994) **117:** 403–5.

78. Epstein RL, Laurence EP, Relative effectiveness of topical ketorolac and topical diclofenac on discomfort after radial keratotomy, *J Cataract Refract Surg* (1995) **21:** 156–9.

79. Hoh H, Local anaesthetic effect and subsequent tolerance of 0.5% levobunolol in normal eyes, *Klin Mbl Augenheilk* (1990) **1:** 20–6.

80. Mather LE, Do the pharmacodynamics of the non-steroidal anti-inflammatory drugs suggest a role in the management of post-operative pain?, *Drugs* (1992) **44:** 1–12.

81. Naidu MUR, Kumar RT, Jagdishchandra US, et al, Evaluation of ketorolac, ibuprofen-paracetamol, and dextropropoxyphene-paracetamol in post-operative pain, *Pharmacotherapy* (1994) **14:** 173–7.

82. Jurna I, Central analgesic effects of non-steroidal anti-rheumatic agents, *Zeitschrift fur Rheumatologie* (1991) **1:** 7–13.

83. Fabbri A, Cruccu G, Sperti P, et al, Piroxicam-induced analgesia: evidence for a central component which is not opioid mediated, *Experientia* (1992) **48:** 1139–42.

84. Frew A, Selected side effects: 13. Non-steroidal anti-inflammatory drugs and asthma, *Prescribers' Journal* (1994) **34:** 74–7.

85. Rapuano CJ, Topical anaesthetic abuse: a case report of bilateral corneal ring infiltrates, *J Ophthal Nursing Technology* (1990) **9:** 94–5.

86. Marr WG, Wood R, Senterfit L, et al, Effect of topical anaesthetics on regeneration of corneal epithelium, *Am J Ophthalmol* (1957) **43:** 606–10.

87. Burstein NL, Corneal cytotoxicity of topically applied drugs, vehicles and preservatives, *Surv Ophthalmol* (1980) **25:** 15–30.

88. (1995–96) *ABPI Data Sheet Compendium*, 1787.

89. (1992) Local anaesthetics *Moorfields Eye Hospital Formulary*, 63.

90. (1995–96) *ABPI Data Sheet Compendium*, 352–3.

91. Stein C, Gramsch C, Herz A, Intrinsic mechanisms of

antinociception in inflammation: local opioid receptors and β-endorphin, *J Neurosci* (1990) **10:** 1292–8.

92. Joris JL, Dubner R, Hargreaves KM, Opioid analgesia at peripheral sites: a target for opioids released during stress and inflammation, *Anesth Analg* (1987) **66:** 1277–81.

93. Stein C, Millan MJ, Yassouridis A, et al, Antinociceptive effects of μ- and ψ-agonists in inflammation are enhanced by a peripheral opioid receptor-specific mechanism, *Eur J Pharmacol* (1988) **155:** 255–64.

94. Stein C, Millan MJ, Shippenberg TS, et al, Peripheral opioid receptors mediating antinociception in inflammation: evidence for involvement of mu, delta and kappa receptors, *J Pharmacol Exp Ther* (1989) **248:** 1269–75.

95. Fanciullacci M, Boccuni M, Pietrini V, et al, The naloxone conjunctival test in morphine addition, *Eur J Pharmacol* (1980) **61:** 319–20.

96. Peyman GA, Rahimy MH, Fernandes ML, Effects of morphine on corneal sensitivity and epithelial wound healing: implications for topical ophthalmic analgesia, *Br J Ophthalmol* (1994) **78:** 138–41.

97. Bergman RH, Spigelman AV, The role of fibroblast inhibitors on corneal healing following photorefractive keratectomy with 193-nanometer excimer laser in rabbits, *Ophthalmic Surgery* (1994) **25:** 170–4.

98. David T, Serdarevic O, Salvoldelli M, et al, Effects of topical corticosteroids and nonsteroidal anti-inflammatory agents on corneal wound healing after myopic photorefractive keratectomy in rabbits, *Refract Corneal Surgery* (1994) **10(Suppl):** S299.

99. Corbett MC, O'Brart DPS, Marshall J, Do topical corticosteroids have a role following excimer laser photorefractive keratectomy? *J Refract Surg* (1995) **11:** 380–7.

100. Gartry DS, Muir MGK, Lohmann CP, et al, The effect of topical corticosteroids on refractive outcome and corneal haze after photorefractive keratectomy: a prospective, randomized, double-blind trial, *Arch Ophthalmol* (1992) **110:** 944–52.

101. Carones F, Brancato R, Venturi E, et al, Efficacy of corticosteroids in postoperative care following photorefractive keratectomies, *Refract Corneal Surg* (1993) **9(Suppl):** S52–S56.

102. Tengroth B, Fagerholm P, Soderberg H, et al, Effect of corticosteroids in postoperative care following photorefractive keratectomies, *Refract Corneal Surg* (1995) **9:** S61–S64.

103. Caubert E, Cause of subepithelial corneal haze over 18 months after photorefractive keratectomy for myopia, *Refract Corneal Surg* (1993) **9:** S65–S70.

104. Morlet N, Gillies MC, Crouch R, et al, Effect of topical interferon-alpha 2b on corneal haze after excimer laser photorefractive keratectomy in rabbits, *Refract Corneal Surg* (1993) **9:** 443–51.

105. Krueger RR, Talamo JH, McDonald MB, et al, Clinical analysis of excimer laser photorefractive keratectomy using a multiple zone technique for severe myopia, *Am J Ophthalmol* (1995) **119:** 263–74.

106. Campos M, Cuevas K, Garbus J, et al, Corneal wound healing after excimer laser ablation. Effects of nitrogen gas blower, *Ophthalmology* (1992) **99:** 893–7.

Chapter 26 Future developments of laser refractive surgery

Stephen L Trokel

FUTURE OF REFRACTIVE SURGERY

While refractive correction of presbyopia has been understood for close to 1000 years, the correction of myopia has been more recent, and the understanding of hyperopia and astigmatism was not fully elucidated until the end of the nineteenth century. The science of refraction took on its modern form and terminology with the work of Donders and others in the middle of the nineteenth century. Publication of *Principles of codified techniques of refraction* became a classic. This text contains one of the earliest references to a refractive surgical procedure that I have been able to document. Donders referred to a procedure in which the pupil is entrapped to form a slit aperture in the anterior segment to treat astigmatism. Nonetheless, he pointed out that the newly available astigmatic spectacle lenses had fewer complications and also produced a satisfactory optical result in the correction of astigmatism. This competition of refractive surgery with optical appliances for correction of vision has therefore been with us in some form for over 150 years. However, it is only with the improved accuracy and precision of surgical techniques over the past decade that refractive surgery has become a serious alternative to optical correction of ametropia.

HISTORICAL CONSIDERATIONS FOR ACCEPTANCE OF REFRACTIVE SURGERY

Incisional techniques, offered initially by Lans at the turn of the century to treat astigmatism, had a complication rate from the outset which was high. Indeed, with refinement in spectacle design, such alternatives to optical correction never developed a wide following until the development of radial keratotomy by Sato and refinement by Fydorov.

It was Fydorov's Microsurgical Institute that gave the impetus to modern refractive surgery with his development of Sato's original techniques for radial keratotomy. This procedure worked well enough to become a popular alternative to the use of glasses and contact lenses in the treatment of myopia. It was, to a large extent, the improved safety that Fydorov demonstrated that allowed this procedure to become more widely accepted. The subsequent evolution of radial keratotomy in the United States, as well as the widespread acceptance of contact lenses over the past 50 years, have focused attention on non-spectacle corrections of refractive error.

The lessons of the past show that each new technique for correction of ametropia has succeeded or failed based upon the patient's perception and the reality of its safety, accuracy, and precision as well as the stability of the results. Considering these factors may allow us to predict the future of evolving technologies. Looking at where current techniques fall short indicates what must be improved upon in relation to these factors and highlights the direction refractive surgery will take in the immediate future.

FUTURE ACCEPTANCE OF REFRACTIVE SURGERY

We wrestle with the question of whether refractive surgery will become accepted as a technique which is a part of each person's growth and development. As adolescents might have teeth straightened at age 13 and get their driver's license at age 16, can we predict that in the near future their refractive error will be corrected at age 22? Will the proven safety, accuracy, and stability of evolving refractive surgical technologies increase the degree to which this technology will be accepted into common use? Indeed, does excimer laser refractive surgery have those properties of accuracy and precision that meet the criteria for broad acceptance? By addressing these questions we can then attempt to predict what changes in refractive surgical technologies will occur to improve these techniques and make some educated guesses as to the extent of their use in the short and medium term future.

PRESENT LASER TECHNOLOGY

LASER THERMAL KERATOPLASTY

Laser thermal keratoplasty (LTK) evolved from other thermal keratoplasty technologies (see Chapter 1). It has undergone broad clinical investigation and it is generally recognized that the precision of induced refractive change is less than the standard accepted for lasers that create myopic refractive changes. The concept and the hardware are simple. Thermal energy is deposited within the corneal stroma in a symmetrical pattern to induce local collagen shrinkage. This shrinkage steepens the central corneal curve in a response to the pattern of deposition of the thermal energy. Persistent problems with this technique have been:

- the high incidence of regression
- induction of irregular astigmatism
- large standard deviation in the results (see Chapter 17).

There have been suggestions that the results of LTK are more stable when done as a secondary procedure after excimer laser PRK overcorrection, and that removal of Bowman's layer eliminates one of the forces that contributes to regression of effect. It has also been noted that the laser energy that falls on the corneal surface is absorbed superficially when using the commonly available holmium laser. This means that little energy is deposited in the deeper layers of the stroma.

I foresee two efforts underway to expand the accuracy and precision of laser thermal keratoplasty. First, new laser designs. The holmium laser produces a pattern of thermal energy absorption where most of the absorption occurs in the superficial two thirds of the cornea. The use of different laser wavelengths and geometries in which the absorption is concentrated in the deepest one third of the cornea may possibly be more effective than the holmium wavelength. This can be done by employing a shorter wavelength and a large beam angle which concentrates the laser energy deep in the cornea at the laser beam focus. It may even be possible, theoretically, to supplement this with light absorbing dyes within the cornea. Secondly, the observation that removal of Bowman's layer improves the effectiveness and stability of laser thermokeratoplasty will surely be pursued. I believe that laser thermal keratoplasty will continue to be evaluated for its ability to steepen the cornea and may find a place for inducing small amounts of corneal steepening. However, I also believe it highly unlikely that this technology will have a role in the treatment of myopia or myopic astigmatism, or for higher degrees of hyperopia.

PHOTOABLATIVE EXCIMER LASERS

Medical excimer laser systems have seen progressive and dramatic developments since the appearance of the first prototypes in 1985. The past was characterized by fragile equipment which had frequent breakdowns and required complex support. Subsequent improvements in hardware have been accompanied by marked advances in our understanding of algorithms that should be applied to the cornea and a substantial change in surgical techniques used.

By far the most commonly used ultraviolet surgical lasers are excimer systems based on an argon fluoride cavity which produces an output of 193 nm. The only alternative ultraviolet source has been a solid state laser harmonic which produces UV light from about 208–213 nm depending upon the system used.

Most excimer systems use a large laser that produces substantial UV output to provide either a large circular beam, centered on the cornea, or a large scanning element, usually a slit, which is moved rapidly across the cornea. In contrast, excimer laser systems based on small spot scanning technology (<1.0 mm diameter) can use a laser that has a much smaller output which can be fired very rapidly. These scanning systems are of relatively recent development and their accuracy and precision, relative to large area lasers and large spot size scanners, has yet to be extensively demonstrated in clinical trials.

The solid state alternative to an argon fluoride excimer laser requires that a scanning system be developed which only requires a small spot. This is because the efficiency of frequency doubling to produce UV light is very low (see Chapter 2). The advantage of the excimer systems are their low cost, technical simplicity, long life, and high outputs of energy. Their disadvantages are the necessity to maintain fresh fills of argon and fluorine gas to maintain laser action, and unevenness of the output both spatially and temporally. The major solid state advantage is the elimination of the necessity for the presence of toxic gas in the environment. However, the doubling crystals are fragile, the amount of energy output is limited, and the design of the laser and optics is intrinsically more complex.

THE FUTURE OF REFRACTIVE LASERS

THE LASER CAVITY

The original excimer systems contained mechanical and electrical elements which interacted with fluorine gas. Because of this interaction frequent gas changes or the use of cryogenic recirculators were required to maintain a constant laser output. Recent design improvements have replaced many of these elements with non-reactive materials, usually ceramics. Entire cavities made of ceramics are currently being developed. This has substantially extended the life of a given gas fill. Indeed we can look forward to glass and ceramic cavities with outputs that will extend for months and several hundred treatments without gas refills. Current improvements in cavity design and materials have already extended the life of each laser gas fill from a few to many patients. It is entirely feasible to anticipate that an argon fluorine cavity can be built that will work reliably over several years, similar to an argon laser tube.

ADVANCES IN SOLID STATE SYSTEMS

There are indications that newer solid state lasers may soon be available which have larger outputs of far ultraviolet light than current systems based on harmonics of infrared laser systems. These lasers may serve as the basis of future refractive laser developments as they become refined. However, what is certain is the appearance of improved excimer lasers, which have longer gas life and far

greater reliability, that will compete with advances in solid state design.

THE OPTICAL DELIVERY SYSTEM

Far ultraviolet laser light is notoriously damaging to lenses, mirrors and prisms. In the early phases of development of this technology, optical elements would be replaced with great frequency and expense. This damage most commonly involved the mirrors, which would often last for only a handful of patients.

Marked improvement in the UV transmission of lenses and prisms have lengthened their life considerably. Similarly, mirror coatings have been improved which allows thousands of patients to be treated without mirror damage. Optical design engineers have learned how to reduce the fluence within the delivery system so that the damage to the optical elements is less. They have also learned how to isolate these optical elements from the environment so that they are less exposed to airborne contaminants which can degrade optical performance.

ENVIRONMENTAL CONSIDERATIONS AND EXCIMER INSTALLATIONS

With increasing experience of clinical excimer laser systems, engineers and biophysicists have recognized that certain environmental variables can affect the accuracy and precision of these lasers as well as their long term performance. Dust particles and volatile organic compounds have been found to be particularly incompatible with the stable long term operation of medical excimer systems. This means that as installations recognize these problems, the excimer surgery suite will come to resemble a 'clean room' with environmental controls of temperature and humidity as well as environmental contaminants.

SYSTEM HARDWARE AND ACTIVE TRACKING SYSTEMS

Ergonomics will continue to improve with greater comfort for the patient and the surgeon. Controls will be developed that can be operated by touch alone. Aiming systems that can be accurately placed with respect to the entrance pupil of the eye during the entire ablation will be the rule, instead of the novel exception, and illumination systems will be refined to allow greater visualization of the anterior segment during the ablation.

SYSTEM SOFTWARE

Algorithms will be developed that maximize optical function of the eye with the least depth of ablation. Corneal analysis with computerized videokeratography has shown us that all corneas are not identical and we anticipate ablations which will be based on local variations in contour. Ultimately we can foresee an ablation which is custom tailored to an optical analysis of the patient's visual needs, a topographical analysis of his cornea and a pupillographic assessment of his pupillary diameter. Excimer laser systems directly linked to corneal topographic analysis are already on the test bench.

INTRASTROMAL ABLATIONS

The suggestion that a laser can be used to remove tissue within the corneal stroma without damaging the anterior surface is powerfully seductive. Photoablation is known to create a breakdown of matter and conversion to small molecular fragments. Unfortunately, the process of photodisruption distorts the optical properties of the cornea as it progresses. This, together with the extremely small amount of tissue that is removed, has made intrastromal ablation ineffective in reprofiling the anterior corneal curve using current technology. It remains an attractive concept but a conceptual breakthrough will be necessary before successful application of the concept can be anticipated.

OTHER TECHNIQUES OF REFRACTIVE SURGERY

Many other refractive surgical techniques exist and will be developed that do not involve laser use to alter corneal structure. Intraocular lenses remain a surgical area that has and will continue to bear fruit. Whether they are used in phakic or pseudophakic eyes, there is much theoretical advantage especially for the higher myopic eye. Other surgical techniques such as intraocular contact lenses, intrastromal rings, and stromal inlays, will continue to evolve and compete in respect to their safety and efficacy relative to existing refractive surgical technologies (see Chapter 20).

FUTURE DEVELOPMENTS IN LASER SURGICAL TECHNIQUES

PATIENT SELECTION

All surgery starts with selection of the patient and we can look forward to a better understanding of those small minority of patients who can be anticipated to react adversely to excimer laser surgery. The current exclusions and relative contraindications will not stand the test of time and will be progressively refined.

PATIENT PREPARATION

It has been apparent for some time that the accuracy of clinical analysis is inadequate to meet the precise needs of the refractive surgeon. This has become critical for those patients being treated for astigmatism. Errors in the alignment of the treatment have been shown to cause a decrease in the accuracy of PRK when astigmatism is treated. Improved tests of clinical refraction will surely evolve as the accuracy and precision of PRK increases for all refractive errors.

EPITHELIAL REMOVAL

A variety of techniques for removing the epithelium have been developed, all with avid proponents. Mechanical techniques using dull, sharp or mechanized devices, chemical techniques using alcohol or other toxic materials, and the laser itself. In the near future we will see refinement of both mechanical and laser epithelial removal techniques with clinical data to support the superiority of a particular technique.

PATIENT POSTOPERATIVE MANAGEMENT

A wide variety of agents, in addition to corticosteroids, have been employed in an attempt to modulate the healing process following PRK (see Chapter 25). At the present time none have withstood the rigours of careful objective analysis. However, with ever increasing interest in this field one might realistically hope that useful adjunctive medical therapies will be identified.

REOPERATIONS

Although only a handful of studies have carefully reviewed aspects of retreatment some early points of consensus have begun to emerge (see Chapter 24) including: delaying treatment to one year or more post PRK in cases of severe corneal haze; transepithelial approaches in asymmetric corrections or where significant haze persists; and avoidance of retreatment with high degrees of regression. Results for retreatment have generally been encouraging, but as more studies emerge, further refinements in technique are likely to produce dividends in terms of predictability of outcome for reoperations.

LASIK

It has been suggested by some that the combination of lamellar refractive and excimer photoablative techniques to produce LASIK has produced a procedure which will be to PRK what phacoemulsification has been to extracapsular surgery over the last 10 years. Whether LASIK will ultimately eclipse PRK is still open to considerable conjecture. Undoubtedly microkeratomes will undergo considerable further refinement and ultimately the lamellar cap may actually be cut by another laser or even a water jet. However, whilst LASIK is rapidly becoming the accepted procedure for higher levels of myopia it remains to be established by ongoing trials whether it will be superior in terms of outcome and safety for the treatment of low to moderate myopia (see Chapters 12 and 18).

THE LIMITS OF EXCIMER REFRACTIVE SURGERY

PHYSICAL LIMITATIONS

The cornea is approximately 11 mm in diameter and 480–560 μm thick. It is within this narrow tissue that photoablative surgery must define its limits. Whether this will ultimately be −15.00D, −20.00D, −25.00D or even greater, will depend on increasing sophistication of algorithms and predictability and accuracy of LASIK. A single cut-off point is unlikely to emerge and PRK, LASIK and other refractive procedures may develop niche positions with upper and lower limits which blur between techniques.

MYOPIA: AN UNPREDICTABLE NATURAL HISTORY

There remain limitations to our knowledge of the natural history of myopia (see Chapter 5). Who are the stable patients and who are the patients who will have slow progressive myopia? Much has been said about the relative contributions of nature versus nurture but little controlled evidence is available that lets us analyse the oft stated problem of myopic progression with any certainty. Clearly, if environmental factors can be identified in the progression of myopia, then measures may ultimately be available to ameliorate the effect.

DIAGNOSTIC TECHNIQUES

It is certain that the demands of increasingly accurate refractive surgery will force associated technology to improve. Computerized videokeratography has gone from the province of a few limited laboratories to a broadly accepted ophthalmic procedure. We can anticipate improved techniques of corneal analysis that will produce true topographic as well as optical power maps of the corneal surface. We can also hope that techniques will evolve that will give us a true measure of both total corneal and epithelial thickness over the entire area of the cornea.

Techniques of refraction are also going to evolve to meet the increasingly accurate needs that refractive surgery demands. The currently tolerated errors in refractive values must be refined. This need is most critical for astigmatism where systematic errors exist in determining both the magnitude and axis of the cylinder. This is of sufficient importance that it continues to limit the inherent accuracy with which astigmatic errors may be surgically treated.

CONCLUSION

THE UNKNOWN

The only thing certain is change and we can anticipate that our view of refractive surgery will be changed by an unknown insight from an unknown quarter. Control of axial length and techniques to change the corneal curve without removing tissue are entirely conceivable.

THE VISION

The excimer laser has served to re-energize the entire field of refractive surgery both in practice and research. Refractive surgery with the excimer laser has, in many parts of the world, at last come of age and developed as a viable alternative to the use of contact lenses and spectacles for the correction of refractive errors.

Index